ATLAS OF TUMOR PATHOLOGY

Third Series
Fascicle 23

TUMORS OF THE OVARY, MALDEVELOPED GONADS, FALLOPIAN TUBE, AND BROAD LIGAMENT

by

ROBERT E. SCULLY, M.D.
Professor of Pathology Emeritus
Massachusetts General Hospital,
Harvard Medical School
Boston, Massachusetts

ROBERT H. YOUNG, M.D., FRCPath
Professor of Pathology
Massachusetts General Hospital,
Harvard Medical School
Boston, Massachusetts

PHILIP B. CLEMENT, M.D.
Professor of Pathology
Vancouver Hospital and Health Sciences Centre
University of British Columbia
Vancouver, Canada

Published by the
ARMED FORCES INSTITUTE OF PATHOLOGY
Washington, D.C.

Under the Auspices of
UNIVERSITIES ASSOCIATED FOR RESEARCH AND EDUCATION IN PATHOLOGY, INC.
Bethesda, Maryland
1998

Accepted for Publication
1996

Available from the American Registry of Pathology
Armed Forces Institute of Pathology
Washington, D.C. 20306-6000
ISSN 0160-6344
ISBN 1-881041-43-3

ATLAS OF TUMOR PATHOLOGY

EDITOR
JUAN ROSAI, M.D.
Department of Pathology
Memorial Sloan-Kettering Cancer Center
New York, New York 10021-6007

ASSOCIATE EDITOR
LESLIE H. SOBIN, M.D.
Armed Forces Institute of Pathology
Washington, D.C. 20306-6000

Tumors of the Ovary, Maldeveloped Gonads, Fallopian Tube, and Broad Ligament

Atlas
of
Tumor Pathology

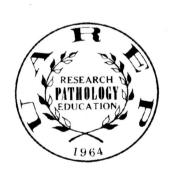

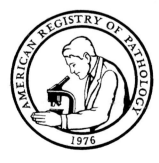

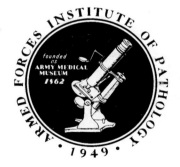

EDITORS' NOTE

The Atlas of Tumor Pathology has a long and distinguished history. It was first conceived at a Cancer Research Meeting held in St. Louis in September 1947 as an attempt to standardize the nomenclature of neoplastic diseases. The first series was sponsored by the National Academy of Sciences-National Research Council. The organization of this Sisyphean effort was entrusted to the Subcommittee on Oncology of the Committee on Pathology, and Dr. Arthur Purdy Stout was the first editor-in-chief. Many of the illustrations were provided by the Medical Illustration Service of the Armed Forces Institute of Pathology, the type was set by the Government Printing Office, and the final printing was done at the Armed Forces Institute of Pathology (hence the colloquial appellation "AFIP Fascicles"). The American Registry of Pathology purchased the Fascicles from the Government Printing Office and sold them virtually at cost. Over a period of 20 years, approximately 15,000 copies each of nearly 40 Fascicles were produced. The worldwide impact that these publications have had over the years has largely surpassed the original goal. They quickly became among the most influential publications on tumor pathology ever written, primarily because of their overall high quality but also because their low cost made them easily accessible to pathologists and other students of oncology the world over.

Upon completion of the first series, the National Academy of Sciences-National Research Council handed further pursuit of the project over to the newly created Universities Associated for Research and Education in Pathology (UAREP). A second series was started, generously supported by grants from the AFIP, the National Cancer Institute, and the American Cancer Society. Dr. Harlan I. Firminger became the editor-in-chief and was succeeded by Dr. William H. Hartmann. The second series Fascicles were produced as bound volumes instead of loose leaflets. They featured a more comprehensive coverage of the subjects, to the extent that the Fascicles could no longer be regarded as "atlases" but rather as monographs describing and illustrating in detail the tumors and tumor-like conditions of the various organs and systems.

Once the second series was completed, with a success that matched that of the first, UAREP and AFIP decided to embark on a third series. A new editor-in-chief and an associate editor were selected, and a distinguished editorial board was appointed. The mandate for the third series remains the same as for the previous ones, i.e., to oversee the production of an eminently practical publication with surgical pathologists as its primary audience, but also aimed at other workers in oncology. The main purposes of this series are to promote a consistent, unified, and biologically sound nomenclature; to guide the surgical pathologist in the diagnosis of the various tumors and tumor-like lesions; and to provide relevant histogenetic, pathogenetic, and clinicopathologic information on these entities. Just as the second series included data obtained from ultrastructural (and, in the more recent Fascicles, immunohistochemical) examination, the third series will, in addition, incorporate pertinent information obtained with the newer molecular biology techniques. As in the past, a continuous attempt will be made to correlate, whenever possible, the nomenclature used in the Fascicles with that proposed by the World Health Organization's International Histological Classification of Tumors. The format of the third series has been changed in order to incorporate additional items and to ensure a consistency of style throughout. Close cooperation between the various authors and their respective liaisons from the editorial board will be emphasized to minimize unnecessary repetition and discrepancies in the text and illustrations.

To its everlasting credit, the participation and commitment of the AFIP to this venture is even more substantial and encompassing than in previous series. It now extends to virtually all scientific, technical, and financial aspects of the production.

The task confronting the organizations and individuals involved in the third series is even more daunting than in the preceding efforts because of the ever-increasing complexity of the matter at hand. It is hoped that this combined effort—of which, needless to say, that represented by the authors is first and foremost—will result in a series worthy of its two illustrious predecessors and will be a suitable introduction to the tumor pathology of the twenty-first century.

Juan Rosai, M.D.
Leslie H. Sobin, M.D.

ACKNOWLEDGMENTS

The authors are grateful to the many pathologists who over the years have submitted interesting cases for consultation, providing the authors with a broad experience in the subject matter of this Fascicle. The reviewers of the initial manuscript offered many helpful suggestions, which have enabled us to improve the clarity of the text. We owe special thanks to Dr. Debra A. Bell and Dr. Judith A. Ferry of the Massachusetts General Hospital and Dr. Arthur L. Herbst of the Chicago Lying-In Hospital for reviewing specific sections of the text. Mrs. Marlene Fairbanks typed the manuscript and Mr. Stephen Conley and Ms. Michelle Forrestall provided photographic assistance. Finally, we wish to thank the editorial staff of UAREP for their support and patience.

Robert E. Scully, M.D.
Robert H. Young, M.D., FRCPath
Philip B. Clement, M.D.

Lippincott-Raven (continued):
    Am J Surg Pathol 1990;14:925–32. For figures 5-39 and 5-40.
    Am J Surg Pathol 1987;11:835–45. For figure 12-13.
    Am J Surg Pathol 1983;7:755–71. For figures 11-10 and 11-30.
    Am J Surg Pathol 1982;6:513–22. For figures 5-33 and 5-37.
    Clin Obstet Gynecol 1984;11:93–134. For figure 10-2.
    Int J Gynecol Pathol 1994;13:259–66. For figure 11-5.
    Int J Gynecol Pathol 1987;6:40–8. For figure 12-16.
    Int J Gynecol Pathol 1984;3:153–78. For figure 22-22.
    Int J Gynecol Pathol 1984;3:77–90. For figure 11-12.
    Int J Gynecol Pathol 1983;2:227–34. For figure 10-20.
    Gynecology and Obstetrics, Vol. 4, 1988. For figure 2-8.

Massachusetts Medical Society:
    N Engl J Med 1977;296:439–44. For figure 21-10.
    N Engl J Med 1976;294:772–7. For figure 20-5.
    N Engl J Med 1972;286:594–600. For figure 19-1.
    N Engl J Med 1969;280:156–60. For figures 2-3 and 4-13.

Masson Publishing:
    Bull du Cancer 1982;69:228–38. For figure 3-12.

Medical Economics:
    Contemp Ob Gyn 1977;9:74–98. For figure 3-3.

Mosby-Year Book:
    Acta Cytol 1974;18:108–17. For figure 2-4.
    Acta Cytol 1973;17:316–9. For figure 2-5.
    Am J Obstet Gynecol 1965;91:251–9. For figures 22-29 and 22-30.
    Am J Obstet Gynecol 1955;59:760–74. For figure 5-17.
    Anderson's Pathology, 3rd ed., 1957. For figure 4-1.
    Endocrine Pathology of the Ovary, 1958. For figure 15-20.

Munksgaard Publishing:
    Acta Pathol Microbiol Scand [A] Suppl 1972;233:56–66. For figures 7-5, 7-6, 7-14,
       7-15, and 7-17.

Springer-Verlag:
    Blaustein's Pathology of the Female Genital Tract, 4th ed., 1994. For figures 9-19,
       18-21, 18-35, and 18-36.
    The Human Yolk Sac and Yolk Sac Tumors, 1993. For figures 13-21, 13-25, and 13-30.
    Histological Typing of Ovarian Tumors, International Histological Classification of
       Tumours No. 9, 1973. For figures 3-10, 3-11, 3-30, 4-11, 4-15, 4-27, 4-39, 5-10, 5-28,
       5-44, 5-45, 6-10, 7-9, 7-12, 10-6, 10-16, 10-17, 13-15, 13-17 through 13-19, 13-36,
       13-37, 14-9, 14-12, 14-13, 14-16 through 14-18, 15-16, 15-18, 16-5, 16-6, 18-20, 18-22,
       22-31, and 22-35.

WB Saunders:

The Pathology of Incipient Neoplasia, 1993. For figures 2-10, 2-11, 3-20A, 5-3, 5-14, and 5-24.

Human Pathol 1990;21:397–403. For figure 3-20B.

Am J Surg Pathol 1985;9:205–14. For figures 5-8 and 5-12.

Human Pathol 1970;1:73–98. For figures 5-6, 14-5, and 18-19.

Human Pathol 1970;16:43–53. For figure 14-8.

Human Pathol 1970;1:73–98. For figures 13-11, 14-3, and 14-5.

Semin Diagn Pathol 1991;8:250–76. For figures 18-8, 18-15, 18-16, 18-23, 18-24, 18-27, 18-29, 18-34, 18-38, 18-39, 18-42, 18-44, 18-45, and 18-51.

Semin Diagn Pathol 1991;8:204–33. For figures 15-1, 20-2, 20-3, and 23-1.

Semin Diagn Pathol 1987;4:275–91. For figure 21-3.

Williams & Wilkins:

Pathology of Reproductive Failure, 1991. For figures 21-1, 21-4, and 21-11.

Progr Gynecol 1963;4:335–47. For figure 13-16.

Yale University Press:

Embryology of the Ovary and Testis, Homo Sapiens and Macaca and Mulatta, 1965. For figures 1-1 through 1-4.

Contents

TUMORS OF THE OVARY, MALDEVELOPED GONADS, FALLOPIAN TUBE, AND BROAD LIGAMENT

1
OVARIAN STRUCTURE AND FUNCTION

DEVELOPMENT

Normal Development

Knowledge of embryology is important in order to understand the origins and microscopic patterns of some ovarian tumors, particularly those in the sex cord–stromal and germ cell categories. Although there is general agreement on the morphologic features of the embryonic and fetal ovary at various stages of development, the dynamic sequence of events determining transition from one stage to the next is less clear.

Also, opinions differ on what designations are most appropriate for various cellular units within the developing ovary. As a result, any classification of ovarian tumors that is based on gonadal development alone will be controversial until embryologists reach agreement.

At approximately 5 weeks' gestation, an indifferent genital ridge is formed by a thickening of the coelomic epithelium (mesothelium) along the medial and ventral borders of the mesonephros (fig. 1-1). Continued proliferation of this epithelium and the subjacent mesenchyme results in

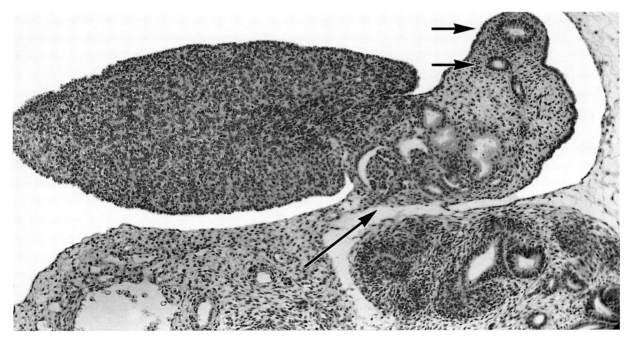

Figure 1-1
UNDIFFERENTIATED GONAD, OVULATION AGE OF 38 DAYS
The gonad lies adjacent to the mesonephros (long arrow) and the wolffian (lower short arrow) and mullerian (upper short arrow) ducts. (Plate 3D from Van Wagenen G, Simpson ME. Embryology of the ovary and testis, Homo sapiens and Macaca mulatta. New Haven: Yale University Press, 1965.)

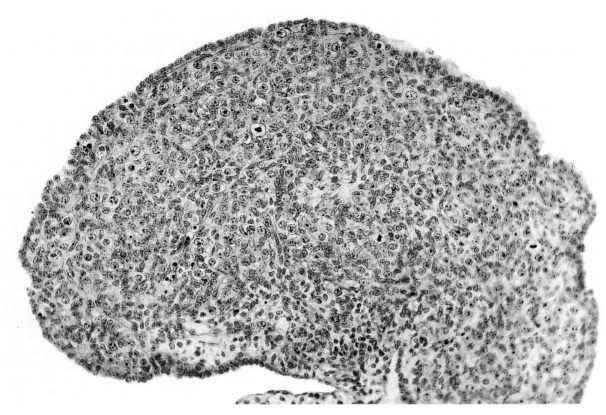

Figure 1-2
OVARY, OVULATION AGE OF 48 DAYS
The surface epithelium is separated focally from the underlying cellular mass by a distinct basement membrane. Scattered large primordial germ cells can be identified throughout. (Plate 4E from Van Wagenen G, Simpson ME. Embryology of the ovary and testis, Homo sapiens and Macaca mulatta. New Haven: Yale University Press, 1965.)

the formation of the gonadal anlage (1). Simultaneously, primordial germ cells migrate toward the gonad from the yolk sac endoderm, reaching the genital ridge during the 5th and 6th weeks of gestation (fig. 1-2) (12). These cells (oogonia) undergo mitotic activity and reach their peak numbers at midgestation; at least two thirds of these cells undergo atresia by term (1,5). At 12 to 15 weeks' gestation, the oogonia begin meiosis and arrest in meiotic prophase, becoming primary oocytes (5,8,11).

At 2 months, the primitive gonad is clearly recognizable as an ovary because it has remained basically unaltered in contrast to the testis, in which sharply defined epithelial cords (the sex cords) and a primitive subepithelial tunica albuginea have developed. At 7 to 9 weeks' gestation, the outer zone of the ovary has enlarged to form the definitive cortex, which consists

of confluent sheets of primitive germ cells and less numerous, smaller pregranulosa cells. Many of the latter are spindle shaped and lack orientation in relation to the oogonia (fig. 1-2) (5,6). At 12 to 15 weeks, vascular connective tissue septa begin to radiate from the mesenchyme of the medulla into the inner portion of the cortex. This process extends into the superficial part of the cortex by 20 weeks (figs. 1-3, 1-4) (6,11). As a result, the cortex becomes divided into cellular groups composed of oocytes and pregranulosa cells (sex cords), which begin to surround individual germ cells to form primordial follicles (fig. 1-4). Folliculogenesis begins in the inner part of the cortex at 14 to 20 weeks' gestation (5,11,12,14), and gradually extends to the outer cortex by the early neonatal period (16). The occasional follicles that mature into preantral and antral follicles in late gestation

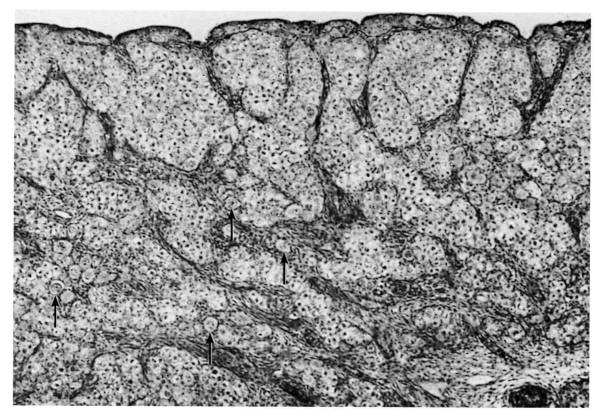

Figure 1-3
OVARY, OVULATION AGE OF 5 MONTHS

Oocytes and pregranulosa cells are forming nests and irregular aggregates. Primordial follicles are forming in deep areas (arrows). (Plate 14A from Van Wagenen G, Simpson ME. Embryology of the ovary and testis, Homo sapiens and Macaca mulatta. New Haven: Yale University Press, 1965.)

become surrounded by a condensation of mesenchymal cells that develop into the theca interna (5,14). The rete ovarii can be detected in the hilus as early as 12 weeks (12).

The origin of the gonadal sex cords (ovarian pregranulosa cells and testicular Sertoli cells) is controversial. Some investigators conclude that they are derived from the coelomic epithelium (3,4,7,11,16), others favor an origin from the "mesenchyme" (13), while some feel that the gonadal blastema is so undifferentiated that it cannot be classified as either epithelial or mesenchymal (9,10). Recent observations indicate that the sex cords are probably of mesonephric origin (2,15,17,18). According to Satoh (15), rudimentary cord-like structures develop from coelomic epithelial cells, but subsequently disappear and do not contribute to the formation of the definitive

sex cords, which are derived from cells that emerge from the mesonephros.

Congenital Malformations

Lobulated, accessory, and supernumerary ovaries are rare. A lobulated ovary is a normally situated ovary divided by one or several fissures into two or more lobes, which may be separated or connected by fibrous tissue or ovarian stroma (29); rarely, both ovaries are affected. A closely related anomaly is an accessory ovary, which is located near a eutopic ovary, with which it has a direct or ligamentous attachment (20,21,29). A supernumerary ovary is similar but is located at a distance from, and not connected to, a eutopic ovary (19,22,25,26,28). A supernumerary ovary may be attached to the uterus, bladder, or pelvic wall, or may be retroperitoneal, within the

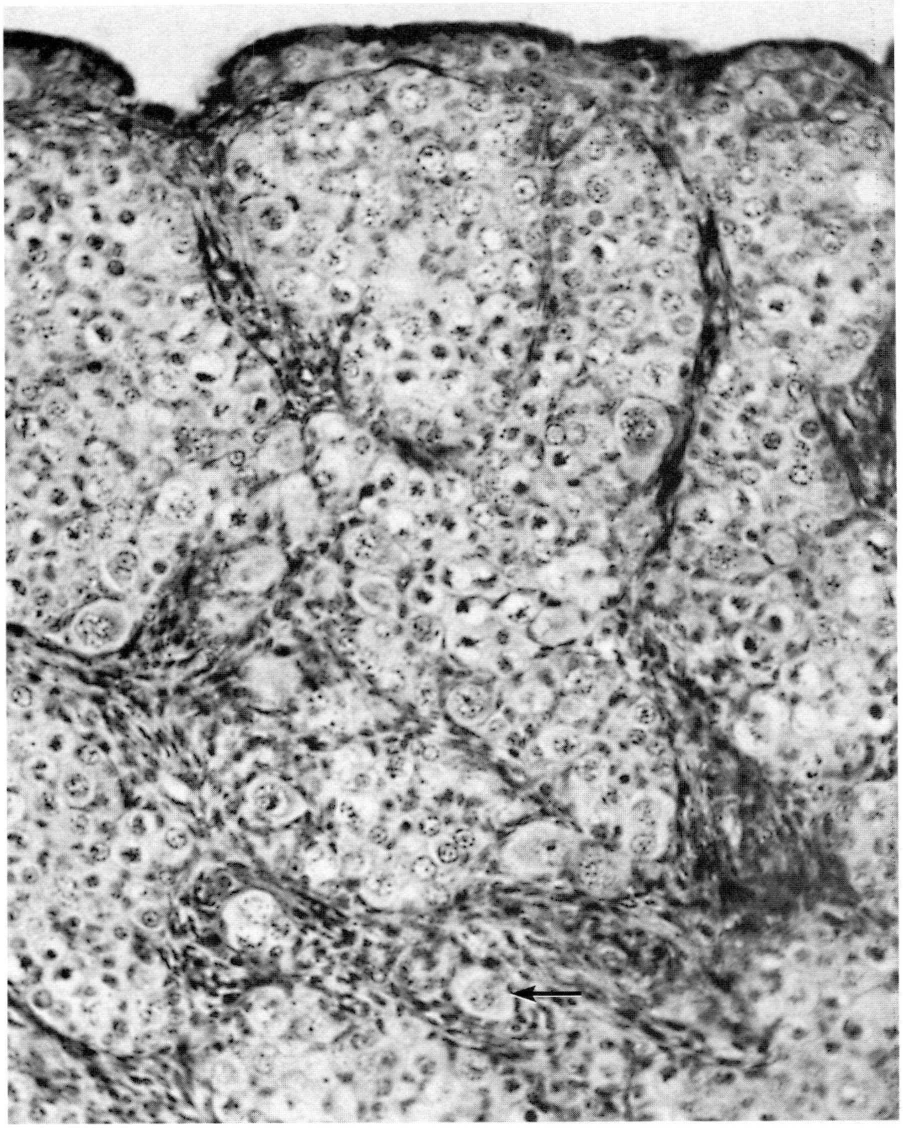

Figure 1-4
OVARY, OVULATION
AGE OF 5 MONTHS
Cortical nests contain oocytes in various stages of prophase of meiosis. A few isolated
primordial follicles have
formed (bottom center). (Plate
14B from Van Wagenen G,
Simpson ME. Embryology of
the ovary and testis, Homo sapiens and Macaca mulatta.
New Haven: Yale University
Press, 1965.)

omentum, in the para-aortic area, or in the mesentery (29). Both accessory and supernumerary
ovaries may be multiple and bilateral (21,22).
Usually they are less than 1 cm in greatest
diameter, and small examples may be overlooked at surgery or autopsy (20,29). Ectopic
ovarian tissue may function, as evidenced by
persistence of menses after bilateral oophorectomy (24), and may undergo pathologic changes
similar to those of normal ovaries (21,23,27). The
presence of a supernumerary ovary provides one
explanation for the development of ovarian-type
tumors in extraovarian sites (see chapter 23). Up

to one third of patients with a lobulated, accessory, or supernumerary ovary have other congenital genitourinary abnormalities.

ANATOMY

Gross Anatomy

The ovaries lie on either side of the uterus
close to the lateral pelvic wall, behind the broad
ligament and anterior to the rectum. Each ovary
is attached to the posterior surface of the broad
ligament along its anterior (hilar) margin by a
double fold of peritoneum, the mesovarium, and

is also attached at its medial pole to the ipsilateral uterine cornu by the ovarian (or utero-ovarian) ligament. Additionally, the infundibulopelvic (suspensory) ligament passes from the superior portion of the lateral pole of the ovary to the lateral pelvic wall.

Prepubertal. The newborn ovary is an elongated, flat structure, 1.3 x 0.5 x 0.3 cm, which lies above the true pelvis (91,95,119). Throughout infancy and childhood, the ovary increases in weight 30-fold, and changes in shape; at puberty it has the size, weight, and shape of an adult ovary, and lies within the true pelvis (95,119). It may contain one or more cystic follicles, particularly during the first few months of life and around the time of puberty (82).

Reproductive Age. Adult ovaries are approximately 3 to 5 x 1.5 to 3 x 0.6 to 1.5 cm in linear dimensions, but their size varies considerably depending on their content of follicular derivatives. They have a pink-white external surface, which is usually smooth in early reproductive life, but becomes increasingly convoluted thereafter. Three ill-defined zones are discernible on the sectioned surfaces: an outer cortex, a central medulla, and the hilus. Follicular structures (cystic follicles, yellow corpora lutea, and white corpora albicantia) are usually visible in the cortex and medulla.

Postmenopausal. After the menopause, the ovaries typically shrink to approximately half their size during the reproductive era. The size varies considerably, however, with the amount of ovarian stromal cells and the number of unresorbed corpora albicantia (38). Most postmenopausal ovaries have a shrunken, gyriform external surface but some have a smooth surface. The cut surface is typically firm and predominantly solid, although occasional cysts measuring several millimeters in diameter (inclusion cysts) may be discernible in the cortex. Small white scars (corpora albicantia) are typically present within the medulla.

Blood Vessels. The ovarian artery, a branch of the aorta, courses along the infundibulopelvic ligament and the mesovarian border of the ovary where it anastomoses with the ovarian branch of the uterine artery. Approximately ten branches arising from this arcade penetrate the ovarian hilus, becoming markedly coiled and branched as they course through the medulla (37,97). At the corticomedullary junction, the medullary arteries and arterioles form a plexus from which smaller, straight cortical arterioles arise and penetrate the cortex in a radial fashion. The cortical arterioles branch and anastomose several times forming sets of interconnected vascular arcades (97), which give rise to the capillaries that form dense networks within the theca layers of the ovarian follicles. Intraovarian veins accompany the arteries, becoming large and tortuous in the medulla. The veins in the hilus form a plexus, which drains into the ovarian veins; the latter traverse the mesovarium and course along the infundibulopelvic ligament (37,97). The ovarian veins also anastomose with tributaries of the uterine veins. The left and right ovarian veins drain into the left renal vein and the inferior vena cava, respectively.

In postmenopausal women, the medullary blood vessels may appear particularly numerous and closely packed as a result of parenchymal atrophy and should not be mistaken for a hemangioma on histologic examination. Many of these vessels may be calcified or have thickened walls and narrowed lumens due to mural deposition of hyaline, amyloid-like material.

Lymphatics. Ovarian lymphatics originate predominantly within the theca layers of the follicles. The granulosa layer of the follicle is devoid of lymphatics in contrast to its counterpart in the corpus luteum, which possesses a rich supply of lymphatics (94). The lymphatics (independent of blood vessels) pass through the ovarian stroma to drain into larger trunks that form a plexus in the hilus (94), where they converge with blood vessels. Four to eight efferent channels pass into the mesovarium where they converge to form the subovarian plexus, which is joined by branches from the fallopian tube and uterine fundus (94). Leaving the plexus, the drainage trunks diminish in number and size, passing along the free border of the infundibulopelvic ligament enmeshed with the ovarian veins. From there they accompany the ovarian vessels and drain into the upper para-aortic lymph nodes at the level of the lower pole of the kidney (51,94). Accessory channels bypass the subovarian plexus and extend through the broad ligament to the internal iliac, external iliac, and interaortic lymph nodes, or in many females, via the round ligament to the iliac and inguinal lymph nodes (51,94). When the pelvic and para-aortic lymph nodes are extensively replaced by tumor, retrograde lymphatic flow may provide a rare route of tumor spread to the ovaries.

Nerves. The nerves of the ovary arise from a sympathetic plexus that is enmeshed with the ovarian vessels in the infundibulopelvic ligament (68). Nerve fibers, which are predominantly nonmyelinated, accompany the ovarian artery, entering the ovary at the hilus. Delicate terminal fibers, many surrounding small arteries and arterioles, penetrate the medulla and cortex to terminate as plexuses surrounding the follicles (68,92). Adrenergic nerve fibers and terminals lie in close contact with smooth muscle cells in the cortical stroma and theca externa.

Microscopic Anatomy

Surface Epithelium. The surface epithelium (modified mesothelium) of the ovary forms a simple, focally pseudostratified layer. The cells vary from flat to cuboidal to columnar, and several types may be seen in different areas of the same ovary; the cells are separated from the underlying stroma by a basement membrane (fig. 1-5). The epithelium is extremely fragile and is often denuded in oophorectomy specimens because of handling by the surgeon and the pathologist, or drying as a result of delayed fixation. Preserved epithelium is often confined to sulci and areas protected by surface adhesions. Histochemical studies have demonstrated glycogen, as well as acid and neutral mucopolysaccharides, within surface epithelial cells (36,81). Activity of 17-beta-hydroxysteroid dehydrogenase, absent in extraovarian mesothelial cells, has also been demonstrated (36). Immunohistochemical staining has revealed positivity for cytokeratin, Ber-EP4, desmoplakin, vimentin, transforming growth factor alpha, and receptors for estrogen, progesterone, and epidermal growth factor (33,44,45,67,70,77,84,99).

Epithelial inclusion glands (EIG) arise from cortical invaginations of the surface epithelium (figs. 1-6, 1-7) and have lost their connection with the surface. Larger examples (epithelial inclusion cysts) may be recognized on macroscopic examination. If an epithelium-lined cyst has a diameter greater than 1 cm it is designated a cystadenoma. Epithelial inclusion glands have

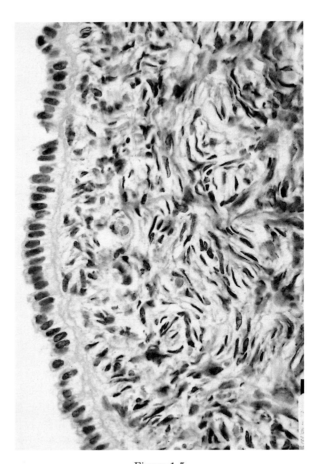

Figure 1-5
SURFACE EPITHELIUM
Low columnar cells are separated from the cortical stroma by a basement membrane.

been identified on microscopic examination of ovaries from all age groups, including fetuses, infants, and adolescents (34,35). With advancing age their frequency increases to the extent that they are common in patients in the late reproductive and postmenopausal age groups. The structures are typically multiple and are scattered singly or in small clusters throughout the superficial cortex (fig. 1-7); less commonly, they extend into the deeper cortical or medullary stroma. They are lined by a single layer of columnar cells, which may be ciliated, mimicking tubal (endosalpingeal) epithelium; psammoma bodies within their lumens or in the adjacent stroma are occasionally present. Similar glands, with or without associated psammoma bodies, encountered on the ovarian surface, within periovarian adhesions,

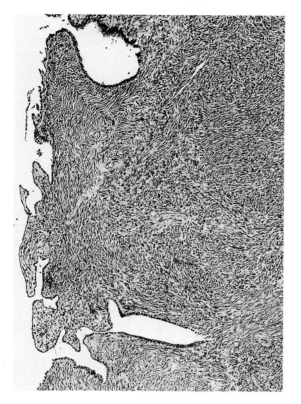

Figure 1-6
FORMATION OF SURFACE EPITHELIAL
INCLUSION GLANDS
The glands are arising from invaginations of the surface epithelium into the cortical stroma.

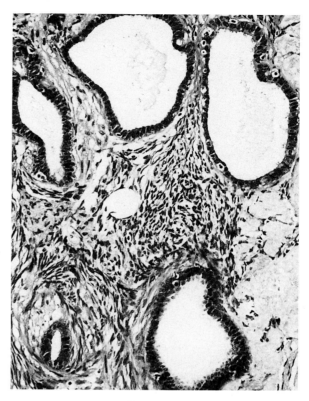

Figure 1-7
SURFACE EPITHELIAL INCLUSION GLANDS
The glands are lined predominantly by columnar cells.

and elsewhere on the peritoneum and in the omentum, have been designated "endosalpingiosis" (110,126). Less frequently, EIGs are lined by other mullerian cell types (endometrioid, mucinous) or by nonspecific columnar or flattened cells (86,121). Urothelial differentiation of the surface epithelium typically takes the form of Walthard nests of transitional cells within the ovarian hilus or superficial cortex (fig. 1-8) (39,47,100,118). The larger nests frequently become cystic and may be lined by columnar mucinous cells.

Stroma. As the stroma of the cortex and medulla is usually continuous, the boundary between these two zones is ill-defined except in some postmenopausal ovaries in which the medulla is composed largely of thick-walled blood vessels. The spindle-shaped stromal cells, which have scanty cytoplasm, are typically arranged in whorls or a storiform pattern (fig. 1-9). Fine droplets of cytoplasmic lipid may be appreciable

with special stains, especially in patients in the late reproductive and postmenopausal age groups (54). Immunohistochemical stains reveal cytoplasmic vimentin, actin, and desmin (33,45, 46,76,84,108). Stromal cells are separated by a dense reticulin network and a variable amount of collagen, which is most abundant in the superficial cortex. Although the latter is sometimes erroneously designated the tunica albuginea, it lacks the densely collagenous, almost acellular appearance and sharp delineation of the tunica albuginea of the testis.

A variety of other cells may be found within the ovarian stroma, most of which are probably of stromal derivation. Luteinized stromal cells, which lie in the stroma at a distance from the follicles, are found singly or in small nests, most often in the medulla. They are characterized by a polygonal shape, abundant eosinophilic to vacuolated cytoplasm containing variable amounts of lipid, a central round nucleus, and a prominent

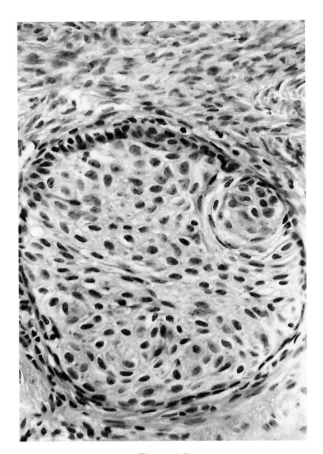

Figure 1-8
WALTHARD NEST
A nest of transitional cells abuts the ovarian stroma.

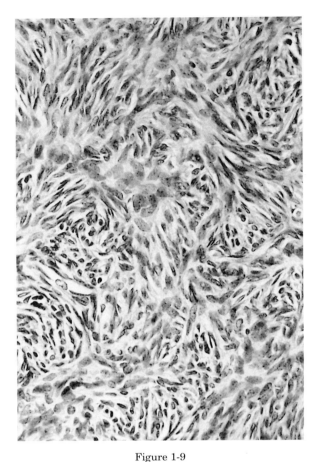

Figure 1-9
OVARIAN STROMA
Spindle cells with scanty cytoplasm are arranged in a storiform pattern.

nucleolus (fig. 1-10). Cytoplasmic immunoreactivity for testosterone has been described (87). The numbers of luteinized stromal cells increase during pregnancy and after menopause, probably secondary to elevated levels of circulating gonadotropins during these periods (38,54). In one autopsy study luteinized stromal cells were demonstrated after diligent searching in 13 percent of women under the age of 55 years and in one third of women over that age; the frequency of their detection increased with increasing degrees of stromal proliferation (38). Although the presence of luteinized cells is usually unaccompanied by clinical evidence of a hormonal disturbance, in some older women but more often in younger patients, more striking degrees of stromal luteinization (stromal hyperthecosis) are frequently associated with androgenic and estro-

genic manifestations. Enzymatically active stromal cells (EASCs) are characterized by oxidative and other enzymatic activity (54,78,88,107). The frequency of their detection and their numbers increase with age; they are detectable in over 80 percent of postmenopausal women, typically in the medulla (78,107). Some EASCs correspond to luteinized stromal cells, but most cannot be distinguished from neighboring nonreactive stromal cells in routine histologic preparations (107). Bundles of smooth muscle may be seen within otherwise unremarkable ovarian stroma, within hyperplastic ovarian stroma such as that typically associated with stromal hyperthecosis or polycystic ovaries (65), and within the stroma surrounding non-neoplastic and neoplastic cysts (106). Nests of cells resembling endometrial stromal cells (stromal endometriosis) occur typically

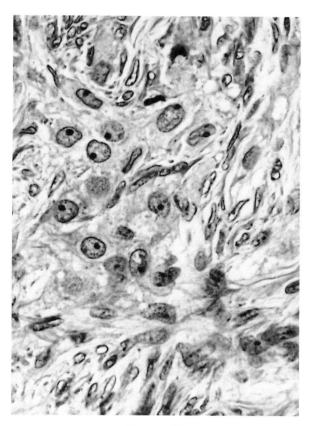

Figure 1-10
LUTEINIZED STROMAL CELLS
The luteinized cells have moderate amounts of (eosinophilic) cytoplasm and a round nucleus with a prominent nucleolus.

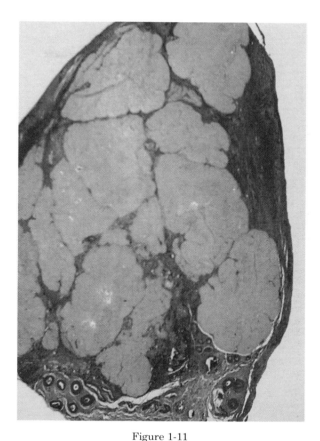

Figure 1-11
POSTMENOPAUSAL ATROPHIC OVARY
The cortical and medullary stroma is scanty. Most of the medulla is occupied by corpora albicantia.

within the cortical stroma, usually in the absence of typical endometriosis (64,66). Foci of mature fat cells occasionally are encountered within the superficial ovarian stroma (59,63); a possible association with obesity was noted in one study (63). Non-neoplastic transformation of ovarian stromal cells to Leydig cells containing Reinke crystals is occasionally seen, typically in association with stromal hyperthecosis or in the stroma within or adjacent to an ovarian neoplasm (see chapter 19) (102,114,125). Ectopic decidua within the ovarian stroma is common during pregnancy.

Although there is typically a gradual increase in the amount of ovarian stroma from the fourth to the seventh decades of life (111), the stroma in postmenopausal women exhibits a wide spectrum of appearances (38,78,111). At one extreme, there is atrophy manifested by a thin cortex and

scanty medullary stroma (fig. 1-11), and at the other extreme, marked stromal proliferation, warranting the designation stromal hyperplasia; generally, however, there are intermediate degrees of nodular or diffuse proliferation of the cortical and medullary stroma, making the normal quantity of ovarian stroma difficult to define (38,78).

Broad irregular areas of cortical fibrosis and fibromatous nodules may be found in perimenopausal and postmenopausal ovaries (38). When they are well-circumscribed, the nodules are designated fibromas if they attain a diameter greater than 1 cm. A similar size designation can be used to distinguish between the foci of surface stromal papillarity that are frequent in this age group and serous surface papillary adenofibromas. Cortical granulomas are occasionally seen in late reproductive and postmenopausal ovaries. These lesions have been demonstrated in up to 45 percent

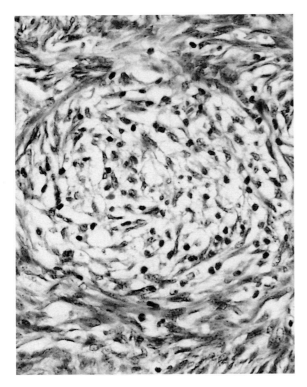

Figure 1-12
CORTICAL GRANULOMA
The granuloma consists of a loose collection of spindle cells, epithelioid cells, and lymphocytes.

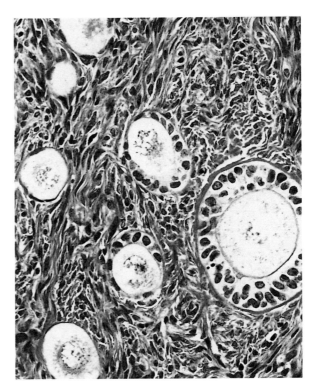

Figure 1-13
PRIMORDIAL AND PRIMARY FOLLICLES
Four primordial follicles (left), two primary follicles (center), and a secondary follicle (right) are present.

of women over the age of 40 years (38,64,66,98, 124) and consist of spherical, usually circumscribed aggregates of epithelioid cells, lymphocytes, and occasionally, multinucleated giant cells (fig. 1-12); anisotropic fat crystals may also be present. Cortical granulomas and the spherical, cloud-like, small hyaline scars present within the superficial stroma of almost all postmenopausal ovaries are of uncertain histogenesis. It has been suggested that the scars may represent regressed foci of stromal endometriosis, ectopic decidua, or luteinized stromal cells.

Follicles and Derivatives. *Primordial Follicles.* The approximately 400,000 primordial follicles that remain in the ovaries at the time of birth occupy most of the ovarian cortex. Subsequently, their numbers continue to decrease progressively by atresia and folliculogenesis until their eventual disappearance, which marks the end of the menopause. Rare follicles may persist for several years after the cessation of menses, however, accounting for sporadic ovulation and

follicle cyst formation accompanied by postmenopausal bleeding (48).

In the reproductive period, primordial follicles are scattered irregularly in clusters throughout a narrow band in the superficial cortex. They consist of a primary oocyte, 40 to 70 μ in diameter, surrounded by a single layer of flat, mitotically inactive granulosa cells resting on a thin basal lamina (fig. 1-13). Rare primordial (and maturing) follicles may contain multiple oocytes, particularly in individuals under 20 years of age (57,79,109, 119). The oocyte is in meiotic prophase at the time of birth, entering an interphase period until preovulatory follicular maturation or degeneration during atresia (31). The large spherical nucleus of the oocyte has finely granular, uniformly dispersed chromatin and one or more dense thread-like nucleoli (31); rare oocytes have multiple nuclei (57,79). The cytoplasm of the oocyte lacks the abundant glycogen and the high alkaline phosphatase activity characteristic of the primordial germ cells of the embryonic gonad.

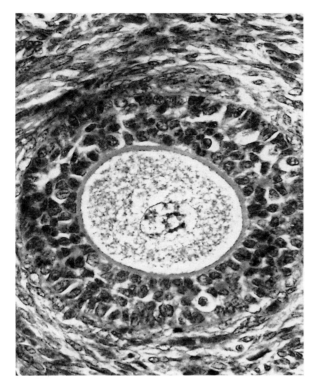

Figure 1-14
SECONDARY FOLLICLE
The stratified granulosa cells surround the oocyte enveloped by its zona pellucida. The theca interna layer is not yet apparent.

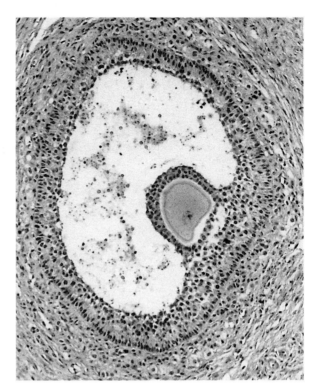

Figure 1-15
GRAAFIAN FOLLICLE
The cumulus oophorus, which contains the oocyte and its zona pellucida, projects into the antrum.

Maturing Follicles. Cohorts of primordial follicles undergo maturation during each menstrual cycle. Follicular maturation begins during the luteal phase and continues throughout the follicular phase of the next cycle. Each month typically only one developing follicle is dominant, achieving complete maturation and release of the oocyte (ovulation). Other developing follicles undergo atresia. Folliculogenesis and atresia also occur prenatally, throughout childhood, and during pregnancy, although maturing follicles rarely reach the preovulatory follicle stage during these periods (43,50,58,61,80,85,89,90,93,119).

The first morphologic evidence of follicular maturation is heightening of the follicular epithelium (composed of granulosa cells) accompanied by enlargement of the oocyte to form a primary follicle (fig. 1-13). The granulosa cells subsequently become stratified to form the secondary or preantral follicle (figs. 1-13, 1-14), in which the oocyte becomes encased by an eosinophilic, periodic acid–Schiff (PAS)-positive, homogeneous, acellular layer, the zona pellucida (fig. 1-14). Preantral follicles are 50 to 400 mm in diameter, and as they increase in size, they migrate into the deeper cortex and medulla. Simultaneously, the surrounding ovarian stromal cells become specialized into an outer ill-defined layer of plump theca externa cells and an inner stratified layer of theca interna cells. Secretion of mucopolysaccharide-rich fluid by the granulosa cells results in their separation by fluid, and the eventual formation of a single antrum lined by several layers of granulosa cells (antral follicle). The first evidence of antrum formation occurs in follicles 200 to 400 mm in diameter, after which the follicles progressively enlarge due to continued fluid secretion into the antrum. Concurrently, the oocyte enlarges to its definitive size and assumes an eccentric position at one pole of the follicle within a proliferation of granulosa cells designated the cumulus oophorus (graafian follicle) (fig. 1-15).

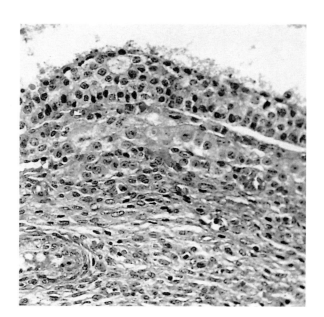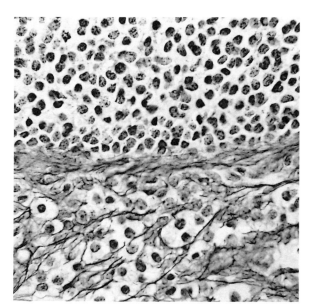

Figure 1-16
LINING OF MATURE FOLLICLE
Left: From the top of the figure to the bottom are the antrum, a layer of granulosa cells with a single Call-Exner body, a layer of luteinized theca interna cells, an ill-defined theca externa, and the ovarian stroma.
Right: Absence of reticulin in the granulosa layer in contrast to abundant reticulin in the theca interna layer. (Reticulin stain)

Late in follicular growth, the oocyte, its zona pellucida, and a single layer of radially disposed columnar granulosa cells (the corona radiata) detach from the cumulus oophorus and float in the antral fluid. The preovulatory follicle reaches a diameter of 15 to 25 mm shortly before ovulation (32). The preovulatory follicle then ruptures, possibly secondary to contraction of perifollicular smooth muscle cells, with liberation of the follicular fluid, oocyte, and surrounding granulosa cells into the peritoneal cavity. Subsequently, the stigma of ovulation is occluded by a mass of coagulated follicular fluid, fibrin, blood, granulosa cells, and connective tissue cells, which is eventually converted to scar tissue.

The granulosa cells within maturing follicles are polyhedral and 5 to 7 μ in diameter; those resting on the basement membrane are often columnar. They have pale scanty cytoplasm, indistinct cell borders, and small, round to oval, hyperchromatic nuclei, which typically lack nuclear grooves (fig. 1-16) (122). Mitotic figures within granulosa cells are usually numerous in maturing follicles, decreasing in number prior to ovulation. Until the onset of luteinization several hours prior to ovulation, cytoplasmic lipid is

absent (or sparse) as are the histochemical patterns characteristic of steroidogenesis (72). The cytoplasm of granulosa cells of primary, secondary, and mature follicles is immunoreactive for cytokeratin, vimentin, and desmoplakin (33,45, 84). Granulosa cells typically surround small cavities, forming Call-Exner bodies (fig. 1-16, left), which are delimited from the granulosa cells by a basal lamina and typically contain deeply eosinophilic, PAS-positive, filamentous material consisting of basal lamina (37,53). The granulosa layer of the maturing follicles is avascular and devoid of a reticulin framework (fig. 1-16, right).

Theca cells differentiate continuously from the stromal cells at the periphery of developing follicles from fetal life to the termination of the menopause. The thecal component of the antral follicle is characterized by a well-developed theca interna and a less defined theca externa. The theca interna layer is three or four cells thick and lies outside the granulosa layer, from which it is separated by a basement membrane (fig. 1-16, left). Unlike the granulosa cells of developing and mature follicles, the theca interna cells typically have a luteinized or partially luteinized appearance and exhibit steroidogenic histochemical patterns (49,54,72). Luteinization of the theca interna of maturing follicles is particularly prominent during pregnancy. The round to polygonal luteinized theca cells are 12 to 20 μ in diameter and have abundant, eosinophilic to vacuolated cytoplasm containing variable amounts of lipid; a central, round, vesicular nucleus typically contains a single prominent nucleolus (fig. 1-16, left). These cells resemble stromal cells in being immunoreactive for vimentin but not cytokeratin (33). Mitotic figures are typically present within the theca cells of maturing follicles and may be numerous. The theca cell layer contains a rich plexus of dilated capillaries and a dense network of reticulin fibrils (fig. 1-16, right). Tangential sections through the luteinized theca interna may result in seemingly isolated nodules of luteinized theca cells, which are misinterpreted occasionally as foci of stromal luteinization.

The theca externa is an ill-defined layer of variable thickness surrounding the theca interna and merging almost imperceptibly with the adjacent ovarian stroma (fig. 1-16, left). It contains plump spindle cells (which lack steroidogenic histochemical features [56]), as well as circumferentially arranged collagen bundles, blood vessels, and lymphatics. The spindle cell layer of the theca externa is typically highly mitotic and has been misinterpreted as early fibrosarcoma, particularly when only the edge of the follicle is seen microscopically (fig. 1-17).

Corpus Luteum of Menstruation. After ovulation on the 14th day of the typical 28-day menstrual cycle and in the absence of fertilization, the collapsed ovulatory follicle becomes the corpus luteum of menstruation (CLM), a 1.5 to 2.5 cm round structure with a festooned contour; a cystic center filled with a gray, focally hemorrhagic coagulum; and a color that changes during the luteal phase from brown to orange-yellow as it acquires more lipid. Occasionally, the CLM may be cystic, but this feature is more characteristic of the corpus luteum of pregnancy. If the cavity exceeds 3 cm, the structure is designated a corpus luteum cyst (page 410), and if smaller, a cystic corpus luteum.

The granulosa cells of the mature CLM are 30- to 35-μ polygonal cells with abundant, pale eosinophilic cytoplasm, which may contain numerous small lipid droplets (56) and spherical nuclei with one or two large nucleoli (fig. 1-18). The histochemical pattern of these cells varies

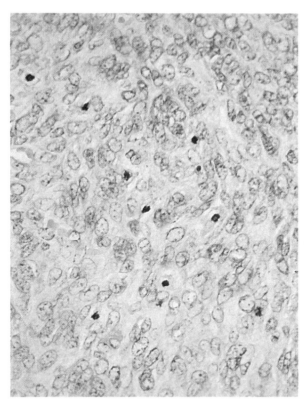

Figure 1-17
THECA EXTERNA OF MATURE FOLLICLE
Numerous mitotic figures are present.

with the age of the CLM, but is generally typical of steroid hormone–producing cells (49,54,123). The cytoplasm of luteinized granulosa cells contains vimentin but little or no cytokeratin (45).

The theca interna forms an irregular outer layer of the CLM several cells in thickness (fig. 1-18) and ensheaths the vascular septa that extend into the center of the structure (56). When these septa are cut in cross section, triangular-shaped wedges of theca cells appear in the sulci of the convoluted, thick granulosa lutein layer. In all but the earliest stages of the CLM, the theca lutein cells are approximately half the size of granulosa lutein cells. They contain a round to oval nucleus with a single prominent nucleolus. The cytoplasm, which is less abundant and more deeply staining than that of the granulosa lutein cells, contains lipid droplets that are usually larger than those in granulosa lutein cells.

During the maturation of the CLM, capillaries originating from the theca interna layer penetrate

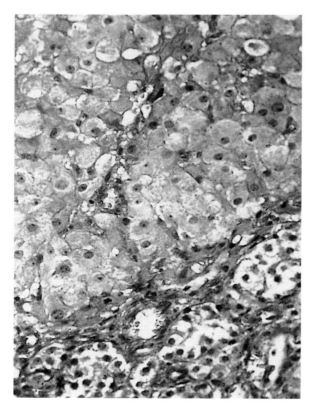

Figure 1-18
CORPUS LUTEUM OF MENSTRUATION
The larger cells are granulosa lutein cells, and the smaller cells with clear (lipid-rich) cytoplasm are theca lutein cells.

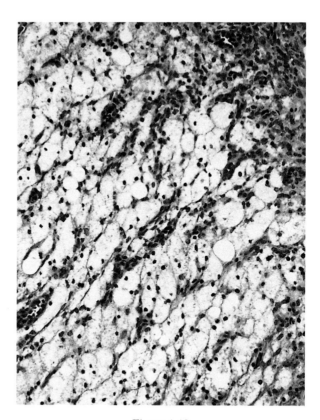

Figure 1-19
INVOLUTING CORPUS LUTEUM OF MENSTRUATION
The granulosa lutein cells are filled with (lipid) vacuoles and contain pyknotic nuclei.

the granulosa layer and reach the central cavity. Fibroblasts, which accompany the vessels, form an increasingly dense reticulin network within the granulosa layer as well as an inner fibrous layer that lines the central cavity. Involutional changes begin on the 8th or 9th day following ovulation (42). The granulosa lutein cells decrease in size, their nuclei become pyknotic, and they accumulate abundant cytoplasmic lipid (fig. 1-19), eventually undergoing dissolution (30). There is progressive fibrosis and shrinkage over a period of several months, with conversion to a corpus albicans and eventual resorption by the ovarian stroma.

Corpus Luteum of Pregnancy. On gross inspection, the corpus luteum of pregnancy (CLP) may be indistinguishable from the CLM, but it is usually larger and bright yellow in contrast to the orange-yellow of the late CLM (60). The larger size, which may account for up to half the ovarian volume, is due primarily to the presence

of a central cystic cavity filled with fluid or a coagulum of fibrin and blood (93,112,120). When the cavity of a CLP is large, typically in the first trimester, the wall may lose its convolutions, becoming stretched and attenuated to the extent that it may consist focally of only the inner fibrous layer (90). Obliteration of the cavity usually begins by the 5th month of gestation and is typically completed by term (90). The CLP thus gradually decreases in size, and by the last trimester, is not conspicuous. During the puerperium, the CLP involutes and converts to a corpus albicans.

The first morphologic evidence within a corpus luteum that conception has occurred is the absence of the normally appearing regressive changes. Instead, the granulosa lutein cells enlarge, reaching their maximum size of 50 to 60 μ by 8 to 9 weeks' gestation. Eosinophilic colloid or hyaline droplets appear within the granulosa cells of a CLP as early as 15 days after ovulation

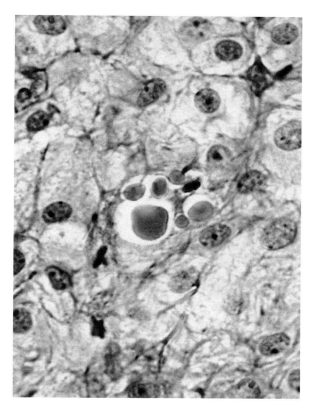

Figure 1-20
CORPUS LUTEUM OF PREGNANCY
Hyaline bodies are present in the center.

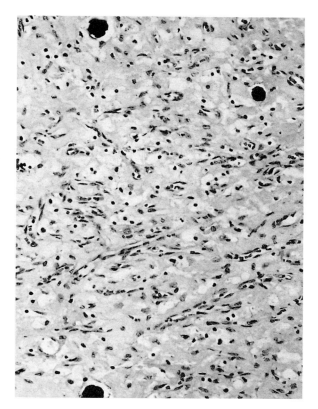

Figure 1-21
INVOLUTING CORPUS LUTEUM OF PREGNANCY
Foci of calcification are visible.

and are almost diagnostic of pregnancy (fig. 1-20), but occur rarely within a CLM (90). They become more numerous as gestation progresses (120), although by term their numbers decrease as they calcify; calcification continues into the puerperium (fig. 1-21) (90,120).

The theca interna is thickest in the early CLP, when it resembles its counterpart in the CLM, surrounding the granulosa lutein layer and forming triangular-shaped vascular septa that extend into the latter. After the 4th month, the theca cells become smaller and fewer in number, with darker, more irregular, oblong to spindle-shaped nuclei, resembling those of fibroblasts (120). By term, the theca interna layer has almost completely disappeared.

As in the mature CLM, the central cystic cavity of the CLP is typically lined by a layer of fibrous tissue composed of variable numbers of fibroblasts, collagen and reticulin fibers, and blood vessels (90). Its thickness varies greatly,

not only within the same CLP, but also from one CLP to another and from one phase of pregnancy to another (120). As gestation advances, the central cyst or coagulum is eventually obliterated by connective tissue, which may exhibit focal hyalinization and calcification (89).

Corpus Albicans. The regressing CLM is invaded by connective tissue, which gradually converts it to a scar, the corpus albicans. The degenerating corpus luteum and the young corpus albicans may contain histiocytes laden with ceroid and hemosiderin pigment (96). The mature corpus albicans is a well-circumscribed structure with convoluted borders composed almost entirely of densely packed collagen fibers with a few admixed fibroblasts. Focal calcification and ossification are occasionally encountered. Most corpora albicantia are eventually resorbed and replaced by ovarian stroma (71), although corpora albicantia often persist in the medulla of postmenopausal women.

Atretic Follicles. Of the original 400,000 primordial follicles present at birth, approximately 400 mature to ovulation. The remaining 99.9 percent undergo atresia, which begins before birth and continues throughout reproductive life, but is most intense immediately after birth and during puberty and pregnancy (40,43,50,58, 61,80,89,93). Factors that initiate atresia and determine which follicles undergo atresia are unknown. Atresia of antral follicles leads to formation of a scar, the corpus fibrosum. Some degenerating follicles may persist as atretic cystic follicles, which along with follicular cysts may persist for several years after the menopause (116). During follicular atresia, the basement membrane between the granulosa and theca interna layers becomes transformed into a thick, wavy, eosinophilic, hyalinized band. The theca interna layer typically persists, often with prominent luteinization, until the late stages of atresia at which time cords and nests of theca cells become surrounded by proliferating connective tissue. Luteinization of the theca layer is particularly striking in atretic follicles during infancy and childhood (74) and pregnancy (90). Microscopic proliferations of persistent granulosa cells within the centers of atretic follicles of pregnant, and less commonly nonpregnant women, may mimic small granulosa cell tumors, or rarely, Sertoli cell tumors (41). Similarly, structures resembling microscopic gonadoblastomas and sex cord tumors with annular tubules have been identified within atretic follicles in up to 35 percent of normal fetuses and infants (73,79,103). There is no evidence to suggest that any of these tumor-like proliferations represent early stages of neoplasia.

Hilus. *Hilus Cells.* Ovarian hilus cells (hilar Leydig cells) are morphologically identical to testicular Leydig cells except for having a female chromatin pattern. Hilus cells are present during fetal life but are not identifiable during childhood. They reappear at the time of puberty and are demonstrable in virtually all postmenopausal women (83,113,115). Their number and location can vary greatly, and they are more numerous during pregnancy, with increasing age after the menopause, and with increasing degrees of ovarian stromal proliferation and stromal luteinization (38).

Hilus cell aggregates of variable size and shape are typically found in the ovarian hilus and adjacent mesovarium (fig. 1-22). They are more numerous in the lateral and medial poles of the hilus and near the junction of the ovarian ligament with the ovary, typically lying close to the junction of the hilus with the medullary stroma (113). The aggregates are closely associated with large hilar veins and lymphatic vessels, and may form nodular protrusions into their lumina (113). Hilus cells characteristically ensheath, or less commonly lie within, nonmedullated nerves (fig. 1-22), and occasionally lie adjacent to the rete ovarii (113). As noted earlier, nests of Leydig cells, probably of ovarian stromal cell origin, may also be present within the medullary stroma near the hilus, or rarely, within the ovarian stroma at a distance from the hilus. Leydig cells are rarely encountered in the perisalpinx and fimbrial endosalpinx (62).

Hilus cells nests are unencapsulated, typically lying within loose connective tissue within the hilus (125). The cells are 15 to 25 μ in diameter; are round to oval, and less commonly elongated; and contain abundant eosinophilic cytoplasm and a spherical vesicular nucleus, which contains one or two prominent nucleoli (fig. 1-23). The cytoplasm may contain crystals of Reinke: homogenous, eosinophilic, nonrefractile, rod-shaped structures, 10 to 35 μ in length, with blunt or occasionally tapered ends (fig. 1-23). The crystals typically lie in a parallel or stacked arrangement within a cell, and often are surrounded by a clear halo; occasionally they appear to extend through or overlie cell membranes. The crystals are unevenly distributed and are typically present in only a minority of cells; frequently they are not identified (69). Their visualization may be facilitated by the use of Masson's trichrome and iron hematoxylin methods, which stain them magenta and black, respectively. Additionally, the crystals exhibit yellow fluorescence when viewed by ultraviolet light in hematoxylin and eosin–stained sections (105). Elongated erythrocytes compressed within capillaries should not be confused with the crystals.

Also present within hilus cells, often in greater numbers than crystals, are spherical or ellipsoidal hyaline globules that may be the precursors of crystals (fig. 1-23). The cytoplasm may also contain perinuclear eosinophilic granules,

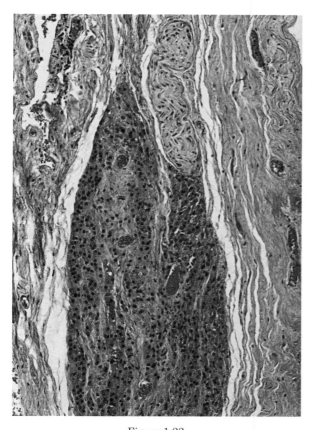

Figure 1-22
HILUS CELLS
A cluster of darkly staining hilus cells lies adjacent to a small nerve fiber (top).

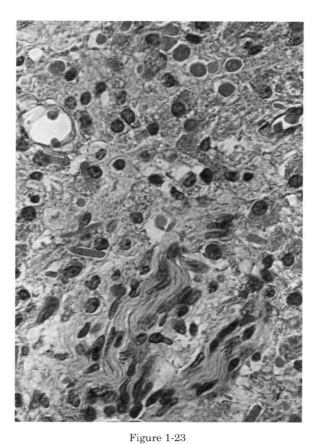

Figure 1-23
HILUS CELLS
Reinke crystals are seen in the lower portion of the field. Rounded hyaline bodies are present in the upper portion. Two parallel strands of a nerve are seen in the lower part of the field.

peripheral lipid vacuoles, and golden brown lipochrome pigment. Delicate collagen fibrils surround each cell. Typically admixed with the hilus cells are fibroblasts and cells intermediate in appearance between the two cell types (75). The hilus and intermediate cells have neural attachments, including true synaptic connections, suggesting that these cells may originate from hilar fibroblasts, possibly under the inductive influence of hilar nerves (75,113). Hilus cells may have bizarre shapes and contain hyperchromatic, pleomorphic nuclei, particularly in postmenopausal women.

Hilus cells should be distinguished from encapsulated adrenal cortical rests. The latter are rare in the ovary (117), and are found most commonly in the mesovarium, and occasionally within the ovarian hilus, in approximately 25 percent of women (fig. 1-24) (52). Their histologic appearance

mimics that of the normal adrenal cortex, with most cells containing numerous lipid vacuoles.

Rete Ovarii. The rete ovarii, the ovarian homologue of the rete testis, which is present in the hilus of all ovaries, consists of a network of tubules with intraluminal polypoid projections, lined by an epithelium that varies from flat to cuboidal to columnar (figs. 1-25, 1-26) (101,104). Solid cords of similar cells may also be seen. The rete is surrounded occasionally by a cuff of spindle cell stroma similar to, but discontinuous from, the ovarian stroma. The rete epithelium is immunoreactive for cytokeratin, vimentin, and desmoplakin (33,45). The rete lies adjacent to and may communicate with mesonephric tubules within the mesovarium (101). The rete epithelium may undergo transitional cell metaplasia (104).

17

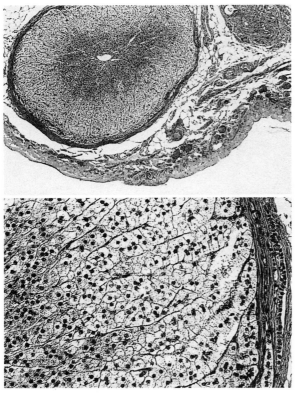

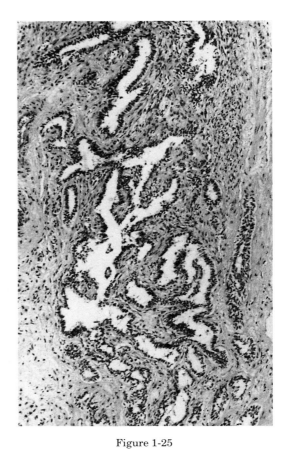

Figure 1-24
ADRENOCORTICAL REST IN MESOSALPINX
Top: A fibrous capsule and zonation into glomerulosa, fasciculata, and reticularis layers are evident.
Bottom: The cells of the zona glomerulosa and zona fasciculata have spongy (lipid-rich) cytoplasm.

Figure 1-25
RETE OVARII
A network of branching tubules lies in a cellular stroma, which may resemble ovarian stroma.

Figure 1-26
RETE OVARII
Polypoid projections with fibrous cores occupy the lumen of a cystically dilated portion. The epithelium varies from flat to cuboidal to columnar.

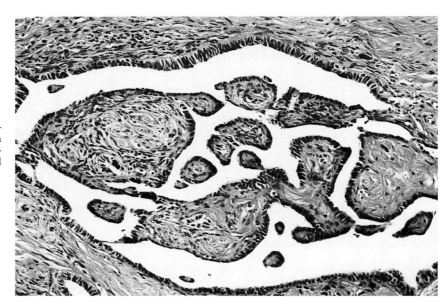

FUNCTION

General Features

The two major functions of the ovary, the release of mature ova at the time of ovulation and the secretion of steroid hormones, depend on the cyclic release of pituitary follicle-stimulating hormone (FSH) and luteinizing hormone (LH). These hormones are regulated by gonadotropin-releasing hormone (GnRH) secreted by the hypothalamus into the pituitary portal circulation. The principal actions of the ovarian steroid hormones are stimulation of growth of the reproductive organs, development of secondary sexual characteristics, and maintenance of the implanted blastocyst. The endocrine functions of the normal ovary can be subdivided into those of its various compartments: the preovulatory follicle, the corpus luteum, the stroma, and the hilus cells.

Preovulatory Follicle

Only the later stages of follicular maturation are under gonadotropin control. As a small antral follicle develops into a preovulatory follicle, the sequence of endocrine events within its fluid differs from most, if not all, other antral follicles (146,147). Early in its development, FSH receptors and intrafollicular FSH increase, accompanied by a rise in estrogen receptors within the granulosa cells of the preovulatory follicle (134, 146,147,159). Estrogen levels within the follicular fluid and serum peak during the mid- to late follicular phase, when plasma FSH falls to a basal level (134,146,147). At this stage the follicle is self-sustaining, continuing to mature under the influence of intrafollicular FSH and estrogen (148). During the late follicular phase, plasma LH rises and LH receptors become apparent within the granulosa cells of the preovulatory follicle but not other follicles (159). In contrast, LH receptors are present within the theca cells of all follicles throughout the follicular phase (159).

Although circulating estrogen is likely derived from both the granulosa cells and the theca cells, intrafollicular estrogen is derived almost exclusively from the granulosa cells by FSH-dependent aromatization of theca-derived androgen (148,149). Aromatase activity is highest in the preovulatory follicle, thereby maintaining a high estrogen:androgen ratio (138,146,147). In contrast, follicles that undergo atresia are FSH and aromatase deficient and have high androgen:estrogen ratios within their fluid.

The granulosa cells also produce the peptide hormone, inhibin, which is secreted into the follicular fluid and ovarian venous effluent in amounts that correlate with steroid levels (135, 163,164). This hormone acts, by negative feedback, to reduce FSH secretion from the hypothalamic-pituitary unit. Also secreted by granulosa cells is mullerian-inhibiting substance (133). High concentrations of prorenin are present within the fluid of mature follicles (158); their granulosa cells, as well as theca and stromal cells, are immunoreactive for renin and angiotensin II (153). The function of the renin-angiotensin system within the ovary is largely unknown.

Corpus Luteum

The formation and function of the CLM is under the control of LH, reflected by the numerous LH receptors within the granulosa lutein cells (135,159). Although progesterone is the major steroid formed by the corpus luteum, it also synthesizes estrone (E1) and estradiol (E2), as well as androgens, mostly androstenedione (141).

After ovulation, LH, FSH, and E2 levels fall, but the LH concentration is sufficient to maintain the CLM (with its increase in LH receptors), producing a midluteal peak in progesterone and E2 concentrations. If fertilization does not occur, the increased levels of progesterone and estrogen result in a fall of LH and FSH to basal levels via a negative feedback mechanism, with a marked decline in progesterone and E2 synthesis after the 22nd day of the cycle (129,134,135, 155,159). These changes are accompanied by morphologic involution of the CLM and the onset of menses. The liver is largely responsible for inactivation of progesterone, which is first reduced to pregnanediol and then conjugated with glucuronic acid for excretion in the urine.

Ovarian Stroma

Numerous studies have demonstrated the steroidogenic potential and the gonadotropin responsiveness of the ovarian stroma in both premenopausal and postmenopausal women (127, 130,132,136,139,140,143,144,148,150,154,165). In vitro incubation of ovarian stromal tissue indicates that it secretes androstenedione, as well as smaller quantities of testosterone and dehydroepiandrosterone (157). In vitro production of androgens is enhanced by human chorionic gonadotropin (hCG), pituitary gonadotropins, and insulin, consistent with the presence of receptors for these hormones within the stromal cells (128,151,152). To what extent the ovarian stroma contributes to the androgen pool in normal premenopausal women is unknown, but it is likely that it is the source of small amounts of testosterone. With cessation of follicular activity at the time of the menopause, the ovarian stroma becomes, together with the adrenal glands, the major source of androgens. Several studies have indicated that testosterone and androstenedione are the major androgens secreted by the ovarian stroma in postmenopausal women (127,130,139,165). Approximately 80 percent of the circulating levels of androstenedione in postmenopausal women, however, is of adrenal origin (130). Despite a cessation of follicular synthesis of E2 after the menopause, small amounts of this hormone are present in the circulation, probably derived from the adrenal glands by peripheral conversion of E1 (130,156), and from the ovarian stroma itself (127,142). E1, however, becomes the major circulating estrogen after the menopause, derived predominantly from the peripheral aromatization of androstenedione, which occurs in fat, muscle, liver, kidney, brain, and adrenal glands (130,137,142). Increased aromatization in postmenopausal women, probably due to their high LH levels, leads to an increase in the production of E1 over that in premenopausal women. In some postmenopausal patients, sufficient estrogen may be elaborated by this mechanism to prevent the clinical manifestations of estrogen withdrawal and play a role in the genesis of endometrial carcinoma (130,160). Indeed, an association between the degree of stromal proliferation and postmenopausal endometrial adenocarcinoma has been noted (160). The variations that exist in the ovarian steroid hormone output from one postmenopausal woman to another may correspond to similar variations in the morphologic appearance of the stroma in this age group, although no correlative functional and structural studies have been performed.

Hilus Cells

The light and electron microscopic appearance and the enzyme content of hilus cells are those of steroid hormone–producing cells, although to what extent hilus cells contribute to the steroid hormone pool in normal females is unknown (145,161). In vitro incubation studies indicate that the major steroid produced by ovarian hilus cells is androstenedione and that it is produced in an amount higher than that secreted by the ovarian stroma (131). Less E2 and progesterone are also produced in vitro. Hilus cells are responsive in vivo to both exogenous and endogenous hCG stimulation, as manifested by increases in cell size, mitotic activity, and cell numbers (162).

LABORATORY EVALUATION OF FUNCTION

Evaluation of the endocrine function of the ovary involves an assessment of its secretion of estrogens, progesterone, and androgens, and assessment of the pituitary gonadotropins. The results of the various tests available for this purpose range from crude estimates to precise measurements.

Estrogens

Inexact, but often clinically useful appraisals of estrogen secretion are based on the cornification or karyopyknotic index of the vaginal epithelium on cytologic examination, the appearance of the endometrium on biopsy, and the ability or inability to induce uterine bleeding by the administration and subsequent withdrawal of progesterone. In the progesterone withdrawal test, bleeding occurs only if the endometrium has already been primed by estrogens. Assays of the various estrogens (E1, E2, and estriol), both free and bound to protein in the plasma, yield more precise information about ovarian estrogen secretion than chemical assays of the urine for estrogens and their metabolites.

Progesterone

Progesterone levels can be estimated by the measurement of urinary pregnanediol, the principal excretory product of progesterone, but this metabolite accounts for less than 20 percent of the secreted hormone. More accurate tests are determinations of plasma progesterone levels by radioimmunoassay, and more recently, enzyme and fluorescence nonisotopic immunoassays.

Androgens

Androgen production is evaluated most often in the course of investigating the cause of anovulation, hirsutism, and virilism. The determination of the urinary 17-ketosteroid level yields little precise information because the value obtained reflects mainly the metabolites of weak androgens, and to some extent those of non-androgenic steroids as well. In addition, the test is too insensitive to detect small, but clinically significant, elevations of the potent androgen, testosterone, which is not a 17-ketosteroid. Functioning ovarian lesions may be associated with the production of the weak androgens, androstenedione and dehydroepiandrosterone, resulting in an elevated 17-ketosteroid level, but high values of the latter, particularly those over 30 mg per 24 hours, are more characteristic of virilism of adrenal origin. Whether of ovarian or adrenal origin, the weak androgens must be present in amounts large enough to cause a marked increase in urinary 17-ketosteroids before virilism appears. More precise evaluation of androgen levels involves radioimmunoassays of free and protein-bound plasma testosterone, androstenedione, and dehydroepiandrosterone.

Since ovarian and most adrenal steroid hormone secretion is under the control of pituitary tropic hormones, an increase in urinary 17-ketosteroids or urinary or plasma androgens after the administration of hCG or adrenocorticotropic hormone (ACTH), or a decline in these values after the administration of an estrogen or dexamethasone, which inhibit the release of gonadotropins or ACTH, respectively, would be expected to provide helpful information in pinpointing the source of excess androgens. Such approaches have occasionally led to erroneous conclusions, however. The most sophisticated diagnostic procedure is catheterization of the ovarian veins, the adrenal veins, or both to assay various hormones and compare the values obtained with the peripheral vein levels. Technical errors and the effects of stress on adrenal secretion, however, have caused difficulties with this approach as well.

Pituitary Gonadotropins

Since ovarian hypofunction or hyperfunction may be either primary or secondary to changes in the levels of pituitary gonadotropins, measurement of the latter by radioimmunoassay may be helpful in identifying the nature of an associated ovarian disorder. Primary ovarian failure with anovulation and a low steroid hormone output is typically accompanied by high gonadotropin levels in both early childhood and adult life because of the failure of the inhibitory feedback mechanisms, while secondary ovarian failure results from low levels of gonadotropins. Secondary ovarian hyperfunction, such as that encountered in central sexual precocity, results from a premature discharge of gonadotropins from the pituitary gland, whereas primary ovarian overproduction of steroid hormones typically inhibits gonadotropin release from the pituitary gland.

REFERENCES

General References

Adashi EY, Leung PC. The ovary. In: Martini L, ed. Comprehensive endocrinology. New York: Raven Press, 1993.

Speroff L, Glass RH, Kase NG. Clinical gynecologic endocrinology and infertility. Baltimore: Williams & Wilkins, 1994.

Development

1. Baker TG, Sum W. Development of the ovary and oogenesis. Clin Obstet Gynecol 1976;3:3–26.
2. Byskov AG. Differentiation of mammalian embryonic gonad. Physiol Rev 1986;66:71–117.
3. Fukuda O, Miyayama Y, Fujimoto T, Okamura H. Electron microscopic study of gonadal development in early human embryos. Prog Clin Biol Res 1989;296:23–9.

4. Gillman J. The development of the gonads in man, with a consideration of the role of fetal endocrines and the histogenesis of ovarian tumors. Contrib Embryol, No 210, 1948;32:81–132.

5. Gondos B. Cellular interrelationships in the human fetal ovary and testis. In: Federoff S, ed. Prog Clin Biol Res, volume 59B. Eleventh international congress of anatomy: Advances in the morphology of cells and tissues. New York: Alan R. Liss Inc, 1981:373–81.

6. Gondos B. Surface epithelium of the developing ovary. Possible correlation with ovarian neoplasia. Am J Pathol 1975;81:303–21.

7. Gondos B. Ultrastructure of the germinal epithelium during oogenesis in the rabbit. J Exp Zool 1969;172:465–79.

8. Gondos B, Bhiraleus P, Hobel CJ. Ultrastructural observations on germ cells in human fetal ovaries. Am J Obstet Gynecol 1971;110:644–52.

9. Gruenwald P. The development of the sex cords in the gonads of man and mammals. Am J Anat 1942;70:359–89.

10. Jirasek JE. Development of the genital system in human embryos and fetuses. In: Development of the genital system and male pseudohermaphroditism. Baltimore: Johns Hopkins Press, 1971:3–41.

11. Hoang-Ngoc M, Smadja A, Herve De Sigalony JP, Orcel L. Etude histologique de la gonade a differenciation ovarienne au cours de l'organogenese. Arch Anat Cytol Pathol 1989;37:201–7.

12. Konishi I, Fujii S, Okamura H, Parmley T, Mori T. Development of interstitial cells and ovigerous cords in the human fetal ovary: an ultrastructural study. J Anat 1986;148:121–35.

13. Pinkerton JH, McKay DG, Adams EC, Hertig AT. Development of the human ovary—a study using histochemical techniques. Obstet Gynecol 1961;18:152–81.

14. Rabinovici J, Jaffe RB. Development and regulation of growth and differentiated function in human and subhuman primate fetal gonads. Endocr Rev 1990;11:532–57.

15. Satoh M. Histogenesis and organogenesis of the gonad in human embryos. J Anat 1991;177:85–107.

16. Van Wagenen G, Simpson ME. Embryology of the ovary and testis, Homo sapiens and Macaca mulatta. New Haven: Yale University Press, 1965.

17. Wartenberg H. Development of the early human ovary and role of the mesonephros in the differentiation of the cortex. Anat Embryol 1982;165:253–80.

18. Wartenberg H. The influence of the mesonephric blastema on gonadal development and sexual differentiation. In: Byskov AG, Peters H, eds. Development and function of reproductive organs. Amsterdam-Oxford-Princeton: Excerpta Medica, 1981:3–12.

Congenital Abnormalities

19. Cruikshank SH, Van Drie DM. Supernumerary ovaries: update and review. Obstet Gynecol 1982;60:126–9.

20. Dillon WP, Dewey M. A case of accessory ovary. Obstet Gynecol 1981;58:660–1.

21. Gabbay-Moore M, Ovadia Y, Neri A. Accessory ovary with bilateral dermoid cysts. Eur J Obstet Gynec Reprod Biol 1982;14:171–3.

22. Hahn-Pedersen J, Larsen PM. Supernumerary ovary. Acta Obstet Gynecol Scand 1984;63:365–6.

23. Heller DS, Harpaz N, Breakstone B. Neoplasms arising in ectopic ovaries: a case of Brenner tumor in an accessory ovary. Int J Gynecol Pathol 1990;9:185–9.

24. Kosasa TS, Griffiths CT, Shane JM, Leventhal JM, Naftolin F. Diagnosis of a supernumerary ovary with human chorionic gonadotropin. Obstet Gynecol 1976; 47:236–8.

25. Lachman MF, Berman MM. The ectopic ovary. A case report and review of the literature. Arch Pathol Lab Med 1991;115:233–5.

26. Lee B, Gore BZ. A case of supernumerary ovary. Obstet Gynecol 1984;63:738–40.

27. Mercer LJ, Toub DB, Cibils LA. Tumors originating in supernumerary ovaries. A report of two cases. J Reprod Med 1987;32:932–4.

28. Printz JL, Choate JW, Townes PL, Harper RC. The embryology of supernumerary ovaries. Obstet Gynecol 1973;41:246–52.

29. Wharton LR. Two cases of supernumerary ovary and one of accessory ovary, with an analysis of previously reported cases. Am J Obstet Gynecol 1959;78:1101–19.

Gross Anatomy and Histology

30. Adams EC, Hertig AT. Studies on the human corpus luteum. I. Observations on the ultrastructure of development and regression of the luteal cells during the menstrual cycle. J Cell Biol 1969;41:696–715.

31. Baca M, Zamboni L. The fine structure of the human follicular oocytes. J Ultrastruct Res 1967;19:354–81.

32. Balboni GC. Structural changes: ovulation and luteal phase. In: Serra GB, ed. The ovary. New York: Raven Press, 1983;123–41.

33. Benjamin E, Law S, Bobrow LG. Intermediate filaments cytokeratin and vimentin in ovarian sex cord-stromal tumours with correlative studies in adult and fetal ovaries. J Pathol 1987;152:253–63.

34. Blaustein A. Surface cells and inclusion cysts in fetal ovaries. Gynecol Oncol 1981;12:222–33.

35. Blaustein A, Kantius M, Kaganowicz A, Pervez N, Wells JK. Inclusions in ovaries of females aged day 1–30 years. Int J Gynecol Pathol 1982;1:145–53.

36. Blaustein A, Lee H. Surface cells of the ovary and pelvic peritoneum: a histochemical and ultrastructural comparison. Gynecol Oncol 1979; 8:34–43.

37. Bloom W, Fawcett DW. A textbook of histology, 10th ed. Philadelphia: WB Saunders, 1975.

38. Boss JH, Scully RE, Wegner KH, Cohen RB. Structural variations in the adult ovary–clinical significance. Obstet Gynecol 1965;25:747–63.

39. Bransilver BR, Ferenczy A, Richart RM. Brenner tumors and Walthard cell nests. Arch Pathol Lab Med 1974;98:76–86.

40. Centola G.M. Structural changes: atresia. In: Serra GB, ed. The ovary. New York: Raven Press, 1983:113–22.

41. Clement PB, Young RH, Scully, RE. Ovarian granulosa cell proliferations of pregnancy: a report of nine cases. Hum Pathol 1988;19:657–62.

42. Corner GW Jr. The histological dating of the human corpus luteum of menstruation. Am J Anat 1956;98:377–401.

43. Curtis EM. Normal ovarian histology in infancy and childhood. Obstet Gynecol 1962;19:444–54.

44. Czernobilsky B, Moll R, Franke WW, Dallenbach-Hellweg G, Hohlweg-Majert P. Intermediate filaments of normal and neoplastic tissues of the female genital tract with emphasis on problems of differential tumor diagnosis. Path Res Pract 1984;179:31–7.

45. Czernobilsky B, Moll R, Levy R, Franke WW. Co-expression of cytokeratin and vimentin filaments in mesothelial, granulosa and rete ovarii cells of the human ovary. Eur J Cell Biol 1985;37:175–90.

46. Czernobilsky B, Shezen E, Lifschitz-Mercer B, et al. Alpha smooth muscle actin (alpha-SM actin) in normal human ovaries, in ovarian stromal hyperplasia and in ovarian neoplasms. Virchows Arch [Cell Pathol] 1989;57:55–61.

47. Danforth DN. Cytologic relationship of Walthard cell rest to Brenner tumor of ovary and the pseudomucinous cystadenoma. Am J Obstet Gynecol 1942;43:984–96.

48. Dawood MY, Strongin M, Kramer EE, Wieche R. Recent ovulation in a postmenopausal woman. Int J Gynaecol Obstet 1980;18:192–4.

49. Deane HW, Lobel BL, Romney SL. Enzymic histochemistry of normal human ovaries of the menstrual cycle, pregnancy, and the early puerperium. Am J Obstet Gynecol 1962;83:281–94.

50. Dekel N, David MP, Yedwab GA, Kraicer PF. Follicular development during late pregnancy. Int J Fertil 1977;22:24–9.

51. Eichner E, Bove ER. In vivo studies on the lymphatic drainage of the human ovary. Obstet Gynecol 1954;3:287–97.

52. Falls JL. Accessory adrenal cortex in the broad ligament. Incidence and significance. Cancer 1955;8:143–50.

53. Ferenczy A, Richart RM. Female reproductive system: dynamics of scan and transmission electron microscopy. New York: John Wiley & Sons, 1974.

54. Fienberg R, Cohen RB. A comparative histochemical study of the ovarian stromal lipid band, stromal theca cell, and normal ovarian follicular apparatus. Am J Obstet Gynecol 1965;92:958–69.

55. Gardner GH, Greene RR, Peckham B. Tumors of the broad ligament. Am J Obstet Gynecol 1957;73:536–55.

56. Gillim SW, Christensen AK, McLennan CE. Fine structure of the human menstrual corpus luteum at its stage of maximum secretory activity. Am J Anat 1969;126:409–27.

57. Gougeon A. Frequent occurrence of multiovular follicles and multinuclear oocytes in the adult human ovary. Fertil Steril 1981;35:417–22.

58. Govan AD. Ovarian follicular activity in late pregnancy. J Endocrinol 1970;48:235–41.

59. Hart WR, Abell MR. Adipose prosoplasia of ovary. Am J Obstet Gynecol 1970;106:929–31.

60. Hertig AT. Gestational hyperplasia of endometrium. A morphologic correlation of ova, endometrium, and corpora lutea during early pregnancy. Lab Invest 1964;13:1153–91.

61. Himelstein-Braw R, Byskov AG, Peters H, Faber M. Follicular atresia in the infant human ovary. J Reprod Fert 1976;46:55–9.

62. Honore LH, O'Hara KE. Ovarian hilus cell heterotopia. Obstet Gynecol 1979;53:461–4.

63. Honore LH, O'Hara KE. Subcapsular adipocytic infiltration of the human ovary: a clinicopathological study of eight cases. Eur J Obstet Gynaecol Reprod Biol 1980;10:13–20.

64. Hughesdon PE. The endometrial identity of benign stromatosis of the ovary and its relation to other forms of endometriosis. J Pathol 1976;119:201–9.

65. Hughesdon PE. Morphology and morphogenesis of the Stein-Leventhal ovary and of so-called "hyperthecosis." Obstet Gynecol Surv 1982;37:59–77.

66. Hughesdon PE. The origin and development of benign stromatosis of the ovary. Br J Obstet Gynaecol 1972;79:348–59.

67. Isola J, Kallioniemi OP, Korte JM, et al. Steroid receptors and Ki-67 reactivity in ovarian cancer and in normal ovary: correlation with DNA flow cytometry, biochemical receptor assay, and patient survival. J Pathol 1990;162:295–301.

68. Jacobowitz D, Wallach EE. Histochemical and chemical studies of the autonomic innervation of the ovary. Endocrinol 1967;81:1132–9.

69. Janko AB. Sandberg EC. Histochemical evidence for the protein nature of the Reinke crystalloid. Obstet Gynecol 1970;35:493–503.

70. Jindal SK, Snoey DM, Lobb DK, Dorrington JH. Transforming growth factor alpha localization and role in surface epithelium of normal human ovaries and in ovarian carcinoma lines. Gynecol Oncol 1994;53:17–23.

71. Joel RV, Foraker AG. Fate of the corpus albicans: a morphologic approach. Am J Obstet Gynecol 1960;80:314–6.

72. Jones GE, Goldberg B, Woodruff JD. Histochemistry as a guide for interpretation of cell function. Am J Obstet Gynecol 1968;100:76–83.

73. Kedzia H. Gonadoblastoma: structures and background of development. Am J Obstet Gynecol 1983;147:81–5.

74. Kraus FT, Neubecker RD. Luteinization of the ovarian theca in infants and children. Am J Clin Pathol 1962;37:389–97.

75. Laffargue P, Adechy-Benkoel L, Valette C. Ultrastructure du stroma ovarien. Ann d'Anat Pathol 1968;13:381–402.

76. Lastarria D, Sachdev RK, Babury RA, Yu HM, Nuovo GJ. Immunohistochemical analysis for desmin in normal and neoplastic ovarian stromal tissue. Arch Pathol Lab Med 1990;114:502–5.

77. Latza U, Niedobitek G, Schwarting R, Nekarda H, Stein H. Ber-EP4: new monoclonal antibody which distinguishes epithelia from mesothelia. J Clin Pathol 1990;43:213–9.

78. Loubet R, Loubet A, Leboutet MJ. The ovarian stroma after the menopause: activity and ageing. In: de Brux J, Gautray JP, eds. Clinical pathology of the ovary. Boston: MTP Press Ltd, 1984:119–41.

79. Manivel JC, Dehner LP, Burke B. Ovarian tumorlike structures, biovular follicles, and binucleated oocytes in children: their frequency and possible pathologic significance. Pediatr Pathol 1988;8:283–92.

80. Maqueo M, Goldzieher JW. Hormone-induced alterations of ovarian morphology. Fertil Steril 1966;17:676–83.

81. McKay DG, Pinkerton JH, Hertig AT, Danziger S. The adult human ovary: a histochemical study. Obstet Gynecol 1961;18:13–39.

82. Merrill JA. The morphology of the prepubertal ovary: relationship to the polycystic ovary syndrome. South Med J 1963;56:225–31.

83. Merrill JA. Ovarian hilus cells. Am J Obstet Gynecol 1959;78:1258–71.

84. Miettinen M, Lehto VP, Virtanen I. Expression of intermediate filaments in normal ovaries and ovarian epithelial, sex cord-stromal, and germinal tumors. Int J Gynecol Pathol 1983;2:64–71.

85. Mikhail G, Allen WM. Ovarian function in human pregnancy. Am J Obstet Gynecol 1967;99:308–12.

86. Mulligan RM. A survey of epithelial inclusions in the ovarian cortex of 470 patients. J Surg Oncol 1976;8:61–6.

87. Nagamani M, Hannigan EV, Van Dinh T, Stuart CA. Hyperinsulinemia and stromal luteinization of the ovaries in postmenopausal women with endometrial cancer. J Clin Endocrinol Metab 1988;67:144–8.

88. Nakano R, Shima K, Yamoto M, Kobayashi M, Nishimori K, Hiraoka J. Binding sites for gonadotropins in human postmenopausal ovaries. Obstet Gynecol 1989;73:196–200.

89. Nelson WW, Greene RR. The human ovary in pregnancy. Int Abstr Surg 1953;97:1–23.

90. Nelson WW, Greene RR. Some observations on the histology of the human ovary during pregnancy. Am J Obstet Gynecol 1958;76:66–89

91. Nicosia SV. Morphological changes of the human ovary throughout life. In: Serra GB, ed. The ovary. New York: Raven Press, 1983:57–81.

92. Owman C, Rosengren E, Sjoberg N. Adrenergic innervation of the human female reproductive organs: a histochemical and chemical investigation. Obstet Gynecol 1967;30:763–73.

93. Peters H, Himelstein-Braw R, Faber M. The normal development of the ovary in childhood. Acta Endocrinol 1976;82:617–30.

94. Plentl AA, Friedman EA. Lymphatic system of the female genitalia: the morphologic basis of oncologic diagnosis and therapy. Philadelphia: WB Saunders, 1971.

95. Pryse-Davies J. The development, structure and function of the female pelvic organs in childhood. Clin Obstet Gynaecol 1974;1:483–508.

96. Reagan JW. Ceroid pigment in the human ovary. Am J Obstet Gynecol 1950;59:433–6.

97. Reeves G. Specific stroma in the cortex and medulla of the ovary. Cell types and vascular supply in relation to follicular apparatus and ovulation. Obstet Gynecol 1971;37:832–44.

98. Roddick JW Jr, Greene RR. Relation of ovarian stromal hyperplasia to endometrial carcinoma. Am J Obstet Gynecol 1957;73:843–52.

99. Rodriguez GC, Berchuk A, Whitaker RS, Schlossman D, Clarke-Pearson DL, Bast RC Jr. Epidermal growth factor receptor expression in normal ovarian epithelium and ovarian cancer. II. Relationship between receptor expression and response to epidermal growth factor. Am J Obstet Gynecol 1991;164:745–50.

100. Roth LM. The Brenner tumor and the Walthard cell nest. An electron microscopic study. Lab Invest 1974;31:15–23.

101. Rutgers JL, Scully RE. Cysts (cystadenomas) and tumors of the rete ovarii. Int J Gynecol Pathol 1988; 7:330–42.

102. Rutgers JL, Scully RE. Functioning ovarian tumors with peripheral steroid cell proliferation: a report of twenty-four cases. Int J Gynecol Pathol 1986;5:319–37.

103. Safneck JR, DeSa DJ. Structures mimicking sex cord-stromal tumours and gonadoblastomas in the ovaries of normal infants and children. Histopathology 1986;10:909–20.

104. Sauramo H. Development, occurrence, function, and pathology of the rete ovarii. Acta Obstet Gynecol Scand 1954;33:29–66.

105. Schmidt WA. Eosin-induced fluorescence of Reinke crystals. Int J Gynecol Pathol 1986;5:88–9.

106. Scully RE. Smooth-muscle differentiation in genital tract disorders [Editorial]. Arch Pathol Lab Med 1981;105:505–7.

107. Scully RE, Cohen RB. Oxidative-enzyme activity in normal and pathologic human ovaries. Obstet Gynecol 1964;24:667–81.

108. Shaw JA, Dabbs DJ, Geisinger KR. Sclerosing stromal tumor of the ovary: an ultrastructural and immunohistochemical analysis with histogenetic considerations. Ultrastruct Pathol 1992;16:363–77.

109. Sherrer CW, Gerson B, Woodruff JD. The incidence and significance of polynuclear follicles. Am J Obstet Gynecol 1977;128:6–12.

110. Sidaway MK, Silverberg SG. Endosalpingiosis in female peritoneal washings: a diagnostic pitfall. Int J Gynecol Pathol 1987;6:340–6.

111. Snowden JA, Harkin PJ, Thornton JG, Wells M. Morphometric assessment of ovarian stromal proliferation—a clinicopathological study. Histopathology 1989;14:369–79.

112. Starup J, Visfeldt J. Ovarian morphology in early and late human pregnancy. Acta Obstet Gynecol Scand 1974;53:211–8.

113. Sternberg WH. The morphology, androgenic function, hyperplasia, and tumors of the human ovarian hilus cells. Am J Pathol 1949;25:493–521.

114. Sternberg WH, Roth LM. Ovarian stromal tumors containing Leydig cells. I. Stromal-Leydig cell tumor and non-neoplastic transformation of ovarian stroma to Leydig cells. Cancer 1973;32:940–51.

115. Sternberg WH, Segaloff A, Gaskill CJ. Influence of chorionic gonadotropin on human ovarian hilus cells (Leydig-like cells). J Clin Endocrinol Metab 1953;13:139–53.

116. Strickler R, Kelly RW, Askin FB. Postmenopausal ovarian follicle cyst: an unusual cause of estrogen excess. Int J Gynecol Pathol 1984;3:318–22.

117. Symonds DA, Driscoll SG. An adrenal cortical rest within the fetal ovary: report of a case. Am J Clin Pathol 1973;60:562–4.

118. Teoh TB. The structure and development of Walthard nests. J Pathol 1953;66:433–9.

119. Valdes-Dapena MA. The normal ovary of childhood. Ann NY Acad Sci 1967;142:597–613.

120. Visfeldt J, Starup J. Histology of the human corpus luteum of early and late pregnancy. Acta Path Microbiol Scand A 1975;83:669–77.

121. Von Numers C. Observations on metaplastic changes in the germinal epithelium of the ovary and on the aetiology of ovarian endometriosis. Acta Obstet Gynecol Scand 1965;44:107–16.

122. White RF, Hertig AT, Rock J, Adams E. Histological and histochemical observations on the corpus luteum of human pregnancy with special reference to corpora lutea associated with early normal and abnormal ova. Contrib Embryol 1951;34:55–74.

123. Wiley CA, Esterly JR. Observations on the human corpus luteum: histochemical changes during development and involution. Am J Obstet Gynecol 1976;125:514–9.

124. Woll E, Hertig AT, Smith GV, Johnson LC. The ovary in endometrial carcinoma. Am J Obstet Gynecol 1948;56:617–33.

125. Zhang J, Young RH, Arseneau J, Scully RE. Ovarian stromal tumors containing lutein or Leydig cells (luteinized thecomas and stromal Leydig cell tumors)—a clinicopathological analysis of fifty cases. Int J Gynecol Pathol 1982;1:270–85.

126. Zinsser KR, Wheeler JE. Endosalpingiosis in the omentum: a study of autopsy and surgical material. Am J Surg Pathol 1982;6:109–17.

Ovarian Function and Laboratory Evaluation

127. Aiman J, Forney JP, Parker CR Jr. Secretion of androgens and estrogens by normal and neoplastic ovaries in postmenopausal women. Obstet Gynecol 1986;68:1–5.

128. Barbieri RL, Makris A, Randall RW, Daniels G, Kistner RW, Ryan KJ. Insulin stimulates androgen accumulation in incubations of ovarian stroma obtained from women with hyperandrogenism. J Clin Endocrinol Metab 1986;62:904–10.

129. Centola GM. Structural changes: follicular development and hormonal requirements. In: Serra GB, ed. The ovary. New York: Raven Press, 1983;95–111.

130. Chang RJ, Judd HL. The ovary after menopause. Clin Obstet Gynaecol 1981;24:181–91.

131. Dennefors BL, Janson PO, Hamberger L, Knutsson F. Hilus cells from human postmenopausal ovaries: gonadotrophin sensitivity, steroid and cyclic AMP production. Acta Obstet Gynecol Scand 1982;61:413–6.

132. Dennefors BL, Janson PO, Knutsson F, Hamberger L. Steroid production and responsiveness to gonadotropin in isolated stromal tissue of human postmenopausal ovaries. Am J Obstet Gynecol 1980;136:997–1002.

133. Donahoe PK, Cate RL, MacLaughlin DT, et al. Mullerian inhibiting substance: gene structure and mechanism of action of a fetal regressor. Recent Prog Horm Res 1987;43:431–67.

134. Erickson GF. Normal ovarian function. Clin Obstet Gynecol 1978;21:31–52.

135. Futterweit W. Polycystic ovarian disease. Clinical perspectives in obstetrics and gynecology. New York: Springer-Verlag, 1985.

136. Greenblatt RB, Colle ML, Mahesh VB. Ovarian and adrenal steroid production in the postmenopausal woman. Obstet Gynecol 1976;47:383–7.

137. Grodin JM, Siiteri PK, MacDonald PC. Source of estrogen production in postmenopausal women. J Clin Endocrinol Metab 1973;36:207–14.

138. Hillier SG. Intrafollicular paracrine function of ovarian androgen. J Steroid Biochem 1987;27:351–7.

139. Judd HL, Judd GE, Lucas WE, Yen SS. Endocrine function of the postmenopausal ovary: concentration of androgens and estrogens in ovarian and peripheral vein blood. J Clin Endocrinol Metab 1974;39:1020–4.

140. Judd HL, Lucas WE, Yen SS. Effect of oophorectomy on circulating testosterone and androstenedione levels in patients with endometrial carcinoma. Am J Obstet Gynecol 1974;118:793–8.

141. LeMaire WJ, Conly PW, Moffett A, Spellacy WN, Cleveland WW, Savard K. Function of the human corpus luteum during the puerperium: its maintenance by exogenous human chorionic gonadotropin. Am J Obstet Gynecol 1971;110:612–8.

142. Longcope C. Metabolic clearance and blood production rates of estrogens in postmenopausal women. Am J Obstet Gynecol 1971;111:778–81.

143. Longcope C, Hunter R, Franz C. Steroid secretion by the postmenopausal ovary. Am J Obstet Gynecol 1980;138:564–8.

144. Mattingly RF, Huang WY. Steroidogenesis of the menopausal and postmenopausal ovary. Am J Obstet Gynecol 1969;103:679–93.

145. McKay DG, Pinkerton JH, Hertig AT, Danziger S. The adult human ovary: a histochemical study. Obstet Gynecol 1961;18:13–39.

146. McNatty KP. Cyclic changes in antral fluid hormone concentrations in humans. Clin Endocrinol Metab 1978;7:577–600.

147. McNatty KP. Follicular determinants of corpus luteum function in the human ovary. Ovarian follicular and corpus luteum function. In: Channing CP, Marsh JM, Sadler WA, eds. Advances in Experimental Medicine and Biology, vol 112. New York: Plenum Press, 1978:465–77.

148. McNatty KP, Makris A, DeGrazia C, Osathanondh R, Ryan KJ. The production of progesterone, androgens, and estrogens by granulosa cells, thecal tissue, and stromal tissue from human ovaries in vitro. J Clin Endocrinol Metab 1979;49:687–99.

149. McNatty KP, Makris A, DeGrazia C, Osathanondh R, Ryan KJ. The production of progesterone, androgens, and oestrogens by human granulosa cells in vitro and in vivo. J Steroid Biochem 1979;11:775–9.

150. McNatty KP, Smith DM, Makris A, et al. The intraovarian sites of androgen and estrogen formation in women with normal and hyperandrogenic ovaries as judged by in vitro experiments. J Clin Endocrinol Metab 1980;50:755–63.

151. Nagamani M, Hannigan EV, Van Dinh T, Stuart CA. Hyperinsulinemia and stromal luteinization of the ovaries in postmenopausal women with endometrial cancer. J Clin Endocrinol Metab 1988;67:144–8.

152. Nakano R, Shima K, Yamoto M, Kobayashi M, Nishimori K, Hiraoka J. Binding sites for gonadotropins in human postmenopausal ovaries. Obstet Gynecol 1989;73:196–200.

153. Palumbo A, Jones C, Lightman A, Carcangiu ML, DeCherney AH, Naftolin F. Immunohistochemical localization of renin and angiotensin II in human ovaries. Am J Obstet Gynecol 1989;160:8–14.

154. Plotz EJ, Wiener M, Stein AA, Hahn BD. Enzymatic activities related to steroidogenesis in postmenopausal ovaries of patients with and without endometrial carcinoma. Am J Obstet Gynecol 1967;99:182–97.

155. Rao CV. Receptors for gonadotropins in human ovaries. Recent advances in fertility research, part A: Developments in reproductive endocrinology. New York: AR Liss, 1982;123–35.

156. Reed MJ, Beranek PA, Ghilchik MW, James VH. Conversion of estrone to estradiol and estradiol to estrone in postmenopausal women. Obstet Gynecol 1985;66:361–5.

157. Rice BF, Savard K. Steroid hormone formation in the human ovary: IV. Ovarian stromal compartment: formation of radioactive steroids from acetate-1-14C and action of gonadotropins. J Clin Endocrinol 1966;26:593–609.

158. Sealey JE, Glorioso N, Itskovitz J, Laragh JH. Prorenin as a reproductive hormone. New form of the renin system. Am J Med 1986;81:1041–6.

159. Shima K, Kitayama S, Nakano R. Gonadotropin binding sites in human ovarian follicles and corpora lutea during the menstrual cycle. Obstet Gynecol 1987;69:800–6.

160. Snowden JA, Harkin PJ, Thornton JG, Wells M. Morphometric assessment of ovarian stromal prolifera-tion—a clinicopathological study. Histopathology 1989;14:369–79.

161. Sternberg WH. The morphology, androgenic function, hyperplasia, and tumors of the human ovarian hilus cells. Am J Pathol 1949;25:493–521.

162. Sternberg WH, Segaloff A, Gaskill CJ. Influence of chorionic gonadotropin on human ovarian hilus cells (Leydig-like cells). J Clin Endocrinol Metab 1953;13:139–53.

163. Tanabe K, Gagliano P, Channing CP, et al. Levels of inhibin-F activity and steroids in human follicular fluid from normal women and women with polycystic ovarian disease. J Clin Endocrinol Metab 1983;57:24–31.

164. Tsonis CG, Messinis IE, Templeton AA, McNeilly AS, Baird DT. Gonadotropic stimulation of inhibin secretion by the human ovary during the follicular and early luteal phase of the cycle. J Clin Endocrinol Metab 1988;66:915–21.

165. Vermeulen A. The hormonal activity of the postmenopausal ovary. J Clin Endocrinol Metab 1976;42:247–53.

2

GENERAL FEATURES OF OVARIAN TUMORS

CLASSIFICATION

Establishing a classification and system of nomenclature for ovarian tumors is difficult because of controversies in gonadal embryology, the diverse or in some cases unknown lineage of a number of these tumors, and the many neoplasms that have overlapping microscopic features. It is important, however, that authors who report their experience, especially with malignant forms of these tumors, use uniform terminology; otherwise, knowledge about epidemiologic features, biologic behavior, and treatment will be compromised. To encourage usage of a standard classification this Fascicle uses the one recently formulated and accepted by the World Health Organization (WHO) and the International Society of Gynecological Pathologists (Table 2-1).

The nomenclature of tumors in the WHO classification is based, whenever possible, on cell types and patterns of growth. Controversial histogenetic designations have been avoided except when they appear to be the most comprehensible terms available. Time-honored and familiar terms, even though not always scientifically optimal, have been retained except when they are seriously misleading. It is important to emphasize that because of the complex and often heterogeneous nature of many ovarian tumors the terms used for them should reflect their entire composition. This approach is particularly desirable for malignant germ cell tumors but is also applicable to other neoplasms: for example, a serous tumor may be composed of both a cystadenoma and an adenofibroma, or a cystadenoma and a carcinoma; in either case, both diagnoses should be reflected in the pathology report, with some indication of their relative quantities and of the relation, if any, between the components.

In addition to the application of specific designations for ovarian tumors grading of most of their malignant forms is important because of its usual correlation with prognosis and occasional therapeutic implications. Also, several pathologic aspects of ovarian tumors other than their type and grade may be important prognostically and therapeutically and should be included in the pathology report. Finally, evaluation of the intrinsic and adjacent stroma of ovarian neoplasms is desirable because stromal cells can assume the morphologic and physiologic attributes of steroid hormone–secreting organs and result in endocrine manifestations. The presence of a stroma compatible with hormone secretion should be acknowledged, therefore, either in the diagnostic statement or in an accompanying comment (see chapter 19).

FREQUENCY

Ovarian tumors account for a considerable proportion of clinically important neoplasms in the female. The figures that follow denote the frequency and age distribution of these tumors, based on several analyses within North America (1,7,8). About two thirds of ovarian tumors occur in women in the reproductive age group, and 80 to 90 percent of them in women between the ages of 20 and 65 years; well under 5 percent occur in children. Seventy-five to 80 percent of ovarian tumors are benign, and 55 to 65 percent of benign tumors occur in women under the age of 40 years; in contrast, 80 to 90 percent of ovarian epithelial cancers, including borderline forms, are detected after the age of 40 years, and 30 to 40 percent of them, after the age of 65 years. The age-specific incidence of ovarian epithelial cancer rises precipitously from approximately 20 to 80 years and subsequently declines (20). From another perspective, the chance that a primary ovarian epithelial tumor is of borderline or invasive malignancy in a patient under the age of 40 years is approximately 1 in 10, but beyond that age it rises to 1 in 3.

Ovarian cancer is the sixth most common form of cancer in females in the United States (based on figures that combine cancers of the uterine corpus and cervix as cancer of the uterus, exclude skin cancer, and include leukemia-lymphoma as a single category); it accounts for 4 percent of all female cancers and 25 percent of cancers of female genital organs (3). Because of its low cure rate of less than 40 percent, ovarian cancer is responsible for 5 percent of cancer

Table 2-1
WORLD HEALTH ORGANIZATION
HISTOLOGICAL CLASSIFICATION OF OVARIAN TUMORS

1. Surface Epithelial–Stromal Tumors
    1.1. Serous Tumors
        1.1.1. Benign
            1.1.1.1. Cystadenoma and papillary cystadenoma
            1.1.1.2. Surface papilloma
            1.1.1.3. Adenofibroma and cystadenofibroma
        1.1.2. Of Borderline Malignancy (of low malignant potential)
            1.1.2.1. Cystic tumor and papillary cystic tumor
            1.1.2.2. Surface papillary tumor
            1.1.2.3. Adenofibroma and cystadenofibroma
        1.1.3. Malignant
            1.1.3.1. Adenocarcinoma, papillary adenocarcinoma, and papillary cystadenocarcinoma
            1.1.3.2. Surface papillary adenocarcinoma
            1.1.3.3. Adenocarcinofibroma and cystadenocarcinofibroma (malignant adenofibroma and cystadenofibroma)
    1.2. Mucinous Tumors, Endocervical-like and Intestinal Types
        1.2.1. Benign
            1.2.1.1. Cystadenoma
            1.2.1.2. Adenofibroma and cystadenofibroma
        1.2.2. Of Borderline Malignancy (of low malignant potential)
            1.2.2.1. Cystic tumor
            1.2.2.2. Adenofibroma and cystadenofibroma
        1.2.3. Malignant
            1.2.3.1. Adenocarcinoma and cystadenocarcinoma
            1.2.3.2. Adenocarcinofibroma and cystadenocarcinofibroma (malignant adenofibroma and cystadenofibroma)
    1.3. Endometrioid Tumors
        1.3.1. Benign
            1.3.1.1. Cystadenoma
            1.3.1.2. Cystadenoma with squamous differentiation
            1.3.1.3. Adenofibroma and cystadenofibroma
            1.3.1.4. Adenofibroma and cystadenofibroma with squamous differentiation
        1.3.2. Of Borderline Malignancy (of low malignant potential)
            1.3.2.1. Cystic tumor
            1.3.2.2. Cystic tumor with squamous differentiation
            1.3.2.3. Adenofibroma and cystadenofibroma
            1.3.2.4. Adenofibroma and cystadenofibroma with squamous differentiation
        1.3.3. Malignant
            1.3.3.1. Adenocarcinoma and cystadenocarcinoma
            1.3.3.2. Adenocarcinoma and cystadenocarcinoma with squamous differentiation
            1.3.3.3. Adenocarcinofibroma and cystadenocarcinofibroma (malignant adenofibroma and cystadenofibroma)
            1.3.3.4. Adenocarcinofibroma and cystadenocarcinofibroma with squamous differentiation (malignant adenofibroma and cystadenofibroma with squamous differentiation)
        1.3.4. Epithelial-Stromal and Stromal
            1.3.4.1. Adenosarcoma, homologous and heterologous
            1.3.4.2. Mesodermal (mullerian) mixed tumor (carcinosarcoma), homologous and heterologous
            1.3.4.3. Stromal sarcoma
    1.4. Clear Cell Tumors
        1.4.1. Benign
            1.4.1.1. Cystadenoma
            1.4.1.2. Adenofibroma and cystadenofibroma

Table 2-1 (continued)
WORLD HEALTH ORGANIZATION
HISTOLOGICAL CLASSIFICATION OF OVARIAN TUMORS

1.4.2.   Of Borderline Malignancy (of low malignant potential)
  1.4.2.1.   Cystic tumor
  1.4.2.2.   Adenofibroma and cystadenofibroma
1.4.3.   Malignant
  1.4.3.1.   Adenocarcinoma
  1.4.3.2.   Adenocarcinofibroma and cystadenocarcinofibroma (malignant adenofibroma and cystadenofibroma)
1.5.   Transitional Cell Tumors
1.5.1.   Brenner Tumor
1.5.2.   Brenner Tumor of Borderline Malignancy (proliferating)
1.5.3.   Malignant Brenner Tumor
1.5.4.   Transitional Cell Carcinoma (non-Brenner type)
1.6.   Squamous Cell Tumors
1.7.   Mixed Epithelial Tumors (specify types)
1.7.1.   Benign
1.7.2.   Of Borderline Malignancy (of low malignant potential)
1.7.3.   Malignant
1.8.   Undifferentiated Carcinoma
2.   Sex Cord–Stromal Tumors
2.1.   Granulosa- Stromal Cell Tumors
2.1.1.   Granulosa Cell Tumor
  2.1.1.1.   Adult
  2.1.1.2.   Juvenile
2.1.2.   Tumors in Thecoma-Fibroma Group
  2.1.2.1.   Thecoma
      typical
      luteinized
  2.1.2.2.   Fibroma
  2.1.2.3.   Cellular fibroma
  2.1.2.4.   Fibrosarcoma
  2.1.2.5.   Stromal tumor with minor sex cord elements
  2.1.2.6.   Sclerosing stromal tumor
  2.1.2.7.   (Stromal luteoma) see 2.6.1.
  2.1.2.8.   Unclassified
  2.1.2.9.   Others
2.2.   Sertoli-Stromal Cell Tumors; Androblastomas
2.2.1.   Well differentiated
  2.2.1.1.   Sertoli cell tumor (tubular androblastoma)
  2.2.1.2.   Sertoli-Leydig cell tumor
  2.2.1.3.   Leydig cell tumor - see 2.6.2.
2.2.2.   Sertoli-Leydig Cell Tumor of Intermediate Differentiation
  2.2.2.1.   Variant - with heterologous elements (specify type)
2.2.3.   Sertoli-Leydig Cell Tumor, Poorly Differentiated (sarcomatoid)
  2.2.3.1.   Variant - with heterologous elements (specify type)
2.2.4.   Retiform
  2.2.4.1.   Variant - with heterologous elements (specify type)
2.3.   Sex Cord Tumor with Annular Tubules
2.4.   Gynandroblastoma
2.5.   Unclassified

Table 2-1 (continued)
WORLD HEALTH ORGANIZATION
HISTOLOGICAL CLASSIFICATION OF OVARIAN TUMORS

2.6. Steroid (Lipid) Cell Tumors
    2.6.1. Stromal Luteoma
    2.6.2. Leydig Cell Tumor
        2.6.2.1. Hilus cell tumor
        2.6.2.1. Leydig cell tumor, nonhilar type
    2.6.3. Unclassified (not otherwise specified)
3. Germ Cell Tumors
    3.1. Dysgerminoma
        3.1.1. Variant - with syncytiotrophoblast cells
    3.2. Yolk Sac Tumor (Endodermal Sinus Tumor)
        3.2.1. Variants - Polyvesicular vitelline tumor
                      - Hepatoid
                      - Glandular (Some glandular yolk sac tumors resemble endometrioid adeno-carcinoma and have been called "endometrioid-like.")
    3.3. Embryonal Carcinoma
    3.4. Polyembryoma
    3.5. Choriocarcinoma
    3.6. Teratomas
        3.6.1. Immature
        3.6.2. Mature
            3.6.2.1. Solid
            3.6.2.2. Cystic (dermoid cyst)
            3.6.2.3. With secondary tumor (specify type)
            3.6.2.4. Fetiform (homunculus)
        3.6.3. Monodermal
            3.6.3.1. Struma ovarii
                3.6.3.1.1. Variant - with secondary tumor (specify type)
            3.6.3.2. Carcinoid tumor
                insular
                trabecular
            3.6.3.3. Strumal carcinoid tumor
            3.6.3.4. Mucinous carcinoid tumor
            3.6.3.5. Neuroectodermal tumors (specify type)
            3.6.3.6. Sebaceous tumors
            3.6.3.7. Others
    3.7. Mixed Germ Cell Tumors (specify types)
4. Gonadoblastoma
    4.1. Variant - with dysgerminoma or other germ cell tumor
5. Germ Cell-Sex Cord-Stromal Tumor of Non-gonadoblastoma Type
    5.1. Variant - with dysgerminoma or other germ cell tumor
6. Tumors of Rete Ovarii
    6.1. Adenoma and Cystadenoma
    6.2. Adenocarcinoma
7. Mesothelial Tumors
    7.1. Adenomatoid Tumor
    7.2. Mesothelioma
8. Tumors of Uncertain Origin and Miscellaneous Tumors
    8.1. Small Cell Carcinomas
    8.2. Tumor of Probable Wolffian Origin
    8.3. Hepatoid Carcinoma
    8.4. Myxoma
    8.5. Others

Table 2-1 (continued)
WORLD HEALTH ORGANIZATION
HISTOLOGICAL CLASSIFICATION OF OVARIAN TUMORS

 9. Gestational Trophoblastic Diseases
10. Soft Tissue Tumors Not Specific to Ovary
11. Malignant Lymphomas and Leukemias
12. Unclassified Tumors
13. Secondary (metastatic) Tumors
14. Tumor-like Lesions
    14.1. Solitary Follicle Cyst
    14.2. Multiple Follicle Cysts (Polycystic Ovarian Disease; Sclerocystic Ovaries)
    14.3. Large Solitary Luteinized Follicle Cyst of Pregnancy and Puerperium
    14.4. Hyperreactio Luteinalis (Multiple Luteinized Follicle Cysts)
        14.4.1. Variant - with corpora lutea (hyperstimulation syndrome)
    14.5. Corpus Luteum Cyst
    14.6. Pregnancy Luteoma
    14.7. Ectopic Pregnancy
    14.8. Stromal Hyperplasia
    14.9. Stromal Hyperthecosis
    14.10. Massive Edema
    14.11. Fibromatosis
    14.12. Endometriosis
    14.13. Cyst, Unclassified (Simple Cyst)
    14.14. Inflammatory Lesions

deaths in females in the United States and over half the deaths due to cancer of the female genital organs. A female's risk at birth of having an ovarian tumor sometime in her life is 6 to 7 percent, of having ovarian cancer, almost 1.5 percent, and of dying from ovarian cancer, almost 1 percent.

CLINICAL MANIFESTATIONS

Ovarian tumors are notorious for the mildness of the early symptoms they produce. The most common initial manifestations are: abdominal distension, which may be due to the tumor itself, ascites, or both; abdominal pain or discomfort; a feeling of pressure in the pelvis; urinary or gastrointestinal tract symptoms; and in occasional cases, particularly if the tumor is functioning or malignant, abnormal vaginal bleeding. Complications such as torsion (fig. 2-1), which most commonly involves nonadherent benign cystic tumors of medium size (9), and rupture (fig. 2-2), which is encountered more frequently if the tumor is malignant and cystic, may produce an acute onset of pain. The ovarian tumors that undergo torsion most often are dermoid cysts and serous cystadenomas (9).

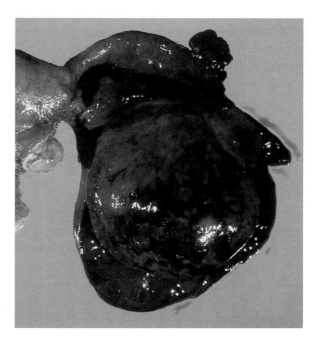

Figure 2-1
TWISTED INFARCTED SOLID OVARIAN TUMOR
The tumor has been bisected, revealing hemorrhagic infarction. The fallopian tube is also infarcted. The uterus is partly shown (Massachusetts General Hospital Case 65-13200).

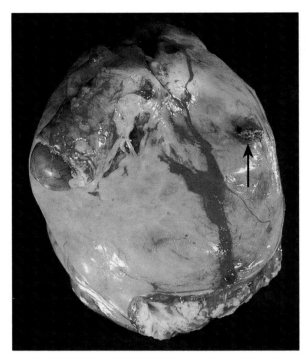

Figure 2-2
RUPTURED OVARIAN CARCINOMA
Arrow points to area of perforation.

Rapid growth or hemorrhage within a tumor also may be associated with pain. Infection of an ovarian tumor (fig. 2-3), which is most commonly secondary to spread of organisms from the genital tract or intestine, is rare. In a small proportion of cases, clinical evidence of a hormonal imbalance, most often related to a high estrogen level (16) but sometimes to androgen excess, is the presenting feature (see chapter 19). Occasionally, paraendocrine or paraneoplastic manifestations (see chapter 20) and, rarely, spread to a distant site herald the presence of an ovarian tumor. Over one fourth of patients with ovarian tumors, most of which are benign, are asymptomatic and the tumors are unexpected findings on abdominal or pelvic examination or at surgery for another indication. If an ovarian tumor in a postmenopausal woman is under 5 cm in diameter (as determined by pelvic examination, ultrasound examination, computer tomographic scanning, pathologic evaluation, or a combination thereof) it is malignant in only 5 percent of the cases; if it is 5 to 10 cm, in 12 percent; and if it is over 10 cm, in over 60 percent of the cases (17). Bilateral ovarian tumors are malignant twice as often as unilateral tumors (10).

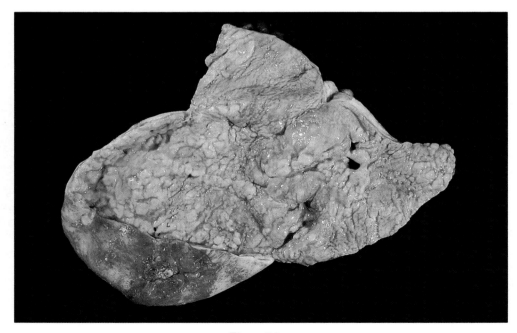

Figure 2-3
OPENED INFECTED MUCINOUS CYSTADENOMA
This tumor communicated by fistulas with both the small and the large intestine. The inner surface is shaggy. (Fig. 4 from Case Records of the Massachusetts General Hospital, Case 3-1969. N Engl J Med 1969;280:156-60.)

EPITHELIAL CANCER

Diagnosis and Screening

Almost all ovarian epithelial cancers (which arise ultimately from the surface epithelium) are diagnosed during or after abdominal exploration to investigate a pelvic or abdominal mass detected on physical examination. By the time of their discovery approximately 70 percent of these tumors have spread beyond the ovary, and in such cases are rarely curable by surgical excision and postoperative chemotherapy, radiation therapy, or both. This dismal prognosis has stimulated research on early detection of ovarian cancer, with the hope that it may lead to improved survival. Annual pelvic examination of women in the cancer age group was proposed initially as a method of early detection, but its yield of ovarian cancers has been very low. Subsequently, cytologic examination of fluid obtained by cul-de-sac puncture was advocated (5), but the rarity of positive findings, the significant risk of complications, such as perforation of the rectum, and poor patient acceptance have caused this method to fall into disuse (13). Currently, the most widely employed approaches to early detection are measurement of tumor markers in the serum, especially CA125, and transvaginal ultrasonography, which is highly effective in evaluating ovarian size and internal structure (15). CA125 is a serous carcinoma antigen, which is elevated in 80 to 85 percent of cases of epithelial cancer, but unfortunately, in only 30 to 50 percent of stage I cases and often in the presence of other neoplasms and non-neoplastic disorders (6). To date, these two approaches have not proved suitable for screening because of the low yield of early cancers, the much greater frequency of detection of benign than malignant lesions (over 10 to 1 in most studies) resulting in many unnecessary operations with their associated morbidity, and the very high cost per case of ovarian cancer detected (12,14). Also, a study of very early epithelial ovarian cancers discovered incidentally only after microscopic examination has shown that some of them have a fatal outcome despite their minute size (2). This finding indicates that an unknown proportion of epithelial cancers spread beyond the ovary before becoming detectable by either measurement of CA125 in the serum or ultrasound examination.

Screening for epithelial ovarian cancer may be improved by measurement of additional tumor markers such as macrophage-colony stimulating factor (M-CSF), ovarian cancer antigens OVX1 and NB/70K, CA15-3, TAG72.3, and numerous other antigens presently under investigation (6); by a combination of tumor marker measurements and transvaginal ultrasonography (19); and possibly by Doppler color flow ultrasonography, which can recognize areas of neovascularization and decreased impedance to blood flow, both of which are features of malignant tumors (11). These additional techniques, however, add considerably to the cost of already expensive approaches, and preliminary experience with Doppler color flow has not been encouraging (4,18).

Cytology

This subject can be divided into four categories for purposes of discussion: 1) specimens from the vagina, endocervix, and endometrium; 2) specimens of ascitic fluid and peritoneal washings; 3) specimens obtained by cul-de-sac puncture; and 4) fine needle aspirates of pelvic, upper abdominal, and other extraovarian masses.

Abnormalities in vaginal, endocervical, and endometrial cytologic specimens may reflect the hormone output of an ovarian tumor, result from the passage of its neoplastic cells into the lumen of the uterus or vagina without invasion of the walls of these organs (32), or reflect the presence of metastatic tumor in the wall of the uterus or vagina. Estrogen-secreting tumors, such as granulosa cell tumors and thecomas, shift the maturation index (based on the relative proportions of parabasal, intermediate, and superficial vaginal epithelial cells) markedly to the right in most of the cases (23); this shift is more often detected in women who are 5 or more years postmenopausal and children who have not yet attained normal puberty. Also, approximately 40 percent of ovarian cancers exclusive of granulosa cell tumors in postmenopausal women are associated with an abnormally high percentage of superficial cells in their cytologic smears (32); this change is assumed to be related to hormone production by the stroma of the tumor and possibly by the neoplastic epithelial cells as well (see

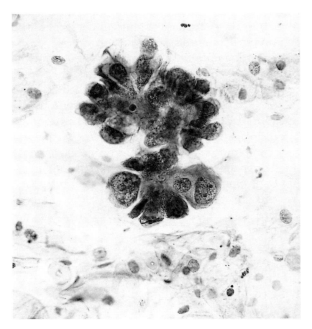

Figure 2-4
OVARIAN CARCINOMA CELLS
IN CERVICAL ASPIRATE
A papillary grouping of poorly differentiated adenocarcinoma cells is seen. Some of the nuclei have multiple nucleoli. There is no tumor diathesis. (Fig. 2 from Ng AB, Teeple D, Lindner EA, Reagan JW. The cellular manifestations of extrauterine cancer. Acta Cytol 1974;18:108-17.)

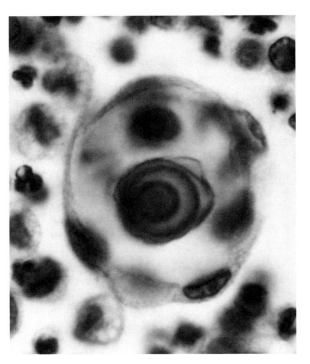

Figure 2-5
OVARIAN TUMOR CELLS AND
PSAMMOMA BODY IN VAGINAL-CERVICAL SMEAR
The primary tumor was a serous surface papillary tumor of borderline malignancy. (Fig. 1A from Masukawa T, Wada Y, Mattingly RF, Kuzma JF. Cytologic detection of minute ovarian, endometrial and breast carcinomas, with emphasis on clinical-pathological approaches. Acta Cytol 1973;17:316-9.)

chapter 19). If an estrogenic ovarian tumor is associated with endometrial hyperplasia, endometrial epithelial cells, which are sometimes atypical, may be present in addition to mature squamous cells. The production of androgens, progesterone, or a mixture of steroid hormones may likewise be reflected by characteristic changes in the vaginal cytologic specimen. The common use of hormone replacement therapy by menopausal and postmenopausal women, however, can negate the validity of drawing conclusions from the above cytologic alterations.

Epithelial cancer of the ovary accounts for approximately three fourths of the cases in which malignant cells within the vaginal or uterine lumen cannot be attributed to primary uterine cancer (29). The presence or absence of several cytologic features suggests an extrauterine source of such cells. A tumor diathesis (the presence of an exudate or transudate, erythrocytes, fibrin, and cellular debris) is observed in only 20 percent of positive smears associated with extra-

uterine cancer in contrast to 90 percent of those attributable to uterine cancer. In the extrauterine cases, the cellular characteristics are typically those of poorly differentiated carcinoma. A papillary arrangement of the neoplastic cells (fig. 2-4) suggests a serous carcinoma as does the presence of psammoma bodies (fig. 2-5), although these features, in themselves, are not diagnostic of either carcinoma in general (25,30) or ovarian carcinoma in particular.

In a review of cytologic preparations from 114 women with clinically documented ovarian epithelial cancer, cervicovaginal smears were found to be positive in 19 percent and endometrial aspiration smears in 42 percent of the cases (36). In most of the cases in which malignant cells are identified cytologically the tumor is growing on the surface of the ovary or has already spread beyond it, but in occasional cases the tumor appears to be confined to the ovary and have an intact surface

(22,29). Rarely, a positive smear is the first clue to the diagnosis of an ovarian cancer (25).

Positive findings on cytologic examination of ascitic fluid or peritoneal washings have been reported in 54 to 96 percent of cases of ovarian epithelial cancer (38). In one series, in which malignant cells were detected in 79 percent of the cases, the figure was 91 percent when the tumor had spread beyond the ovary and 36 percent when it was confined to one ovary and had an intact surface (24). The latter figure might be related to a failure to use strict criteria for the cytologic diagnosis of carcinoma, inadequacy of histologic sampling of the surface of the ovarian tumor, or shedding of tumor cells into the peritoneal cavity unrelated to invasion of the surface of the tumor. The last mechanism is possible in view of the occasional finding of epithelial cells from intact benign ovarian tumors in peritoneal fluid (26). Several authors have reported a 20 to 70 percent frequency of negative cytologic findings in patients with histologically demonstrated peritoneal disease (31,33,35,38); peritoneal washings are falsely negative more often than ascitic fluid (31). Although the results of cytologic examination of peritoneal fluid are incorporated into the staging of ovarian epithelial cancer, their significance remains elusive. There is no convincing evidence at present that a positive finding is predictive of outcome independent of other prognostic factors (38). Subdivision of International Federation of Gynecology and Obstetrics (FIGO) stages Ic and IIc carcinomas into cases in which those stages depend on growth on the external surface, rupture, positive cytologic examinations, or combinations of these findings would be necessary to establish a prognostically independent value of peritoneal cytology.

Features of malignant cells in peritoneal effusions that are very suggestive of an ovarian origin are an arrangement in balls or tight clusters (fig. 2-6), which is seen in almost all the cases, and vacuolization of many of the cells (fig. 2-7), which is observed in over two thirds of the cases (28). The cells of ovarian carcinomas must be distinguished from those of borderline tumors and endosalpingiosis on the basis of the architectural complexity of the cell clusters and the degree of nuclear atypia (34).

Several features aid in distinguishing carcinoma cells from reactive mesothelial cells. The

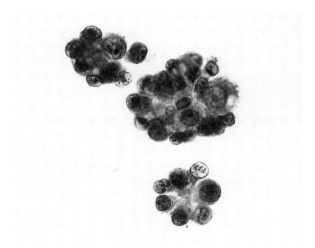

Figure 2-6
OVARIAN CARCINOMA CELLS
IN PERITONEAL FLUID
The cells are arranged in rosettes. (Fig. 4 from Murphy WM, Ng AB. Determination of primary site by examination of cancer cells in body fluids. Am J Clin Pathol 1972;58:479-88.)

cellular clustering and vacuolization that are highly suggestive of carcinoma are also seen occasionally in reactive mesothelial cells. Nuclear abnormalities, such as variations in size and shape, chromatin irregularities, and large, often irregular nucleoli, are characteristic of carcinoma, while the presence of intercellular windows is typical of mesothelial cells. Immunocytochemical staining may be helpful in difficult cases (page 73).

Almost all specimens of peritoneal fluid are obtained at the time of laparotomy in the course of staging an ovarian cancer or performing a second-look operation. Only rarely is fluid obtained as the initial diagnostic procedure either by abdominal paracentesis in a patient who has inoperable disease or is a poor operative risk, or by cul-de-sac aspiration. In the first reported series of cases in which the latter procedure was used for screening, atypical or malignant cells were identified in 22 of 840 subjects investigated (2 to 3 percent); only 2 of these women proved to have carcinoma, which was interpreted as "microinvasive," and 20 had "borderline proliferation" of the surface epithelium of undetermined significance (21). Although generally abandoned for screening purposes, cul-de-sac puncture is still used occasionally to confirm recurrence of ovarian cancer, thereby avoiding a more extensive diagnostic approach.

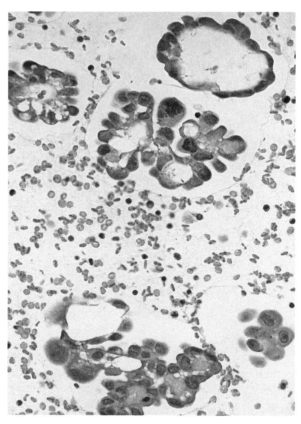

Figure 2-7
OVARIAN CARCINOMA CELLS IN ASCITIC FLUID
Papillary clusters of vacuolated carcinoma cells in cell block.

Fine needle aspiration of ovarian tumors and cysts has been introduced recently as a diagnostic procedure, performed preoperatively with ultrasonographic guidance or during laparoscopy, but a number of gynecologic oncologists consider it contraindicated because of suboptimal accuracy (27) and the possible complication of spilling malignant tumor cells into the peritoneal cavity (37). An occasional cause of an erroneous diagnosis of carcinoma is the aspiration of granulosa cells, which are often mitotically active, from cystic follicles or corpora lutea; the distinctive features of granulosa cell nuclei and awareness of the gross appearance of the cyst, however, generally facilitate the correct interpretation. Fine needle aspiration is used more appropriately in the diagnosis of inoperable ovarian cancer and for confirmation of suspected recurrent disease.

Spread and Staging

Ovarian epithelial cancer is generally stated to be bilateral in one third to half of the cases, but if the analysis of laterality is restricted to those cases in which there is no extraovarian extension (stage I cases) to exclude participation of the contralateral ovary in generalized spread, the figure for bilateral involvement is less than 20 percent (48). Since lymphatic pathways between the ovaries have been considered of minor importance in the spread of ovarian cancer, bilaterality in most stage I cases has been assumed to reflect independent origin of tumor in each ovary. Recent molecular genetic and karyotypic studies, which have shown identical or almost identical findings in both ovaries in most stage III cases with bilateral involvement, however, have suggested that only one of the ovarian cancers is primary and the other, metastatic (49,52,56). Future investigations of stage IB ovarian cancers should provide interesting information regarding the clonality of bilateral tumors, but the results must be correlated with the survival rates of patients with clonal and nonclonal carcinomas for optimal evaluation of whether the two tumors are the same or of independent primary origin.

The routes of spread of epithelial ovarian cancer are reflected in its staging systems, of which the most widely used is that of FIGO (53). The current FIGO staging system and the parallel Tumor, Node, Metastasis (TNM) system are presented in Table 2-2. These systems reflect the direct spread of ovarian cancers to adjacent pelvic organs and the pelvic wall; implantation on the peritoneum, especially in the right paracolic gutter, on the right undersurface of diaphragm, and on the omentum (fig. 2-8); metastasis to pelvic (iliac, obturator, and hypogastric) lymph nodes via broad ligament lymphatics and to para-aortic lymph nodes via infundibulopelvic ligament lymphatics (fig. 2-9) (44,47,55); and hematogenous spread. The frequencies of the stages of ovarian carcinomas and borderline tumors (distinguished by WHO criteria) (page 52) are shown in Table 2-3.

Ovarian cancers are often understaged by inexperienced surgeons, who may fail to sample adequately the peritoneum and lymph nodes. The importance of careful staging is emphasized by the finding that operative reevaluation of

Table 2-2

TUMOR-NODE-METASTASIS AND INTERNATIONAL FEDERATION OF GYNECOLOGY AND OBSTETRICS STAGING SYSTEMS FOR OVARIAN CANCER*

Primary Tumor (T)

TNM	FIGO	DEFINITION
TX	—	Primary tumor cannot be assessed
T0	—	No evidence of primary tumor
T1	I	Tumor limited to ovaries (one or both)
T1a	IA	Tumor limited to one ovary; capsule intact, no tumor on ovarian surface, no malignant cells in ascites or peritoneal washings
T1b	IB	Tumor limited to both ovaries; capsules intact, no tumor on ovarian surface, no malignant cells in ascites or peritoneal washings
T1c	IC	Tumor limited to one or both ovaries with any of the following: capsule ruptured, tumor on ovarian surface, malignant cells in ascites or peritoneal washings
T2	II	Tumor involves one or both ovaries with pelvic extension
T2a	IIA	Extension and/or implants on the uterus and/or tube(s); no malignant cells in ascites or peritoneal washings
T2b	IIB	Extension to other pelvic tissues; no malignant cells in ascites or peritoneal washings
T2c	IIC	Pelvic extension (IIa or IIb) with malignant cells in ascites or peritoneal washings
T3 and/or N1	III	Tumor involves one or both ovaries with microscopically confirmed peritoneal metastasis outside the pelvis and/or regional lymph node metastasis
T3a	IIIA	Microscopic peritoneal metastasis beyond the pelvis
T3b	IIIB	Macroscopic peritoneal metastasis beyond the pelvis 2 cm or less in greatest dimension
T3c and/or N1	IIIC	Peritoneal metastasis beyond the pelvis more than 2 cm in greatest dimension and/or regional lymph node metastasis
M1	IV	Distant metastasis (excludes peritoneal metastasis)

Note: Liver capsule metastasis is T3/stage III; liver parenchymal metastasis, M1/stage IV. Pleural effusion must have positive cytology for M1/stage IV.

Regional Lymph Nodes (N)

NX	Regional lymph nodes cannot be assessed
N0	No regional lymph node metastasis
N1	Regional lymph node metastasis

Distant Metastasis (M)

TNM	FIGO	DEFINITION
MX	—	Presence of distant metastasis cannot be assessed
M0	—	No distant metastasis
M1	IV	Distant metastasis (excludes peritoneal metastasis)

Note: The presence of nonmalignant ascites is not classified. The presence of ascites does not affect staging unless malignant cells are present.

pTNM Pathologic Classification

The pT, pN, and pM categories correspond to the T, N, and M categories.

STAGE GROUPING

AJCC/UICC**				FIGO
Stage IA	T1a	N0	M0	Stage IA
Stage IB	T1b	N0	M0	Stage IB
Stage IC	T1c	N0	M0	Stage IC
Stage IIA	T2a	N0	M0	Stage IIA
Stage IIB	T2b	N0	M0	Stage IIB
Stage IIC	T2c	N0	M0	Stage IIC
Stage IIIA	T3a	N0	M0	Stage IIIA
Stage IIIB	T3b	N0	M0	Stage IIIB
Stage IIIC	T3c	N0	M0	Stage IIIC
	Any T	N1	M0	
Stage IV	Any T	Any N	M1	Stage IV

*From: Manual for Staging of Cancer, 4th ed. Beahrs OH, Henson DE, Hutter RV, Kennedy BJ, eds. Philadelphia: JB Lippincott Company, 1992, and TNM Classification of Malignant Tumors, 5th ed. Sobin LH, Wittekind C, eds. New York: John Wiley & Sons, 1997.
**AJCC = American Joint Committee on Cancer; UICC = Union Internationale Contre le Cancer.

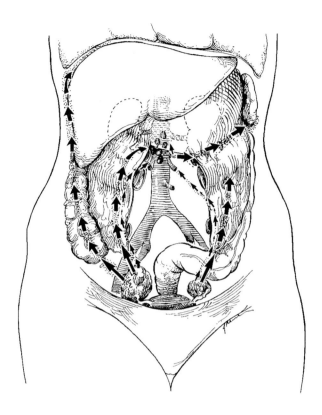

Figure 2-8
PERITONEAL ROUTE OF SPREAD
OF OVARIAN CANCER
Portions of the omentum, small intestine, and transverse colon are not illustrated. (From Knapp RC, Berkowitz RS, Leavitt P Jr, Bast RC Jr. Natural history and detection of ovarian cancer. In: Buchsbaum HG, ed. Gynecology and Obstetrics, vol. 4. Philadelphia: Lippincott, 1988.)

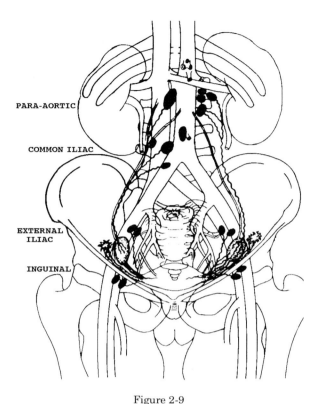

Figure 2-9
LYMPH NODES DRAINING OVARIES
Pelvic and para-aortic lymph nodes are illustrated. (Courtesy of Dr. Renato Musumeci, Milan, Italy.)

suboptimally staged tumors by experienced surgeons elevates the stage in almost one third of the cases (51). If one includes all stages of ovarian cancer, the pelvic or para-aortic lymph nodes or both are involved by tumor in 50 to 60 percent of the cases (40,41,57). The frequency of lymph node involvement according to stage as determined without consideration of lymphadenectomy findings is presented in Table 2-4. The most common sites of distant metastasis at the time of staging are the lung and pleura and the liver. Additional distant sites that are occasionally involved at presentation are bone, skin, and brain, although a wide variety of other rare sites of spread have been reported as well (45,46,50).

Autopsy studies, reflecting mainly the end-stages of the disease, have added another dimension to the knowledge of the spread of ovarian cancer (39,42,54). In addition to peritoneal and lymph node spread, which are found in 75 to 88 percent and 70 to 87 percent of the cases at autopsy, respectively, a number of organs may be involved, as listed in Table 2-5 (42,54). The lymph nodes that are found to contain tumor most frequently are pelvic and abdominal (para-aortic and mesenteric), but thoracic, cervical, supraclavicular, axillary, and inguinal lymph nodes are often involved as well. Abdominal viscera are frequently invaded by tumor as a result of direct extension, spread from the peritoneum, or lymphatic spread. The most common cause of death from ovarian cancer is carcinomatosis, followed by infection and pulmonary embolism; chemotherapy toxicity is a contributory factor in some cases (43) and the major factor in occasional cases.

Table 2-3

STAGE DISTRIBUTION OF OVARIAN CANCER*

Stage		Carcinoma (%)	Borderline (%)
I		24	73
	A	13	53
	B	3	11
	C	8	9
II		13	9
	A	3	2
	B & C	10	7
III		47	17
IV		16	1

* Adapted from reference 53. FIGO accepts the WHO criteria for the distinction between borderline tumors and carcinomas.

Treatment

The treatment of ovarian cancer is complicated and controversial in several of its aspects. The approach that follows is currently the most widely used although exceptions are made in individual cases (59–62,64,65). In the absence of widespread dissemination and inoperability, the initial management of ovarian cancer includes abdominal exploration, careful staging, and removal of all or almost all grossly identifiable disease (bulk resection), if this can be accomplished technically without the risk of serious complications. The standard treatment for stage I ovarian epithelial cancer is bilateral salpingo-oophorectomy with total hysterectomy. An exception may be made, however, in the management of a child or a young woman with a unilateral tumor in whom preservation of fertility is desirable. In that situation it is justifiable to restrict the operation to a unilateral oophorectomy or salpingo-oophorectomy if the cancer is of low-grade malignancy, if it is one that is rarely bilateral, or if it is almost always curable by chemotherapy. If such an approach is chosen, careful follow-up is essential, and the residual adnexa and uterus may be removed after the patient has completed her childbearing. The postoperative management of women with stage I ovarian cancer differs with the tumor type. Patients with most types of primitive germ cell tumor are treated routinely with combination chemotherapy (66,67). Those with grade 3 epi-

Table 2-4

FREQUENCY OF LYMPH NODE METASTASIS ACCORDING TO STAGE

Stage*	Series 1**	Series 2[†]	Series 3[‡]
I	27%	22%	24%
II	30%	50%	50%
III	55%	67%	74%
IV	100%	44%	73%
Total	53%	58%	62%

* Stage as determined before lymphadenectomy findings.
**Epithelial cancers; adapted from reference 41.
[†]All cancers; adapted from reference 57.
[‡]Cancer; adapted from reference 40.

Table 2-5

AUTOPSY ORGAN INVOLVEMENT*

Organ	Percent	
	Series 1**	Series 2[†]
Large intestine	55	49
Small intestine	52	48
Liver	45	48
Lung	39	34
Fallopian tubes	23	—
Pancreas	21	11
Spleen	15	20
Adrenal gland	15	21
Thyroid gland	2	14
Stomach	12	19
Bone	11	11
Uterus	10	—
Kidney	10	7
Brain	6	3
Skin	5	5
Breast	1	2

*Excludes serosal involvement only.
**From reference 42.
[†]From reference 54.

thelial cancers usually receive postoperative chemotherapy even though their tumors are stage IA or IB. Preoperative rupture of many forms of ovarian cancer is considered an indication for postoperative chemotherapy, external beam radiation therapy, or intra-abdominal installation of radioactive colloids. Patients with stage II ovarian cancers and densely adherent stage I tumors require a more extensive surgical procedure than otherwise to remove all tumor if possible, followed by chemotherapy in some cases. Women with stage III ovarian cancer are treated by most gynecologists by bulk resection of the tumor even though uncertainty exists whether the operation itself or the low aggressiveness of tumors that lend themselves to successful bulk resection accounts for the improved prognosis following this procedure. In cases of stage III ovarian cancer postoperative chemotherapy is usually administered; many authorities, however, believe that most stage III borderline tumors are an exception to this generalization.

The chemotherapeutic agents that are most commonly used for epithelial ovarian cancers are platinum compounds (cisplatin and carboplatin), various alkylating agents, and taxol and related drugs, but a wide variety of other agents (doxorubicin, hexamethylmelamine) have been used, particularly in combination with the above drugs (63). Progesterone and tamoxifen have occasionally been administered for low-grade carcinomas, with sporadically encouraging results. Numerous drugs, including cisplatin, dactinomycin, the vinca alkaloids, etoposide (VP-16), bleomycin, and cyclophosphamide in various combinations, have been used to treat primitive germ cell tumors (58,66,67); the most commonly employed combinations at the present time are BEP (bleomycin, etoposide, and cisplatin) and PVB (cisplatin, vinblastine, and bleomycin). Sex cord–stromal tumors that are of high grade, have ruptured, have spread beyond the ovary, or have recurred are often treated with chemotherapeutic regimens similar to those used for germ cell tumors (67).

External beam radiation therapy is currently used much less often than chemotherapy in the management of advanced ovarian cancer because of an association with a higher frequency of complications than the latter and the inadvisability of delivering tumoricidal doses to the renal and hepatic regions. Radiation therapy is most effective for radiosensitive tumors, such as dysgerminoma and granulosa cell tumor, for minimal or localized disease, and as salvage therapy after chemotherapy, mostly for undetectable or minimal residual disease. Intra-abdominal administration

Table 2-6

FIVE-YEAR SURVIVAL RATE BY STAGE: EPITHELIAL CANCERS

Stage		FIGO (%)*		NCDB (%)**	
I		79		89	
	A		84		92
	B		79		85
	C		70		82
II		57		57	
	A		61		67
	B		56†		56
	C				51
III		23		24	
	A		49		39
	B		32		26
	C		19		17
IV		8		12	

*Adapted from reference 84.
**National cancer data base, reference 82.
†IIB and IIC.

of P32 has likewise been used in the treatment of potential or minimal peritoneal spread.

Prognosis

Five-year survival rates for patients with ovarian epithelial cancer have varied widely, with most recorded figures presently ranging between 30 and 40 percent. The differences in reported results from various institutions may depend less on the mode of therapy utilized than on the differing proportions of cases within each stage, the inclusion or exclusion of tumors of borderline malignancy, and the diagnostic criteria of the pathologist. The stage of an ovarian epithelial cancer is generally considered the most reliable indicator of its prognosis, with the survival rate three to four times higher for patients with stage I than with stage III tumors (Table 2-6) (68,69,74,82,84). Other clinical, operative, and laboratory findings associated with, or possibly associated with, a reduced survival are listed in Table 2-7. The independent prognostic significance of some of these findings is clouded by inadequate appraisal of other prognostic features in the reported investigations.

A wide variety of microscopic features of epithelial ovarian cancers have been investigated for their prognostic significance in numerous

Table 2-7

OPERATIVE, CLINICAL, AND LABORATORY FINDINGS INDEPENDENTLY ASSOCIATED WITH REDUCED SURVIVAL OTHER THAN STAGE, GRADE, AND DNA PLOIDY

1. Large volume of residual tumor after cytoreduction
2. Ascites, particularly if high volume
3. Rupture, preoperative or intraoperative*
4. Dense adhesion of tumor**
5. Increasing age[†]
6. High serum level of CA125 postoperatively
7. High serum level of CA125 preoperatively[‡]

*Controversial (88,89,91,92). Spontaneous preoperative rupture—reduced survival; intraoperative puncture or rupture—no impact on survival (91).
**Controversial (73,94).
[†]Controversial (80,83).
[‡]Preliminary evidence (81).

reports, many of which are flawed for various reasons (90). Histologic grade has been studied most extensively. Various grading systems have been used, with most based on architectural features, the degree of various nuclear abnormalities, or a combination of both. Some investigators, however, have included other findings in their grading systems, such as the appearance of the tumor margin, the amount of round cell infiltration and the quantity of stroma within the tumor, and the presence or absence of vascular space invasion (72). Still other authors have not specified their criteria for grading, or in multicenter studies, have allowed participating pathologists to utilize their own criteria (77). Almost all the reported studies of grading have shown a correlation with prognosis, at least at a univariate level, indicating that pathologists using a variety of grading methods can stratify ovarian cancers into several prognostic groups. The success in achieving this result is probably based on the existence of a subset of easily diagnosable grades 1, 2, and 3 (or 4) tumors. The poor reproducibility of grading, as shown by analysis of individual cases circulated among pathologists, however, indicates that disagreement exists on tumors with borderline grades (70). The unfortunate conclusion is that unless a tumor is judged to belong indisputably within a grade, the grade

assigned is an unreliable criterion on which to base therapy of an individual patient.

Some investigators have concluded that morphometric analysis of features such as mitotic figures per volume index, volume percentage of neoplastic epithelium, nuclear density, nuclear area, and nuclear shape is more objective and reproducible than grading, and a more accurate indicator of prognosis (70,76,79). This approach warrants further investigation in carefully designed studies. In most investigations of ovarian cancer, aneuploidy and in some studies, a high S-phase fraction, correlate with a higher tumor grade, a higher stage, more bulky postoperative residual disease, a shorter survival time, and a reduced survival rate in comparison to diploidy and a low S-phase fraction (71,75,93). In some of these investigations the DNA findings were shown to be independent prognostic indicators. Authors of reviews of the literature, however, have concluded that DNA ploidy is not yet established as a reproducible prognostic indicator independent of other parameters of outcome (85,88). The independent prognostic significance of tumor cell type, which will be covered in the chapters to follow, amplification and overexpression of various oncogenes and tumor-suppressor genes (86, 88) (page 46), and estrogen and progesterone receptor levels (78) also remains controversial.

Epidemiology

Clues to the causes of ovarian epithelial cancer have been provided by epidemiologic data, which can be divided into those that are generally accepted and those that remain controversial and require further investigation (Table 2-8) (99, 113). Nulliparity has been shown in several studies to be associated with a 1.5 to 3.2 times greater risk of the development of ovarian cancer than parity, with most investigators reporting a progressive decrease in risk with increasing parity and increasing duration of lactation. Women who have never used oral contraceptives have a risk 1.4 to 2.5 times greater than that of women who have ever used these drugs; also, the risk of ovarian cancer decreases with increasing duration of usage (103). A controversial finding is the suggestion of an increased risk of development of ovarian cancer in women who have been exposed to ovulation-inducing drugs and have not

Table 2-8

ACCEPTED AND PROPOSED RISK FACTORS FOR OVARIAN EPITHELIAL CANCER

Generally Accepted	Preliminary or Controversial
Nulliparity	Exposure to ovulation-inducing drugs
No oral contraceptive usage	High fat diet
	High galactose diet
	Talc exposure
No breast feeding	
Family history, especially if hereditary	Subclinical mumps oophoritis
	Unopposed estrogen administration
Radiation exposure	Prior tubal ligation or hysterectomy

succeeded in becoming pregnant (130); conclusions drawn from studies of this possible association have been flawed, however, by major components of borderline epithelial and granulosa cell tumors among the cancers found in the treated groups since such tumors appear to have little in common biologically (129). The associations with nulliparity and never-usage of oral contraceptives support strongly the incessant ovulation theory of development of ovarian cancer. According to this theory ovulation causes a loss of integrity of the ovarian surface epithelium followed by regeneration, multiple mutations, and eventual transformation to carcinoma. Because the surface epithelial cells are not stem cells that give rise to fully differentiated cells like the stem cells of the basal layer of the epidermis and those in intestinal crypts, the regenerated ovarian surface epithelial cells are similar to their forebears, retaining the capacity to proliferate after additional trauma by subsequent ovulations (104). Multiple reparative events may be associated with mutations in these cells, with activation of oncogenes and inactivation of tumor-suppressor genes, eventually resulting in the development of a carcinoma (104). A second component of the incessant ovulation theory, which is espoused by some investigators, is that surface epithelial regeneration is accompanied by a downgrowth of the reparative epithelium into the stigmata of ovulation, with the formation of surface epithelial inclusion glands. Most ovarian carcinomas,

which are basically cystic, appear to arise from these glands rather than directly from the surface epithelium. The mechanism of development of these inclusions, however, is not entirely clear. Although the stigmata of ovulation have not been carefully studied histologically, no convincing evidence has been advanced that the surface epithelium invades them to form intraparenchymal epithelial inclusions. In an unpublished study of over 900 ovaries removed surgically, there was no association of surface epithelial inclusion glands with sites of ovulation; also, the number of these inclusions increased with patient age, and they were significantly more common in parous than nulliparous women (R.E.S., unpublished data, 1980). Finally, women with polycystic ovarian disease, who do not ovulate or ovulate only rarely, have inclusion cysts in their ovaries much more often than women without this disorder (121).

Alternative explanations for the association between incessant ovulation and the increased risk of ovarian epithelial cancers are hormonal. One proposed hormonal explanation is that pituitary gonadotropic hormones affect the surface epithelium and its inclusion glands in the direction of malignancy. It is known that both pregnancy and oral contraceptive intake cause a reduction in pituitary gonadotropins, and it is postulated additionally that an unknown proportion of nulliparous women, who are at high risk for ovarian cancer, may be nulliparous because of ovarian hypofunction, which results in a secondary increase in pituitary gonadotropin levels. A second proposed hormonal explanation for the pathogenetic role of incessant ovulation is that follicular rupture exposes the surface epithelium to high concentrations of estrogens and possibly other constituents in the follicular fluid. The existence of receptors for various hormones in the ovarian surface epithelium strengthens the possibility that these substances may have a role in the development of ovarian epithelial cancer.

Approximately 7 percent of women with ovarian epithelial cancer have one or more relatives with the disease (familial ovarian cancer). These women are estimated to have a risk for the development of ovarian cancer slightly over three times that of women without a family history. It has been estimated that less than 1 to 3 percent of ovarian cancer patients have a germline genetic abnormality that greatly increases their risk of development of ovarian cancer (hereditary ovarian cancer) (107). Three hereditary types of ovarian cancer with autosomal dominant modes of inheritance from either the mother or father have been described: the ovary-specific syndrome; the breast-ovary syndrome; and the Lynch II syndrome, in which cancer may appear in the ovary, endometrium, colon, and occasionally other organs with variable degrees of frequency (114). The gene that is most frequently mutated in the hereditary breast-ovary form (*BRCA*1) is present on the long arm of chromosome 17 at locus 21. Carriers of *BRCA*1 have a lifetime risk of 50 percent for ovarian cancer.

Dietary composition has been linked to ovarian epithelial cancer by some investigators, either directly on the basis of case-control studies or indirectly on the basis of differences in ovarian cancer incidence in various countries with dietary differences (Table 2-9). Diets high in meat and animal fats, dairy products, and specifically galactose have been implicated by several groups of investigators. Although diet may be responsible for the international differences observed, other factors such as family size and environmental exposure may also have important roles.

Women with ovarian epithelial cancer have been shown in some studies to use talcum powder, which may contain asbestos particles, on the perineum almost twice as often as controls. Since particles introduced into the vagina may pass upward in the female genital tract and be recovered in the peritoneal cavity, it is postulated that talc may travel that route and result in malignant transformation of the ovarian surface epithelium. Other factors that have been implicated in the development of ovarian cancer but are either controversial or if generally accepted, account for only a small proportion of the cases are subclinical mumps oophoritis, radiation exposure, and unopposed estrogen replacement therapy for menopausal symptoms. Finally, prior tubal ligation and prior hysterectomy have been shown in several studies to reduce the risk of ovarian cancer by unknown mechanisms (105). Prevention of upward passage of talc or other possible carcinogens in the female genital tract has been suggested as an explanation for the apparent protective effect of these operations (127).

Table 2-9

AGE-ADJUSTED ANNUAL INCIDENCE RATES PER 100,000 POPULATION OF OVARIAN CANCER*

Sweden	14.9
United States (white)	9.4 to 13.3
Germany	11.8
England	11.1
United States (black)	8.6 to 9.9
Israel (native Jews)	8.7
Finland	7.9
India	4.6
Japan	2.7

*Adapted from Table 8-1, reference 113.

Pathogenesis

At present it is not known what proportion of ovarian epithelial cancers develop de novo from the surface epithelium or its inclusion glands and what proportion originate in preexisting benign epithelial tumors or non-neoplastic disorders such as endometriosis. There is abundant evidence that ovarian carcinomas in the epithelial-stromal category can arise de novo from the surface epithelium and its inclusions. Borderline tumors and carcinomas of microscopic dimensions have been observed to arise directly in these sites (figs. 2-10, 2-11) and are commonly associated with dysplasia in similar sites elsewhere in the same or contralateral ovary (figs. 2-12, 2-13) (95,100,106, 125). Tubal metaplasia of surface epithelial inclusion glands in ovaries contralateral to those containing epithelial cancers (fig. 2-14) is significantly more common than in control ovaries, suggesting that mullerian differentiation may be an early step in carcinogenesis (95,117,121). Since more ovarian epithelial-stromal tumors are located within the ovarian stroma than on its surface, at least in their early stages, it is logical to conclude that such tumors arise principally from epithelial inclusion glands rather than directly from the surface epithelium. Also, morphologic and immunohistochemical characteristics (tubal metaplasia; immunostaining for CA125, CA19-9, human milk fat globule protein, and placental-like alkaline phosphatase; expression of *HER*-2 *neu*/gene) that are often found in epithelial cancers, are either absent or much less frequent in the surface epithelium than in glandular

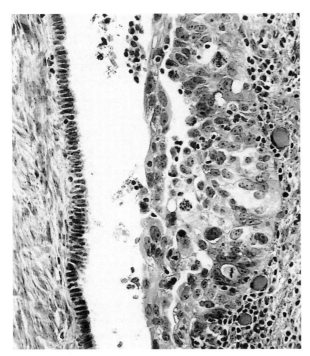

Figure 2-10
HIGH-GRADE OVARIAN CARCINOMA
ARISING ON SURFACE OF OVARY
The tumor occupies one wall of a crevice on the ovarian surface. The opposite wall of the crevice is lined by normal-appearing surface epithelium. (Fig. 15-3 from Scully RE. Ovary. In: Henson DE, Albores-Saavedra J, eds. The pathology of incipient neoplasia. Philadelphia: WB Saunders, 1993:285.)

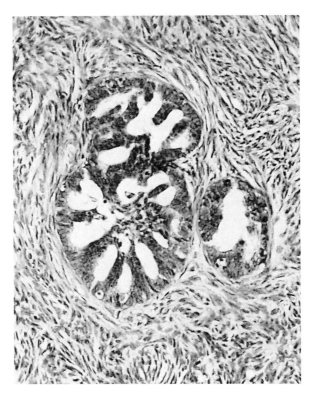

Figure 2-11
GRADE 1 ADENOCARCINOMA
Tumor occupies the site of a surface epithelial inclusion gland. (Fig. 15-5 from Scully RE. Ovary. In: Henson DE, Albores-Saavedra J, eds. The pathology of incipient neoplasia. Philadelphia: WB Saunders, 1993:286.)

inclusion epithelium, consistent with a greater tendency of the latter to undergo neoplasia. Possibly the greater contact of the inclusions with ovarian stroma is partly responsible for the differences between their epithelium and that of the ovarian surface in this respect.

Evidence for the development of carcinomas from preexisting benign epithelial lesions include: 1) an average mean age of patients with epithelial cancers 12 years older than that of patients with benign epithelial tumors (126); 2) the five-times greater frequency of benign epithelial tumors in first- and second-degree relatives of patients with ovarian cancer than in controls (98); and 3) the identification of benign-appearing epithelium in a high proportion of cases of epithelial cancer by retrospective study of routinely sampled tumors (120,125). In one study, the association of carcinoma with benign-appearing epithelium was highest in cases of mucinous carcinoma,

intermediate in cases of endometrioid and clear cell carcinomas, and lowest in cases of serous and transitional cell carcinomas (125). The benign epithelium was found in cystadenomas, adenofibromas, and endometriosis, the last of which is frequently associated with clear cell and endometrioid carcinomas. Although the presence of benign-appearing epithelium in association with both borderline tumors and carcinomas suggests an origin of these tumors from this epithelium, in some cases the latter may be part of a collision lesion and in others it may be malignant epithelium that has undergone maturation to the extent that it appears indistinguishable from benign epithelium on routine staining. Such maturation is frequently observed in metastatic adenocarcinomas from the intestine and pancreas (see chapter 18). These alternative explanations for the association of benign-appearing and malignant epithelium in the same specimen (origin versus

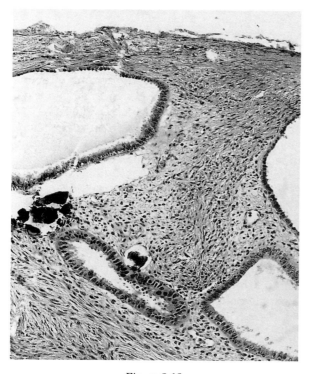

Figure 2-12
EPITHELIAL INCLUSION GLANDS
Four surface epithelial inclusion glands and cysts, one of which is lined by dysplastic epithelium (center).

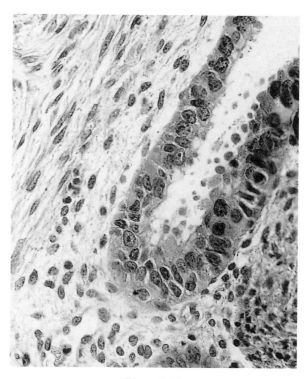

Figure 2-13
EPITHELIAL INCLUSION GLAND
Severe dysplasia of the lining of the epithelial inclusion gland illustrated in figure 2-12.

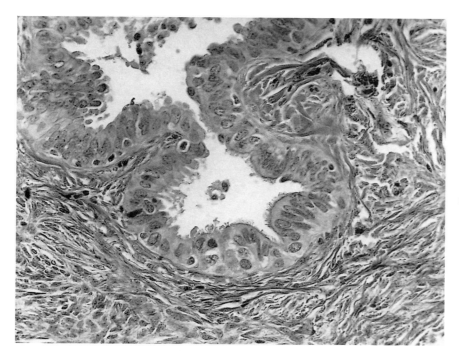

Figure 2-14
TUBAL METAPLASIA
OF SURFACE EPITHELIAL
INCLUSION GLAND
Some of the lining cells are ciliated.

maturation) make it impossible to obtain an accurate figure at the present time for the frequency of cancer development in preexisting benign epithelial lesions. Solution of this problem requires further investigation in specifically designed prospective studies and the additional use of evolving techniques such as immunohistochemistry, molecular genetics, and DNA image analysis applied to the epithelial cells of all the types encountered in these tumors.

Chromosomal and Genetic Abnormalities

Simple changes in the karyotypes of ovarian tumors, consisting of numerical changes only, a single structural change, or both, are largely confined to benign, borderline, and low-grade malignant forms. The most common simple change is trisomy 12, which is seen most frequently in fibromas, juvenile granulosa cell tumors, and borderline epithelial tumors (118,119).

Moderately and poorly differentiated ovarian carcinomas almost always have complex changes in their karyotypes, with numerous numerical as well as structural alterations (101,112,118). The most common numerical changes are chromosome losses, involving particularly chromosomes X, 22, 17, 13, and 8. Structural abnormalities are more numerous with increasing grade and stage of the carcinoma. Chromosomes that have been shown to be structurally abnormal most often are: 1, 3, 6, 11, 12, 13, 17, 18, and 19.

Relatively little is known about the role of oncogenes, tumor suppressor genes, and DNA repair genes in the development of ovarian carcinoma since only a few of these genes have been studied by more than a few investigators, and the results have not always agreed (96,123). Human epidermal growth factor receptor-2/neuroblastoma (*HER*-2 /*neu*) gene, also referred to as c-*erb*B-2 and located on chromosome 17q, has been shown to be amplified in 0 to 32 (average, 18) percent and overexpressed in 0 to 72 (average, 27) percent of ovarian carcinomas (128), but whether amplification or overexpression is an independent prognostic indicator remains controversial (115,116,122,128). Epidermal growth factor receptor (*erb*B-1) gene is often overexpressed in ovarian carcinomas but whether overexpression correlates with survival is also controversial (110,124). Rat sarcoma (*ras*) genes, chicken myelocytomatosis (c-*myc*), *fos* (a member of the *myc* family), and macrophage-colony stimulating factor receptor (*fms*) genes have been demonstrated to be amplified or overexpressed in differing percentages of cases in several small series, but clear-cut relations to tumor behavior have not been shown (96,101A, 103). The only tumor suppressor gene that has been investigated extensively in ovarian carcinoma is p53, which is located on chromosome 17. Immunohistochemical staining indicating overexpression of this gene has been demonstrated in 50 to 79 percent of ovarian carcinomas (111), more often in poorly differentiated than well-differentiated forms (97), twice as often in aneuploid as in diploid tumors (108), and three times as frequently in stages IC and II carcinomas as in stages IA and IB carcinomas (109); in some studies, a correlation of p53 overexpression with rate or length of survival has been demonstrated (97,108).

REFERENCES

Frequency, Clinical Manifestations, and Diagnosis and Screening

1. Beck RP, Latour JP. Review of 1019 benign ovarian neoplasms. Obstet Gynecol 1960;16:479–81.
2. Bell DA, Scully RE. Early de novo ovarian carcinoma: a study of fourteen cases. Cancer 1994;73:1859–64.
3. Boring CC, Squires TS, Tong T, Montgomery S. Cancer statistics, 1994. CA Cancer J Clin 1994;44:7–26.
4. Bromley B, Goodman H, Benacerraf BR. Comparison between sonographic morphology and doppler waveform for the diagnosis of ovarian malignancy. Obstet Gynecol 1994;83:434–7.
5. Graham JB, Graham RM. Cul-de-sac puncture in the diagnosis of early ovarian cancer. J Obstet Gynaecol Br Commonw 1967;74:371–8.
6. Jacobs IJ, Oram DH, Bast RC Jr. Strategies for improving the specificity of screening for ovarian cancer with tumor-associated antigens CA 125, CA 15-3, and TAG 72.3. Obstet Gynecol 1992;80:396–9.
7. Katsube Y, Berg JW, Silverberg SG. Epidemiologic pathology of ovarian tumors: a histopathologic review of primary ovarian neoplasms diagnosed in the Denver standard metropolitan statistical area, 1 July—31 December 1969 and 1 July—31 December 1979. Int J Gynecol Pathol 1982;1:3–16.
8. Koonings PP, Campbell K, Mishell DR Jr, Grimes DA. Relative frequency of primary ovarian neoplasms: a 10-year review. Obstet Gynecol 1989;74:921–6.
9. Koonings PP, Grimes DA. Adnexal torsion in postmenopausal women. Obstet Gynecol 1989;73:11–2.
10. Koonings PP, Grimes DA, Campbell K, Sommerville M. Bilateral ovarian neoplasms and the risk of malignancy. Am J Obstet Gynecol 1990;162:167–9.
11. Kurjak A, Schulman H, Sosic A, Zalud I, Shalan H. Transvaginal ultrasound, color flow, and doppler waveform of the postmenopausal adnexal mass. Obstet Gynecol 1992;80:917–21.
12. Look KY. Epidemiology, etiology, and screening of ovarian cancer. In: Rubin SC, Sutton GP, eds. Ovarian cancer. New York: McGraw-Hill, 1992:175–87.
13. McGowan L, Bunnag B, Arias LB. Peritoneal fluid cytology associated with benign neoplastic ovarian tumors in women. Am J Obstet Gynecol 1972;113:961–6.
14. NIH Consensus Conference. Ovarian cancer. Screening, treatment, and follow-up. JAMA 1995;273:491–7.
15. Ozols RF, Rubin SC, Dembo AJ, Robboy SJ. Epithelial ovarian cancer. In: Hoskins WJ, Perey CA, Young RC, eds. Principles and practice of gynecologic oncology. Philadelphia: JB Lippincott, 1992:731–81.
16. Rome RM, Laverty CR, Brown JB. Ovarian tumours in postmenopausal women. Clinicopathological features and hormonal studies. J Obstet Gynaecol Br Commonw 1973;80:984–91.
17. Rulin MC, Preston AL. Adnexal masses in postmenopausal women. Obstet Gynecol 1987;70:578–81.
18. Valentin L, Sladkevicius P, Marsàl K. Limited contribution of Doppler velocimetry to the differential diagnosis of extrauterine pelvic tumors. Obstet Gynecol 1994;83:425–33.
19. van Nagell JR Jr. Methods to improve the diagnostic accuracy of ultrasound in the detection of ovarian cancer [Editorial]. Gynecol Oncol 1994;54:115–6.
20. Yancik R, Ries LG, Yates JW. Ovarian cancer in the elderly: an analysis of surveillance, epidemiology and end results program data. Am J Obstet Gynecol 1986;154:639–47.

Cytology

21. Graham JB, Graham RM. Cul-de-sac puncture in the diagnosis of early ovarian cancer. J Obstet Gynaecol Br Commonw 1967;74:371–8.
22. Graham RM, van Niekerk WA. Vaginal cytology in cancer of the ovary. Acta Cytol 1962;6:496–9.
23. Johnston WW, Goldston WR, Montgomery MS. Clinicopathologic studies in feminizing tumors of the ovary. III. The role of genital cytology. Acta Cytol 1971;15:334–8.
24. Keettel WC, Pixley EE, Buchsbaum HJ. Experience with peritoneal cytology in the management of gynecological pathology. Am J Obstet Gynecol 1974;120:174–82.
25. Koss LG. Diagnostic cytology and its histopathologic bases, 4th edition. Philadelphia: JB Lippincott, 1992.
26. McGowan L, Bunnag B, Arias LB. Peritoneal fluid cytology associated with benign neoplastic ovarian tumors in women. Am J Obstet Gynecol 1972;113:961–6.
27. Moran O, Menczer J, Ben-Baruch G, Lipitz S, Goor E. Cytologic examination of ovarian cyst fluid for the distinction between benign and malignant tumors. Obstet Gynecol 1993;82:444–6.
28. Murphy WM, Ng AB. Determination of primary site by examination of cancer cells in body fluids. Am J Clin Pathol 1972;58:479–88.
29. Ng AB, Teeple D, Lindner EA, Reagan JW. The cellular manifestations of extrauterine cancer. Acta Cytol 1974;18:108–17.
30. Picoff RC, Meeker CI. Psammoma bodies in the cervicovaginal smear in association with benign papillary structures of the ovary. Acta Cytol 1970;14:45–7.
31. Pretorius RG, Lee KR, Papillo J, Baker S, Belinson J. False-negative peritoneal cytology in metastatic ovarian carcinoma. Obstet Gynecol 1986; 68:619–23.
32. Rubin DK, Frost JK. The cytologic detection of ovarian cancer. Acta Cytol 1963;7:191–5.
33. Rubin SC, Dulaney ED, Markman M, Hoskins WJ, Saigo PE, Lewis JL Jr. Peritoneal cytology as an indicator of disease in patients with residual ovarian carcinoma. Obstet Gynecol 1988;71:851–3.
34. Sneige N, Fanning CV. Peritoneal washing cytology in women: diagnostic pitfalls and clues for correct diagnosis. Diagn Cytopathol 1992;8:632–42.
35. Spinelli P, Pilotti S, Luini A, Spatti GB, Pizzetti P, De Palo G. Laparoscopy combined with peritoneal cytology in staging and restaging ovarian carcinoma. Tumori 1979;65:601–10.
36. Takashima T, Oma M, Kanda Y, Sagae S, Hayakawa O, Ito E. Cervicovaginal and endometrial cytology in ovarian cancer. Acta Cytol 1988;32:159–62.
37. Trimbos JB, Hacker NF. The case against aspirating ovarian cysts. Cancer 1993;72:828–31.
38. Yoshimura S, Scully RE, Taft PD, Herrington JB. Peritoneal fluid cytology in patients with ovarian cancer. Gynecol Oncol 1984;17:161–7.

Spread and Staging of Ovarian Cancer

39. Bergman F. Carcinoma of the ovary. A clinicopathological study of 86 autopsied cases with special reference to mode of spread. Acta Obstet Gynecol Scand 1966;45:211–31.

40. Burghardt E, Girardi F, Lahousen M, Tamussino K, Stettner H. Patterns of pelvic and paraaortic lymph node involvement in ovarian cancer. Gynecol Oncol 1991;40:103–6.

41. Chen SS, Lee L. Incidence of para-aortic and pelvic lymph node metastases in epithelial carcinoma of the ovary. Gynecol Oncol 1983;16:95–100.

42. Dvoretsky PM, Richard KA, Angel C, et al. Distribution of disease at autopsy in 100 women with ovarian cancer. Hum Pathol 1988;19:57–63.

43. Dvoretsky PM, Richards KA, Angel C, Rabinowitz L, Beecham JB, Bonfiglio TA. Survival time, causes of death, and tumor/treatment-related morbidity in 100 women with ovarian cancer. Hum Pathol 1988;19:1273–9.

44. Feldman GB, Knapp RC. Lymphatic drainage of the peritoneal cavity and its significance in ovarian cancer. Am J Obstet Gynecol 1974;119:991–4.

45. Frauenhoffer EE, Ro JY, Silva EG, El-Naggar A. Well-differentiated serous ovarian carcinoma presenting as a breast mass: a case report and flow cytometric DNA study. Int J Gynecol Pathol 1991;10:79–87.

46. Izquierdo MA, Ojeda B, Pallarés C, Alonso MC, Matias-Guiu X. Ovarian carcinoma preceded by cerebral metastasis: review of the literature. Gynecol Oncol 1992;45:206–10.

47. Knapp RC, Friedman EA. Aortic lymph node metastasis in early ovarian cancer. Am J Obstet Gynecol 1974;119:1013–7.

48. Kottmeier HL. Surgical management-conservative surgery. Indications according to the type of the tumour. In: Gentil F, Junqueira AC, eds. UICC monograph series, vol. 11. Ovarian cancer. Berlin: Springer-Verlag: 1968:157–64.

49. Li S, Han H, Resnik E, Carcangiu ML, Schwartz PE, Yang-Feng TL. Advanced ovarian carcinoma: molecular evidence of unifocal origin. Gynecol Oncol 1993;51:21–5.

50. McGonigle KF, Dudzinski MR. Endometrioid carcinoma of the ovary presenting with an enlarged inguinal lymph node without evidence of abdominal carcinomatosis. Gynecol Oncol 1992;45:225–8.

51. Ozols RF, Rubin SC, Dembo AJ, Robboy S. Epithelial ovarian cancer. In: Hoskins WJ, Perez CA, Young RC, eds. Principles and practice of gynecologic oncology. Philadelphia: JB Lippincott, 1992:731–81.

52. Pejovic T. Genetic changes in ovarian cancer. Ann Med 1995;27:73–8.

53. Pettersson F. Annual report of the results of treatment in gynecological cancer. Stockholm: International Federation of Gynecology and Obstetrics, 1991.

54. Rose PG, Piver MS, Tsukada Y, Lau T. Metastatic patterns in histologic variants of ovarian cancer. An autopsy study. Cancer 1989;64:1508–13.

55. Rubin SC. Surgery for ovarian cancer. In: Ozols RF, ed. Hematology/Oncology Clinics of North America. Ovarian cancer. Philadelphia: WB Saunders, 1992:851–65.

56. Tsao SW, Mok CH, Knapp RC, et al. Molecular genetic evidence for a unifocal origin for human serous ovarian carcinomas. Obstet Gynecol 1993;48:5–10.

57. Wu PC, Qu JY, Lang JH, Huang RL, Tang MY, Lian LJ. Lymph node metastasis of ovarian cancer: a preliminary survey of 74 cases of lymphadenectomy. Am J Obstet Gynecol 1986;155:1103–8.

Treatment of Ovarian Cancer

58. Gershenson DM. Update on malignant ovarian germ cell tumors. Cancer 1993;71:1581–90.

59. Hoskins WJ. Primary surgical management of advanced ovarian cancer. In: Rubin SC, Sutton FP, eds. Ovarian cancer. New York: McGraw-Hill, 1992:241–53.

60. McGuire WP. Primary chemotherapy of epithelial ovarian cancer. In: Rubin SC, Sutton FP, eds. Ovarian cancer. New York: McGraw-Hill, 1992:255–68.

61. Mychalczak BR, Fuks Z. The current role of radiotherapy in the management of ovarian cancer. In: Ozols RF, ed. Hematology/Oncology Clinics of North America. Ovarian cancer. Philadelphia: WB Saunders, 1992:895–913.

62. NIH Consensus Conference. Ovarian cancer. Screening, treatment, and follow-up. JAMA 1995;273:491–7.

63. Ozols RF. Chemotherapy for advanced epithelial ovarian cancer. In: Ozols RF, ed. Hematology/Oncology Clinics of North America. Ovarian cancer. Philadelphia: WB Saunders, 1992:879–94.

64. Rubin SC. Surgery for ovarian cancer. In: Ozols RF, ed. Hematology/Oncology Clinics of North America. Ovarian cancer. Philadelphia: WB Saunders, 1992:851–65.

65. Schilder RJ, Young RC. Management of early-stage ovarian cancer. In: Ozols RF, ed. Hematology/Oncology Clinics of North America. Ovarian Cancer. Philadelphia: WB Saunders, 1992:867–77.

66. Williams SD. Germ cell tumors. In: Ozols RF, ed. Hematology/Oncology Clinics of North America. Ovarian cancer. Philadelphia: WB Saunders, 1992:967–81.

67. Williams SD, Gershenson DM, Horowitz CJ, Scully RE. Ovarian germ cell and stromal tumors. In: Hoskins WJ, Perez CA, Young RC, eds. Principles and practice of gynecologic oncology. Philadelphia: JB Lippincott, 1992:715–30.

Prognosis of Epithelial Cancer

General References

68. Baak JP, Chan KK, Stolk JG, Kenemans P. Prognostic factors in borderline and invasive ovarian tumours of the common epithelial type. Path Res Pract 1987;182:755–74.

69. Haapasalo H, Collan Y, Atkin NB. Major prognostic factors in ovarian carcinomas. Int J Gynecol Cancer 1991;1:155–62.

Specific References

70. Baak JP, Wisse-Brekelmans EC, Langley FA, Talerman A, Delemarre JF. Morphometric data to FIGO stage and histological type and grade for prognosis of ovarian tumours. J Clin Pathol 1986;39:1340–6.
71. Bell DA. Flow cytometry of ovarian neoplasms. In: Sasano N, ed. Current topics in pathology. Gynecological tumors. Recent progress in diagnostic pathology. Berlin: Springer-Verlag, 1992:85:337–56.
72. Bichel P, Jakobsen A. A new histologic grading index in ovarian carcinoma. Int J Gynecol Pathol 1989;8:147–55.
73. Dembo AJ, Davy M, Stenwig AE, Berle EJ, Bush RS, Kjorstad K. Prognostic factors in patients with Stage 1 epithelial ovarian cancer. Obstet Gynecol 1990;75:263–73.
74. deSouza PL, Friedlander ML. Prognostic factors in ovarian cancer. In: Ozols RF, ed. Hematology/Oncology Clinics of North America. Ovarian Cancer. Philadelphia: WB Saunders, 1992:6:761–81.
75. Gajewski WH, Fuller Jr AF, Pastel-Ley C, Flotte TJ, Bell DA. Prognostic significance of DNA content in epithelial ovarian cancer. Gynecol Oncol 1994;53:5–12.
76. Haapasalo H, Collan Y, Seppa A, Gidland AL, Atkin NB, Pesonen E. Prognostic value of ovarian carcinoma grading methods—a method comparison study. Histopathology 1990;16:1–7.
77. Henson DE. The histological grading of neoplasms. Arch Pathol Lab Med 1988;112:1091–6.
78. Kommoss F, Pfisterer J, Geyer H, Thome M, Sauerbrei W, Pfleiderer A. Estrogen and progesterone receptors in ovarian neoplasms: discrepant results of immunohistochemical and biochemical methods. Int J Gynecol Cancer 1991;1:147–53.
79. Ludescher C, Weger AR, Lindholm J, et al. Prognostic significance of tumor cell morphometry, histopathology, and clinical parameters in advanced ovarian carcinoma. Int J Gynecol Pathol 1990;9:343–51.
80. Markman M, Lewis JL Jr, Saigo P, et al. Impact of age on survival of patients with ovarian cancer. Gynecol Oncol 1993;49:236–9.
81. Nagele F, Petru E, Medl M, Kainz C, Graf AH, Sevelda P. Preoperative CA 125: an independent prognostic factor in patients with Stage I epithelial ovarian cancer. Obstet Gynecol 1995;86:259–64.
82. Nguyen HN, Averette HE, Hoskins W, Sevin BU, Penalver M, Steren A. National survey of ovarian carcinoma VI. Critical assessment of current International Federation of Gynecology and Obstetrics staging system. Cancer 1993;72:3007–11.
83. Park RC. Age—is it a risk factor in ovarian cancer? [Editorial]. Cancer 1994:73:245–6.
84. Pettersson F. Annual report of the results of treatment in gynecological cancer. Stockholm: International Federation of Gynecology and Obstetrics, 1991.
85. Rice LW, Mark SD, Berkowitz RS, Goff BA, Lage JM. Clinicopathologic variables, operative characteristics, and DNA ploidy in predicting outcome in ovarian epithelial carcinoma. Obstet Gynecol 1995;86:379–85.
86. Rubin SC, Finstad CL, Wong GY, Almadrones L, Plante M, Lloyd KO. Prognostic significance of HER-2/neu expression in advanced epithelial ovarian cancer: a multivariate analysis. Am J Obstet Gynecol 1993;168:162–9.
87. Sainz de la Cuesta R, Goff BA, Fuller AF Jr., Nikrui N, Eichhorn JH, Rice LW. Prognostic importance of intraoperative rupture of malignant ovarian epithelial neoplasms. Obstet Gynecol 1994;84:1–7.
88. Scully RE, Silva E. Pathology of ovarian cancer. In: Gershenson DM, McGuire WP, eds. Controversies in the management of ovarian cancer. New York: Churchill Livingstone, 1998:425–44.
89. Sevelda P, Dittrich C, Salzer H. Prognostic value of the rupture of the capsule in Stage I epithelial ovarian carcinoma. Gynecol Oncol 1989;35:321–2.
90. Silverberg SG. Prognostic significance of pathologic features of ovarian carcinoma. In: Nogales F, ed. Current topics in pathology. Ovarian pathology. Berlin: Springer-Verlag, 1989:85–109.
91. Sjövall K, Nilsson B, Einhorn N. Different types of rupture of the tumor capsule and the impact on survival in early ovarian carcinoma. Int J Gynecol Cancer 1994;4:333–6.
92. Trimbos JB, Hacker NF. The case against aspirating ovarian cysts. Cancer 1993;72:828–31.
93. Tropé C, Kaern J. DNA ploidy in epithelial ovarian cancer: a new independent prognostic factor? [Editorial]. Gynecol Oncol 1994;53:1–4.
94. Vergote IB, Kaern J, Abeler VM, Pettersen EO, DeVos LN, Tropé CG. Analysis of prognostic factors in Stage 1 epithelial ovarian carcinoma: importance of degree of differentiation and deoxyribonucleic acid ploidy in predicting relapse. Am J Obstet Gynecol 1993;169:40–52.

Epidemiology and Pathogenesis of Epithelial Cancer

95. Bell DA, Scully RE. Early de novo ovarian carcinoma. A study of fourteen cases. Cancer 1994;73:1859–64.
96. Berchuck A, Kohler MF, Bast RC Jr. Oncogenes in ovarian cancer. In: Ozols RF, ed. Hematology/Oncology Clinics of North America. Philadelphia: WB Saunders, 1992:6:813–27.
97. Bosari S, Viale G, Radaelli U, Bossi P, Bonoldi E, Coggi G. p53 accumulation in ovarian carcinomas and its prognostic implications. Hum Pathol 1993;24:1175–9.
98. Bourne TH, Whitehead MI, Campbell S, et al. Ultrasound screening for familial ovarian cancer. Gynecol Oncol 1991;43:927.
99. Daly MB. The epidemiology of ovarian cancer. In: Ozols RF, ed. Hematology/Oncology Clinics of North America. Ovarian cancer. Philadelphia: WB Saunders, 1992;6:729–38.
100. Deligdisch L, Gil J. Characterization of ovarian dysplasia by interactive morphometry. Cancer 1989;63:748–55.
101. Gallion HH, Powell DE, Smith LW, Vaugh CC, Case EA. Cytogenetic changes in human epithelial ovarian cancer. In: Sharp F, Mason WP, Creasman E, eds. Ovarian cancer 2. Biology, diagnosis and management. London: Chapman Hall, 1992:17–22.
102. Godwin AK, Schultz DC, Hamilton TC, Knudson AG Jr. Oncogenes and tumor suppressor genes. In: Hoskins WJ, Perez CA, Young RC, eds. Principles and practice of gynecologic oncology, 2nd ed. Philadelphia: Lippincott-Raven, 1966:107–48.
103. Gross TP, Schlesselman JJ. The estimated effect of oral contraceptive use on the cumulative risk of epithelial ovarian cancer. Obstet Gynecol 1994;83:419–24.

104. Hamilton TC. Ovarian cancer, part 1: Biology. In: Ozols RF, ed. Current problems in cancer. 1992;16:3–57.

105. Hankinson SE, Colditz GA, Hunter DJ, et al. Tubal ligation, hysterectomy, and risk of ovarian cancer. A prospective study. JAMA 1993;270:2813–8.

106. Hutson R, Ramsdale J, Wells M. p53 protein expression in putative precursor lesions of epithelial ovarian cancer. Histopathology 1995;27:367–71.

107. Kerlikowske K, Brown JS, Grady DG. Should women with familial ovarian cancer undergo prophylactic oophorectomy? Obstet Gynecol 1992;80:700–7.

108. Kihana T, Tsuda H, Teshima S, et al. High incidence of p53 gene mutation in human ovarian cancer and its association with nuclear accumulation of p53 protein and tumor DNA aneuploidy. Jpn J Cancer Res 1992;83:978–84.

109. Kohler MF, Kerns BJ, Humphrey PA, Marks JR, Bast RC Jr, Berchuck A. Mutation and overexpression of p53 in early-stage ovarian cancer. Obstet Gynecol 1993;81:643–50.

110. Kommoss F, Bauknecht T, Birmelin G, et al. Oncogene and growth factor expression in ovarian cancer. Acta Obstet Gynecol Scand 1992;71(Suppl 155):19–24.

111. Kupryjanczyk J, Thor AD, Beauchamp R, et al. p53 gene mutations and protein accumulation in human ovarian cancer. Proc Natl Acad Sci USA 1993;90:4961–5.

112. Leary JA, Doris CP, Boltz EM, Houghton CR, Kefford RF, Friedlander ML. Investigation of loss of heterozygosity at specific loci on chromosomes 3p, 6q, 11p, 17p and 17q in ovarian cancer. Int J Gynecol Cancer 1993;3:293–8.

113. Look KY. Epidemiology, etiology, and screening of ovarian cancer. In: Rubin SC, Sutton GP, eds. Ovarian cancer. New York: McGraw-Hill, 1992:175–87.

114. Lynch HT, Lynch JF, Conway TA. Hereditary ovarian cancer. In: Rubin SC, Sutton GP, eds. Ovarian cancer. New York: McGraw-Hill, 1992:189–217.

115. Makar AP, Holm R, Kristensen GB, Nesland JM, Tropé CG. The expression of c-erbB-2 (HER-2/neu) oncogene in invasive ovarian malignancies. Int J Gynecol Cancer 1994;4:194–99.

116. Meden H, Marx D, Rath W, et al. Overexpression of the oncogene c-erb B2 in primary ovarian cancer: evaluation of the prognostic value in a Cox proportional hazards multiple regression. Int J Gynecol Pathol 1994;13:45–53.

117. Mittal KR, Zeleniuch-Jacquotte A, Cooper JL, Demopoulos RI. Contralateral ovary in unilateral ovarian carcinoma: a search for preneoplastic lesions. Int J Gynecol Pathol 1993;12:59–63.

118. Pejovic T. Genetic changes in ovarian cancer. Ann Med 1995;27:73–8.

119. Persons DL, Hartmann LC, Herath JH, Keeney GL, Jenkins RP. Fluorescence in situ hybridization analysis of trisomy 12 in ovarian tumors. Am J Clin Pathol 1994;102:775–9.

120. Puls LE, Powell DE, DePriest PD, et al. Transition from benign to malignant epithelium in mucinous and serous ovarian cystadenocarcinoma. Gynecol Oncol 1992;47:53–7.

121. Resta L, Russo S, Colucci GA, Prat J. Morphologic precursors of ovarian epithelial tumors. Obstet Gynecol 1993;82:181–6.

121a. Risch HA. Estrogen replacement therapy and risk of epithelial ovarian cancer. Gynecol Oncol 1996;63:254–7.

122. Rubin SC, Finstad CL, Federici MG, Scheiner L, Lloyd KO, Hoskins WJ. Prevalence and significance of HER-2/neu expression in early epithelial ovarian cancer. Cancer 1994;73:1456–9.

123. Sasano H, Garrett CT. Oncogenes in gynecological tumors. In: Sasano N, ed. Current topics in pathology. Gynecological tumors. Recent progress in diagnostic pathology. Berlin: Springer-Verlag, 1992:85:357–72.

124. Scambia G, Panici PB, Battaglia F, et al. Significance of epidermal growth factor receptor in advanced ovarian cancer. J Clin Oncol 1992;10:529–35.

125. Scully RE. Early de novo ovarian cancer and cancer developing in benign ovarian lesions. Int J Gynecol Obstet 1995;49:9-15.

126. Scully RE. Ovary. In: Henson DE, Albores-Saavedra J, eds. Pathology of incipient neoplasia. Philadelphia: WB Saunders, 1993:283–300.

127. Silver AL. Tubal ligation, hysterectomy, and risk of ovarian cancer [Editorial]. J Am Med Assn 1994;271:1235.

128. Singleton TP, Perrone T, Oakley G, et al. Activation of c-erb B-2 and prognosis in ovarian carcinoma. Comparison with histologic type, grade, and stage. Cancer 1994;73:1460-6.

129. Whittemore AS. The risk of ovarian cancer after treatment for infertility. N Engl J Med 1994;331:805–6.

130. Whittemore AS, Harris R, Ithyre J. Characteristics relating to ovarian cancer risk: collaborative analysis on 12-case control studies. II. Invasive epithelial ovarian cancers in white women. Collaborative Ovarian Cancer Group. Am J Epidemiol 1992;136:1184–203.

❖❖❖

3

SURFACE EPITHELIAL–STROMAL TUMORS
SEROUS TUMORS

SURFACE EPITHELIAL–STROMAL TUMORS

These tumors are so designated because, with occasional exceptions, they are considered to be derived ultimately from the ovarian surface epithelium (modified mesothelium) and the adjacent ovarian stroma. The evidence for a surface epithelial origin is strongest for the serous, endometrioid, and clear cell subtypes, and is substantial but weaker for other forms such as mucinous and squamous cell tumors, some of which originate from epithelial elements within germ cell tumors. Nevertheless, because of the frequency with which the six specific subtypes of these tumors are admixed and the similarities in their biologic behavior and treatment, it is convenient and practical to include all of them except those that are clearly of germ cell lineage within the surface epithelial–stromal category. The word "stroma" is included in the terminology of this group of tumors because stroma is present in variable amounts in all the subtypes and is the predominant neoplastic element in some of them. Additionally, unlike the stroma of tumors elsewhere in the body, the stroma of these neoplasms is derived in most cases from the distinctive ovarian stroma and can secrete steroid hormones, resulting in endocrine manifestations that may dominate the clinical presentation (see chapter 19).

Surface epithelial–stromal tumors account for 50 to 55 percent of all ovarian tumors, and their malignant forms for approximately 90 percent of all ovarian cancers in the western world (4,5). The corresponding figures for Japan are 46 to 50 percent and 70 to 75 percent, respectively (6,8). Surface epithelial cancers account for only 58 percent of ovarian cancers in Nigeria (9).

These tumors are subclassified pathologically according to four criteria: 1) the epithelial cell type(s); 2) the relative amounts of epithelial and stromal components; 3) the location of the epithelial elements: surface (exophytic), cystic (endophytic), or both; and 4) the histologic patterns and nuclear features, which determine whether the tumor is benign, borderline (of low malignant potential), or carcinoma, and which generally correlate with clinical behavior. The six epithelial cell types are serous, mucinous, endometrioid, clear (including hobnail and other rarer cell types), transitional (urothelial), and squamous.

The Brenner subtype of transitional cell tumor is the only neoplasm in the surface epithelial–stromal category that typically contains a larger stromal than epithelial component. When the stroma of tumors of the other cell types occupies an area greater than that of the cysts and their contents, the suffix "-fibroma" is added to the diagnostic designation, e.g., serous adenofibroma; the presence of more than a rare cyst over 1 cm in diameter in such tumors warrants use of the prefix "cyst-" before "adenofibroma."

The epithelial components of intraovarian surface epithelial–stromal tumors are thought to arise from surface epithelial inclusion glands and cysts (see figs. 1-6, 1-7) rather than directly from the surface epithelium (see figs. 2-11–2-13). These glands and cysts, which are commonly encountered in the ovaries of adult women, but may also develop earlier in life, are derived from the surface epithelium, probably as a result of an interplay of stromal and surface epithelial proliferation or the formation of surface adhesions. The cysts are almost always lined by epithelial cells that appear indifferent, serous (ciliated), or endometrioid; rarely, they are lined by mucinous or clear cells. Solid nests of transitional cells (Walthard nests) are also encountered occasionally in the superficial ovarian stroma or the ovarian hilus, and may be the source of some transitional cell tumors.

The subclassification of surface epithelial–stromal tumors that is most important from a clinical viewpoint is their division into benign, borderline, and carcinomatous forms. Tumors in which the patterns of growth and cytologic features are intermediate between those of obviously benign and obviously malignant tumors of the same cell type(s) are associated with a far better prognosis, stage for stage, than that of ovarian carcinomas and have been designated by the World Health Organization (WHO) as "tumors of borderline malignancy" or "tumors of low malignant potential." These neoplasms have been the subject of considerable controversy among both pathologists and gynecologists with regard to their diagnostic features, terminology, and therapy (66a). The WHO recommends the presence or absence of "obvious invasion" of the stroma of the tumor as the distinction between carcinomas and borderline tumors. Some pathologists, however, do not require obvious stromal invasion for a diagnosis of carcinoma if the neoplastic epithelial cells are malignant cytologically. Other pathologists have introduced alternative designations for various subtypes of borderline tumors such as "proliferating," "atypical," and "atypical proliferating" (3,7). Another problem unique to the mucinous category of neoplasms is controversy as to whether the "borderline" tumors that are associated with peritoneal spread in the form of pseudomyxoma are always primary ovarian tumors, always metastatic tumors from the appendix or elsewhere, or include examples of both (page 99). From a clinical viewpoint, some gynecologists manage high-stage borderline tumors conservatively, removing as much tumor as technically feasible but withholding chemotherapy and radiation therapy, while others administer additional radiation or chemotherapy. As a result of these problems, the literature on borderline tumors is confusing, particularly when the diagnostic criteria used are not clearly defined and important clinical or pathologic data are missing.

The microscopic features of malignant epithelial-stromal tumors (borderline tumors and carcinomas) that have been shown to have prognostic significance are: the presence or absence of obvious stromal invasion (strong evidence), the extent of the invasion if present (strong evidence), and in the absence of obvious invasion, whether the noninvasive cells are only atypical or carcinomatous (suggestive evidence). Because of tumor heterogeneity, particularly in mucinous tumors, the extent of sampling of the neoplasm is important for assessment of the validity of authors' conclusions. Although a large body of data has accumulated on serous and mucinous borderline tumors, criteria for their classification and nomenclature remain controversial. Much less information exists on the value of various criteria for distinguishing the much

rarer borderline tumors from carcinomas in the other epithelial categories.

To promote uniformity of terminology throughout the world, we propose usage of the WHO basic diagnostic criterion for distinguishing between borderline tumors and carcinomas, with amplification and explanations as follows:

Borderline Tumor (no obvious invasion)
   Variant
   With intraepithelial carcinoma (the extent of the carcinomatous epithelium should be noted)

Carcinoma (obvious invasion)*
   Disorderly penetration of the cyst wall or the stromal component of a predominantly fibromatous tumor by carcinoma cells, with or without a stromal reaction** or

   Confluence of carcinoma cells in the cyst wall or in the stromal component of a predominantly fibromatous tumor**

*Strict adherence to the criterion of obvious invasion for the diagnosis of carcinoma without consideration of other microscopic features will result in underdiagnosis of a small number of otherwise obvious carcinomas. For example, some serous papillary carcinomas characterized by large areas of obvious carcinoma may have a sharp border with the adjacent stroma, or the latter may not be present in available sections. Also, exophytic intraepithelial carcinomas (serous surface papillary tumors of borderline malignancy with intraepithelial carcinoma) must be assumed to have a guarded prognosis regardless of their extent, since their cells are exposed to the peritoneal cavity, and microscopic carcinomas on or near the surface of the ovary are commonly associated with a malignant course (19).

**The extent of the obvious invasion should be noted. We use the term "microinvasion" for the presence of one or more separate foci 10 sq mm or less in area. Microinvasive carcinoma must be distinguished from microinvasive borderline tumor, in which a distinctive pattern is present and the invasive cells do not have the cytologic features of carcinoma cells (page 61).

The alternative terms for borderline tumors, proliferating, atypical, and atypical proliferating

(3,7), are undesirable because of their divergence from current generally accepted terminology, and are misleading since borderline tumors are capable of spread beyond the ovary, occasionally to distant sites, and can be fatal. Use of the alternative terms (except possibly in the case of borderline Brenner tumors) would not transmit the malignant potential of these neoplasms to the patients' physicians; would result in a failure of physicians to report them to cancer registries, such as that of FIGO, eliminating important avenues for further investigation; and would confuse many pathologists, clinicians, and epidemiologists by engendering nosologic disarray.

SEROUS TUMORS

Definition. These tumors are characterized in their benign forms and in well-differentiated areas within some of their borderline forms by ciliated epithelial cells and occasionally other cell types resembling those of the fallopian tube. In less differentiated tumors the epithelial elements lose the characteristic cytologic features of tubal epithelium but grow in distinctive patterns including: extensive, often complex papillarity with prominent cellular budding; the formation of glands with irregular, often slit-like lumens; and solid nests and sheets. Psammoma bodies and larger calcific deposits are common, especially in serous carcinomas.

General Features. In the western world serous tumors account for about 30 percent of all ovarian neoplasms; of these, approximately 60 percent are benign; 10 percent, borderline; and 30 percent, carcinomatous (42,44,62). In Asians, in whom epithelial neoplasms are less common than in Caucasians, serous tumors account for 20 to 25 percent of all ovarian tumors (38,57,69). Borderline and invasive serous tumors together account for 40 to 45 percent of all ovarian cancers (59). Serous carcinomas are among the most common cancers in the female associated with paraneoplastic phenomena (see chapter 20). Occasionally, the stroma of serous tumors is activated to produce steroid hormones, with accompanying endocrine manifestations (see chapter 19). The serum level of CA125 is elevated in over 80 percent of cases of serous carcinoma (30,48); a variety of other markers may be elevated as well.

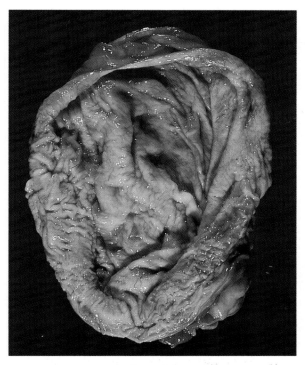

Figure 3-1
SEROUS CYSTADENOMA
The lining of the thin-walled cyst is smooth and glistening.

Benign serous tumors occur at any age, but are most common in women in the reproductive age group. Borderline tumors are rare before the age of 20 years but the incidence increases thereafter, with an average patient age of 46 years (44,64,69). Serous carcinoma is exceedingly rare in the first two decades but there is a progressively increasing rise in age-specific incidence subsequently, with an average patient age of 56 years (64).

Gross Findings. Serous cystadenoma is composed of one or more thin-walled cysts filled with watery fluid (fig. 3-1). The cyst lining may bear polypoid excrescences composed almost entirely of stroma (fig. 3-2, left) and characterized by a firm consistency if the stroma is dense and fibrous, or a soft consistency if it is edematous (fig. 3-2, right). Tumors containing stromal "polyps" cannot be distinguished with certainty from serous borderline cystic tumors on gross examination alone, but the latter tumors typically have a lush growth of fine papillae as well as polypoid excrescences (fig. 3-3). Serous cystadenomas can be large but only occasionally reach the huge dimensions that are more

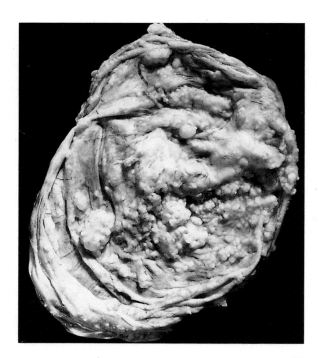
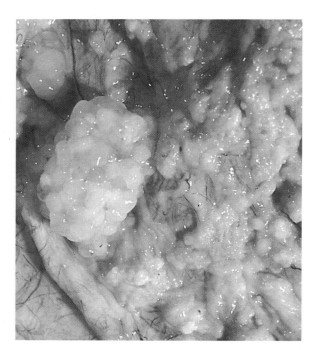

Figure 3-2
SEROUS PAPILLARY CYSTADENOMA
Left: The inner surface of the large cyst bears numerous polypoid projections, which were composed predominantly of stroma.
Right: The polypoid projections were soft and edematous.

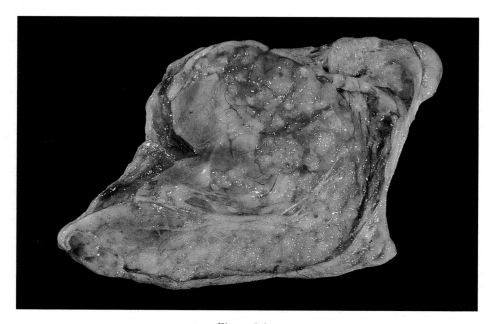

Figure 3-3
SEROUS PAPILLARY CYSTIC TUMOR OF BORDERLINE MALIGNANCY
A large portion of the inner surface of the cyst is covered by both large polypoid excrescences and small papillae. (Fig. 1 from Richart RM, Boronow RC, Norris HJ, Scully RE, Woodruff JD. Diagnosing borderline tumors of the ovary. Contemp Ob Gyn 1977;9:74–98.)

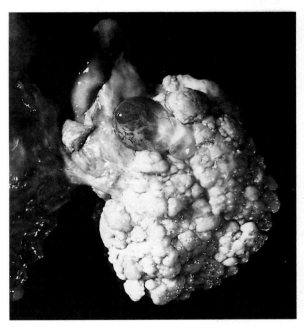

Figure 3-4
SEROUS SURFACE PAPILLARY ADENOFIBROMA
The external surface of the ovary is covered by confluent large polypoid excrescences and small granular papillae.

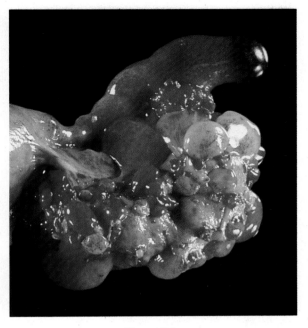

Figure 3-5
SEROUS SURFACE PAPILLARY ADENOFIBROMA
Some of the polypoid excrescences are edematous, resembling vesicles.

often attained by mucinous cystadenomas, which are on average almost twice the diameter of the former. Serous cystadenomas are bilateral in 7 to 20 percent of the cases (42,57,62,72).

Serous surface papillary adenofibromas appear as warty excrescences, which are usually limited in extent but may be widespread on the outer surface of one or both ovaries (fig. 3-4). Exceptionally, these tumors are characterized by large, edematous, polypoid excrescences resembling the vesicles of a hydatidiform mole (fig. 3-5). Benign serous surface tumors may be impossible to distinguish from borderline forms on gross examination alone.

Serous adenofibromas and cystadenofibromas are typically hard, white to yellow-white, predominantly solid, fibromatous tumors that contain glands or cysts filled with clear fluid. The cyst linings may bear polypoid excrescences, and their presence in combination with the hard consistency of the stromal component may lead to an erroneous gross impression of carcinoma, particularly when the tumors are bilateral in postmenopausal women.

In serous tumors of borderline malignancy polypoid excrescences accompanied by finer papillae occupy part or all of the lining of one or more cysts, the outer surface of the ovary (serous surface papillary tumor of borderline malignancy), or both (fig. 3-3). Some serous cystic borderline tumors secrete thick mucinous fluid, which should not lead to an erroneous gross diagnosis of a mucinous cystic tumor. Serous cystadenofibromas of borderline malignancy contain solid, white to yellow-white fibromatous components. Serous borderline tumors are bilateral in 25 to 30 percent of the cases (59).

Serous carcinomas range from predominantly cystic papillary tumors to entirely solid, soft or hard masses, often having papillary surfaces (figs. 3-6, 3-7). The tumor may be entirely exophytic (serous surface carcinoma) but most often, the underlying ovary is at least focally replaced by neoplastic tissue as well. Serous surface carcinomas may appear as one or more soft, white to red, velvety patches or hard plaques on the ovarian surface (fig. 3-8). Most poorly differentiated serous carcinomas cannot be distinguished grossly from other types of

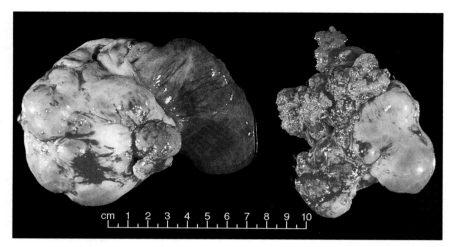

Figure 3-6
SEROUS PAPILLARY
CARCINOMA, BILATERAL
The tumors are partly solid
and partly cystic. The rough-sur-
faced polypoid tumor has extended through the capsule.

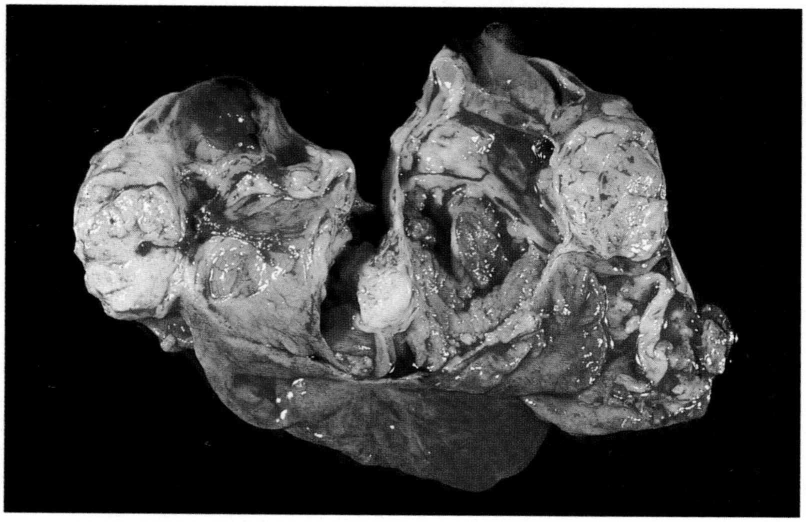

Figure 3-7
SEROUS PAPILLARY
CARCINOMA
The tumor has solid and cystic compo-
nents.

Figure 3-8
SEROUS SURFACE
PAPILLARY CARCINOMA
Small, hemorrhagic, polypoid excrescenses oc-
cupy part of the external surface of the ovary.

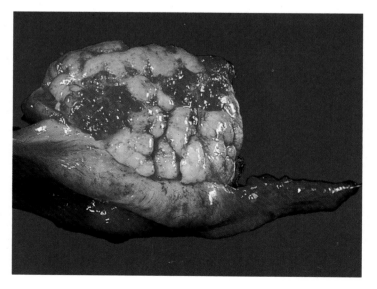

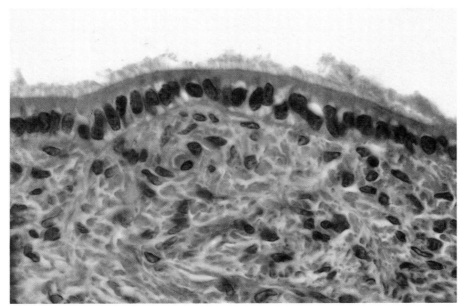

Figure 3-9
SEROUS CYSTADENOMA
The cyst is lined by ciliated epithelium without significant nuclear atypia.

poorly differentiated ovarian cancer, sharing with them nonspecific characteristics of cancer, such as friability, necrosis, cystic degeneration, and hemorrhage. Focal or diffuse calcific deposits suggest the serous nature of the tumor. Serous carcinomas are bilateral in about two thirds of all cases, but in only 25 to 30 percent of stage I cases (calculated by relative numbers of stage IA and stage IB cases) (59).

Microscopic Findings. *Benign Tumors.* Benign serous tumors are typically lined by an epithelium similar to that of the fallopian tube (fig. 3-9), with ciliated cells and much less often nonciliated secretory cells. Tumors lined entirely by nonciliated, cuboidal or columnar epithelium that resembles the surface epithelium of the ovary have been customarily classified as serous as well, even though they lack specific serous features (page 72) (fig. 3-10). Psammoma bodies may be present, but are generally inconspicuous. Polypoid excrescences are composed almost entirely of stroma, which ranges from dense and collagenous to markedly edematous (fig. 3-11).

Borderline Tumors. 1. Primary Tumors. Serous borderline tumors are characterized by polypoid excrescences and papillae occupying a variable extent of a cyst lining, the outer surface of the ovary, or both. The lining cells typically exhibit mild to marked nuclear atypia, rare to occasional mitotic figures, and stratification (figs. 3-12, 3-13).

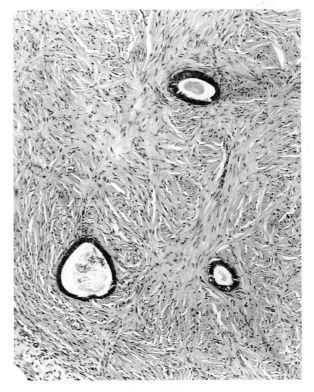

Figure 3-10
SEROUS ADENOFIBROMA
Gland-like structures lined by indifferent cuboidal epithelium are distributed within a slightly hyalinized fibromatous stromal component. (Fig. 5 from Serov SF, Scully RE, Sobin LH. Histological typing of ovarian tumours. International Histological Classification of Tumours No. 9. Geneva: World Health Organization, 1973.)

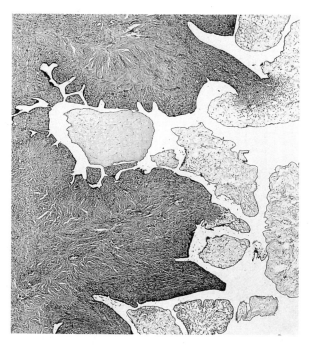

Figure 3-11
SEROUS PAPILLARY CYSTADENOMA
The lining of the cyst is polypoid, with some of the excrescences composed predominantly of dense stroma and others, of loose edematous stroma. (Fig. 6 from Serov SF, Scully RE, Sobin LH. Histological typing of ovarian tumours. International Histological Classification of Tumours No. 9. Geneva: World Health Organization, 1973.)

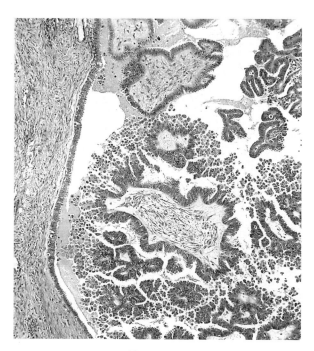

Figure 3-12
SEROUS PAPILLARY CYSTIC TUMOR
OF BORDERLINE MALIGNANCY
In addition to large polypoid excrescences on the inner surface of a cyst lined by stratified epithelium, there are many small papillae, some of which appear to lack a stromal core. (Fig. 2 from Scully RE. Common epithelial tumors of borderline malignancy (carcinomas of low malignant potential). Bull du Cancer 1982;69:228–38.)

The three most characteristic features, which are essential for the diagnosis, are the formation of cellular buds that appear to float in the intracystic fluid or off the surface of the ovary, some degree of nuclear atypia, and a lack of "obvious" invasion of the stromal component of the tumor. The stroma of the generally bulbous polypoid excrescences may resemble ovarian stroma but is more often edematous or fibromatous. The tumor cells typically have scanty cytoplasm but, particularly in the cellular buds, may contain abundant eosinophilic cytoplasm (fig. 3-14); cells of the latter type are more numerous if the patient is pregnant. Psammoma bodies may be present. In some cases the neoplastic cells secrete abundant mucin (fig. 3-15) but mucin is barely recognizable in the superficial portion of the cytoplasm and does not fill the cytoplasm of the cells, as it typically does in mucinous borderline tumors of endocervical-like type.

A common and sometimes confusing finding in a serous borderline tumor is an orderly, often

extensive penetration of its stroma by tubular structures and microcysts with papillae, without elicitation of a stromal reaction (fig. 3-16). This feature reflects the complexity of the epithelial and stromal proliferation and should not be misinterpreted as stromal invasion. Another microscopic pattern that is occasionally seen in serous borderline tumors and may lead to an erroneous diagnosis of carcinoma is so-called autoimplantation (18), the presence of sharply delimited desmoplastic plaques usually on the outer surface but occasionally on the inner (cystic) surface of the tumor (fig. 3-17), resembling the noninvasive desmoplastic implants that may occur on the extraovarian peritoneum (page 64).

Three additional uncommon and controversial variations of epithelial proliferation within serous borderline tumors may be encountered focally or diffusely: 1) an intracystic or less often, surface cribriform pattern (fig. 3-18); 2) an intracystic or

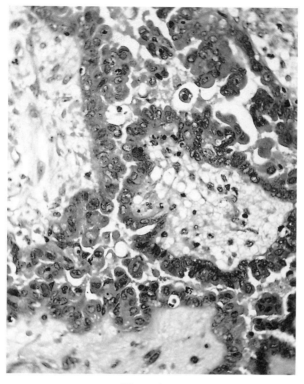

Figure 3-13
SEROUS PAPILLARY CYSTIC TUMOR
OF BORDERLINE MALIGNANCY
The lining cells are stratified with cellular budding. The nuclei are moderately atypical and the cytoplasm is moderately abundant.

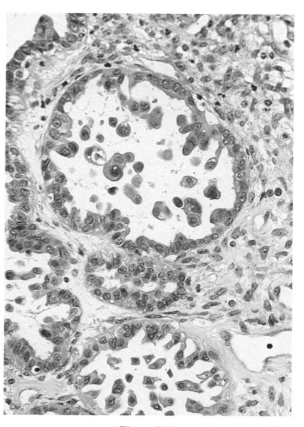

Figure 3-14
SEROUS PAPILLARY CYSTIC TUMOR OF
BORDERLINE MALIGNANCY
Tumor cells with abundant eosinophilic cytoplasm are evident.

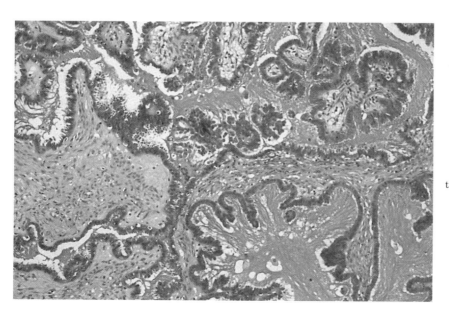

Figure 3-15
SEROUS PAPILLARY
CYSTIC TUMOR OF
BORDERLINE MALIGNANCY
Abundant basophilic mucin fills the lumen of the cyst.

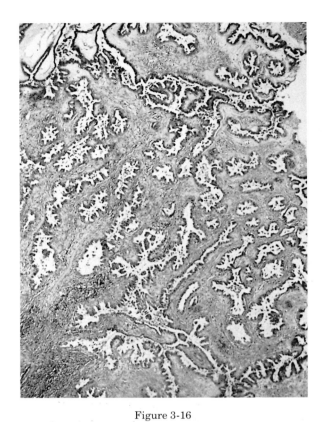

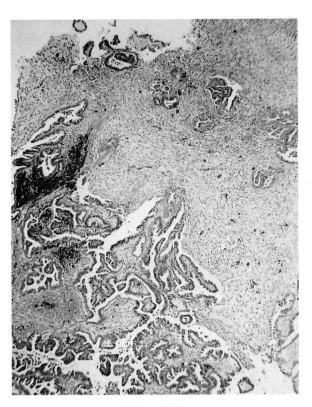

Figure 3-16
SEROUS PAPILLARY CYSTIC TUMOR
OF BORDERLINE MALIGNANCY
Tubule-like structures with papillae are distributed in
an orderly arrangement in the stromal component of the
tumor without a stromal reaction.

Figure 3-17
SEROUS PAPILLARY CYSTIC TUMOR
OF BORDERLINE MALIGNANCY
WITH AUTOIMPLANTATION
The upper and right portions of the figure contain
desmoplastic tissue in which scattered tumor cell units and
psammoma bodies create an appearance similar to that of a
desmoplastic peritoneal implant.

Figure 3-18
SEROUS PAPILLARY CYSTIC
TUMOR OF BORDERLINE
MALIGNANCY WITH
CRIBRIFORM PATTERN

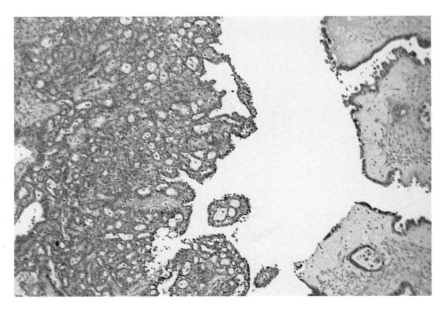

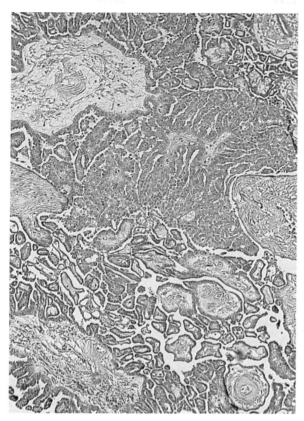

Figure 3-19
SEROUS PAPILLARY CYSTIC TUMOR OF
BORDERLINE MALIGNANCY WITH
MICROPAPILLARY PATTERN

surface micropapillary pattern, characterized by delicate branching filiform cellular papillae (fig. 3-19); and 3) a solid or almost solid intracystic proliferation. These patterns have not been described in large numbers of cases with long-term follow-up data and their significance is as yet unclear. Burks et al. (23) concluded that the first two patterns are associated with a poorer prognosis than the typical patterns of serous borderline tumors in cases with peritoneal involvement because of a higher frequency of invasive implants (65a). Katzenstein et al. (42a), however, had found in an earlier study that neither an extensive micropapillary pattern nor a surface or stromal cribriform pattern worsened the prognosis in cases of serous borderline tumor. Finding any of these unusual patterns in a borderline tumor should lead to more extensive sampling as well as careful evaluation of peritoneal im-

plants, if present, to exclude invasion. We continue to classify tumors with these unusual patterns in the borderline category, but note their presence and extent and inform the clinician regarding their poorer prognosis if accompanied by invasive implants. Further investigation of tumors with these patterns is desirable.

A cumulative analysis of the literature has shown that 14 percent of serous borderline tumors are aneuploid (17). When fresh tumor tissue has been used for flow cytometric studies, however, these tumors have been diploid almost without exception (47).

2. Microinvasion. A variant of the serous borderline tumor that must be distinguished from serous carcinoma is the subtype with microinvasion of the stroma, which is characterized by the presence of one or more discrete foci of tumor cells with borderline features in the stroma, none of which exceed 10 sq mm in area (fig. 3-20) (20,70). The foci typically consist of single epithelial cells, which may have abundant eosinophilic cytoplasm, and small clusters of such cells, sometimes accompanied by psammoma bodies, generally lying in empty spaces that have probably been produced by the secretion of serous fluid by the tumor cells. A stromal reaction characteristic of invasion by carcinoma is lacking. Invasion of vascular spaces (fig. 3-21) has been observed in 10 percent of the 39 reported cases of microinvasive borderline tumor (20,70). Stromal microinvasion may be present in 10 percent or more of serous borderline tumors; it is identified more easily by examination of slides stained for cytokeratins than by examination of routinely stained sections (35). In occasional cases of microinvasion neoplastic cells are present in cribriform nests or in rounded islands with a microcystic pattern (fig. 3-22). Experience with these patterns of invasion is limited.

3. Implants. Microscopic evaluation of the peritoneal lesions in stage II and III cases is much more important for prognosis and therapy than evaluation of the primary ovarian tumor since the latter is almost always completely removed, leaving only the peritoneal lesions for the gynecologist to manage. These lesions range from foci of benign-appearing serous epithelium forming glands, cysts, and sometimes papillae with psammoma bodies (endosalpingiosis) (figs. 3-23, 3-24) (75), to noninvasive deposits of borderline

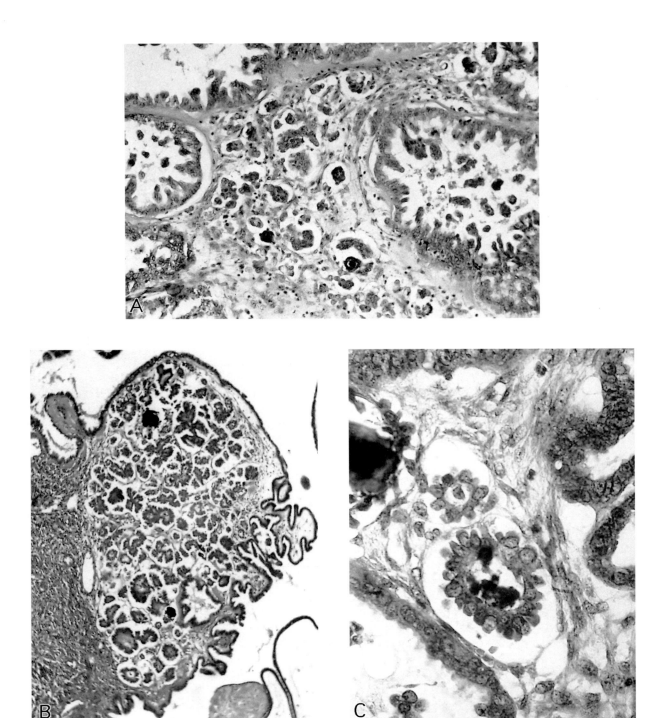

Figure 3-20
SEROUS PAPILLARY CYSTIC TUMOR OF BORDERLINE MALIGNANCY WITH MICROINVASION

A: In the stroma separating several cysts are numerous small clusters of tumor cells and psammoma bodies lying within clear spaces. (Fig. 15-13 from Scully RE. Ovary. In: Henson DE, Albores-Saavedra J, eds. Pathology of incipient neoplasia. Philadelphia: WB Saunders, 1986:287.)

B: The oval area in the center is composed of closely packed clusters of tumor cells surrounded by clear spaces. (Fig. 5 from Bell DA, Scully RE. Ovarian serous borderline tumors with microinvasion. A report of 21 cases. Human Pathol 1990;21:397–403.)

C: Two papillae lie in spaces that are not lined by endothelium.

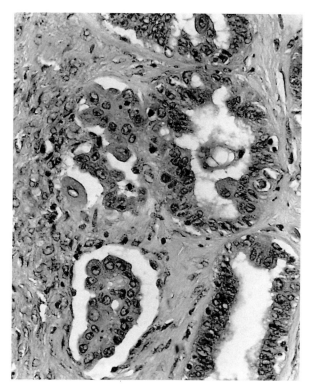

Figure 3-21
SEROUS PAPILLARY CYSTIC TUMOR
OF BORDERLINE MALIGNANCY
WITH MICROINVASION
A lymphatic vessel in the lower portion of the figure contains a cluster of tumor cells.

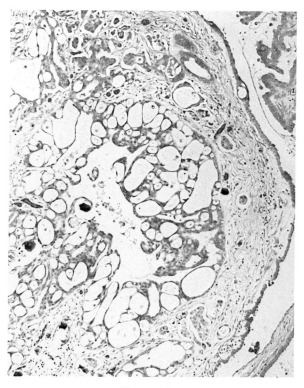

Figure 3-22
SEROUS PAPILLARY CYSTIC TUMOR
OF BORDERLINE MALIGNANCY
WITH MICROINVASION
The invasive tumor has a cribriform, microcystic pattern.

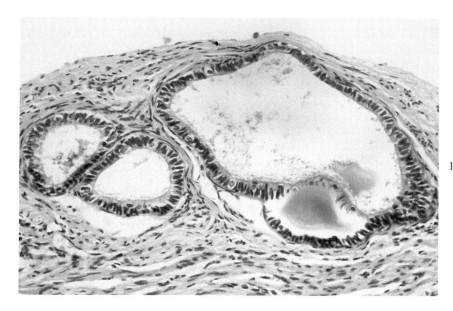

Figure 3-23
ENDOSALPINGIOSIS
OF PERITONEUM
Glands lined by ciliated epithelium lie in fibrous stroma.

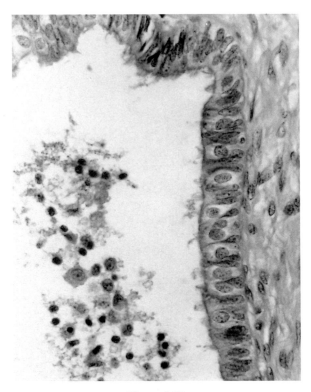

Figure 3-24
ENDOSALPGINGIOSIS
Ciliated, secretory and intercalated cells line the cystic space.

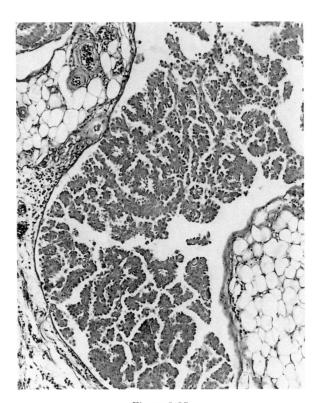

Figure 3-25
NONINVASIVE EPITHELIAL IMPLANT OF
SEROUS BORDERLINE TUMOR ON PERITONEUM
The implant extends between lobules of greater omentum.

epithelium and stroma, to invasive implants indistinguishable from low-grade serous carcinoma. Endosalpingiosis, which often accompanies ovarian serous borderline tumors, and may occasionally be the source of a peritoneal serous borderline tumor or carcinoma, is a benign process, the presence of which should not cause up-staging of an accompanying ovarian borderline tumor from I to II or III. Noninvasive implants of ovarian serous borderline tumors may be composed predominantly of neoplastic epithelial cells (epithelial implants) or of stroma, which is typically desmoplastic (desmoplastic implants) (21). Noninvasive epithelial implants resemble the papillary proliferations of the primary ovarian tumor (fig. 3-25). Noninvasive desmoplastic implants form sharply circumscribed plaques or nodules that appear to be plastered on the surface of the peritoneum, often extending as septa between lobules of omentum (fig. 3-26). These lesions may be encountered at several stages of development.

Early forms may be characterized by massive necrosis and acute inflammation (fig. 3-27). Late lesions are composed of dense fibrous stroma resembling the desmoplastic stroma of a carcinoma and containing, typically in small numbers, disorderly, often jagged nests of tumor cells, individual tumor cells, and psammoma bodies accompanied by a subacute inflammatory cell reaction and often focal hemorrhage (fig. 3-28). When underlying tissue is absent in the biopsy specimen, we classify the lesion as noninvasive on the assumption that it has been stripped away with ease. Invasive implants, which in our experience are found in 12 percent of the cases (21), infiltrate underlying tissue in a disorderly fashion. When present in the omentum, they usually have an irregular border, with replacement and destruction of the adipose tissue (figs. 3-29, 3-30), in contrast to the sharp border of a desmoplastic noninvasive implant, which respects the integrity of the omental lobules.

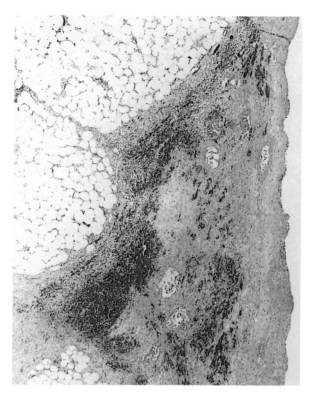

Figure 3-26
NONINVASIVE DESMOPLASTIC IMPLANT
OF SEROUS BORDERLINE TUMOR
The implant coats the surface of the omentum and extends
as a septum between adjacent lobules. Scattered nests of tumor
cells and foci of hemorrhage are present within the implant.

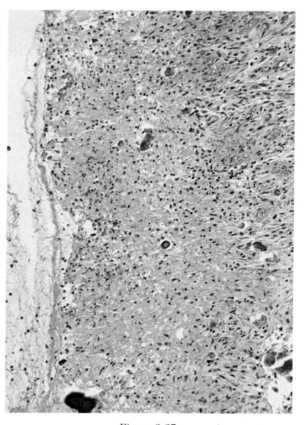

Figure 3-27
EARLY STAGE OF NONINVASIVE DESMOPLASTIC
IMPLANT OF SEROUS BORDERLINE TUMOR
The implant has undergone massive necrosis.

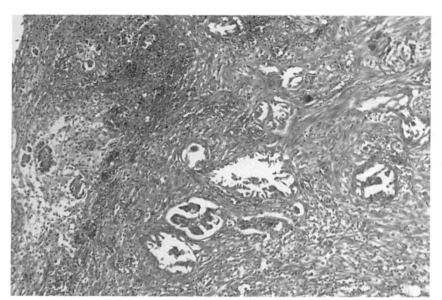

Figure 3-28
NONINVASIVE DESMOPLASTIC
IMPLANT OF SEROUS
BORDERLINE TUMOR
Disorderly groups of tumor cells lie
in dense, focally hemorrhagic stroma.

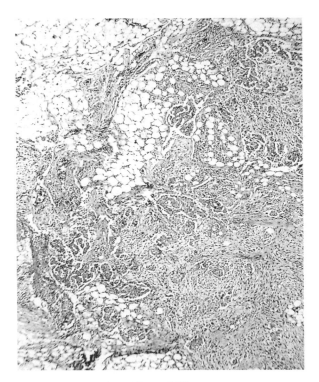

Figure 3-29
INVASIVE IMPLANT OF
SEROUS BORDERLINE TUMOR
The desmoplastic implant invades omental tissue in an
irregular fashion.

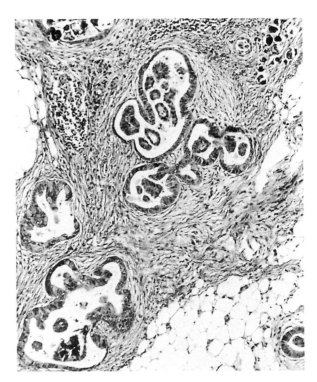

Figure 3-30
INVASIVE IMPLANT OF
SEROUS BORDERLINE TUMOR
The tumor has the appearance of grade 1 serous carci-
noma. The invasive nature of this implant was recognizable
from its low-power pattern. (Fig. 11 from Serov SF, Scully
RE, Sobin LH. Histological typing of ovarian tumours. In-
ternational Histological Classification of Tumours No. 9.
Geneva: World Health Organization, 1973.)

Implants of ovarian borderline tumors should
be sampled as extensively as technically feasible
since noninvasive and invasive implants may
coexist at different sites. Also, some implants of
serous carcinoma may be noninvasive and resemble noninvasive desmoplastic implants of serous borderline tumors. Unlike the latter, however, in which the neoplastic epithelium is
usually relatively minor in extent, the epithelial
component in desmoplastic carcinomatous implants typically occupies 25 percent or more of the
area of the lesion and exhibits a higher degree of
epithelial nuclear atypia than seen in the noninvasive implant of a borderline tumor (fig. 3-31).
The differential diagnosis is a problem mainly
when the primary ovarian tumor is not removed
and only one or two of its implants are available
for microscopic examination.

The occasional discrepant appearance of the
ovarian and peritoneal lesions in stages II and III
serous borderline tumors and the evidence that
extraovarian peritoneal mesothelium has the
ability to give rise to endosalpingiosis and serous
neoplasms have led some observers to favor the
interpretation that the peritoneal implants associated with ovarian serous borderline tumors are
independent foci of primary neoplasia instead of
true implants (63). Other investigators favor the
implantation explanation for the peritoneal lesions, based on their finding that almost two thirds
of ovarian serous borderline tumors with an exophytic component are associated with implants in
contrast to less than 5 percent of those lacking an
exophytic component (65). Molecular genetic
clonality studies may be helpful in the eventual
resolution of this problem. The important considerations from the viewpoint of management, however, are the quantity and microscopic features of
the peritoneal lesions and not their site of origin.

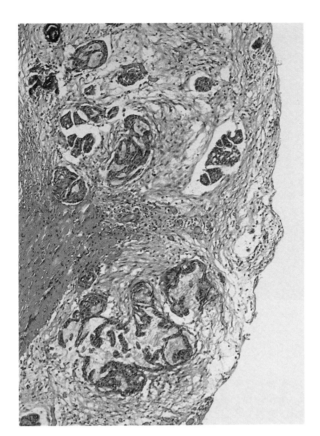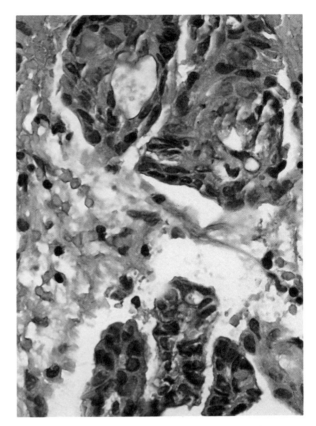

Figure 3-31
DESMOPLASTIC NONINVASIVE IMPLANT OF SEROUS CARCINOMA
Left: Large numbers of epithelial cell islands are present.
Right: The tumor cells are too severely atypical for the usual serous borderline tumor.

Carcinoma. Serous carcinomas are characterized by more extensive cellular budding, more confluent cellular growth, and almost always greater nuclear atypia than serous borderline tumors, as well as by obvious invasion of the stromal component of the tumor in most cases (figs. 3-32–3-43). The extent of papillarity in serous carcinomas varies greatly. At least a few papillae are present in most tumors, many tumors have a prominent papillary component, and occasional tumors are predominantly or exclusively papillary. The papillae are typically small but are occasionally large with prominent vessels in their stromal cores. Tumors that are poorly differentiated architecturally are generally characterized by solid sheets of cells (fig. 3-35) or almost solid masses that may contain tubular glands, but more often contain irregular, typically slit-like spaces (figs. 3-32, 3-33). Another pattern of serous

carcinoma is that of small, oval nests of moderately to well-differentiated epithelial cells or tubules lined by similar cells within a collagenous stroma (figs. 3-36–3-38). Laminated psammoma bodies may be present in variable numbers in such tumors and often coalesce to form larger, amorphous, calcific aggregates (figs. 3-36–3-38). Psammoma bodies in large numbers are particularly characteristic of a highly differentiated form of serous carcinoma, the psammocarcinoma (figs. 3-39, 3-40). This tumor, which is almost always stage III, has been defined as an invasive serous tumor characterized by cells with no more than moderate nuclear atypia lying in nests, at least 75 percent of which contain psammoma bodies and none of which contain cells greater than 15 in number along the longest dimension of the nest (33). Psammoma calcification in a serous carcinoma may be sufficiently

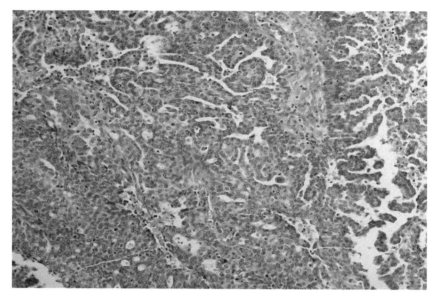

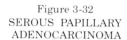
Figure 3-32
SEROUS PAPILLARY
ADENOCARCINOMA
The tumor is characterized by high cellularity, extensive formation of cellular papillae, and irregular slit-like spaces.

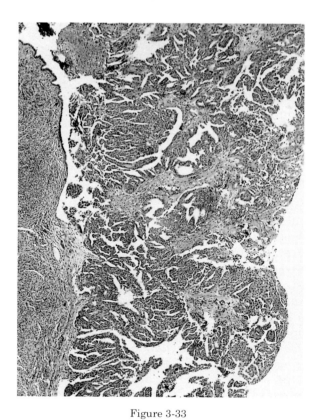

Figure 3-33
SEROUS SURFACE PAPILLARY ADENOCARCINOMA
The tumor is characterized by an exophytic proliferation of cellular papillae and the formation of slit-like glandular spaces. (Fig. 30 from Young RH, Clement PB, Scully RE. Pathology of the ovary. In: Sternberg SS, ed. Diagnostic surgical pathology, Vol 2, 1st ed. New York: Raven Press, 1989:1674.)

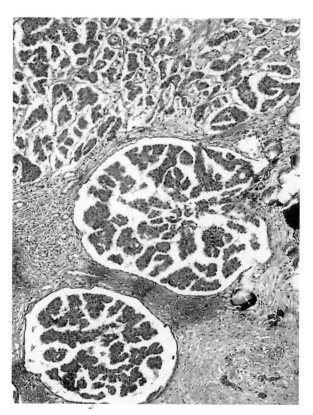

Figure 3-34
SEROUS PAPILLARY ADENOCARCINOMA
Complex papillae form glomeruloid structures.

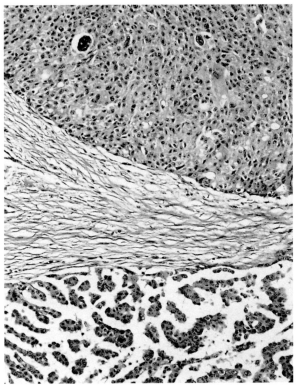

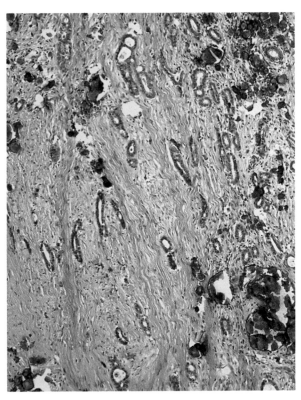

Figure 3-35
SEROUS PAPILLARY ADENOCARCINOMA,
POORLY DIFFERENTIATED
One nodule is characterized by cellular papillae. The larger
nodule is composed of a solid proliferation of tumor cells.

Figure 3-36
SEROUS PAPILLARY ADENOCARCINOMA
The tumor is composed of thin tubular glands lying in
dense stroma. Many psammoma bodies and larger calcific
deposits are present.

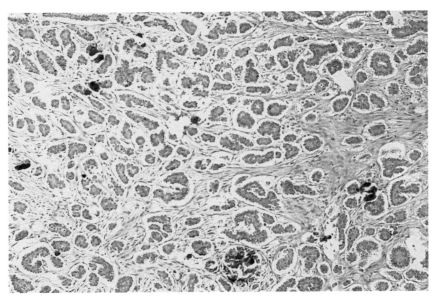

Figure 3-37
SEROUS PAPILLARY
ADENOCARCINOMA
The tumor is composed of small
nests of well-differentiated epithelial
cells lying in a fibrous stroma, with
occasional psammoma body formation.

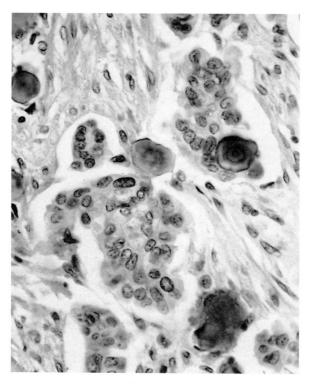

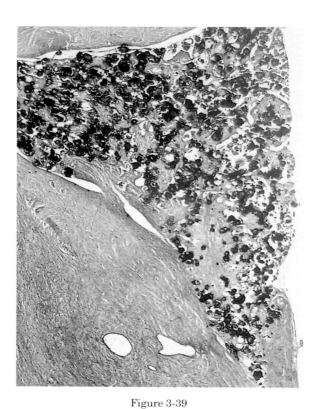

Figure 3-38
SEROUS PAPILLARY CARCINOMA
The tumor cells are slightly pleomorphic and focally hyperchromatic, but nucleoli are not prominent. Occasional psammoma bodies are present.

Figure 3-39
SEROUS PSAMMOCARCINOMA
ON SURFACE OF OVARY
Most of the tumor is made up of psammoma bodies lying in dense stroma. Invasion is not seen in this area.

Figure 3-40
SEROUS
PSAMMOCARCINOMA
IN LYMPHATICS
OF MYOMETRIUM

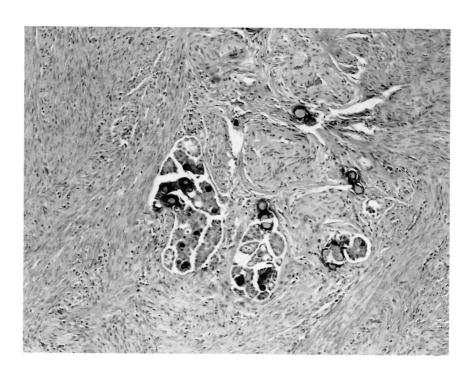

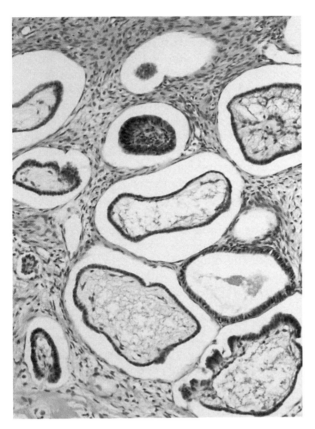

Figure 3-41
SEROUS PAPILLARY ADENOCARCINOMA, LOW GRADE
The papillae lie within nonlymphatic spaces separated
by stroma derived from ovarian stroma.

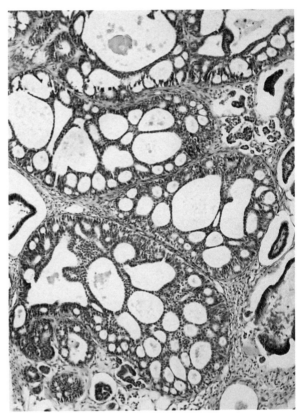

Figure 3-42
ADENOID CYSTIC-LIKE COMPONENT
OF SEROUS CARCINOMA

prominent to be visible on an X-ray film of the abdomen, typically in the form of small, hazy, granular opacities, or on computed tomographic scans (54). Adequate sampling (arbitrarily defined as five or more sections in biopsy material) is important in making a diagnosis of psammocarcinoma as its characteristic features may be seen focally in carcinomas that are elsewhere more cellular and diagnostic of more typical serous carcinoma. A rarer pattern of well-differentiated serous carcinoma is characterized by papillae lined by tumor cells lying in spaces without an endothelial lining, probably created by secretion of serous fluid by the tumor cells (fig. 3-41). Rare serous carcinomas have an adenoid cystic carcinoma-like component (fig. 3-42) (page 322); undergo focal squamous differentiation (73); have microcysts; contain multinucleated giant cells, which can resemble syncytiotrophoblast cells and

may stain for human chorionic gonadotropin (hCG) (fig. 3-43); or have a focal reticular pattern simulating that of a yolk sac tumor. Serous surface carcinomas range from highly papillary to poorly differentiated forms that have an almost solid architecture; they usually invade the underlying ovarian stroma. The cells in most serous carcinomas have nonspecific features; confusing features that are present in some tumors are small foci of hobnail cells or of cells with abundant eosinophilic cytoplasm.

Serous carcinomas are typically malignant-appearing throughout but in some cases have components of what appear to be benign or borderline serous neoplasia. The nature of the association of these various components in individual specimens merits further study with newer techniques to determine whether the more benign-or borderline-appearing elements are the sites of

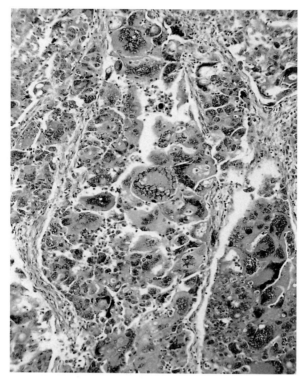

Figure 3-43
SEROUS CARCINOMA, GRADE 4,
RESEMBLING CHORIOCARCINOMA
Many of the cells are multinucleated and resemble syncytiotrophoblast cells.

origin of the more malignant-appearing components or represent maturation of the latter into the former.

Although the architectural and cytologic features of serous carcinomas generally parallel one another as far as grading is concerned, nuclear grading is probably preferable to architectural grading in the determination of prognosis since some nuclear grade 1 carcinomas composed of small solid nests of cells embedded in stroma may be associated with an indolent clinical course.

A cumulative review of the literature has revealed that 65 percent of serous carcinomas are aneuploid (17).

Several cases of single or multiple nodules of sarcoma or anaplastic carcinoma as well as larger solitary masses of sarcoma have been described in association with benign, borderline, or carcinomatous serous cystic tumors (15). In a few cases the sarcomas have been heterologous.

Differential Diagnosis. *Benign Tumors.* The distinction between an epithelial inclusion cyst with serous features and a small serous cystadenoma is based arbitrarily on whether the diameter of the lesion is 1 cm or less or larger, respectively. Serous cystadenomas must be distinguished from rare rete cystadenomas (page 326), which arise in the ovarian hilus, commonly have a layer of smooth muscle or a proliferation of hilus cells in their walls, typically exhibit shallow crevices along their inner surfaces, and are lined by cells that contain few or no cilia. Rarely, a struma ovarii is characterized by widespread cystic dilatation of follicles to the extent that it resembles closely a serous cystadenoma. In such cases the finding of small follicles containing colloid in the wall or septa of the cyst enables one to make the diagnosis, which in some cases is necessary to confirm with immunostaining for thyroglobulin (page 290). Tumors that are interpreted as nonciliated serous adenofibromas when encountered in pure form are often present as a component of a tumor containing endometrioid carcinoma, raising the question whether this type of adenofibroma is endometrioid instead of serous (37). Except in cases in which the epithelial cells are either predominantly ciliated or predominantly nonciliated and stratified with endometrioid features (which may include squamous differentiation) it may be impossible to distinguish these two forms of adenofibroma, justifying a diagnosis of "adenofibroma, question serous or endometrioid" in such cases.

Serous surface papillary adenofibromas must be distinguished from the relatively common tiny warty excrescences that may be encountered on the outer surface of the ovary of adult women. The latter are scattered and do not form a confluent mass over 1 cm in diameter (page 440).

Borderline Tumors. Serous borderline tumors that secrete abundant mucin into their lumens differ from endocervical-like mucinous borderline tumors (page 88) by a lack of more than apical intracellular mucin. Serous borderline tumors may also be simulated by retiform Sertoli-Leydig cell tumors (page 211). Ovarian serous borderline tumors must be differentiated from similar tumors arising from an extraovarian site, particularly the extraovarian peritoneum (page 452), and the implants of ovarian borderline tumors should not be confused with noninvasive implants of serous carcinoma (page 66) and foci of florid mesothelial hyperplasia (page 439).

Carcinoma. An endometrioid adenocarcinoma may be difficult to distinguish from a serous carcinoma, particularly when the tumor is poorly differentiated. The papillae in serous carcinomas are characteristically complex, and are associated with cellular budding, whereas those of endometrioid carcinomas are larger and have a more uniform villous pattern, generally with little or no cellular budding. When cellular budding occurs in endometrioid carcinomas the buds are typically composed of well-differentiated cells of endometrioid type, which may show squamous differentiation. The irregular and slit-like glands of serous carcinoma contrast with the more orderly tubular glands of endometrioid carcinoma. Squamous differentiation is common in endometrioid carcinomas but rare in serous carcinomas; in contrast, psammoma bodies are much more common and extensive in serous than endometrioid carcinomas. When poorly differentiated adenocarcinomas have intermediate or overlapping features it is preferable to interpret them as serous carcinomas because such tumors behave like the latter clinically. This practical approach should increase the reproducibility of the differential diagnosis and avoid expanding an undesirable heterogenous category of unclassified carcinomas.

When clear cell carcinomas have a papillary pattern they can closely resemble serous papillary carcinomas. Usually, the presence of other patterns of either tumor or of clear, hobnail, or oxyphilic cells in the clear cell carcinoma facilitates the diagnosis; rarely, however, hobnail-type cells and oxyphilic cells may be seen in small foci in serous carcinomas. Other features that are helpful in the differential diagnosis are the greater regularity of the complex, fine papillae, and the presence of hyalinization of the papillary cores in clear cell carcinomas; the latter finding is unusual and, when present, is only focal in serous papillary carcinomas. The rare retiform subtype of Sertoli-Leydig cell tumor may be difficult to distinguish from a serous carcinoma on the basis of its histologic features alone, but the diagnosis of the former is strongly suggested by the youth of the patient (average age, 15 years) and the occasional presence of androgenic manifestations, which are extremely rare in cases of serous neoplasia. The diagnosis of a retiform tumor is confirmed by its distinctive patterns and the presence in most cases of other more familiar patterns of Sertoli-Leydig cell tumor (page 211).

The rare primary ependymoma of the ovary (page 300) may have a papillary pattern that simulates that of a serous carcinoma, even to the point of conspicuous psammoma body formation. The presence of perivascular pseudorosettes, columnar cells with apical nuclei, and basal fibrillary cytoplasm stainable immunohistochemically for glial fibrillary acidic protein, and occasional true rosettes confirms the diagnosis of ependymoma.

Serous carcinomas must be distinguished from the rare primary and more common diffuse malignant epithelial mesotheliomas involving the surface of the ovary (page 329). In addition to the usual differences in the distribution of these tumors, their distinctive patterns and cytologic features almost always permit a confident distinction. The typical tubular and papillary patterns of mesotheliomas are unlike the more disorderly patterns of serous carcinomas. The typically cuboidal mesothelioma cells, which are usually accompanied by few or no psammoma bodies, contrast with malignant serous cells, which characteristically have less cytoplasm and more irregular nuclei than neoplastic mesothelial cells and are often associated with a desmoplastic stromal reaction and abundant psammoma body formation. Cytoplasmic staining with periodic acid–Schiff after diastase digestion (PAS-D) is observed in many cases of serous carcinoma but rarely in malignant mesotheliomas (22). In difficult cases, results of staining with a panel of antibodies (to Leu-M1, TAG-72 [antibody B72.3], and carcinoembryonic antigen [CEA]) and with antibody BER-EP4 are positive in cases of serous carcinoma and usually or always negative in cases of epithelial mesothelioma (22,31,43,66).

Primary serous carcinoma of the ovary must be distinguished from secondary involvement by serous carcinoma of the fallopian tube (page 471), endometrium, and extraovarian peritoneum. In some cases of serous carcinoma of the endometrium in which there is vascular space invasion in the myometrium and tumor is present in the ovarian parenchyma or hilus within vascular spaces, the diagnosis of metastasis from the endometrial carcinoma is clear-cut; in other cases, however, in which the ovarian tumor has the typical features of a primary serous carcinoma, either the ovarian tumor is an independent primary tumor or is the sole primary tumor with endometrial spread; and in still other cases surface involvement of the ovary with or without involvement of the extraovarian peritoneum could reflect a multifocal field change or result from implantation from the endometrial carcinoma. In many cases the problem of distinguishing unifocal and multifocal origin of serous carcinoma involving the endometrium and ovary is insoluble; molecular genetic investigation in a few cases has supported the concept of spread from one organ to the other rather than a field change (45). The distinction between high-stage ovarian serous carcinomas and serous carcinomas arising from the extraovarian peritoneum is discussed on page 451.

Another secondary tumor that may be confused with a serous carcinoma is the occasional metastatic poorly differentiated carcinoma from the breast that lacks histologic features distinctive of breast cancer and may be papillary (page 350). In most such cases a history of breast carcinoma and a comparison of its microscopic features with those of the ovarian carcinoma facilitate the diagnosis. If the differential diagnosis remains a problem immunohistochemical staining with several antibodies may be helpful. CA125 is demonstrable much more often in ovarian than in mammary carcinomas (52), and staining for gross cystic disease fluid protein-15 strongly favors metastatic breast carcinoma over primary ovarian carcinoma (25,55,74).

Frozen Section. Frozen section interpretation of serous tumors that have gross features suggesting either borderline or invasive malignancy should be based on examination of one to three microscopic sections that sample those areas most suspicious for the higher degree of malignancy. Since a diagnosis of at least borderline malignancy is almost always followed by surgical staging, and a diagnosis of carcinoma is generally followed by hysterectomy and bilateral salpingo-oophorectomy with more extensive staging, including lymph node sampling, the pathologist should be conservative in his interpretation; and the surgeon should be cautious in his decision regarding the extent of the operation to avoid overtreatment, particularly if the patient is young and desires to preserve her reproductive capacity. Also, the surgeon should be advised that more extensive sampling of the specimen postoperatively may alter a preliminary diagnosis of benign to borderline or borderline to carcinoma and warrant reoperation in some cases.

Cytology. Cytologic examination of ascitic fluid or peritoneal washings in cases of borderline and invasive serous tumors can be difficult because atypical mesothelial cells and the cells of endosalpingiosis may simulate those of serous borderline neoplasia, and the latter cells may be difficult to distinguish from those of serous carcinoma. Both the architecture and the nuclear features are important in making the differential diagnosis (67) (page 35). A panel of immunocytochemical stains (epithelial membrane antigen [EMA], B72.3, and CEA) helps distinguish between mesothelial cells and serous tumor cells in difficult cases (29) (page 73). Although the results of cytologic examination of peritoneal fluid may alter the staging of ovarian cancer they rarely influence management in the absence of histologic confirmation.

Spread and Metastases. Serous borderline tumors are confined to one or both ovaries in 68 percent of the cases; they have spread to the pelvis by the time of their discovery in 11 percent, to the upper abdomen, lymph nodes, or both in 21 percent, and more distantly in less than 1 percent of the cases (59). Parallel figures for serous carcinomas are 16, 11, 55, and 18 percent. In addition to local and peritoneal spread both types of tumor can metastasize by lymphatics and the blood stream (42a), although hematogenous metastases are rare in cases of serous borderline tumors. Sampling of pelvic lymph nodes, para-aortic lymph nodes, or both has shown involvement in up to 63 percent of cases of serous carcinoma (34). The frequency of lymph node involvement by serous borderline tumors has not been investigated extensively. Sampling of pelvic lymph nodes, para-aortic lymph nodes, or both has revealed involvement in 23 percent of the cases in one study (49), and in another investigation of all types of ovarian borderline tumor, of which 70 percent were serous and in which both pelvic and para-aortic lymph nodes were sampled, involvement was detected in 9 of 18 cases (27). On rare occasions, serous borderline tumors extend to extra-abdominal lymph nodes, including cervical nodes. Tan et al. (68) reported that lymph node involvement in some patients with serous borderline tumors may not be detected until years after the primary tumor has been removed. In such cases those authors found that

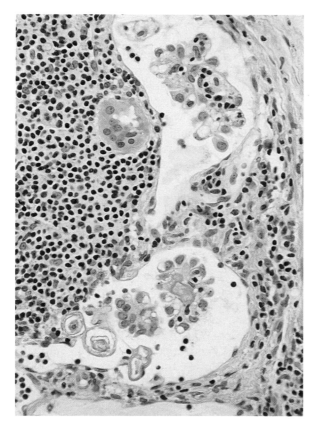

Figure 3-44
SEROUS BORDERLINE TUMOR LYING
WITHIN A LYMPHATIC OF A LYMPH NODE
The tumor cells form papillary clusters. Their presence
was associated with a serous borderline tumor of the ovary.

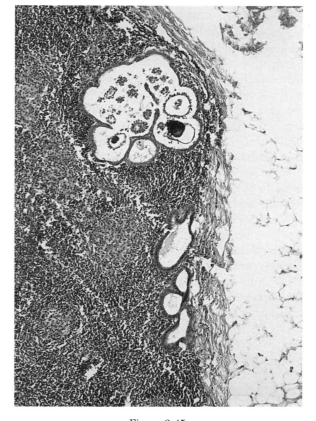

Figure 3-45
SEROUS PAPILLARY BORDERLINE TUMOR
ARISING IN PARENCHYMA OF LYMPH NODE
The tumor is in the upper portion of the figure. Mullerian
inclusion glands that do not contain tumor are present in the
lower portion.

some of the nodes were replaced by poorly differentiated serous neoplasia and some of the involved nodes were extra-abdominal.

The surprisingly high frequency of abdominal lymph node "metastasis" in cases of serous borderline neoplasia may be spurious. One reason is that nodal involvement in such cases can have two patterns. One is obviously metastatic, with tumor cells occupying sinusoids (fig. 3-44); the other is primary, with the tumor originating within mullerian inclusion glands (endosalpingiosis) and occupying predominantly the parenchyma or capsule of the lymph node (fig. 3-45) (28,41a). Mullerian inclusions have been found in up to 41 percent of women who have had a lymphadenectomy as part of the treatment of squamous cell carcinoma of the cervix (41). A

second phenomenon that can cause confusion in the identification of metastatic tumor in abdominal lymph nodes and may account partly for its reported high frequency is the intrasinusoidal presence of cytokeratin-positive mesothelial cells, singly or in groups (25a). Immunohistochemical staining is most helpful in the differential diagnosis in such cases (page 73). In our limited experience the presence of mesothelial cells in abdominal lymph nodes is associated with marked proliferation of these cells in response to peritoneal involvement by tumor. Future investigators of the prevalence of lymph node metastasis in cases of serous borderline neoplasia must exclude the above phenomenon as well as an origin in mullerian inclusion glands to arrive at an accurate figure for true metastatic spread.

Treatment and Prognosis. Serous carcinomas are treated as described for epithelial cancers in general (page 39). The therapy for serous borderline tumors is more controversial. In women who are menopausal or postmenopausal or have completed their childbearing, the surgical treatment is generally similar to that for serous carcinomas. In young women who have a unilateral tumor with a normal-appearing contralateral ovary and wish to preserve their reproductive capacity a unilateral oophorectomy is usually performed, with careful follow-up examination and the option of a hysterectomy with residual salpingo-oophorectomy after the patient has completed her childbearing. In such cases a similar tumor develops in the contralateral conserved ovary in 10 to 15 percent of the cases (50,71). In cases in which unilateral or bilateral oophorectomy would sterilize a young patient, unilateral or bilateral cystectomy has been performed successfully in a number of cases, with recurrences in the residual ovarian tissue in 12 percent of the cases (50). Persistent or recurrent tumor in the ovary subjected to cystectomy was encountered in one series only when more than one cyst was removed or the resection margin of the cyst was positive for tumor (50). Postoperative management of stages II, III, and IV borderline neoplasia has varied from no therapy to various forms of chemotherapy and radiation therapy. There is no clear evidence in the literature that such treatment alters the course of the disease (42b,51,56), and both radiation therapy and chemotherapy can be associated with both morbidity (32) and a mortality that may be higher than that associated with untreated tumor (46). Several investigators have found that noninvasive implants on the peritoneum, whether predominantly epithelial or desmoplastic, are associated with an excellent prognosis in contrast to the poor prognosis accompanying implants that are invasive of underlying tissue (21,26,53,61). These findings suggest that only patients with invasive implants should receive additional therapy. One of the above groups of investigators (21) found severe nuclear atypia within implants to be a significant adverse prognostic feature, but a far less powerful predictor of a poor outcome than invasion. Other pathologists have placed greater emphasis on the cytologic features of the implants (51) or their DNA ploidy (26,58) than on the presence or absence of invasion to divide the patients into good-prognosis and poor-prognosis groups. Additional investigations of implants are desirable to confirm the impact of their various features on prognosis.

Although only about 40 patients with serous borderline tumors with microinvasion of the stroma have been followed for 2 or more years, the results suggest that these tumors are associated with a prognosis similar to that of tumors lacking microinvasive foci (20,42b,57a,70). For that reason, the former tumors should not be designated "microinvasive carcinoma." The prognostic significance of lymph node involvement in cases of serous borderline neoplasia is still unclear. Although few patients with this complication have been followed for many years, several reports in the literature (27,49,60,68) and our limited experience to date have not demonstrated any effect on survival.

According to the 1991 annual report of the International Federation of Gynecology and Obstetrics (FIGO) (59), the 5-year survival figures for patients with stages I, II, and III serous borderline tumors are between 90 and 95 percent although the previous annual report and most other sources report a much lower 5-year survival figure (approximately 70 percent) for patients with stage III tumors (56). Barnhill et al. (16) have reported a survival rate of over 99 percent for patients with stage I serous borderline tumors based on a review of many recent series in the literature. Patients with spread beyond the ovary may die of their disease after more than 10 years of follow-up examination (14,39). In one large study (14) the survival rate dropped from 97 to 76 percent in the follow-up interval between 5 and 20 years. Kaern et al. (40) have demonstrated a significantly poorer prognosis associated with aneuploid borderline tumors of all types, but no figures for the specific significance of aneuploidy in cases of serous borderline neoplasia were given; analysis of those authors' data suggests that their results apply predominantly to mucinous borderline tumors. Also, Harlow et al. (36) were unable to duplicate the results of that study in a smaller series of cases. FIGO 5-year survival figures for patients with serous carcinoma are: stage I, 76 percent; stage II, 56 percent; stage III, 25 percent; and stage IV, 9 percent (59). Even incidentally detected microscopic serous carcinomas are associated with a guarded prognosis (19). Architectural grading has been shown by one group of investigators to be a strong independent indicator of prognosis (24). Silva, however, found nuclear grading more reliable than architectural grading (64a).

REFERENCES

Surface Epithelial–Stromal Tumors

General References

1. Hendrickson MR. State of the art reviews. Pathology, surface epithelial neoplasms of the ovary. Philadelphia: Hanley & Belfus, 1992.

2. Russell P, Bannatyne P. Surgical pathology of the ovaries. Edinburgh: Churchill Livingstone, 1989.

Specific References

3. Barnhill DR, Kurman RJ, Brady MF, et al. The behavior of stage I ovarian serous tumors of low malignant potential. A Gynecologic Oncology Group Study. Trans Am Gynecol Obstet Soc 1995;12:35–42.
4. Katsube Y, Berg JW, Silverberg SG. Epidemiologic pathology of ovarian tumors: a histopathologic review of primary ovarian neoplasms diagnosed in the Denver standard metropolitan statistical area, 1 July–31 December 1969 and 1 July–31 December 1979. Int J Gynecol Pathol 1982;1:3–16.
5. Koonings PP, Campbell K, Mishell DR Jr, Grimes DA. Relative frequency of primary ovarian neoplasms: a 10-year review. Obstet Gynecol 1989;74:921–6.
6. Nakashima N, Nagasaka T, Fukata S, et al. Study of ovarian tumors treated at Nagoya University Hospital, 1965–1988. Gynecol Oncol 1990;37:103–11.

7. Russell P. Surface epithelial-stromal tumors of the ovary. In: Kurman RJ, ed. Blaustein's pathology of the female genital tract, 4th ed. New York: Springer-Verlag, 1994:705–82.
8. Tateno H, Sasano N. Ovarian tumours in Sendai, Japan. General hospital material. In: Stalsberg H, ed. An international survey of distributions of histologic types of tumours of the testis and ovary. UICC technical report series, vol 75., Geneva: UICC, 1983:291–6.
9. Williams AO, Junaid TA. Ovarian tumours in Nigerian Africans. In: Stalsberg H, ed. An international survey of distributions of histologic types of tumours of the testis and ovary. UICC technical report series, vol 75. Geneva: UICC, 1983:143–6.

Serous Tumors

General References

10. Bell DA, Rutgers JL, Scully RE. Ovarian epithelial tumors of borderline malignancy. In: Damjanov I, Cohen AE, Mills SE, Young RH, eds. Progress in reproductive and urinary tract pathology. New York: Field & Wood Medical Publishers, 1989:1–29.
11. Bell DA, Scully RE. Clinical perspectives on borderline tumors of the ovary. In: Stenchever MA, ed. Current topics in obstetrics and gynecology. New York: Elsevier Science Publishing, 1991:119–34.
12. Hendrickson MR. State of the art reviews. Pathology, surface epithelial neoplasms of the ovary. Philadelphia, Hanley & Belfus, 1992.
13. Russell P, Bannatyne P. Surgical pathology of the ovaries. Edinburgh: Churchill Livingstone, 1989.

Specific References

14. Aure JC, Hoeg K, Kolstad P. Clinical and histologic studies of ovarian carcinoma. Long-term follow-up of 990 cases. Obstet Gynecol 1971;37:1–9.
15. Baergen RN, Rutgers JL. Mural nodules in common epithelial tumors of the ovary. Int J Gynecol Pathol 1994;13:62–72.
16. Barnhill DR, Kurman RJ, Brady MF, et al. The behavior of stage I ovarian serous tumors of low malignant potential. A Gynecologic Oncology Group Study. Trans Am Gynecol Obstet Soc 1995;12:35–42.
17. Bell DA. Flow cytometry of ovarian neoplasms. In: Sasano N, ed. Current topics in pathology. Gynecological tumors, recent progress in diagnostic pathology. Berlin: Springer-Verlag, 1992;337–56.
18. Bell DA. Ovarian serous cystadenoma of borderline malignancy with stromal microinvasion. ASCP Check Sample, Anatomic Pathology AP92-1 1992;215:1–4.

19. Bell DA, Scully RE. Early de novo ovarian carcinoma: a study of fourteen cases. Cancer 1994;73:1859–64.
20. Bell DA, Scully RE. Ovarian serous borderline tumors with stromal microinvasion: a report of 21 cases. Hum Pathol 1990;21:397–403.
21. Bell DA, Weinstock MA, Scully RE. Peritoneal implants of ovarian serous borderline tumors. Histologic features and prognosis. Cancer 1988;62:2212–22.
22. Bollinger DJ, Wick MR, Dehner LP, Mills SE, Swanson PE, Clarke RE. Peritoneal malignant mesothelioma vs. serous papillary adenocarcinoma. A histochemical and immunohistochemical comparison. Am J Surg Pathol 1989;659–70.
23. Burks RT, Sherman ME, Kurman RJ. Micropapillary serous carcinoma of the ovary. A distinctive low-grade carcinoma related to serous borderline tumors. Am J Surg Pathol 1996;20:319–30.

24. Carey MS, Dembo AJ, Simm JE, Fyles AW, Treger T, Bush RS. Testing the validity of a prognostic classification in patients with surgically optimal ovarian carcinoma: a 15-year review. Int J Gynecol Cancer 1993;24–35.

25. Chaubert P, Hurlimann J. Mammary origin of metastases. Immunohistochemical determination. Arch Pathol Lab Med 1992;116:1181–8.

25a. Clement PB, Young RH, Oliva E, Summer HW, Scully RE. Hyperplastic mesothelial cells within abdominal lymph nodes: mimic of metastatic ovarian carcinoma and serous borderline tumor—a report of two cases associated with ovarian neoplasms. Mod Pathol 1996;9:879–86.

26. deNictolis M, Montironi R, Tommasoni S, et al. Serous borderline tumors of the ovary. A clinicopathologic, immunohistochemical, and quantitative study of 44 cases. Cancer 1992;70:152–60.

27. DiRe F, Paladini D, Fontanelli R, Feudale EA, Raspagliesi F. Surgical staging for epithelial ovarian tumors of low malignant potential. Int J Gynecol Cancer 1994;4:310–4.

28. Ehrmann RL, Federschneider JM, Knapp RC. Distinguishing lymph node metastases from benign glandular inclusions in low-grade ovarian carcinoma. Am J Obstet Gynecol 1980;136:737–46.

29. Esteban JE, Yokota S, Husain S, Battifora H. Immunocytochemical profile of benign and carcinomatous effusions. A practical approach to difficult diagnosis. Am J Clin Pathol 1990;94:698–705.

30. Gadducci A, Ferdeghini M, Prontera C, et al. The concomitant determination of different tumor markers in patients with epithelial ovarian cancer and benign ovarian masses: relevance for differential diagnosis. Gynecol Oncol 1992;44:147–54.

31. Gaffey MJ, Mills SE, Swanson PE, Zarbo RJ, Shah AR, Wick MR. Immunoreactivity for BER-EP4 in adenocarcinomas, adenomatoid tumors, and malignant mesotheliomas. Am J Surg Pathol 1992;16:593–9.

32. Gershenson DM, Silva EG. Serous ovarian tumor of low malignant potential with peritoneal implants. Cancer 1990;65:578–85.

33. Gilks CB, Bell DA, Scully RE. Serous psammocarcinoma of the ovary and peritoneum. Int J Gynecol Pathol 1990;9:110–21.

34. Goldberg GL, Scheiner J, Friedman A, O'Hanlan KA, Davidson SA, Runowicz CD. Lymph node sampling in patients with epithelial ovarian carcinoma. Gynecol Oncol 1992;47:143–5.

35. Hanselaar AG, Vooijs GP, Mayall B, Ras-Zeijlmans GJ, Chadha-Ajwani S. Epithelial markers to detect occult microinvasion in serous ovarian tumors. Int J Gynecol Pathol 1993;12:20–7.

36. Harlow BL, Fuhr JE, McDonald TW, Schwartz SM, Beuerlein FJ, Weiss NS. Flow cytometry as a prognostic indicator in women with borderline epithelial ovarian tumors. Gynecol Oncol 1993;50:305–9.

37. Hughesdon P. Benign endometrioid tumours of the ovary and the mullerian concept of ovarian epithelial tumours. Histopathology 1984;8:977–90.

38. Isarangkul W. Ovarian epithelial tumors in Thai women: a histological analysis of 291 cases. Gynecol Oncol 1984;17:326–39.

39. Kaern J, Tropé CG, Abeler VM. A retrospective study of 370 borderline tumors of the ovary treated at the Norwegian Radium Hospital from 1970 to 1982. Cancer 1993;71:1810–20.

40. Kaern J, Tropé CG, Kristensen GB, Abeler VM, Pettersen EO. DNA ploidy: the most important prognostic factor in patients with borderline tumors of the ovary. Int J Gynecol Oncol 1993;3:349–58.

41. Karp LA, Czernobilsky B. Glandular inclusions in pelvic and abdominal para-aortic lymph nodes. Am J Clin Pathol 1969;52:212–8.

41a. Kadar N, Krumerman M. Possible metaplastic origin of lymph node "metastases" in serous ovarian tumor of low malignant potential (borderline serous tumor). Gynecol Oncol 1995;59:394–7.

42. Katsube Y, Berg JW, Silverberg SG. Epidemiologic pathology of ovarian tumors: a histopathologic review of primary ovarian neoplasms diagnosed in the Denver standard metropolitan statistical area, 1 July–31 December 1969 and 1 July–31 December 1979. Int J Gynecol Pathol 1982;1:3–16.

42a. Katzenstein AL, Mazur MT, Morgan TE, Kao MS. Proliferative serous tumors of the ovary. Am J Surg Pathol 1978;2:339–55.

42b. Kennedy AW, Hart WR. Ovarian papillary serous tumors of low malignant potential (serous borderline tumors). A long-term follow-up study, including patients with microinvasion, lymph node metastasis, and transformation to invasive serous carcinoma. Cancer 1996;78:278–86.

43. Khoury N, Raju U, Crissman JD, Zarbo RJ, Greenawald KA. A comparative immunohistochemical study of peritoneal and ovarian serous tumors, and mesotheliomas. Hum Pathol 1990;21:811–9.

44. Koonings PP, Campbell K, Mishell DR Jr, Grimes DA. Relative frequency of primary ovarian neoplasms: a 10-year review. Obstet Gynecol 1989;74:921–6.

45. Kupryjanczyk J, Thor AD, Beauchamp R, Polemba C, Scully RE, Yandell DW. Ovarian, peritoneal and endometrial serous carcinoma: p53 analysis supports a clonal origin of multifocal disease. Mod Pathol 1996;9:166–73.

46. Kurman RJ, Trimble CL. The behavior of serous tumors of low malignant potential: are they ever malignant? Int J Gynecol Pathol 1993;12:120–7.

47. Lage JM, Weinberg DS, Huettner PC, Mark SD. Flow cytometric analysis of nuclear DNA content in ovarian tumors. Association of ploidy with tumor type, histologic grade, and clinical stage. Cancer 1992;69:2668–75.

48. Leake J, Woolas RP, Daniel J, Oram DH, Brown CL. Immunocytochemical and serological expression of CA 125: a clinicopathological study of 40 malignant ovarian epithelial tumours. Histopathology 1994;24:57–64.

49. Leake JF, Rader JS, Woodruff JD, Rosenshein NB. Retroperitoneal lymphatic involvement with epithelial ovarian tumors of low malignant potential. Gynecol Oncol 1991;42:124–30.

50. Lim-Tan SK, Cajigas HE, Scully RE. Ovarian cystectomy for serous borderline tumors: a follow-up study of 35 cases. Obstet Gynecol 1988;72:775–81.

51. Longacre TA, Kempson RL, Hendrickson MR. Well-differentiated serous neoplasms of the ovary. In: State of the art reviews. Pathology, surface epithelial neoplasms of the ovary. Philadelphia: Hanley & Belfus, 1992;1:255–306.

52. Loy TS, Quesenberry JT, Sharp SC. Distribution of CA 125 in adenocarcinomas. An immunohistochemical study of 481 cases. Am J Clin Pathol 1992;98:175–9.

53. McCaughey WT, Kirk ME, Lester W, Dardick I. Peritoneal epithelial lesions associated with proliferative serous tumours of ovary. Histopathology 1984;8:195–208.

54. Mitchell DG, Hill MC, Hill S, Zaloudek C. Serous carcinoma of the ovary: CT identification of metastatic calcified implants. Radiology 1986;158:649–52.

55. Monteagudo C, Merino MJ, LaPorte N, Neumann RD. Value of gross cystic disease fluid protein-15 in distinguishing metastatic breast carcinoma among poorly differentiated neoplasms involving the ovary. Hum Pathol 1991;22:368–72.

56. Morrow CP. Malignant and borderline epithelial tumors of ovary: clinical features, staging, diagnosis, intraoperative assessment and review of management. In: Coppleson M, ed. Gynecologic oncology, vol 2, 2nd ed. Edinburgh: Churchill Livingstone, 1992:889–915.

57. Nakashima N, Nagasaka T, Fukata S, et al. Study of ovarian tumors treated at Nagoya University Hospital, 1965-1988. Gynecol Oncol 1990;37:103–11.

57a. Nayar R, Siriaunkgul S, Robbins KM, McGowan L, Ginzan S, Silverberg SG. Microinvasion in low malignant potential tumors of the ovary. Hum Pathol 1996;27:521–7.

58. Padberg BC, Stegner HE, von Sengbusch S, Arps H, Schröder S. DNA-cytophotometry and immunohistochemistry in ovarian tumours of borderline malignancy and related peritoneal lesions. Virchows Arch [A] 1992;421:497–503.

59. Pettersson F. Annual report of the results of treatment in gynecological cancer. Stockholm, International Federation of Gynecology and Obstetrics, 1991.

60. Rice LW, Berkowitz RS, Mark SD, Yavner DL, Lage JM. Epithelial ovarian tumors of borderline malignancy. Gynecol Oncol 1990;39:195–8.

61. Russell P. Borderline epithelial tumours of the ovary: a conceptual dilemma. Clin Obstet Gynaecol 1984;11:259–77.

62. Russell P. The pathological assessment of ovarian neoplasms. 1: Introduction to the common "epithelial" tumours and analysis of benign "epithelial" tumours. Pathology 1979;11:5–26.

63. Russell P, Bannatyne PM, Solomon HJ, Stoddard LD, Tattersall MH. Multifocal tumorigenesis in the upper female genital tract—implications for staging and management. Int J Gynecol Pathol 1985;4:192–210.

64. Scully RE. Ovary. In: Henson DE, Albores-Saavedra J, eds. The pathology of incipient neoplasia. Philadelphia: WB Saunders, 1986:279–93.

64a. Scully RE, Silva E. Pathology of ovarian cancer. In: Gershenson DM, McGuire WP, eds. Ovarian cancer. Controversies in management. New York: Churchill Livingstone, 1998:425–44.

65. Segal GH, Hart WR. Ovarian serous tumors of low malignant potential (serous borderline tumors). The relationship of exophytic surface tumor to peritoneal "implants." Am J Surg Pathol 1992;16:577–83.

65a. Seidman JD, Kurman RJ. Subclassification of serous borderline tumors of the ovary into benign and malignant types. A clinicopathologic study of 65 advanced stage cases. Am J Surg Pathol 1996;20:1331–45.

66. Sheibani K. Immunopathology of malignant mesothelioma [Editorial]. Hum Pathol 1994;25:219–20.

66a. Silva EG, Kurman RJ, Russell P, Scully RE. Symposium: Ovarian tumors of borderline malignancy. Int J Gynecol Pathol 1996;15:281–302.

67. Sneige N, Fanning CV. Peritoneal washing cytology in women: diagnostic pitfalls and clues for correct diagnosis. Diagn Cytopathol 1992;8:632–40.

68. Tan LK, Flynn SD, Carcangiu ML. Ovarian serous borderline tumors with lymph node involvement. Clinicopathologic and DNA content study of seven cases and review of the literature. Am J Surg Pathol 1994;18:904–12.

69. Tateno H, Sasano N. Ovarian tumours in Sendai, Japan. General hospital material. In: Stalsberg H, ed. An international survey of distribution of histologic types of tumours of the testis and ovary. UICC technical report series, vol 75. Geneva: UICC, 1983:291–6.

70. Tavassoli FA. Serous tumor of low malignant potential with early stromal invasion (serous LMP with microinvasion). Mod Pathol 1988;1:407–14.

71. Tazelaar HD, Bostwick DG, Ballon SC, Hendrickson MR, Kempson RL. Conservative treatment of borderline ovarian tumors. Obstet Gynecol 1985;66:417–22.

72. Tiltman AJ, Sweerts M. Ovarian neoplasms in the Western Cape. S Afr Med J 1982;61:343–5.

73. Ulbright TM, Roth LM, Sutton GP. Papillary serous carcinoma of the ovary with squamous differentiation. Int J Gynecol Pathol 1990;9:86–94.

74. Wick MR, Lillemore TJ, Copland GT, Swanson PE, Manivel JC, Kiang DT. Gross cystic disease fluid protein-15 as a marker for breast cancer: immunohistochemical analysis of 690 human neoplasms and comparison with alpha-lactalbumin. Hum Pathol 1989;20:281–7.

75. Zinsser KR, Wheeler JE. Endosalpingiosis in the omentum: a study of autopsy and surgical material. Am J Surg Pathol 1982;6:109–17.

❖ ❖ ❖

4

MUCINOUS TUMORS AND PSEUDOMYXOMA PERITONEI

MUCINOUS TUMORS

Definition. Mucinous tumors are characterized by glands and cysts lined by epithelial cells, some or all of which contain abundant intracytoplasmic mucin. The neoplastic cells may resemble those of the endocervix, gastric pylorus, or intestine; in occasional tumors only scattered goblet cells, which may be accompanied by other cells of intestinal type, are present in an otherwise nonmucinous lining epithelium. Borderline tumors that are composed predominantly of cells resembling endocervical cells have clinical and pathologic features that differ from those containing intestinal-type cells (page 88).

General Features. Mucinous tumors account for 12 to 15 percent of all ovarian tumors in the western world (28,30,59), 8 percent of ovarian tumors in Uganda (25), and 20 to 23 percent in Japan (36,56), possibly due to a lower prevalence of serous tumors in the latter country. Approximately 75 percent of mucinous tumors are benign; 10 percent, borderline; and 15 percent, carcinomatous (28,30). Mucinous cystadenomas account for 12 percent of benign ovarian tumors, and mucinous carcinomas, for 9 percent of ovarian cancers (30). In most series (28,30,40) mucinous borderline tumors are less common than serous borderline tumors by percents ranging from 20 to over 100, but in Japan (36,56) and Norway (26) the two types of tumor are equally prevalent, and in Thailand, mucinous borderline tumors are more common than serous borderline tumors (24). The variations in the relative frequencies of these tumors may be related to epidemiologic factors or to differences in the criteria used for distinguishing borderline tumors from carcinomas. Mucinous cystadenomas can occur at any age but are diagnosed most often in women in the fourth to sixth decades. Mucinous borderline tumors and carcinomas generally occur in older women, with mean ages of 51 to 52 years for patients with borderline tumors and 53 to 54 for those with carcinomas (49,53). Although rare in the first two decades, benign, borderline, and carcinomatous mucinous tumors are more common during that age period than analogous serous tumors (36,39,56).

Although mucinous metaplasia of the surface epithelium and mucinous epithelial inclusion glands and cysts (fig. 4-1) are rare, mucinous neoplasms are classified as surface epithelial–stromal

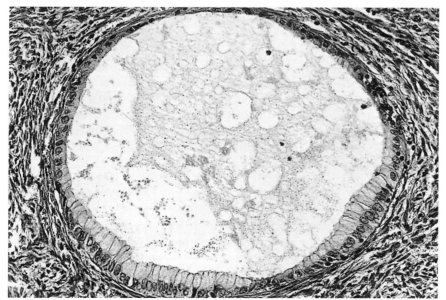

Figure 4-1
SURFACE EPITHELIAL
INCLUSION CYST
The cyst is partly lined by mucinous epithelium. (Fig. 950 from Hertig AT, Mansell H. In: Anderson WA, ed. Pathology, 3rd ed. St.Louis: CV Mosby, 1957.)

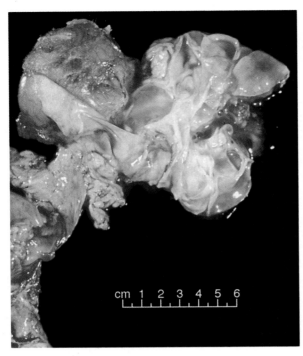

Figure 4-2
MUCINOUS CYSTADENOMA ASSOCIATED
WITH DERMOID CYST
The ovarian tumor has been sectioned. It is attached to the uterus, only part of which is shown.

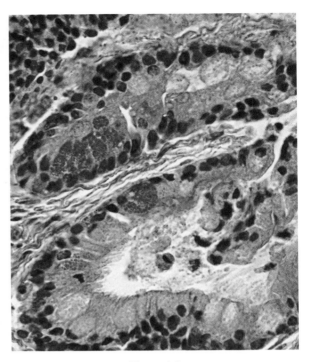

Figure 4-3
MUCINOUS CYSTIC TUMOR
The epithelial lining contains Paneth cells with eosinophilic cytoplasmic granules.

tumors because transitions have been observed between them and serous and endometrioid tumors, both of which belong in that category. Evidence exists, however, that some mucinous tumors may be of germ cell derivation. Mucinous glands and cysts are common constituents of teratomas, and 3 to 5 percent of mucinous tumors develop in association with dermoid cysts (fig. 4-2) (3,8,45), a more frequent association than exists with other surface epithelial–stromal tumors. Also, many mucinous tumors contain intestinal-type cells that are recognizable with routine (figs. 4-3, 4-4) or special stains (fig. 4-5) and have immunohistochemical and ultrastructural features that are more characteristic of gastrointestinal and pancreatic than endocervical epithelium (page 86). None of these observations, however, establishes a germ cell origin for all mucinous tumors, since neometaplasia (change from one cell type to another in neoplastic transformation or within a neoplasm) of ovarian surface-epithelial derivatives provides an alternative explanation for

the development of mucinous tumors with gastrointestinal features. This explanation is supported by the occasional observation of a continuous transition from the epithelial lining of an endometriotic cyst through an endocervical-like or pyloric-like epithelium of a mucinous cystic tumor to an intestinal-type lining of the cyst.

The frequent presence within Brenner tumors of mucinous epithelium that resembles ultrastructurally the type that may be encountered in the urinary tract (31), as well as the rare occurrence of Brenner tumors in the walls of mucinous cystic tumors (8), suggests that the urothelial-like cells of a Brenner tumor are a rare source of mucinous neoplasia. The terminology of mixtures of mucinous and Brenner neoplasia is discussed on page 165.

Mucinous ovarian tumors may be associated with mucinous tumors of other organs. The most common of these associations is with mucinous tumors of the appendix, almost always accompanied by pseudomyxoma peritonei. Because of

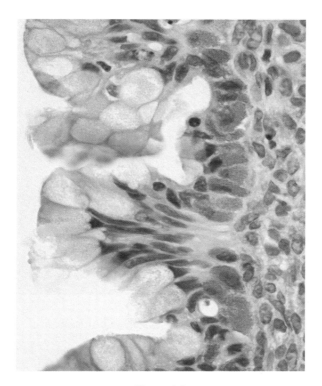

Figure 4-4
MUCINOUS CYSTIC TUMOR
The epithelial lining contains both goblet cells and argentaffin cells with coarse orange-red granules in their basal cytoplasm.

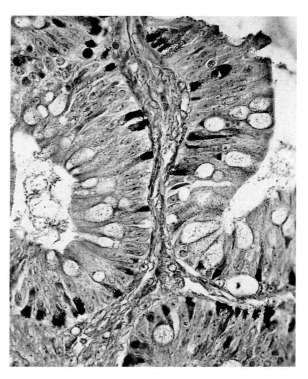

Figure 4-5
MUCINOUS CYSTIC TUMOR
This mucinous cystic tumor has an epithelial lining containing goblet cells and argyrophil cells containing black granules. (Grimelius stain)

controversy regarding the origin of the latter condition (63,77) this association is discussed in detail on page 100.

Mucinous ovarian tumors may be accompanied also by mucinous adenocarcinomas of the cervix, particularly those of the adenoma malignum (minimal deviation adenocarcinoma) type (64). This association may occur in patients with the Peutz-Jeghers syndrome, in whom both tumors appear to be increased in prevalence (page 387). Because of the high degree of differentiation of the tumors at both sites in such cases it may be very difficult or impossible to determine whether the ovarian tumor is an independent primary tumor or a highly differentiated metastatic tumor of cervical origin (page 361).

Mucinous ovarian tumors are among the most common neoplasms in the nonendocrine cell category to be accompanied by hormonal manifestations. The most frequent clinical syndromes are those caused by the secretion of steroid hormones,

which are probably produced predominantly in the stroma within or surrounding the tumor (see chapter 19). Less common manifestations are the Zollinger-Ellison syndrome, caused by gastrin production by neuroendocrine cells in the lining epithelium of the cysts (page 381), and very rarely, the carcinoid syndrome (page 291).

CA125 is elevated in 35 to 67 percent of cases of mucinous carcinoma (17,32,58), carcinoembryonic antigen is above normal in 88 percent (58), and carbohydrate antigen (CA19-9) in 83 percent (17). The serum level of inhibin, a hormone normally produced by granulosa cells that inhibits the secretion of follicle-stimulating hormone by the anterior pituitary gland, has been reported to be a tumor marker for primary mucinous borderline tumors and carcinomas (elevated in 89 and 77 percent of the cases, respectively) (22).

Gross Findings. Mucinous neoplasms tend to be the largest of all ovarian tumors. Many of them are 15 to 30 cm in diameter and weigh

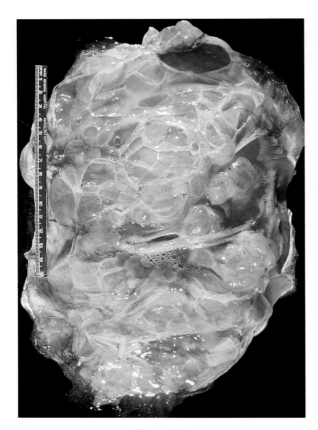

Figure 4-6
MUCINOUS CYSTADENOMA
The sectioned surface reveals numerous thin-walled locules.
(Fig. 32 from Young RH, Clement PB, Scully RE. Pathology
of the ovary. In: Sternberg SS, ed. Diagnostic surgical pa-
thology, Vol 2, 1st ed. New York: Raven Press, 1989:1675.)

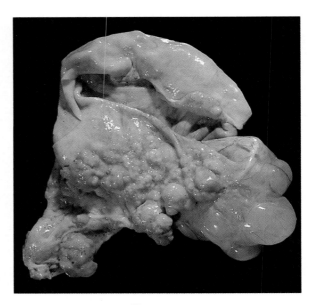

Figure 4-7
MUCINOUS CYSTIC TUMOR OF BORDERLINE
MALIGNANCY, INTESTINAL TYPE
Part of the lining of the large cyst is smooth but most of
it is covered by confluent papillae.

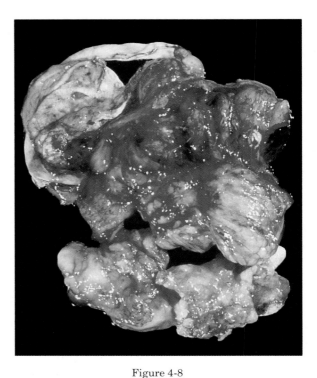

Figure 4-8
MUCINOUS ADENOCARCINOMA
The sectioned surface appears gelatinous, with extensive
hemorrhage and necrosis.

2,000 to 4,000 g. Several huge tumors have been
recorded; the largest documented example was
a mucinous cystadenoma with benign teratomatous components weighing 303 pounds (38). The
mucinous cystadenoma may be unilocular, but
more often has many locules, which typically
have thin walls and contain thick to watery
mucinous fluid (fig. 4-6). Borderline and invasive
mucinous tumors (figs. 4-7–4-9) often contain
papillae and solid areas, which may be soft and
mucoid or firm. Occasional mucinous carcinomas
are predominantly solid. The stromal component
of a mucinous adenofibroma is also solid and
firm. Borderline tumors characterized microscopically by endocervical-like epithelium are
smaller and contain fewer locules than those
lined by intestinal-type epithelium. Necrosis and
hemorrhage are more common in invasive than

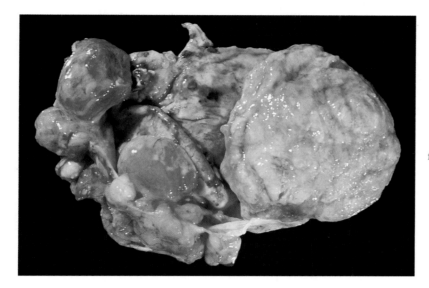

Figure 4-9
MUCINOUS
CYSTADENOCARCINOMA
In addition to cysts the sectioned sur-
face contains a large solid nodule.

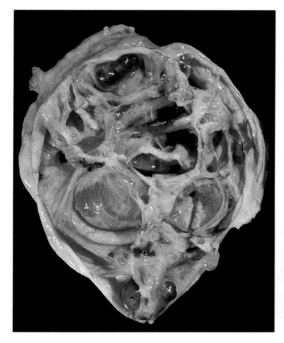
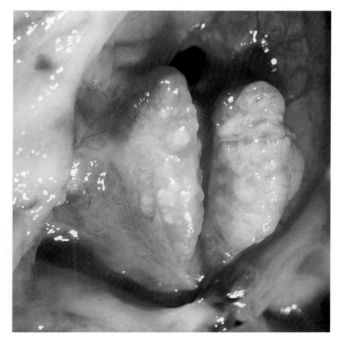

Figure 4-10
MUCINOUS CYSTIC TUMOR WITH BENIGN, BORDERLINE, AND CARCINOMATOUS COMPONENTS
Left: Bisected solid nodule of carcinoma protrudes into a cyst in the lower right portion of the specimen.
Right: Mucinous carcinoma component. (Higher magnification of bisected nodule shown on the left.)

in borderline and benign mucinous tumors but may be seen in the latter tumors, sometimes giving them a deceptively alarming appearance on gross inspection. Borderline or invasive neoplasia may be diffuse within a mucinous tumor, or involve only a small portion of it (fig. 4-10),

and, therefore, the pathologist should examine carefully all portions of the specimen, opening each cyst and sampling the tumor extensively and judiciously for microscopic examination. Optimal sampling of a mucinous borderline tumor with intraepithelial carcinoma to exclude stromal

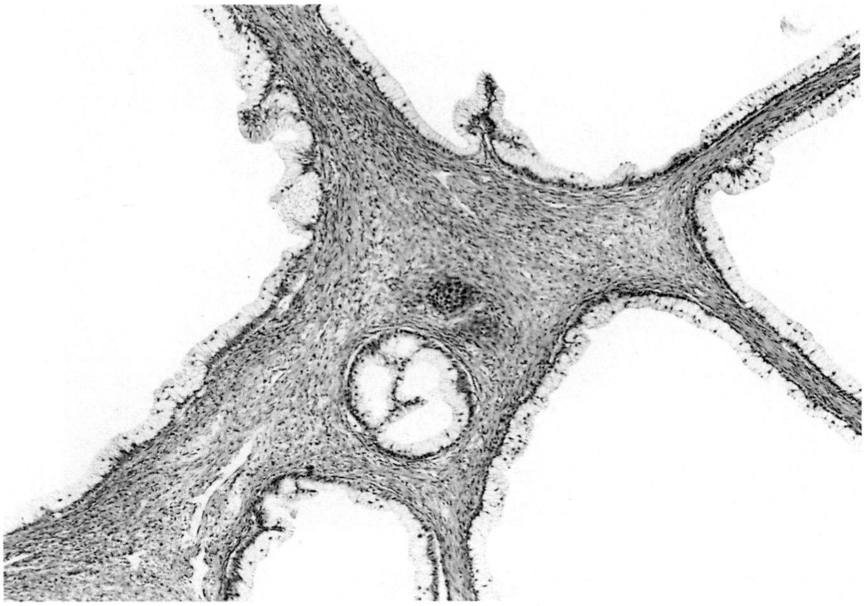

Figure 4-11
MUCINOUS CYSTADENOMA
Multiple locules are lined by "picket-fence" columnar epithelium. The cytoplasm is filled with mucin. (Fig. 17 from Serov SF, Scully RE, Sobin LH. Histological typing of ovarian tumours. International Histological Classification of Tumours No. 9. Geneva: World Health Organization, 1973.)

invasion may require two sections for every centimeter of diameter of the tumor (18). Also, a locule that has ruptured should be sampled and designated separately as its lining may differ from that of other components of the specimen.

The mucinous tumors of the ovary that are present in most cases of pseudomyxoma peritonei (page 99) may have the same gross characteristics as those unassociated with that complication. However, some have a distinctive appearance of one or more thin-walled sacs filled with jelly-like material.

Benign mucinous tumors are bilateral in 2 to 5 percent of cases, borderline tumors in 6 percent of stage I cases, and carcinomas in 7 percent of stage I cases (40). The relatively uncommon endocervical-like mucinous borderline tumors (page 88), however, are bilateral in 40 percent of the cases (48).

Microscopic Findings. *Mucinous Cystadenoma.* This tumor is composed of glands and cysts that occasionally contain papillae with fibrovascular cores. The epithelial lining typically resembles endocervical epithelium at the light microscopic level, consisting of a single row of uniform mucin-filled columnar cells with basal nuclei (figs. 4-11, 4-12). The common finding of goblet cells (figs. 4-13, 4-14), argyrophil cells (fig. 4-5), serotonin-containing cells, and peptide hormone–containing cells, and the less frequent

identification of argentaffin cells (fig. 4-4) and Paneth cells (fig. 4-3) in mucinous tumors, however, attest to the gastrointestinal rather than endocervical nature of the neoplastic cells in at least some cases (50,57). Also, tumors composed of endocervical-like epithelium often express gastric epithelial markers (cathepsin E, periodic acid-concanavalin A, mucin antigen M2) and have an epithelium that is more characteristic of gastric-pyloric than endocervical epithelium on ultrastructural examination (31,57). Rarely, foci of squamous differentiation are seen in mucinous tumors, particularly in those composed predominantly of endocervical-like cells.

The stroma of mucinous cystadenomas usually resembles ovarian stroma but typically contains more collagen; in the rare mucinous adenofibroma (4), the stroma predominates and has an appearance similar to that of a fibroma (fig. 4-15). The stroma of mucinous tumors is occasionally luteinized, particularly during pregnancy (see chapter 19), and often contains irregular spicules of calcification. Bands of smooth muscle may also develop in the stroma, usually parallel to the lining of a large cyst. In 5 percent of mucinous cystadenomas mucin escapes from the glands or cysts to form pools in the stroma, typically eliciting a histiocytic and foreign body giant cell response (45). Occasionally, necrosis with associated inflammation results in a

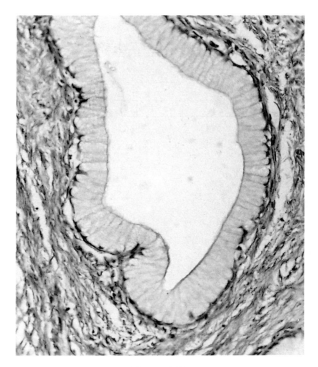

Figure 4-12
MUCINOUS CYSTADENOMA
The cytoplasm is full of mucin and the nuclei are small and basal.

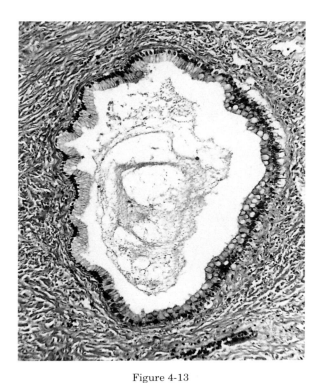

Figure 4-13
MUCINOUS CYSTADENOMA
The small cyst is lined by epithelium, part of which is endocervical-like and part of which (right) is of intestinal type, with goblet cells. (Fig. 5 from Case records of the Massachusetts General Hospital. Case 3-1969. N Eng J Med 1969;280:156–60.)

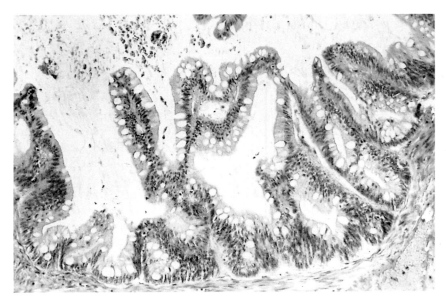

Figure 4-14
MUCINOUS CYSTIC TUMOR OF BORDERLINE MALIGNANCY, INTESTINAL TYPE
The cyst is lined by mucinous epithelium with filiform papillae. Goblet cells and nuclear stratification are evident.

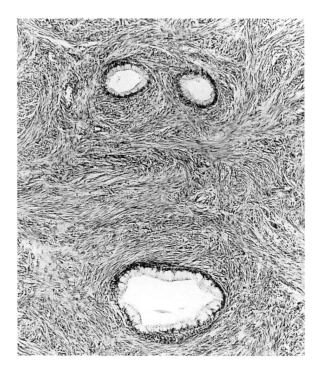

Figure 4-15
MUCINOUS ADENOFIBROMA
The tumor is composed predominantly of fibromatous tissue. (Fig. 21 from Serov SF, Scully RE, Sobin LH. Histological typing of ovarian tumours. International Histological Classification of Tumours No. 9. Geneva: World Health Organization, 1973.)

Table 4-1

**DIFFERENCES BETWEEN
ENDOCERVICAL-LIKE AND
INTESTINAL-TYPE
MUCINOUS BORDERLINE TUMORS***

	EMBT	IMBT
Average age (years)	34	41
Bilaterality (%)	40	6
Diameter (mean cm)	8	19
Multilocularity (%)	20	72
Argyrophil cells (%)	3	91
Acute inflammation (%)	100 (diffuse)	22 (focal)
Endometriosis, either ovary (%)	30	6
Endometriosis, ipsilateral ovary (%)	20	0
Pseudomyxoma peritonei (%)	0	17

*From reference 48.

desmoplastic stromal response, which should not be misinterpreted as the desmoplastic stroma of a carcinoma.

Borderline Tumors and Carcinomas. Most borderline mucinous cystic tumors are characterized by more obvious and extensive intestinalization of their epithelial lining than their benign counterparts, but a minority of these tumors (15 percent in a consultation series [48], 19 percent in a combined consultation and hospital series [51], and 5 percent in a tumor registry series [18]) lack obviously intestinal-type epithelium and have been designated "endocervical-like" or "of mullerian type" (Table 4-1).

Endocervical-like mucinous borderline tumors have an architecture similar to that of serous borderline tumors, with both large, bulbous papillae and smaller papillae with prominent cellular budding. The papillae are lined by slightly to moderately atypical epithelial cells, which may attain a height of over 20 cells (figs. 4-16, 4-17). Most of the neoplastic cells contain abundant cytoplasmic mucin, but some may be mucin-free and contain large amounts of eosinophilic cytoplasm. A diffuse, acute inflammatory infiltrate is almost always present in the stroma, among the neoplastic epithelial cells, and in the luminal mucin (fig. 4-18). This type of mucinous borderline tumor is associated with endometriosis in the ipsilateral ovary, often in continuity, in 20 percent of the cases (48). Intestinal-type mucinous borderline tumors, in contrast, either lack papillae or have branching filiform papillae (fig. 4-14). The cysts and papillae are lined by atypical epithelium that contains variable numbers of goblet cells and other intestinal cell types.

The diagnostic criteria that distinguish mucinous borderline tumors of the intestinal type from mucinous carcinomas are controversial, resulting in considerable confusion in the literature. According to the World Health Organization (WHO) classification, the distinction depends entirely on the demonstration of obvious invasion of the stroma of the tumor in carcinomas, as defined on page 52. Many authors, however, while accepting obvious invasion as a valid criterion for the diagnosis of mucinous carcinoma, do not require its presence; some accept in its absence a criterion

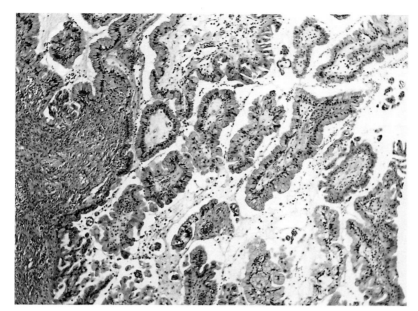

Figure 4-16
MUCINOUS CYSTIC
TUMOR OF
BORDERLINE MALIGNANCY,
ENDOCERVICAL-LIKE

The architecture of the papillae is similar to that seen in a serous borderline tumor. (Fig. 1 from Rutgers JL, Scully RE. Mullerian mucinous papillary cystadenomas of borderline malignancy: a clinicopathological analysis of 30 cases. Cancer 1988;61:340–8.)

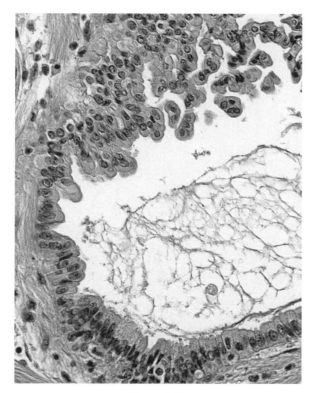

Figure 4-17
MUCINOUS CYSTIC TUMOR OF BORDERLINE
MALIGNANCY, ENDOCERVICAL-LIKE

Stratification with cellular budding is evident. (Fig. 4 from Rutgers JL, Scully RE. Mullerian mucinous papillary cystadenomas of borderline malignancy: a clinicopathological analysis of 30 cases. Cancer 1988;61:340–8.)

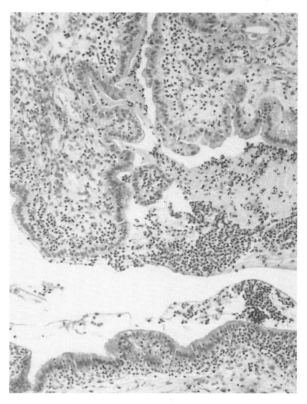

Figure 4-18
MUCINOUS CYSTIC TUMOR OF BORDERLINE
MALIGNANCY, ENDOCERVICAL-LIKE

The stroma of the papillae is diffusely infiltrated with polymorphonuclear leukocytes, which are also present in the lumen of the cyst.

Table 4-2

**DIFFERENTIAL MICROSCOPIC FEATURES OF TWO SUBTYPES OF
INTESTINAL-TYPE MUCINOUS BORDERLINE TUMORS**

	Typical	**With Intraepithelial Carcinoma**
Tumor cells	Atypical nuclear features	Malignant nuclear features
Intracystic growth patterns that may be present	1. No papillarity or Short and blunt to filiform, often branching papillae, which have at least minimal stromal support	1. No papillarity or Stroma-free cellular papillae
	2. Secondary gland formation with at least minimal stromal support and intracytoplasmic mucin in some glandular cells	2. Cribriform (cyst linings thickened by stroma-free bridges of nonmucin-containing tumor cells)
	3. Cellular stratification, usually with 3 or fewer vertical rows of nuclei	3. Cellular stratification, usually with 4 or more vertical rows of nuclei

of Hart and Norris (20) (stratification of the neoplastic cell nuclei to four or greater in thickness) or modifications thereof that place greater emphasis on other architectural findings and carcinomatous nuclear features (Table 4-2) (5,19,23). Resolution of the controversy is best accomplished by maintaining the diagnostic criteria of the WHO and additionally dividing the borderline category of mucinous tumors into typical forms with epithelial atypia (fig. 4-14) and variants with intraepithelial carcinoma (figs. 4-19, 4-20) (page 52). In diagnosing the latter we place greater reliance on the cytologic than the architectural features.

Mucinous carcinomas (i.e., invasive) may contain only endocervical-like cells, only intestinal-type cells, or a combination of the two, but are usually composed of cells that are not specifically suggestive of either endocervical or intestinal-type mucinous cells (figs. 4-21–4-28). Therefore, the distinction between endocervical-like and intestinal-type mucinous carcinomas is not clear-cut in most cases. The occasional carcinomas in the endocervical-like category resemble the endocervical types of mucinous carcinoma that are encountered in the cervix, composed of cells that are uniformly rich in mucin or cells that are stratified with little or no intracytoplasmic mucin (fig. 4-22). The latter cells resemble those of well-differentiated endometrioid adenocarcinoma, but typically are more stratified and have nuclei that are taller and more slender. Some mucinous carcinomas resemble typical adenocarcinomas of

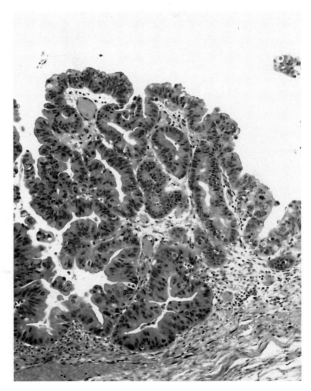

Figure 4-19

MUCINOUS CYSTIC TUMOR OF
BORDERLINE MALIGNANCY WITH
INTRAEPITHELIAL CARCINOMA

Obviously malignant mucinous epithelium, from which most of the mucin has disappeared, lines a portion of a locule in a tumor that had a predominantly benign appearance.

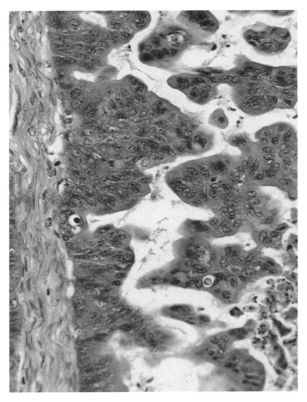

Figure 4-20
MUCINOUS CYSTIC TUMOR OF
BORDERLINE MALIGNANCY WITH
INTRAEPITHELIAL CARCINOMA
The lining of a locule is characterized by stroma-free cellu-
lar papillae and marked nuclear atypia. Most of the locules
were lined by epithelium that was benign or typical borderline.

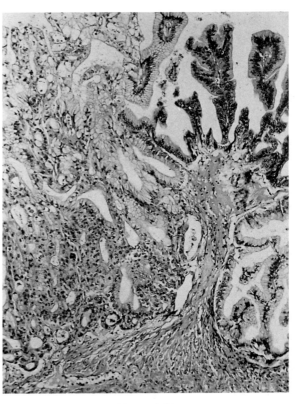

Figure 4-21
MUCINOUS ADENOCARCINOMA
The tumor is well differentiated, with a cribriform pattern.
A villous portion of the tumor in the right upper corner has the
appearance of a borderline tumor.

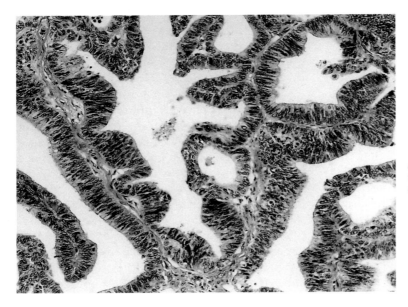

Figure 4-22
MUCINOUS ADENOCARCINOMA
RESEMBLING ENDOMETRIOID
ADENOCARCINOMA
In this area of the tumor almost no intra-
cellular mucin remains in the stratified epi-
thelium, which is characterized by cells with
elongated nuclei.

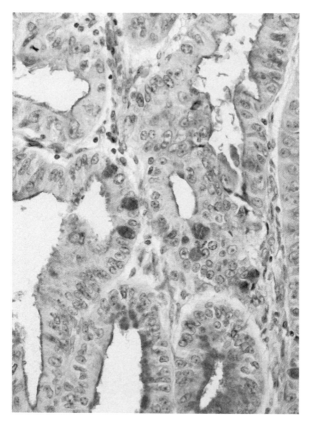

Figure 4-23
MUCINOUS ADENOCARCINOMA
Much of the mucin is apical but several goblet cells
containing red mucin are evident. (Mucicarmine stain)

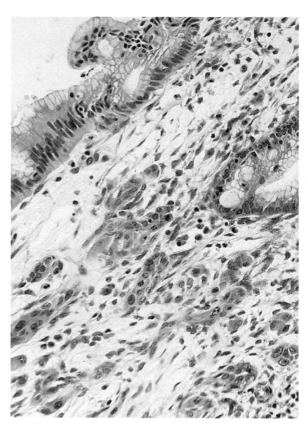

Figure 4-24
MUCINOUS ADENOCARCINOMA
WITH MICROINVASION OF STROMA
This tumor, which appeared mostly benign and borderline, contained foci of intraepithelial carcinoma as well as
this tiny invasive focus composed of irregular small groups
of malignant cells and single similar cells.

the large intestine; such tumors may contain
only occasional goblet cells as evidence of their
intestinal nature (fig. 4-23). Occasionally, a signet-ring cell carcinoma is present focally in a
mucinous adenocarcinoma, supporting the concept of a rare primary Krukenberg tumor of the
ovary. The existence of such a tumor is very
difficult to prove, however, since primary signet-
ring cell carcinomas in other organs may remain
occult for years after metastasizing to the ovary,
requiring long-term (at least 10 years') follow-up
or an exhaustive autopsy to exclude their presence. A small number of mucinous carcinomas of
the ovary resemble colloid carcinoma of the large
intestine (fig. 4-28). Many mucinous carcinomas
contain cysts with or without papillae, which
often contain "dirty" necrotic material; irregular
small glands with jagged margins (fig. 4-25);
solid clusters of mucinous cells; or single mucin-

ous cells in the stroma (fig. 4-26). Rarely, a
mucinous carcinoma belongs in the microinvasive category (fig. 4-24) (36a).

The stroma of mucinous carcinomas may be
desmoplastic, extensively infiltrated by inflammatory cells, or both, or it may resemble ovarian
stroma and contain clusters of lutein cells (see
chapter 19). Borderline and malignant mucinous
tumors are associated with an escape of pools of
mucin from the glands and cysts into the stroma
in 25 and 30 percent of the cases, respectively (46,
47). This process may be focal, with the mucin often
containing histiocytes and occasionally inciting a
foreign body giant cell reaction (fig. 4-29). Dissection of mucin into the stroma is especially common
and extensive in cases of pseudomyxoma peritonei

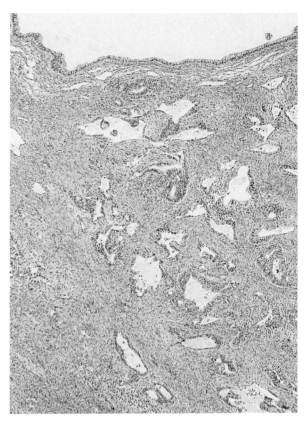

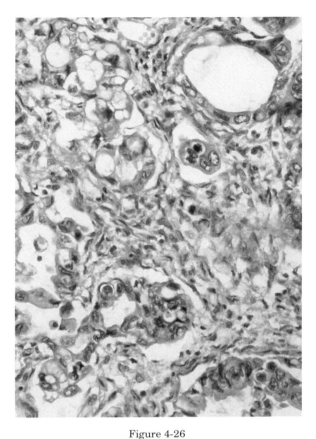

Figure 4-25
MUCINOUS ADENOCARCINOMA
The tumor is characterized by a disorderly arrangement
of cysts and glands of irregular shapes.

Figure 4-26
MUCINOUS ADENOCARCINOMA
The tumor is characterized by invasive small glands and
small collections of signet-ring cells.

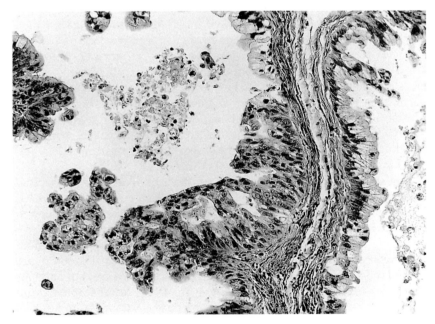

Figure 4-27
MUCINOUS
ADENOCARCINOMA
The cysts are lined by cells, some of
which are highly stratified and some
of which contain abundant mucin. The
nuclei are highly atypical and necrotic
debris is present in the lumens. (Fig. 25
from Serov SF, Scully RE, Sobin LH.
Histological typing of ovarian tumours.
International Histological Classification of Tumours No. 9. Geneva: World
Health Organization, 1973.)

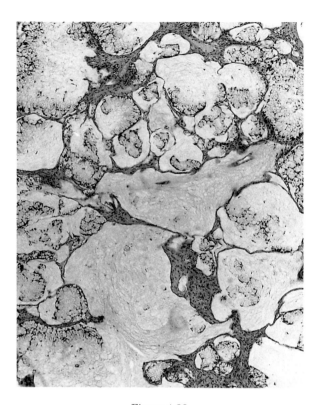

Figure 4-28
MUCINOUS ADENOCARCINOMA
The tumor resembles mucinous (colloid) carcinoma of the intestine.

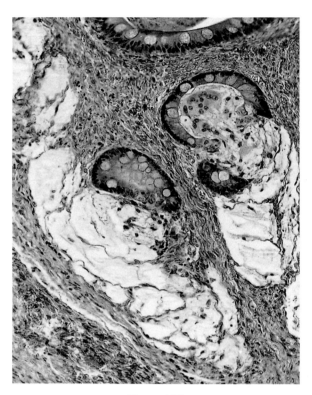

Figure 4-29
MUCINOUS CYSTIC TUMOR OF BORDERLINE
MALIGNANCY, INTESTINAL TYPE
Small cysts have ruptured, with extrusion of mucin into adjacent stroma and an associated inflammatory cell reaction.

and is designated "pseudomyxoma ovarii." In this form of stromal dissection the mucin is typically unassociated with a significant inflammatory cell or foreign body giant cell response and often contains or is partly lined by neoplastic epithelial cells (fig. 4-30). Michael and associates (35) have interpreted ovarian tumors associated with pseudomyxoma ovarii as a form of mucinous carcinoma because of its association in some cases with pseudomyxoma peritonei, but there is no evidence that stage I tumors with that feature have a worse prognosis than stage I mucinous tumors without it. Also, as discussed on page 100, there is controversy whether many of the ovarian tumors with pseudomyxoma ovarii and pseudomyxoma peritonei are metastatic from the appendix or elsewhere in the gastrointestinal tract instead of originating in the ovary.

Rare mucinous carcinomas are admixed with solid carcinomas with neuroendocrine features (15a,15b) (page 321).

Mural Nodules in Mucinous Tumors. An unusual feature of mucinous cystic tumors, which is exceptionally rare in other ovarian tumors (12, 15), is the occurrence of a puzzling, heterogeneous group of mural nodules, which differ markedly in their histologic features from the mucinous tumors themselves (41–43). These nodules have been classified as: 1) anaplastic carcinomas; 2) sarcomas of various types; 3) carcinosarcoma; 4) sarcoma-like nodules; 5) mixed nodules; and 6) leiomyomas (33,37).

Approximately 16 cases of anaplastic-carcinomatous nodules have been reported (1,2,11,21, 37,52). Grossly, one or more nodules are seen in the walls of mucinous cystic tumors, which are mostly borderline or carcinomatous. The nodules vary from 0.5 to 12 cm in diameter, are generally yellow, and often have areas of necrosis and hemorrhage (fig. 4-31). Microscopic examination reveals typically solid sheets or nests of

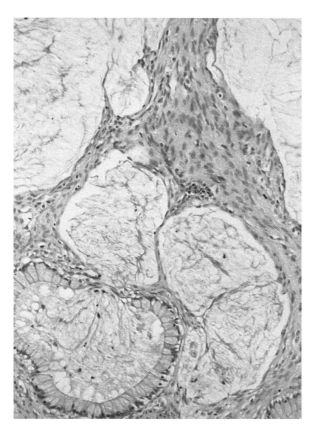

Figure 4-30
MUCINOUS CYSTIC TUMOR WITH
PSEUDOMYXOMA OVARII
Large pools of almost acellular mucin are evident. There
is no inflammatory cell response.

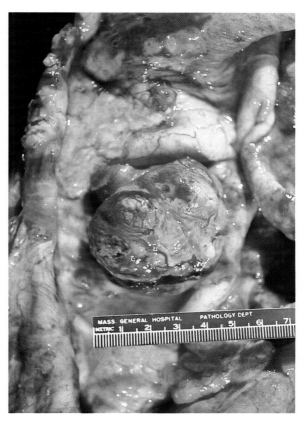

Figure 4-31
ANAPLASTIC CARCINOMA IN
MUCINOUS CYSTIC TUMOR
A nodule of anaplastic carcinoma (center) protrudes into
one of the locules.

large, rounded epithelial cells with poorly differentiated nuclei and often abundant eosinophilic cytoplasm (figs. 4-32, 4-33), poorly differentiated spindle-shaped epithelial cells, or both; occasionally focal glandular differentiation is present. The nodules are typically ill-defined and the tumor cells may invade vessels.

Sarcomas form yellow, pink, or red nodules of various sizes, often with areas of necrosis. Microscopic diagnoses have included fibrosarcoma (6,42), rhabdomyosarcoma (60), and undifferentiated sarcoma (42), all of which tend to be ill-defined and may invade vessels. In addition to discrete nodules, large masses of sarcoma have been reported in association with mucinous cystic tumors (1,2,44). A single case of a carcinosarcomatous nodule in the wall of a mucinous cystadenocarcinoma has been reported (55).

Approximately 16 cases of "sarcoma-like" nodules have been reported in patients with mucinous cystadenomas, borderline cystic tumors, and cystadenocarcinomas. These nodules are 0.6 to 6 cm in diameter, and may be single or multiple and soft or firm; they are usually red-brown or brown. Microscopic examination discloses sharply circumscribed nodules composed typically of varying numbers of pleomorphic cells with bizarre nuclei and atypical mitotic figures (mitotic activity may be as high as 10 per 10 high-power fields), spindle cells, epulis-type giant cells, and acute and chronic inflammatory cells. Hemorrhage and necrosis are common, but vascular invasion is absent (figs. 4-34, 4-35). The pathogenesis and nature of these nodules are unclear although they are considered reactive because of their associated benign clinical course. Perplexing features are focal

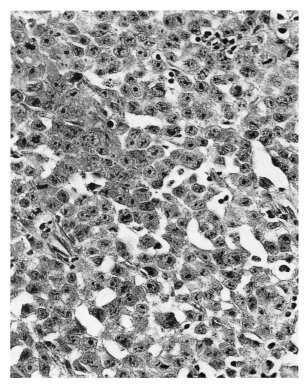

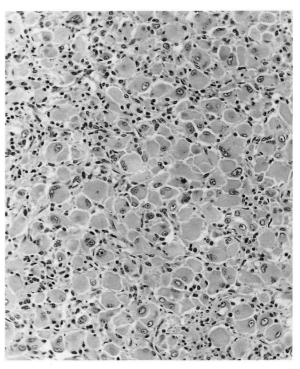

Figure 4-32
ANAPLASTIC CARCINOMA ARISING
IN MUCINOUS CYSTIC TUMOR

The tumor is characterized by a diffuse arrangement of
uniform cells with moderate amounts of cytoplasm and
malignant-appearing nuclei with prominent nucleoli.

Figure 4-33
ANAPLASTIC CARCINOMA ARISING
IN MUCINOUS CYSTIC TUMOR

The tumor is characterized by a diffuse arrangement of cells
with abundant (eosinophilic) cytoplasm and malignant-appearing nuclei. Many nucleoli are prominent.

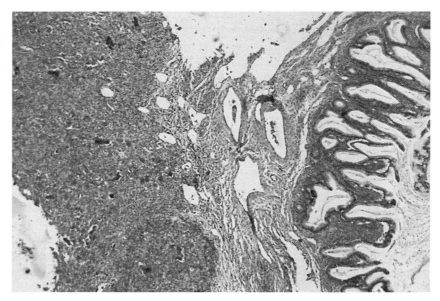

Figure 4-34
SARCOMA-LIKE NODULE
IN WALL OF MUCINOUS
CYSTIC TUMOR OF
BORDERLINE MALIGNANCY

The cellular nodule is well demarcated.

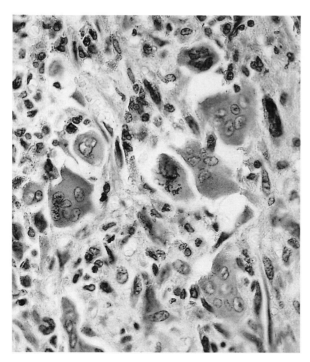

Figure 4-35
SARCOMA-LIKE NODULE IN WALL
OF MUCINOUS CYSTIC TUMOR

The cells of the nodule include osteoclast-like giant cells and smaller mononuclear cells. An atypical mitotic figure is present in the center. (Fig. 5 from Prat J, Scully RE. Ovarian mucinous tumors with sarcoma-like mural nodules: a report of seven cases. Cancer 1979;44:1332–44.)

staining of the pleomorphic cells for cytokeratin (34) and the occasional finding of adenocarcinoma or anaplastic carcinoma within the nodule (mixed nodule) (16,29).

Usually, examination of routine sections enables one to differentiate among the several types of nodules; immunohistochemical staining may be helpful in difficult cases (37). Strong and extensive staining for cytokeratin warrants a diagnosis of carcinoma; weak or focal staining for this antigen in occasional cases of sarcoma-like nodules is difficult to interpret but does not, in itself, indicate a carcinomatous component. Diffuse vimentin staining is not helpful in distinguishing the heterogeneous sarcoma-like nodules from the more homogeneous sarcoma. Immunohistochemical investigation of more cases, in addition to longer follow-up data, will be necessary to differentiate clearly among these various types of mural nodules.

Differential Diagnosis. The differentiation of mucinous carcinomas from serous and endometrioid carcinomas with abundant luminal mucin depends on the presence of at least occasional goblet cells with mucin-rich cytoplasm in the former tumors in contrast to an absence of more than minimal cytoplasmic accumulation in most of the cells in the latter two tumors. Very small foci of benign-appearing endocervical-type epithelium may be seen, however, in endometrioid carcinomas. Vimentin staining of serous and endometrioid carcinomas may prove helpful in distinguishing them from the typically negative mucinous adenocarcinomas (13,61); also, cytoplasmic staining for carcinoembryonic antigen (CEA) favors strongly a mucinous carcinoma (13).

Most heterologous Sertoli-Leydig cell tumors contain glands and cysts lined by mucinous epithelium, which may have benign, borderline, or occasionally, carcinomatous features (page 213). In some cases the mucinous element is the predominant component and the tumor is grossly indistinguishable from a mucinous cystic tumor. Careful microscopic examination, however, reveals foci of typical Sertoli-Leydig cell tumor, usually of the intermediate type. Differentiation of mucinous cystic tumors from mucinous carcinoid tumors is discussed on page 299.

The most difficult problem in the differential diagnosis of mucinous carcinomas of the ovary is their distinction from metastatic adenocarcinomas from the gastrointestinal tract, biliary tract, pancreas, and uterine cervix. These differential diagnoses are discussed in chapter 18.

Frozen Section. The pathologist should be careful not to overdiagnose a benign mucinous tumor as borderline or a borderline tumor as carcinoma on frozen section examination, particularly in a young woman who wishes to preserve her reproductive capacity. The surgeon should also be aware that the more extensive microscopic sampling that is done postoperatively may disclose a tumor with a more malignant component than that identified on frozen section examination. Finally, any ovarian mucinous tumor, particularly if it is malignant or bilateral, or in an older woman, should raise the possibility of metastatic mucinous adenocarcinoma, and a history of a primary mucinous carcinoma elsewhere should be sought; if the history is negative, the abdomen should be explored for a possible source of metastasis.

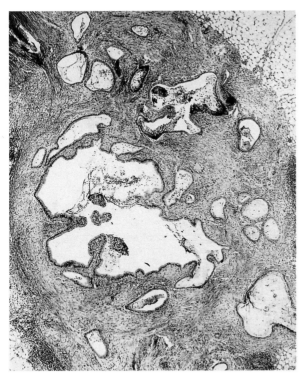

Figure 4-36
OMENTAL IMPLANT OF MUCINOUS BORDERLINE
TUMOR OF ENDOCERVICAL-LIKE TYPE

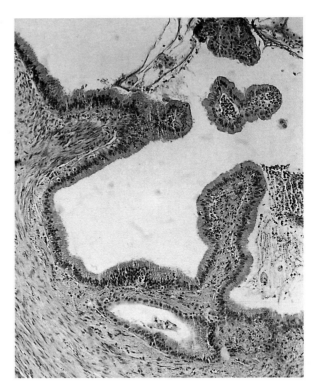

Figure 4-37
OMENTAL IMPLANT OF MUCINOUS BORDERLINE
TUMOR OF ENDOCERVICAL-LIKE TYPE
The epithelial lining of the cysts and their papillae is well differentiated.

Spread and Metastasis. According to the International Federation of Gynecology and Obstetrics (FIGO) annual report, mucinous borderline tumors are confined to one or both ovaries in 82 percent of the cases, are stage II in 6 percent, stage III in 10 percent, and stage IV in 2 percent (40). The parallel figures for mucinous carcinoma are 49, 11, 29, and 10 percent of the cases. Almost all so-called stage II and stage III mucinous borderline tumors of intestinal type, however, have spread in the form of pseudomyxoma peritonei, and, as mentioned earlier, many of these tumors may be secondary to mucinous tumors of the appendix or another intestinal site instead of primary in the ovary (page 99). Isolated implants on the peritoneum are rare in cases of intestinal-type mucinous borderline tumors but have been reported in 23 percent of the cases of endocervical-like mucinous borderline tumors (figs. 4-36, 4-37) (48).

Treatment. Stage I mucinous borderline tumors are generally treated like serous borderline tumors (page 76). Except in cases of endocervical-like mucinous borderline tumors, which are bilateral in approximately 40 percent of the cases, there is relatively little concern about performing only a unilateral oophorectomy in a young woman with a mucinous borderline tumor since less than 10 percent of the intestinal-type tumors are bilateral. If the contralateral normal-appearing ovary is conserved, however, the patient should be followed carefully for many years because of the possible development of a similar tumor in it. The treatment of pseudomyxoma peritonei consists mainly of removal of as much tumor as technically feasible and attempts to relieve symptoms by withdrawal of abdominal fluid. Such treatment has generally been unsatisfactory from the viewpoint of cure. Mucinous carcinomas are managed as outlined in the general section on therapy of ovarian carcinomas (page 39).

Prognosis. According to the FIGO annual report the 5-year survival rate for patients with stage I mucinous borderline tumors is 92 percent; stage II, 100 percent; and stage III, 51 percent (40). The parallel figures for mucinous carcinomas are 83 percent, 55 percent, and 21 percent, and for stage IV tumors, 9 percent. The survival rate of patients with mucinous borderline tumors (all stages) drops from approximately 95 to 87 percent if the follow-up period extends to 15 years because of late recurrences according to Kaern et al. (26). If cases with pseudomyxoma peritonei and appendiceal tumors are excluded from the ovarian borderline category, however, an analysis of those authors' data shows that a smaller portion of their patients died during the 15-year follow-up period. Kaern and associates (27) concluded that ploidy is an important prognostic factor, but the extent to which it is significant is difficult to ascertain from their publication because their survival statistics refer to borderline tumors of all cell types as a group and include cases of mucinous borderline tumors with pseudomyxoma peritonei and synchronous appendiceal mucinous tumors.

It is difficult to determine from the literature whether intestinal-type borderline tumors with intraepithelial carcinoma are associated with a worse prognosis than those with epithelial atypia. An analysis of a literature review (51) that lists series of stage I mucinous borderline tumors in which follow-up information was available, reveals an almost identical survival rate in seven series in which tumors with intraepithelial carcinoma were included in the borderline category and seven other series in which such tumors were excluded. Also, some authors who have specifically addressed in their studies the prognostic differences among borderline mucinous tumors with epithelial atypia, those with intraepithelial carcinoma, and (invasive) mucinous carcinomas have found either presentation at a higher stage (10,62) or decreasing survival in stage I cases (10,20,54) with increasing extent of malignancy, while others (14,18,51) have not. Differences in microscopic interpretation, the extent of sampling of the tumors, and the interpretation of the origin of pseudomyxoma peritonei in the above series of cases probably account for some of these disparate results. Architectural grading of mucinous carcinomas has been demonstrated by some authors to have independent prognostic significance (7).

Despite the presence of extraovarian spread in the form of discrete peritoneal implants or lymph node metastasis in almost a quarter of the cases of endocervical-like mucinous borderline tumors, no deaths of patients with these tumors have been recorded as yet. Long-term follow-up data are not available in a large number of cases, however (48).

No patients with sarcoma-like mural nodules have been reported to have a malignant clinical course, and the seven patients with those lesions who had been followed for 5 or more years were alive and free of tumor. In contrast, most patients with mural nodules of anaplastic carcinoma have had a malignant, often rapid course. Too few cases of sarcomatous nodules have been published to warrant a conclusion regarding their prognosis.

PSEUDOMYXOMA PERITONEI

Pseudomyxoma peritonei, the presence of masses of jelly-like mucus in the pelvis, and in many cases, the upper abdomen as well, has been reported as an occasional complication of mucinous tumors involving the ovary. In such cases the disease has been interpreted as stage II or III ovarian borderline tumor or carcinoma in most reported studies. There is widespread disagreement in the recent literature, however, whether that interpretation is warranted. The major questions regarding the relation of mucinous ovarian tumors to pseudomyxoma peritonei are listed in Table 4-3.

It is impossible to ascertain with certainty from the literature how many cases of mucinous cystic tumors of the ovary accompanied by pseudomyxoma peritonei are associated with appendiceal tumors because in many cases the appendix has not been removed for microscopic examination or even visualized at operation. In six recent series of cases of pseudomyxoma peritonei in which cystic ovarian tumors were characterized microscopically and the microscopic findings in the appendix were also recorded (Table 4-4), 25 of the 37 ovarian tumors were interpreted as borderline and in 15 of the 25 cases some type of mucinous lesion was found in the appendix. The appendiceal lesions were characterized as benign in 12 of the ovarian "borderline" cases. Although no statement about the extent of microscopic sampling of the appendix

Table 4-3

QUESTIONS IN CASES OF "PSEUDOMYXOMA PERITONEI" ASSOCIATED WITH CYSTIC OVARIAN TUMORS

1. How often is an ovarian tumor an isolated primary tumor in cases of pseudomyxoma peritonei?

2. If an ovarian tumor is judged to be primary after a careful microscopic examination of the appendix is negative, is it benign, borderline, or malignant?

3. If an appendiceal tumor is also found, is it benign, borderline, or malignant?

4. If tumors of both organs are present are they independent primary tumors or is the ovarian tumor metastatic from the appendix?

5. Is the peritoneal tumor metastatic from the ovary, appendix, or both, or independently primary?

6. What are the features of the intra-abdominal mucin (free; superficial, organizing; dissecting with fibrosis) (cell-free; with benign-appearing cells; with atypical cells; with carcinoma cells)?

Table 4-4

MICROSCOPIC FEATURES OF MUCINOUS CYSTIC OVARIAN TUMORS AND APPENDIX IN PSEUDOMYXOMA PERITONEI

Reference	Ovary	Appendix
Kaern (71)	16 borderline	9 benign 7 normal
Costa (68)	3 borderline	1 borderline 2 normal
Prayson (74)	3 borderline	2 benign 1 carcinoma
	1 benign	1 benign
Kahn (72)	3 borderline	1 benign 1 carcinoma 1 normal
	2 benign	2 benign
Ronnett (75)	3 benign 2 carcinoma	3 benign 2 benign
Michael (73)	4 carcinoma	3 benign 1 normal
	37 cystic tumors	26 mucinous lesions 11 normal
	25 borderline tumors	15 mucinous lesions 10 normal

was made in the normal-appendix cases, raising the possibility that small mucinous lesions were overlooked because of inadequate sampling, it appears highly probable from these studies that at least some cases of pseudomyxoma peritonei are secondary to a primary ovarian mucinous cystic tumor. One has to assume also the possibility in the normal-appendix cases that the ovarian tumor interpreted as borderline was not a well-differentiated metastatic tumor originating elsewhere in the gastrointestinal tract or at another site (75).

The terms used for appendiceal and ovarian tumors associated with pseudomyxoma peritonei have varied considerably from one author to another (66,70,77,79). The appendiceal lesions have been designated as benign (mucocele, adenoma, cystadenoma, villous adenoma), borderline, and carcinoma; some authors have used terms such as "moderately atypical villous adenoma" and "severely atypical villous adenoma." The ovarian tumors associated with pseudomyxoma peritonei have been designated mostly as borderline but occasionally as benign or carcinoma. Different diagnostic criteria and variations in the extent of sampling of both the appendiceal and ovarian tumors probably account for this terminologic confusion.

When mucinous lesions of both the ovary and the appendix are present there is disagreement whether they are independently primary or whether the ovarian tumor is metastatic from the appendix. Arguments advanced for the independent primary nature of the ovarian tumor are: 1) reports of a normal appendix or an unruptured mucinous lesion of the appendix in some cases of pseudomyxoma peritonei associated with ovarian mucinous tumors; 2) differences in the observed degree of malignancy of the appendiceal and ovarian tumors on microscopic examination; 3) immunohistochemical differences between the two tumors in many cases; and 4) reports of the occasional coexistence of ovarian and appendiceal mucinous tumors in the absence of peritoneal involvement (72,77,78).

Arguments supporting the spread of a primary appendiceal tumor to the ovary and peritoneum in cases of pseudomyxoma peritonei are: 1) the common finding of an appendiceal tumor in association with ovarian mucinous tumors in cases of pseudomyxoma peritonei in which the appendix has been investigated microscopically in contrast to its far lower frequency in the absence of peritoneal involvement; 2) the usual histologic similarity of the appendiceal and ovarian tumors that is evident when both are adequately sampled; 3) the much higher frequency of bilaterality of ovarian mucinous tumors in the presence of appendiceal and peritoneal involvement than in its absence, correlating with the much greater frequency of bilaterality of metastatic than primary mucinous tumors in general; 4) the higher frequency of involvement of the right ovary when the ovarian tumor is unilateral in cases of appendiceal and peritoneal involvement (in contrast to a similar frequency of involvement of both ovaries in its absence); and 5) differences in the microscopic appearance of mucinous ovarian tumors in the presence of appendiceal and peritoneal involvement and in its absence (specifically, the common finding of unusually tall mucinous epithelium and extensive pseudomyxoma ovarii in the former and their usual absence in the latter) (74,75,79,80).

Those who espouse the appendiceal primary tumor explanation for pseudomyxoma peritonei with ovarian mucinous tumors argue that the finding of a "normal" appendix in association with the ovarian tumors establishes an ovarian source of the pseudomyxoma only in cases in which the appendix has been sampled adequately to exclude a small mucinous tumor (74,75,79,80). Appendiceal tumors in cases of pseudomyxoma peritonei may be small, and sites of rupture may be sealed by periappendiceal mucin and require careful gross and microscopic sampling to identify (65). Differences in the microscopic appearance of the appendiceal and ovarian tumors may reflect tumor heterogeneity or inadequate sampling of either tumor. Also, mucinous tumors metastatic to the ovary from various other sites often exhibit a much higher degree of differentiation than the primary tumors, even appearing histologically benign in some areas. Differences in immunohistochemical staining between the appendiceal and ovarian tumors may also reflect tumor heterogeneity or inadequate sampling of either or both neoplasms.

Recent molecular genetic studies have not resolved the problem of the relation of ovarian and appendiceal tumors in cases of pseudomyxoma peritonei. Study of loss of heterozygosity on chromosomes 17q and 5q in 12 cases showed divergent findings in the two tumors in some cases, supporting the independent primary tumor explanation, and similar findings in other cases, supporting metastasis from the appendix to the ovary (67). Cuatrecases et al. (69), however, demonstrated an identical pattern of c-Ki-ras mutation in synchronous ovarian and appendiceal tumors in five cases with pseudomyxoma peritonei and an absence of that mutation in both tumors in a sixth case, findings that strongly suggest that all the tumors in that series were clonal.

Ronnett et al. (76) have provided strong evidence for the appendiceal origin of most accompanying mucinous cystic tumors of the ovary in cases of pseudomyxoma peritonei. Those investigators have shown that when the two tumors coexist they have identical immunostaining reactions in the great majority of the cases, including negative results for HAM 56 and CK 7. The latter reactions are typical for intestinal primary tumors in contrast to positive findings characteristic of isolated mucinous borderline tumors unaccompanied by pseudomyxoma peritonei.

Some investigators who espouse the independent primary appendiceal and ovarian tumor explanation for pseudomyxoma peritonei also believe that the peritoneal tumor is a third site of independent primary neoplasia (77,78). This conclusion is based on the occasional origin of serous tumors of ovarian type from extraovarian peritoneal mesothelial cells and the speculation that mucinous tumors may arise in a similar fashion. In opposition, a primary origin of the peritoneal tumor is considered very unlikely by others in view of the great rarity of mucinous metaplasia of the peritoneal mesothelium and the observation that abdominal mucinous tumors that do not involve the ovary or appendix but resemble primary ovarian mucinous tumors are retroperitoneal rather than intracavitary (page 452). Also, preliminary molecular genetic studies and karyotypic analyses have suggested that the peritoneal tumor has the same clonality as the ovarian and appendiceal tumors (67).

A final problem in cases of pseudomyxoma peritonei is the definition of the term. Extraovarian intra-abdominal mucus associated with mucinous ovarian tumors may be of several

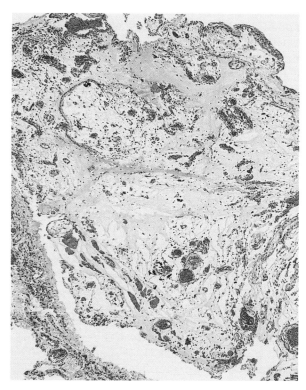

Figure 4-38
MUCIN SPILLAGE FROM
OVARIAN MUCINOUS TUMOR
The mucin is attached to the serosa of the fallopian tube and has been organized by an ingrowth of capillaries.

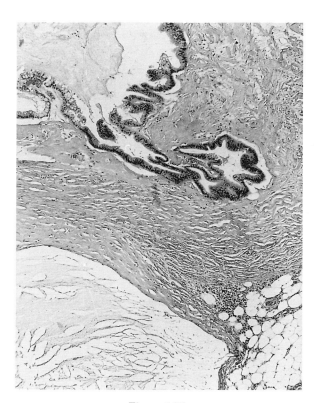

Figure 4-39
DISSECTING MUCIN WITH FIBROSIS IN OMENTUM
Two cysts, one with and the other without a borderline mucinous lining, are separated by hyalinized collagenous tissue. (Fig. 27 from Serov SF, Scully RE, Sobin LH. Histological typing of ovarian tumours. International Histological Classification of Tumours No. 9. Geneva: World Health Organization, 1973.)

types, all of which have been included in case reports and series of "pseudomyxoma peritonei." These types comprise: free mucin in the abdominal cavity (mucinous ascites); small or large deposits of mucin adherent to peritoneal surfaces, containing inflammatory and mesothelial cells and sometimes organizing capillaries and fibroblasts, but usually lacking neoplastic epithelial cells (fig. 4-38); and masses composed of pools of mucin, which may or may not contain neoplastic cells, surrounded by dense collagenous tissue (dissecting mucin) (fig. 4-39). There is no consensus in the literature as to how many of these types of intra-abdominal mucus warrant the designation pseudomyxoma peritonei.

Obviously, many questions about the nature of the ovarian, appendiceal, and peritoneal tumors in cases of pseudomyxoma peritonei will be answered only by prospective study of new cases with as extensive sampling of all the lesions as technically feasible in addition to further studies with special techniques such as immunohistochemistry and molecular biology. From the viewpoint of reporting pathology specimens we believe that the ovarian and appendiceal tumors, which show the same range of histologic and cytologic features, should be designated in a similar manner according to the degree of atypia of the epithelium as benign, borderline (atypical), or malignant. We do not regard dissection of mucin containing only benign or atypical cells as true invasion warranting a diagnosis of carcinoma. Until generally accepted criteria for determining whether the ovarian cystic tumors are independent primary tumors or metastatic from the appendix are available those that are associated with pseudomyxoma peritonei should continue to be staged as ovarian tumors, with the realization that their clinical behavior may not reflect accurately that of mucinous tumors of unquestionable ovarian origin. Finally, the term pseudomyxoma peritonei, which is a clinical and surgical designation, should not appear as a diagnosis in the pathology report. The report should contain an accurate appraisal of the ovarian and appendiceal tumors as benign, borderline, or malignant, with a notation of the presence or absence of rupture, and the peritoneal lesions should be diagnosed specifically as mucinous ascites (free fluid in abdomen), organizing mucinous fluid, or mucin dissection with fibrosis. Since there appears to be a correlation between the presence or absence of tumor cells in the peritoneal mucin and the cytologic features of the cells, if present, with the prognosis (68,74,75,79), their presence or absence and whether they appear benign, borderline (atypical), or malignant should also be included in the report.

REFERENCES

Mucinous Tumors

1. Baergen RN, Rutgers JL. Classification of mural nodules in common epithelial tumors of the ovary. Adv Anat Pathol 1995;2:346–51.

2. Baergen RN, Rutgers JL. Mural nodules in common epithelial tumors of the ovary. Int J Gynecol Pathol 1994;13:62–72.

3. Beck RP, Latour JP. A review of 1019 benign ovarian neoplasms. Obstet Gynecol 1960;16:479–82.

4. Bell DA. Mucinous adenofibromas of the ovary. A report of 10 cases. Am J Surg Pathol 1991;15:227–32.

5. Bell DA, Rutgers JL, Scully RE. Ovarian epithelial tumors of borderline malignancy. In: Damjanov I, Cohen AE, Mills SE, Young RH, eds. Progress in reproductive and urinary tract pathology. New York: Field and Wood Medical Publishers, 1989:1–29.

6. Bruijn JA, Smit VT, Que DG, Fleuren GJ. Immunohistology of a sarcomatous mural nodule in an ovarian mucinous cystadenocarcinoma. Int J Gynecol Pathol 1987;6:287–93.

7. Carey MS, Dembo AJ, Simm JE, Fyles T, Treger T, Bush RS. Testing the validity of a prognostic classification in patients with surgically optimal ovarian carcinoma: a 15-year review. Int J Gynecol Cancer 1993;3:24–35.

8. Cariker M, Dockerty M. Mucinous cystadenomas and mucinous cystadenocarcinomas of the ovary. A clinical and pathological study of 355 cases. Cancer 1954;7:302–10.

9. Carr NJ, Sobin LH. Unusual tumors of the appendix and pseudomyxoma peritonei. Semin Diagn Pathol 1996;13:314–25.

10. Chaitin BA, Gershenson DM, Evans HL. Mucinous tumors of the ovary. A clinicopathologic study of 70 cases. Cancer 1985;55:1958–62.

11. Chan YF, Ho HC, Yau SM, Ma L. Ovarian mucinous tumor with mural nodules of anaplastic carcinoma. Gynecol Oncol 1989;35:112–9.

12. Clarke TJ. Sarcoma-like mural nodules in cystic serous ovarian tumours. J Clin Pathol 1987;40:1443–8.

13. Dabbs DJ, Sturtz K, Zaino RJ. The immunohistochemical discrimination of endometrioid adenocarcinomas. Hum Pathol 1996;27:172–7.

14. DeNictolis M, Montironi R, Tommasoni S, et al. Benign, borderline, and well-differentiated malignant intestinal mucinous tumors of the ovary: a clinicopathologic, histochemical, immunohistochemical, and nuclear quantitative study of 57 cases. Int J Gynecol Pathol 1994;13:10–21.

15. DeRosa G, Donofrio V, De Rosa N, Fulciniti F, Zeppa P. Ovarian serous tumor with mural nodules of carcinomatous derivation (sarcomatoid carcinoma): report of a case. Int J Gynecol Pathol 1991;10:311–8.

15a. Eichhorn JH, Lawrence WD, Young RH, Scully RE. Ovarian neuroendocrine carcinomas of non-small-cell type associated with surface epithelial adenocarcinomas. A study of five cases and review of the literature. Int J Gynecol Pathol 1996;15:304–14.

15b. Eichhorn JH, Young RH, Scully RE. Primary ovarian small cell carcinoma of pulmonary type. A clinicopathologic, immunohistologic, and flow cytometric analysis of 11 cases. Am J Surg Pathol 1992;16:926–38.

16. Fujii S, Konishi I, Kobayashi F, Okamura H, Yamabe H, Mori T. Sarcoma-like mural nodules combined with a microfocus of anaplastic carcinoma in mucinous ovarian tumor. Gynecol Oncol 1985;20:219–33.

17. Gadducci A, Ferdeghini M, Prontera C, et al. The concomitant determination of different tumor markers in patients with epithelial ovarian cancer and benign ovarian masses: relevance for differential diagnosis. Gynecol Oncol 1992;44:147–54.

18. Guerrieri C, Hogberg T, Wingren S, Fristedt S, Simonsen E, Boeryd B. Mucinous borderline and malignant tumors of the ovary: a clinicopathologic and DNA ploidy study of 92 cases. Cancer 1994;74:2329–40.

19. Hart WR. Ovarian epithelial tumors of borderline malignancy (carcinomas of low malignant potential). Hum Pathol 1977;8:541–9.

20. Hart WR, Norris HJ. Borderline and malignant mucinous tumors of the ovary. Histologic criteria and clinical behavior. Cancer 1973;31:1031–45.

21. Hayman JA, Östör AG. Ovarian mucinous tumour with a focus of anaplastic carcinoma: a case report. Pathology 1985;17:591–3.

22. Healy DL, Burger HG, Mamers P, et al. Elevated serum inhibin concentrations in postmenopausal women with ovarian tumors. N Engl J Med 1993;329:1539–42.

23. Hendrickson MR, Kempson RL. Well-differentiated mucinous neoplasms of the ovary. In: State of the art reviews. Pathology: surface epithelial neoplasms of the ovary. Philadelphia: Hanley & Belfus, 1992:1–27.

24. Isarangkul W. Ovarian epithelial tumors in Thai women: a histological analysis of 291 cases. Gynecol Oncol 1984;17:326–39.

25. James PD, Taylor CW, Templeton AC. Tumors of the female genitalia. In: Templeton AC, ed. Tumours in a tropical country. A survey of Uganda 1964-1968. Berlin: Springer-Verlag, 1973:101–31.

26. Kaern J, Tropé CG, Abeler VM. A retrospective study of 370 borderline tumors of the ovary treated at the Norwegian Radium Hospital from 1970 to 1982. A review of clinicopathologic features and treatment modalities. Cancer 1993;71:1810–20.

27. Kaern J, Tropé CG, Kristensen GB, Abeler VM, Pettersen EO. DNA ploidy: the most important prognostic factor in patients with borderline tumors of the ovary. Int J Gynecol Cancer 1993; 3:349-58.

28. Katsube Y, Berg JW, Silverberg SG. Epidemiologic pathology of ovarian tumors: a histopathologic review of primary ovarian neoplasms diagnosed in the Denver standard metropolitan statistical area, 1 July–31 December 1969 and 1 July–31 December 1979. Int J Gynecol Pathol 1982;1:3–16.

29. Kessler E, Halpern M, Koren R, Dekel A, Goldman J. Sarcoma-like mural nodules with foci of anaplastic carcinoma in ovarian mucinous tumor: clinical, histological, and immunohistochemical study of a case and review of the literature. Surg Pathol 1990;3:211–9.

30. Koonings PP, Campbell K, Mishell DR Jr, Grimes DA. Relative frequency of primary ovarian neoplasms: a 10-year review. Obstet Gynecol 1989;74:921–6.

31. Langley FA, Cummins PA, Fox H. An ultrastructural study of mucin secreting epithelia in ovarian neoplasms. Acta Path Microbiol Scand [A] 1972;233:76–86.

32. Leake J, Woolas PR, Daniel J, Oram DH, Brown CL. Immunohistochemical and serological expression of CA 125: a clinicopathological study of 40 malignant ovarian epithelial tumours. Histopathology 1994;24:57–64.

33. Lifschitz-Mercer B, Dgani R, Jacob N, Fogel M, Czernobilsky B. Ovarian mucinous cystadenoma with leiomyomatous mural nodule. Int J Gynecol Pathol 1990;9:80–5.

34. Matias-Guiu X, Aranda I, Prat J. Immunohistochemical study of sarcoma-like mural nodules in a mucinous cystadenocarcinoma of the ovary. Virchows Arch [A] 1991;419:89–92.

35. Michael H, Sutton G, Roth LM. Ovarian carcinoma with extracellular mucin production: reassessment of "pseudomyxoma ovarii et peritonei." Int J Gynecol Pathol 1987;6:298–312.

36. Nakashima N, Nagasaka T, Fukata S, et al. Study of ovarian tumors treated at Nagoya University Hospital, 1965-1988. Gynecol Oncol 1990;37:103–11.

36a.Nayar R, Siriaunkgul S, Robbins KM, McGowan L, Ginzan S, Silverberg SG. Microinvasion in low malignant potential tumors of the ovary. Hum Pathol 1996;27:521–7.

37. Nichols GE, Mills SE, Ulbright TM, Czernobilsky B, Roth LM. Spindle cell mural nodules in cystic ovarian mucinous

38. tumors. A clinicopathologic and immunohistochemical study of five cases. Am J Surg Pathol 1991;15:1055–62.

38. O'Hanlan KA. Resection of a 303.2-pound ovarian tumor. Gynecol Oncol 1994;54:365–71.

39. Ong HC, Chan WF. Mucinous cystadenoma, serous cystadenoma and benign cystic teratoma of the ovary. Clinico-pathologic differences observed in a Malaysian hospital. Cancer 1978;41:1538–42.

40. Pettersson F. Annual report of the results of treatment in gynecological cancer. Stockholm, International Federation of Gynecology and Obstetrics, 1991.

41. Prat J, Scully RE. Ovarian mucinous tumors with sarcoma-like mural nodules: a report of seven cases. Cancer 1979;44:1332–44.

42. Prat J, Scully RE. Sarcomas in ovarian mucinous tumors: a report of two cases. Cancer 1979;44:1327–31.

43. Prat J, Young RH, Scully RE. Ovarian mucinous tumors with foci of anaplastic carcinoma. Cancer 1982; 50:300–4.

44. Rahilly MA, Candlish W, Al-Nafussi A. Fibrosarcoma arising in an ovarian mucinous tumor:a case report. Int J Gynecol Cancer 1994;4:211–4.

45. Russell P. The pathological assessment of ovarian neoplasms: I: introduction to the common epithelial tumours and analysis of benign epithelial tumours. Pathology 1979;11:5–26.

46. Russell P. The pathological assessment of ovarian neoplasms: II: the proliferating epithelial tumours. Pathology 1979;11:251–82.

47. Russell P. The pathological assessment of ovarian neoplasms: III: the malignant epithelial tumours. Pathology 1979;11:493–532.

48. Rutgers JL, Scully RE. Ovarian mullerian mucinous papillary cystadenomas of borderline malignancy. A clinicopathologic analysis. Cancer 1988;61:340–8.

49. Scully RE. Ovary. In: Henson DE, Albores-Saavedra J, eds. The pathology of incipient neoplasia. Philadelphia: WB Saunders, 1993:283–300.

50. Scully RE, Aguirre P, DeLellis RA. Argyrophilia, serotonin, and peptide hormones in the female genital tract and its tumors. Int J Gynecol Pathol 1984;3:51–70.

51. Siriaunkgul S, Robbins KM, McGowan L, Silverberg SG. Ovarian mucinous tumors of low malignant potential: a clinicopathologic study of 54 tumors of intestinal and mullerian type. Int J Gynecol Pathol 1995;14:198–208.

52. Sondergaard G, Kaspersen P. Ovarian and extraovarian mucinous tumors with solid mural nodules. Int J Gynecol Pathol 1991;10:145–55.

53. Stalsberg H, Bjarnason O, DeCarvalho AR, et al. International comparisons of histologic types of ovarian cancer in Cancer Registry Material. In: Stalsberg H, ed. An international survey of distributions of histologic types of tumours of the testis and ovary. UICC technical report series, vol. 75. Geneva: UICC, 1983:247–80.

54. Sumithran E, Susil BJ, Looi LM. The prognostic significance of grading in borderline mucinous tumors of the ovary. Hum Pathol 1988;19:15–8.

55. Suurmeijer AJ. Carcinosarcoma-like mural nodule in an ovarian mucinous tumour. Histopathology 1991;18:268–71.

56. Tateno H, Sasano N. Ovarian tumours in Sendai, Japan. General hospital material. In: Stalsberg H, ed. An international survey of distribution of histologic types of tumours of the testis and ovary. UICC technical report series, vol. 75. Geneva: UICC, 1983;291–6.

57. Tenti P, Aguzzi A, Riva C, et al. Ovarian mucinous tumors frequently express markers of gastric, intestinal, and pancreatobiliary epithelial cells. Cancer 1992;69:2131–42.

58. Tholander B, Taube A, Lindgren A, et al. Pretreatment serum levels of CA 125, carcinoembryonic antigen, tissue polypeptide antigen and placental alkaline phosphate in patients with ovarian carcinoma, borderline tumors or benign adnexal masses: relevance for differential diagnosis. Gynecol Oncol 1990;39:16–25.

59. Tiltman AJ, Sweerts M. Ovarian neoplasms in the Western Cape. S Afr Med J 1982;61:343–5.

60. Tsujimura T, Kawano K. Rhabdomyosarcoma coexistent with ovarian mucinous cystadenocarcinoma: a case report. Int J Gynecol Pathol 1992;11:58–62.

61. Viale G, Gambacorta M, Dell'Orto P, Coggi G. Co-expression of cytokeratins and vimentin in common epithelial tumors of the ovary: an immunocytochemical study of eighty-three cases. Virchows Arch [A] 1988;413:91–101.

62. Watkin W, Silva EG, Gershenson DM. Mucinous carcinoma of the ovary. Pathologic prognostic factors. Cancer 1992;208–12.

63. Young RH, Gilks CB, Scully RE. Mucinous tumors of the appendix associated with mucinous tumors of the ovary and pseudomyxoma peritonei. A clinicopathological analysis of 22 cases supporting an origin in the appendix. Am J Surg Pathol 1991;15:415–29.

64. Young RH, Scully RE. Mucinous ovarian tumors associated with mucinous adenocarcinoma of the cervix. A clinicopathological analysis of 16 cases. Int J Gynecol Pathol 1988;7:99–111.

Pseudomyxoma Peritonei

65. Campbell JS, Lou P, Ferguson JP, et al. Pseudomyxoma peritonei et ovarii with occult neoplasms of appendix. Obstet Gynecol 1973;42:897–902.

66. Carr NJ, Sobin LH. Unusual tumors of the appendix and pseudomyxoma peritonei. Semin Diagn Pathol 1996;13:314–25.

67. Chuaqui RF, Zhuang Z, Emmert-Buck MR, et al. Genetic analysis of synchronous mucinous tumors of the ovary and appendix. Hum Pathol 1996;27:165–71.

68. Costa MJ. Pseudomyxoma peritonei. Histologic predictors of patient survival. Arch Pathol Lab Med 1994;118:1215–9.

69. Cuatrecasas M, Matias-Guiu X, Prat J. Synchronous mucinous tumors of the appendix and the ovary associated with pseudomyxoma peritonei. A clinicopathologic study of six cases with comparative analysis of c-Ki-ras mutations. Am J Surg Pathol 1996;20:739–46.

70. Higa E, Rosai J, Pizzimbono CA, Wise L. Mucosal hyperplasia, mucinous cystadenoma, and mucinous cystadenocarcinoma of the appendix. A re-evaluation of appendiceal "mucocele." Cancer 1973;6:1525–41.

71. Kaern J, Tropé CG, Abeler VM. A retrospective study of 370 borderline tumors of the ovary treated at the Norwegian Radium Hospital from 1970 to 1982. Cancer 1993;71:1810–20.

72. Kahn MA, Demopoulos RI. Mucinous ovarian tumors with pseudomyxoma peritonei: a clinicopathological study. Int J Gynecol Pathol 1992;11:15–23.

73. Michael H, Sutton G, Roth LM. Ovarian carcinoma with extracellular mucin production: reassessment of "pseudomyxoma ovarii et peritonei." Int J Gynecol Pathol 1987;6:298–312.

74. Prayson RA, Hart WR, Petras RE. Pseudomyxoma peritonei. A clinicopathologic study of 19 cases with emphasis on site of origin and nature of associated ovarian tumors. Am J Surg Pathol 1994;18:591–603.

75. Ronnett BM, Kurman RJ, Zahn CM, et al. Pseudomyxoma peritonei in women: a clinicopathologic analysis of 30 cases with emphasis on site of origin, prognosis, and relationship to ovarian mucinous tumors of low malignant potential. Human Pathol 1995;56:509–24.

76. Ronnett BM, Shmookler BM, Diener-West M, Sugarbaker PH, Kurman RJ. Immunohistochemical evidence supporting the appendiceal origin of pseudomyxoma peritonei in women. Int J Gynecol Pathol 1997;16:1–9.

77. Seidman JD, Elsayed AM, Sobin LH, Tavassoli FA. Association of mucinous tumors of the ovary and appendix. A clinicopathologic study of 25 cases. Am J Surg Pathol 1993;17:22–34.

78. Seidman JD, Elsayed AM, Sobin LH, Tavassoli FA. Authors' reply to the editor. Am J Surg Pathol 1993;17:1070–1.

79. Young RH, Gilks CB, Scully RE. Mucinous tumors of the appendix associated with mucinous tumors of the ovary and pseudomyxoma peritonei. A clinicopathological analysis of 22 cases supporting an origin in the appendix. Am J Surg Pathol 1991;15:415–29.

80. Young RH, Gilks CB, Scully RE. Pseudomyxoma peritonei [Letter]. Am J Surg Pathol 1993;17:1068–70.

✧✧✧

5
ENDOMETRIOID TUMORS

Endometrioid tumors are characterized by the presence of epithelial elements, stromal elements, or both that closely resemble similar components of tumors encountered more commonly in the endometrium. These include endometrioid carcinomas, stromal sarcomas, mullerian adenosarcomas, and malignant mullerian mixed tumors (carcinosarcomas). An origin from endometriosis is demonstrable in some of the cases but is not required for the diagnosis. Moreover, since tumors of other cell types also arise from endometriosis, albeit less often (28), such an origin, per se, does not establish a tumor as endometrioid. Most endometrioid tumors probably arise directly from surface epithelial inclusions, the ovarian stroma, or both.

Although some pathologists (6) regard endometriosis as a neoplasm and a recent investigation has shown a monoclonal X-chromosome inactivation pattern in some endometriotic cysts consistent with neoplasia (29), this text will follow the more widely accepted viewpoint that this disorder reflects a non-neoplastic ectopia of endometrial-type tissue. Therefore, except for its precancerous alterations, endometriosis will be discussed under tumor-like disorders (page 430). The first section discusses epithelial endometrioid tumors and the following section, those that are partly or entirely sarcomatous.

EPITHELIAL TUMORS

General Features. Endometrioid epithelial tumors account for 2 to 4 percent of all ovarian tumors. Less than 1 percent of benign ovarian neoplasms are endometrioid, and almost all of them are adenofibromas (18,24); only 2 to 3 percent of borderline epithelial tumors are endometrioid; and endometrioid carcinomas account for 10 to 20 percent of ovarian carcinomas in most series (18,23,24,31,36).

Benign, borderline, and malignant endometrioid epithelial tumors occur most commonly in women in the older reproductive and postmenopausal age groups, with mean ages of 56, 51, and 56 years, respectively (2,34,42,43). The tumors are often accompanied by endometriosis in the

same ovary or at any site in the pelvis (11,15,28); the frequencies of these associations in cases of benign and borderline endometrioid tumors are 28 and 38 percent, respectively (2,42). Endometrioid carcinoma is accompanied by ipsilateral ovarian endometriosis in 11 to 42 percent of the cases, and by pelvic endometriosis in general in 11 to 28 percent (11,13a,28). A transition to endometriotic epithelium has been reported in 5 to 10 percent of ovarian endometrioid carcinomas. Women with endometrioid carcinoma and endometriosis in the same ovary are 5 to 10 years younger on average than women without associated ovarian endometriosis (39).

The entire spectrum of endometrial hyperplastic lesions, both simple and complex, typical and atypical, has been encountered sporadically in ovarian endometriosis (figs. 5-1, 5-2) (41). In addition to atypical glandular lesions simulating those seen in the endometrium, the lining epithelium of endometriotic cysts is occasionally composed of large cells with abundant eosinophilic cytoplasm and large, hyperchromatic, often smudgy nuclei (fig. 5-3) (41). Although this

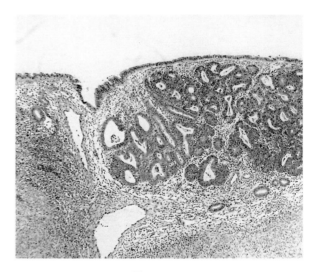

Figure 5-1
ATYPICAL COMPLEX HYPERPLASIA
IN WALL OF AN ENDOMETRIOTIC CYST
The glands are closely packed.

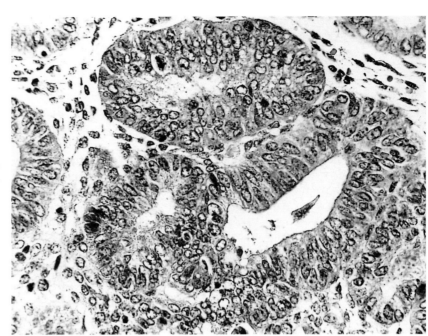

Figure 5-2
ATYPICAL
COMPLEX HYPERPLASIA
In this high-power view of figure 5-1, the glands are lined by stratified, highly atypical cells.

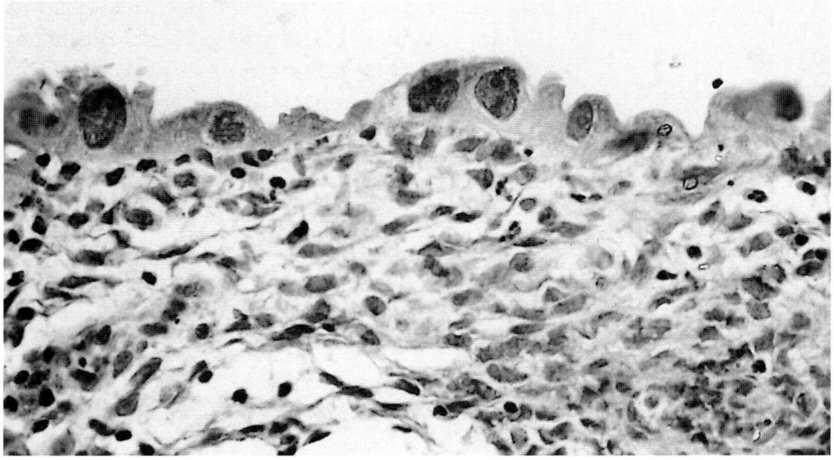

Figure 5-3
ATYPIA OF LINING
EPITHELIUM OF
ENDOMETRIOTIC CYST
The atypical cells have pleomorphic, hyperchromatic, occasionally smudgy nuclei with prominent nucleoli and abundant cytoplasm, which was eosinophilic. (Fig. 15-10 from Scully RE. Ovary. In: Henson DE, Albores-Saavedra J, eds. The pathology of incipient neoplasia. Philadelphia: WB Saunders, 1993:289.)

change is often seen in cysts from which a carcinoma has arisen its cancerous potential is unknown since it may occur in the absence of carcinoma as well. A final change occasionally seen in an endometriotic cyst is a stroma-free papillary hyperplasia of the lining, sometimes with mucinous metaplasia. It is possible that this type of proliferation is a precursor of the endocervical-like or mixed mullerian type of borderline tumor, each of which is often accompanied by endometriosis.

The precancerous significance of atypical endometriosis is unclear since foci of it are often completely resected, eliminating the possibility of meaningful follow-up data. The findings that 15 percent of epithelial cancers of the ovary, including 23 percent of endometrioid carcinomas, were associated with atypical ipsilateral endometriosis and that 63 percent of the endometriotic lesions accompanying the epithelial cancers were atypical in contrast to a 2 percent frequency of atypicality in cases of ovarian endometriosis in the absence of an ovarian tumor, however, strongly suggest a role of atypical endometriosis in the evolution of malignancy (13a).

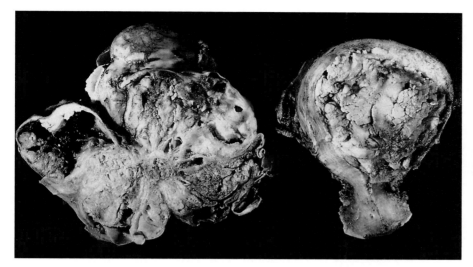

Figure 5-4
ENDOMETRIOID
CARCINOMA OF OVARY
AND ENDOMETRIUM
Endometrioid carcinoma is
shown on the sectioned surface
of the ovary and in the opened
uterus.

Another association of endometrioid carcinoma of the ovary is with carcinoma of the endometrium (fig. 5-4), which has been reported to be present in 15 to 20 percent of the cases (22,23, 26,54); in a few of these cases the association is metachronous. Criteria for distinguishing ovarian endometrioid carcinoma with spread to the uterus, a vice-versa situation, and independent primary neoplasia of both organs are presented on page 125. Finally, ovarian endometrioid carcinoma is accompanied rarely by atypical hyperplasia or carcinoma arising in extraovarian endometriosis (41).

The association of a significant number of ovarian endometrioid carcinomas with endometriosis, endometrial carcinoma, or both, and the known response of endometriotic tissue to steroid hormones suggest that some endometrioid carcinomas of the ovary may have the same risk factors for their development as endometrial carcinomas. Several, but not all, epidemiologic studies support this conclusion (8).

The clinical manifestations of ovarian endometrioid carcinomas are similar in general to those of other ovarian cancers. Endometrioid carcinomas are, in addition, among the most common primary ovarian tumors of nonendocrine cells that are associated with endocrine manifestations caused by steroid hormone secretion (see chapter 19). CA125 is elevated in the serum in over 80 percent of cases of endometrioid carcinoma (14,25).

Gross Findings. Endometrioid tumors have no gross features that distinguish them from other neoplasms in the surface epithelial–stromal category except for the more frequent presence in the same ovary of recognizable small foci of endometriosis or an endometriotic cyst within which the tumor may have arisen (figs. 5-5, 5-6). Endometrioid adenofibromas, including those of borderline malignancy, are predominantly solid tumors, which may contain variable numbers of cysts (fig. 5-7). The carcinomas range from solid with a soft, friable, or fibrous consistency (fig. 5-4) to cystic with a thin, velvety or soft papillary lining, or with a fungating mass protruding into the lumen, which may contain chocolate-colored fluid or mucus (fig. 5-6). Endometrioid adenofibromas and borderline tumors are almost always unilateral; stage I endometrioid carcinoma is bilateral in 17 percent of the cases (31).

Microscopic Findings. *Benign Tumors.* Endometrioid cystadenomas are rare. They are lined by stratified, typically nonciliated, nonmucin-containing epithelium. Absent are an underlying endometrial-type stroma; pseudoxanthoma cells containing hemofuscin, hemosiderin, or both; and the distinctive stroma containing small spindle-shaped fibroblasts that often develops in the wall of an endometriotic cyst. Extensive sampling of a cyst of this type, however, may reveal foci in which these stromal findings are present, establishing the diagnosis of an endometriotic cyst and suggesting that a pure endometrioid cystadenoma may not even exist.

The endometrioid adenofibroma is characterized typically by glands lined by stratified non-mucin-containing epithelium lying within a predominantly fibromatous stromal component (fig. 5-8) (2,42). Occasionally, the epithelium is simple columnar, cuboidal, or flat, creating a problem in differentiation from a serous adenofibroma (fig. 5-9) (17) (page 72). Squamous differentiation in the form of morules, which may exhibit central necrosis, may be present within some glands (fig. 5-9). The morules occasionally incite a myxoid fibroblastic response in the adjacent stromal component, which should not in itself be regarded as evidence of borderline malignancy. Rare intracystic polypoid and papillary tumors containing bland-appearing endometrioid epithelium also belong in the benign endometrioid category (figs. 5-10, 5-11).

Borderline Tumors. There is no agreement on the criteria for diagnosing endometrioid tumors of borderline malignancy (2,19,30,34,42), with some authors including in this category tumors with small foci that fulfill the criteria for carcinoma. Most endometrioid tumors that have been designated "borderline" have an adenofibromatous pattern. Our present diagnostic criteria for

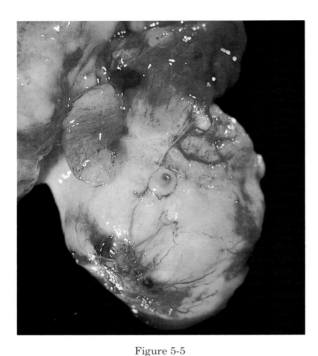

Figure 5-5
ENDOMETRIOSIS ON SURFACE OF
ENDOMETRIOID ADENOFIBROMA
The endometriosis is characterized by the presence of blueberry-like nodules surrounded by hemorrhage.

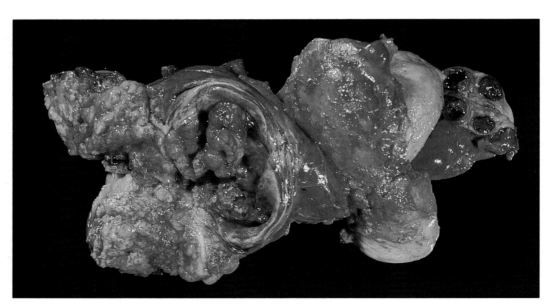

Figure 5-6
ENDOMETRIOID CARCINOMA ARISING IN ENDOMETRIOTIC CYST
The tumor is a polypoid mass protruding from the dark brown lining of the opened cyst. Endometriosis is also present on the posterior surface of the uterus. (Fig. 6 from Scully RE. Recent progress in ovarian cancer. Hum Pathol 1970;1:73–98.)

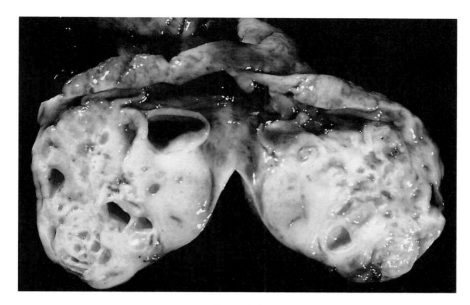

Figure 5-7
ENDOMETRIOID ADENOFIBROMA

The sectioned surfaces are predominantly fibromatous but contain small and medium-sized cysts as well. This figure depicts the sectioned surfaces of the tumor shown in figure 5-5.

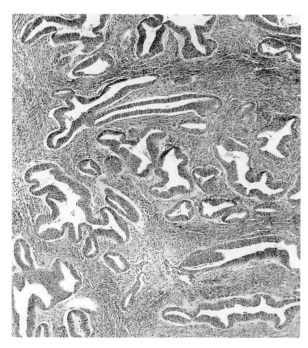

Figure 5-8
ENDOMETRIOID ADENOFIBROMA

The glands are irregularly shaped and are lined by stratified epithelium, which was not atypical. The fibromatous stroma was the predominant component of the tumor. (Fig. 3 from Bell DA, Scully RE. Atypical and borderline endometrioid adenofibromas of the ovary. A report of 27 cases. Am J Surg Pathol 1985;9:205–14.)

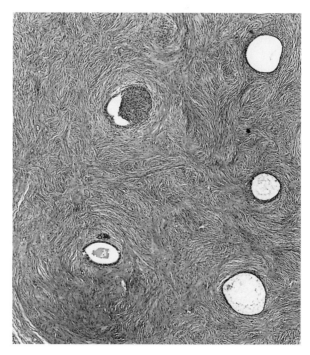

Figure 5-9
ENDOMETRIOID ADENOFIBROMA
WITH SQUAMOUS DIFFERENTIATION

The tumor is composed predominantly of hyalinized fibromatous tissue containing small cysts lined by indifferent epithelium. The squamous differentiation in one cyst provides evidence of the endometrioid nature of the tumor.

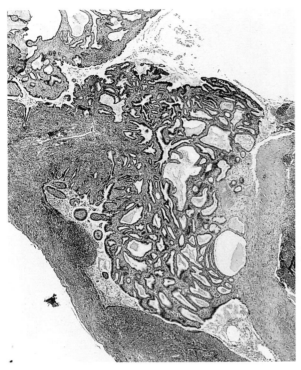

Figure 5-10
ENDOMETRIOID POLYP ARISING
IN ENDOMETRIOTIC CYST
The tumor resembles an endometrial polyp with irregular, closely packed glands (complex hyperplasia). (Fig. 31 from Serov SF, Scully RE, Sobin LH. Histological typing of ovarian tumours. International Classification of Tumours No. 9. Geneva: World Health Organization, 1973.)

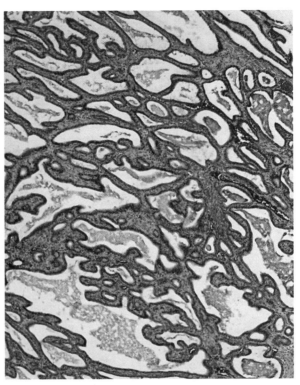

Figure 5-11
ENDOMETRIOID POLYP
The glands are lined by benign epithelium and are separated by small amounts of fibrous stroma.

this form of borderline tumor follow the World Health Organization (WHO) criteria, namely the presence of atypical to cytologically malignant endometrioid-type cells lying within epithelial aggregates or lining glands or cysts (fig. 5-12) and an absence of obvious stromal invasion. The latter is characterized by a disorderly penetration of the stroma, often with a stromal reaction, or a back-to-back arrangement of the glands (i.e., without even minimal intervening stroma recognizable at the light microscopic level). We further state whether the epithelial component is atypical or carcinomatous. If it is the latter, we grade it 1 to 3 according to criteria used for grading endometrioid carcinoma of the uterine corpus (fig. 5-13) (40). If stromal invasion is present, we distinguish arbitrarily between microinvasion (one or more foci 10 sq mm or less in area) and more extensively invasive carcinoma, which may

coexist with a benign or borderline adenofibroma and which we designate "carcinoma in (or with) an adenofibroma" (fig. 5-14). Because of the rarity of borderline endometrioid adenofibromas, as well as those with microinvasion, and the clinically benign behavior of the relatively few reported cases in these categories, recognition of features that may predict malignant behavior requires additional experience with these tumors; for the present, the gynecologist should be aware of the apparently excellent prognosis associated with all these neoplasms.

When an entirely intracystic villoglandular tumor is lined by malignant endometrioid epithelium, we designate it "borderline with intraepithelial carcinoma."

Carcinoma. Most endometrioid carcinomas of the ovary closely resemble the common subtypes of endometrioid carcinoma of the uterine corpus; rare examples resemble the secretory, ciliated cell, or oxyphilic variants of the latter (11b,16,32).

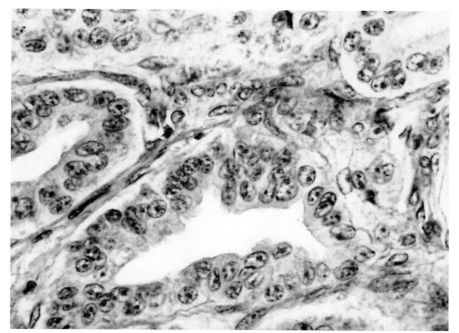

Figure 5-12
ENDOMETRIOID
ADENOFIBROMA
OF BORDERLINE
MALIGNANCY
Atypical endometrioid glands
are separated by stroma, which
was the predominant element of
the tumor. (Fig. 8 from Bell DA,
Scully RE. Atypical and borderline
endometrioid adenofibromas of the
ovary. A report of 27 cases. Am J
Surg Pathol 1985;9:205–14.)

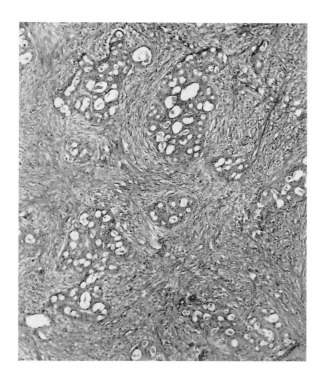

Figure 5-13
ENDOMETRIOID ADENOFIBROMA OF
BORDERLINE MALIGNANCY WITH
INTRAEPITHELIAL CARCINOMA, GRADE 1
Well-demarcated cribriform islands are uniformly dis-
tributed in an abundant fibromatous stroma.

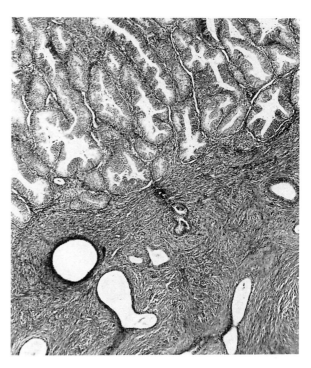

Figure 5-14
ENDOMETRIOID ADENOCARCINOMA
Endometrioid adenocarcinoma (top), arising in association with endometrioid adenofibroma (bottom). (Fig. 15-12
from Scully RE. Ovary. In: Henson DE, Albores-Saavedra J,
eds. Pathology of incipient neoplasia. Philadelphia: WB
Saunders, 1993:292.)

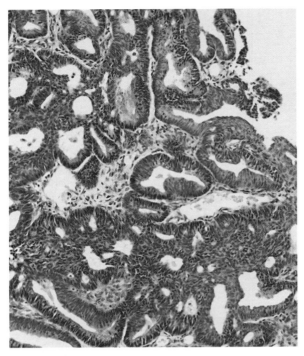

Figure 5-15
ENDOMETRIOID ADENOCARCINOMA

In its well-differentiated form and in well-differentiated areas of higher grade tumors the typical endometrioid adenocarcinoma is characterized by invasive round, oval, or tubular glands lined by stratified nonmucin-containing epithelium (fig. 5-15). A typically orderly, cribriform pattern of glandular differentiation may be present. A villoglandular pattern is encountered frequently, with the villous papillae projecting into one or more cysts (fig. 5-16). In occasional cases the tumor cells are confined largely to the lining of a cyst (fig. 5-17). Abundant mucin may fill the glandular lumens and occupy the apex of the cytoplasm of the tumor cells in the so-called mucin-rich form (fig. 5-18). Minor foci of epithelium resembling the lining of a mucinous cystadenoma are present in some endometrioid carcinomas and should not lead to an erroneous diagnosis of mucinous carcinoma. Occasionally, the glands contain eosinophilic colloid-like material, and if they are cystically dilated, may simulate the follicles of struma ovarii (fig. 5-19). In the secretory endometrioid adenocarcinoma the lining cells of the glands are vacuolated,

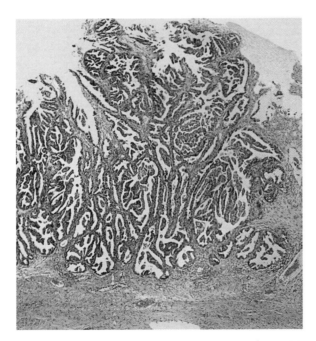

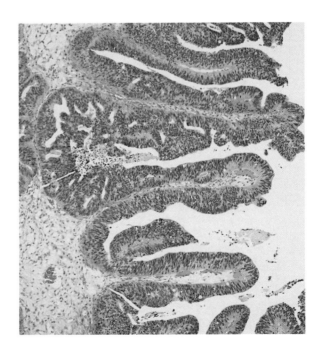

Figure 5-16
ENDOMETRIOID ADENOCARCINOMA
Left: A villoglandular pattern is seen. More obvious stromal invasion was present elsewhere.
Right: The villi and glands are lined by stratified, nonmucin-containing endometrioid epithelium. Note the absence of cellular budding.

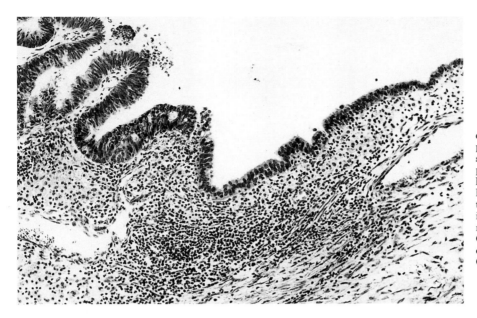

Figure 5-17
ENDOMETRIOID
ADENOCARCINOMA
LINING
ENDOMETRIOTIC CYST

Well-differentiated, stratified endometrioid carcinoma lines part of an endometriotic cyst; the stroma contains numerous lymphocytes. The epithelial lining has a cribriform pattern in the left portion of the field. This tumor was invasive of the stroma in other areas. (Fig. 6 from Corner GW Jr, Ho CY, Hertig HT. Ovarian carcinoma arising in endometriosis. Am J Obstet Gynecol 1955;59: 760–74.)

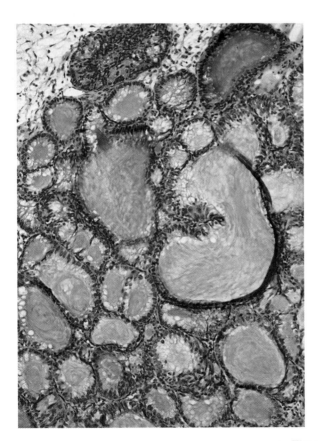
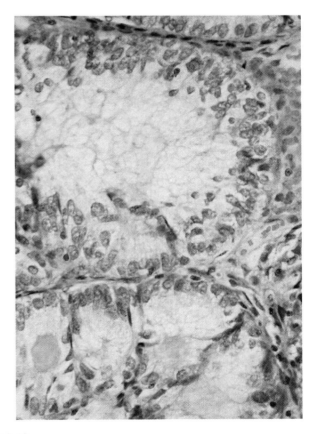

Figure 5-18
ENDOMETRIOID ADENOCARCINOMA
Left: The glands are filled with mucin.   Right: There is little or no intracellular mucin.

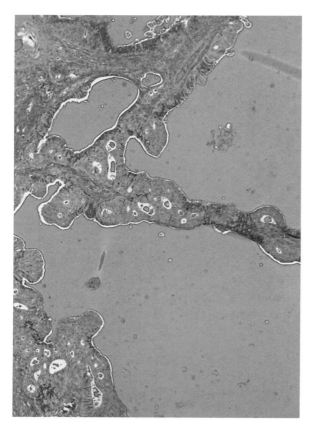

Figure 5-19
ENDOMETRIOID ADENOCARCINOMA
The cystic glands are distended by colloid-like material.

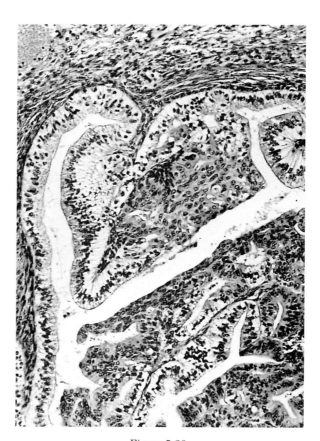

Figure 5-20
ENDOMETRIOID ADENOCARCINOMA,
SECRETORY VARIANT, WITH FOCAL
SQUAMOUS DIFFERENTIATION
Both basal and supranuclear vacuoles are present in the glandular epithelium.

resembling the glandular cells of a 16-day secretory endometrium (fig. 5-20). In the oxyphilic endometrioid adenocarcinoma, the glandular linings and solid areas of the tumor are composed of oxyphil cells with abundant cytoplasm (fig. 5-21), and in the ciliated cell endometrioid adenocarcinoma (fig. 5-22) a cribriform pattern is characteristic and most of the glandular lining cells bear cilia (11b). Rare endometrioid carcinomas contain scattered balloon-like, presumably hydropic, vacuoles in well-differentiated glandular cells (fig. 5-23), or similar vacuoles may occupy the basal portion of the cytoplasm, displacing the nuclei to the apices of the cells.

Some endometrioid carcinomas are characterized by solid areas punctured by variable numbers of tubular or round glands (figs. 5-24, 5-25) or occasionally by tiny rosette-like glands (microglandular pattern), simulating on low-power examination the microfollicular pattern of an adult granulosa cell tumor (fig. 5-26). Rarely, an insular or trabecular pattern of solid or microglandular aggregates enhances the resemblance to the latter tumor. Solid areas in endometrioid carcinoma may be characterized by uniform cells with variable amounts of cytoplasm and small, uniformly round, hyperchromatic nuclei (fig. 5-25). Such areas may prove to be neuroendocrine carcinomas on special staining (11a,11c) (pages 320 and 321).

Squamous differentiation in endometrioid carcinomas has been reported in one third (37) to half of the cases. It may be in the form of morules composed of small, immature but cytologically benign-appearing squamous cells (figs. 5-27, 5-28), which occasionally contain balloon-like, hydropic vacuoles (fig. 5-29); or nests or diffuse areas of cytologically malignant squamous epithelium

116

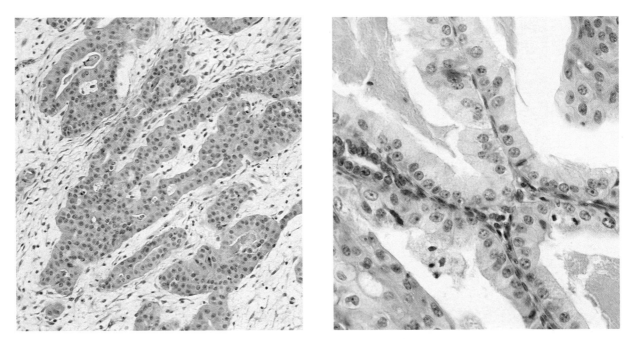

Figure 5-21
ENDOMETRIOID ADENOCARCINOMA, OXYPHILIC VARIANT
Left: A few glands are present in addition to solid trabeculae separated by stroma.
Right: The glands are lined by cells with abundant eosinophilic cytoplasm.

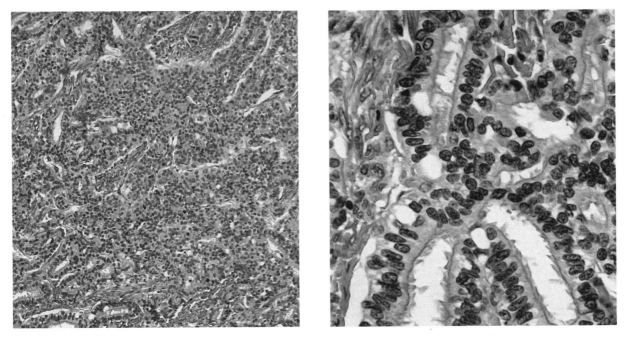

Figure 5-22
ENDOMETRIOID ADENOCARCINOMA, CILIATED-CELL VARIANT
Left: Occasional tubular glands are present within otherwise solid masses of tumor cells.
Right: The glands are lined by epithelial cells bearing cilia.

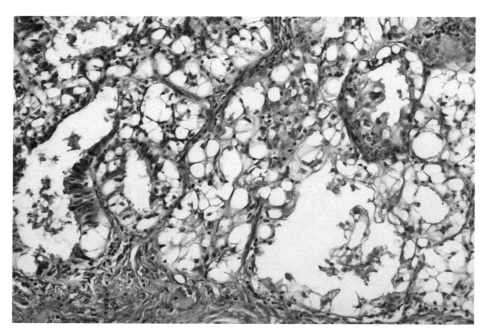

Figure 5-23
ENDOMETRIOID ADENOCARCINOMA
Balloon-type vacuoles are in the cytoplasm of most of the cells.

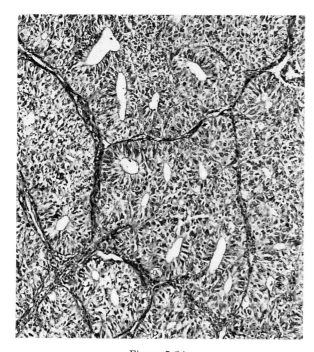

Figure 5-24
ENDOMETRIOID ADENOCARCINOMA
Over half the tumor is solid. (Fig. 15-9 from Scully RE. Ovary. In: Henson DE, Albores-Saavedra J, eds. The pathology of incipient neoplasia. Philadelphia: WB Saunders, 1993:289.)

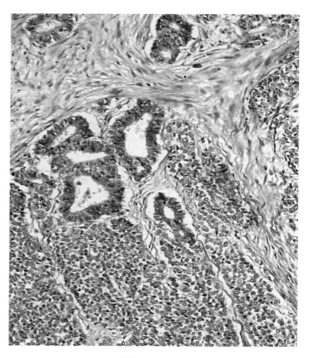

Figure 5-25
ENDOMETRIOID ADENOCARCINOMA
A few glands were found in this tumor, which was predominantly undifferentiated.

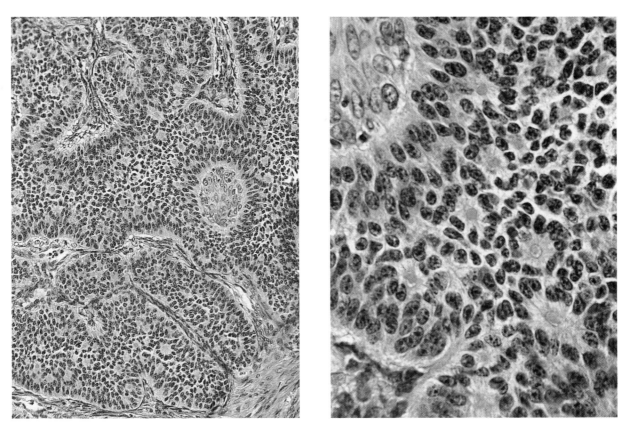

Figure 5-26
ENDOMETRIOID ADENOCARCINOMA SIMULATING GRANULOSA CELL TUMOR
Left: The tumor cells are arranged in insular and trabecular patterns and line microglands, simulating Call-Exner bodies.
Right: The small spaces appear as glands containing eosinophilic secretion. The nuclei are round and hyperchromatic instead of pale and oval or angular as in a granulosa cell tumor.

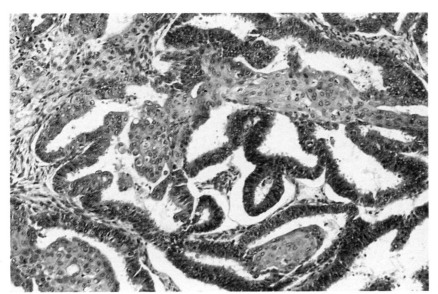

Figure 5-27
ENDOMETRIOID
ADENOCARCINOMA
WITH SQUAMOUS
DIFFERENTIATION
The squamous cells are growing in the form of morules.

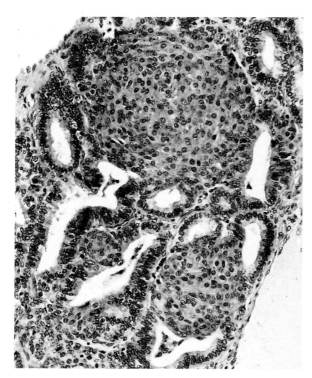

Figure 5-28
ENDOMETRIOID ADENOCARCINOMA
WITH SQUAMOUS DIFFERENTIATION

The squamous cells are immature but cytologically benign. (Fig. 37 from Serov SF, Scully RE, Sobin LH. Histological typing of ovarian tumours. International Histological Classification of Tumours No. 9. Geneva: World Health Organization, 1973.)

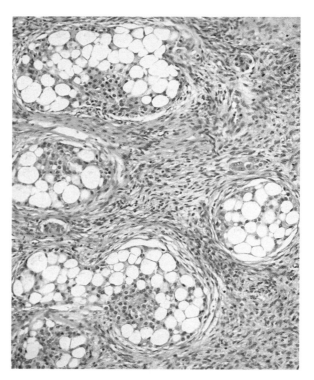

Figure 5-29
ENDOMETRIOID ADENOCARCINOMA
WITH SQUAMOUS DIFFERENTIATION

The squamous cells contain large numbers of balloon-type vacuoles.

(figs. 5-30, 5-31). As in the endometrium, some authors (13) have divided these carcinomas accordingly into "adenoacanthomas" and "adenosquamous carcinomas"; those authors concluded that the latter are three times as common as the former and are associated with a much poorer prognosis. Other observers (7,37) however, state that adenoacanthomas are more frequent than adenosquamous carcinomas.

The WHO classification favors the generic designation "endometrioid adenocarcinoma with squamous differentiation" followed by the grade of the tumor instead of using the above two terms (40). The squamous epithelium may show extensive keratinization and calcification and elicit a foreign body giant cell reaction (fig. 5-32). An occasional finding in endometrioid carcinomas is focal or extensive formation of aggregates of spindle-shaped epithelial cells (fig. 5-33), which may

appear to transform into fibroblasts with collagen production, both within the aggregates and at their periphery (46,49). Occasionally, spindle cell nests undergo transition to clearly recognizable squamous cells, suggesting that the spindle cells represent abortive squamous differentiation. A rare pattern of endometrioid carcinoma related to the type showing squamous differentiation has a basaloid nonglandular component (fig. 5-34) (page 322).

Approximately 10 percent of endometrioid carcinomas contain argyrophil cells of neuroendocrine type (47), but the designation "argyrophil cell carcinoma" is inappropriate since such cells may be present in many other types of ovarian epithelial neoplasia. Rare endometrioid carcinomas are admixed with undifferentiated carcinomas with neuroendocrine staining features (11a, 11c) (pages 320 and 321).

An unusual microscopic feature of endometrioid carcinomas of the ovary that is shared only rarely by similar tumors in the endometrium is the

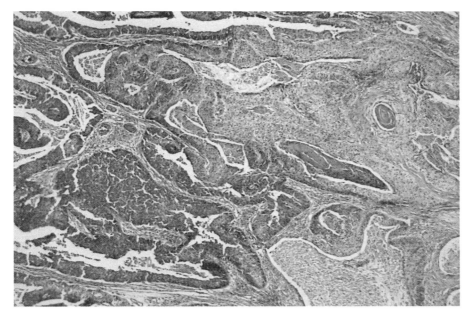

Figure 5-30
ENDOMETRIOID
ADENOCARCINOMA
WITH SQUAMOUS
DIFFERENTIATION
Keratinizing squamous cell
carcinoma (right) merges with
adenocarcinoma (left).

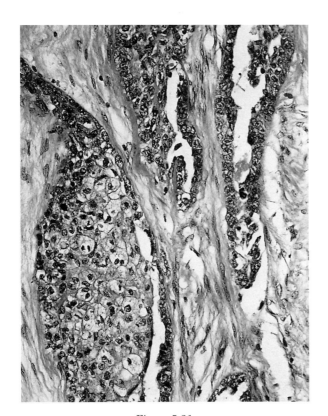

Figure 5-31
ENDOMETRIOID ADENOCARCINOMA
WITH SQUAMOUS DIFFERENTIATION
The squamous cells are cytologically malignant and were
independently invasive of the stroma.

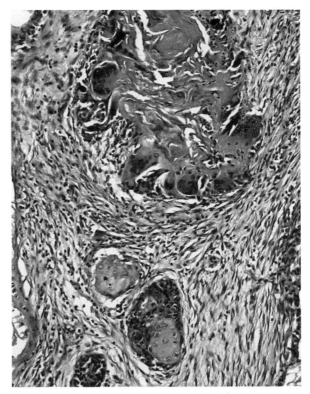

Figure 5-32
ENDOMETRIOID ADENOCARCINOMA
WITH SQUAMOUS DIFFERENTIATION
A foreign body reaction to keratin is present in addition
to viable-appearing squamous nests.

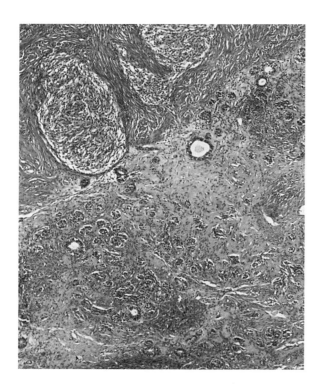 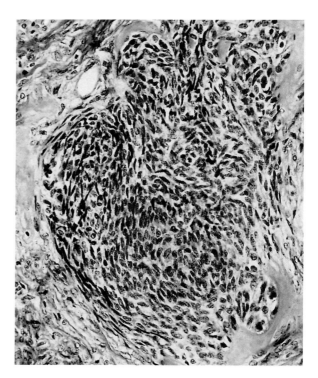

Figure 5-33
ENDOMETRIOID ADENOCARCINOMA

Left: The neoplastic epithelial cells are spindle shaped (top) and form small tubular glands simulating the tubules of a well-differentiated Sertoli cell tumor (bottom).

Right: The epithelial cells have become spindle shaped and appear to merge with collagen-producing spindle cells at the periphery. (Fig. 8 from Young RH, Prat J, Scully RE. Ovarian endometrioid carcinomas resembling sex-cord stromal tumors. A clinicopathological analysis of 13 cases. Am J Surg Pathol 1982;6:513–22.)

Figure 5-34
ENDOMETRIOID
CARCINOMA

The tumor has the pattern
of an adenoid basal carcinoma.

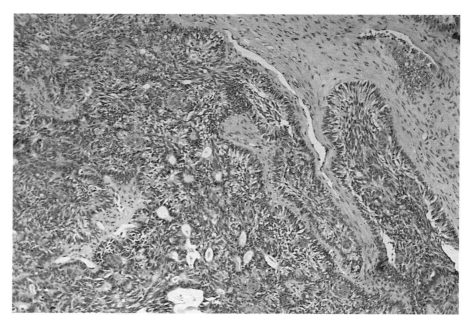

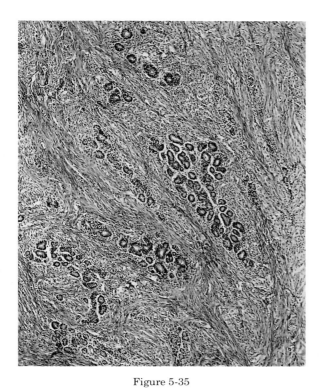

Figure 5-35
ENDOMETRIOID ADENOCARCINOMA
SIMULATING SERTOLI CELL TUMOR
The small glands simulate the small tubules of a well-differentiated Sertoli cell or Sertoli-Leydig cell tumor.

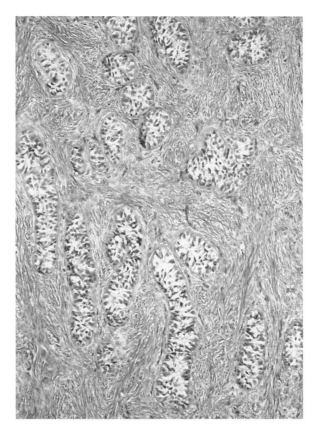

Figure 5-36
ENDOMETRIOID ADENOCARCINOMA
SIMULATING SERTOLI CELL TUMOR
The carcinoma cells form solid tubules indistinguishable from those of a Sertoli cell tumor.

presence of focal to extensive areas resembling Sertoli cell and Sertoli-Leydig cell tumors (35, 49). Some endometrioid carcinomas contain small, well-differentiated glands in a lobular arrangement, suggesting the hollow tubules of a well-differentiated Sertoli cell tumor (fig. 5-35). In other cases there may be solid tubular structures containing cells with pale oval nuclei and a central, pale, cytoplasmic pseudosyncytium (figs. 5-36, 5-37); such tubular structures resemble the solid tubules of a Sertoli cell tumor, particularly of the type seen in the testis of patients with the androgen insensitivity syndrome (page 404). The cells of the hollow or solid tubule-like structures in endometrioid carcinomas may be vacuolated and lipid rich (fig. 5-38), and difficult to distinguish from those of a lipid-rich Sertoli cell tumor (page 203). Rarely, thin cords resembling sex cords are present. If there is, in addition, luteinization of the stroma of the endometrioid carcinoma accompanied by virilization of the patient, the likeli-

hood of misdiagnosing a Sertoli-Leydig cell tumor is even greater.

Differential Diagnosis. The differentiation of endometrioid tumors from serous and mucinous neoplasms has been discussed with those neoplasms. Occasionally, an endometrioid adenofibroma with squamous morular differentiation is confused with a Brenner tumor, but when the latter has a glandular component it is most commonly mucinous and occasionally serous; also, nuclear grooves, which are typically prominent in the transitional cells of a Brenner tumor, are not a conspicuous feature of squamous morules. Endometrioid adenocarcinoma of the secretory type may be mistaken for a clear cell adenocarcinoma composed exclusively of clear cells. In the secretory adenocarcinoma, however, the better differentiated areas contain glands with basal

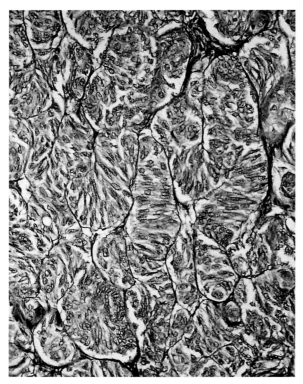

Figure 5-37
ENDOMETRIOID ADENOCARCINOMA
SIMULATING SERTOLI CELL TUMOR

The carcinoma cells are well differentiated and form solid tubular structures simulating those of a Sertoli cell tumor. (Fig. 2 from Young RH, Prat J, Scully RE. Ovarian endometrioid carcinomas resembling sex-cord stromal tumors. A clinicopathological analysis of 13 cases. Am J Surg Pathol 1982;6:513–22.)

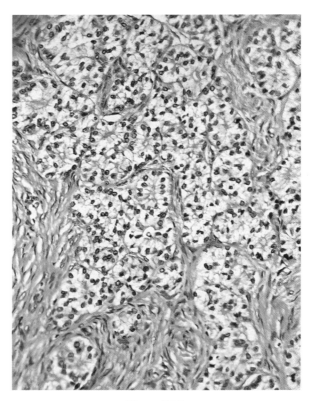

Figure 5-38
ENDOMETRIOID ADENOCARCINOMA SIMULATING
SERTOLI CELL TUMOR OF LIPID-RICH TYPE

The carcinoma cells form solid tubular structures and contain cytoplasmic vacuoles that were positive for fat on special staining.

and supranuclear vacuoles; cells with completely vacuolated cytoplasm and eccentric nuclei are typically absent. Occasionally, however, endometrioid and clear cell carcinoma are intermixed, and in such cases a diagnosis of a mixed carcinoma is warranted if the minor component accounts for 10 percent or more of the tumor. The very rare ovarian tumor of probable wolffian origin (52) (page 324) may contain tubular glands resembling those of well-differentiated endometrioid adenocarcinoma. The glands of endometrioid carcinoma, however, commonly contain intraluminal mucin, which is absent or scanty in wolffian tumors. Additionally, other characteristic patterns of endometrioid carcinomas or wolffian tumors, such as the sieve-like and adenomatoid-like patterns of the latter, are usually also present in the specimen and are

helpful clues in the differential diagnosis. Finally, if the differentiation cannot be made by routine staining, the much higher frequency of staining for epithelial membrane antigen and TAG72 (with antibody B72.3) in endometrioid tumors can facilitate the diagnosis (10,45).

The rare endometrioid-like glandular variant of the yolk sac tumor (4) (page 249) is characterized by the formation of glands and often villous papillae lined by cells that resemble closely those of a proliferative or secretory endometrium. Additionally, there may be a solid intraluminal proliferation of hepatoid cells that simulates the morule of an endometrioid adenocarcinoma with squamous differentiation. Finally, the presence of a fibromatous stroma in some endometrioid-like yolk sac tumors may suggest an endometrioid adenofibromatous tumor. However, glandular yolk sac tumors occur typically in young women, in whom endometrioid carcinomas are infrequent. Microscopic features that are helpful in the differential diagnosis are the additional presence of other more common patterns of yolk sac tumor and immunohistochemical staining for alpha-fetoprotein. A positive staining result almost always confirms the diagnosis of a yolk sac tumor of germ cell origin but exceptionally, yolk sac neometaplasia, like choriocarcinomatous neometaplasia, develops in tumors of somatic cell origin, such as endometrioid carcinoma (29a,38). In such a situation, however, features diagnostic of endometrioid carcinoma, which may be accompanied by endometriosis, are also present.

The very rare ovarian ependymoma (page 300) (21), which may have solid, gland-like, and papillary patterns, can be confused occasionally with an endometrioid carcinoma, particularly a rare subtype of the latter in which many of the cells have apical nuclei. Perivascular pseudorosettes, occasional true rosettes, and the basal fibrillary cytoplasm of the tumor cells, which can be stained immunohistochemically for glial fibrillary acidic protein, establish the diagnosis of ependymoma in such cases (page 302). In one study (27), however, occasional cells in 3 of 8 endometrioid carcinomas were positive for glial fibrillary acidic protein.

The distinction between an endometrioid carcinoma with a pattern that is insular, trabecular, or microglandular and an insular, trabecular, or microfollicular granulosa cell tumor is based on the coexistence of other characteristic patterns of either tumor, on the different appearances of microglands and Call-Exner bodies, and on the different nuclear features of the two tumors. The nuclei of endometrioid carcinoma cells are typically round and hyperchromatic and those of granulosa cell tumors are characteristically round, oval, or angular, pale, and often grooved (49). Sertoli-stromal cell tumors and the endometrioid adenocarcinomas that simulate them morphologically have very different age distributions, with endometrioid carcinomas occurring mostly in postmenopausal women, Sertoli-Leydig cell tumors at an average age of 25 years (51), and pure Sertoli cell tumors at an average age of 35 years (50). Bilaterality is more common in cases of endometrioid carcinoma of this type than in those of Sertoli-stromal cell tumors (12 versus 2 percent) (49). Microscopic

examination usually provides the definitive answer. Although glands resembling those of typical endometrioid adenocarcinoma are seen rarely, and then, usually only focally, in Sertoli-stromal cell tumors (9), typical patterns of endometrioid adenocarcinoma are seen additionally in 75 percent of endometrioid carcinomas resembling Sertoli-stromal cell tumors. Intraluminal mucin is much more common and extensive in endometrioid carcinomas than in Sertoli-stromal cell tumors; squamous differentiation is present in 75 percent of endometrioid carcinomas resembling Sertoli-stromal cell tumors but has not been reported in the latter; and an adenofibromatous component has been encountered in three quarters of the cases of endometrioid carcinoma in contrast to its absence in Sertoli cell or Sertoli-Leydig cell tumors. In the rare case in which the differential diagnosis cannot be made immunohistochemical staining may prove decisive. Epithelial membrane antigen can be demonstrated in almost all endometrioid carcinomas but is absent in granulosa cell tumors and is rarely present in Sertoli cells, and then only in isolated cells (1,5). Also, α-inhibin staining is usually positive in Sertoli cells and negative in endometrioid carcinoma cells (54a).

A special problem in differential diagnosis arises when a carcinoma of the ovary is accompanied by a carcinoma of the uterine corpus. This occurrence has been reported in 15 to 20 percent of cases of ovarian cancer, and in the majority of such cases both tumors are of the endometrioid type (12,48,54). In many cases there is strong evidence in favor of synchronous primary neoplasia of both organs or of metastasis from one organ to the other, but in some cases interpretation of the relation of the two tumors is difficult or impossible. The features that favor one or the other, or both sites of origin in cases of synchronous endometrioid carcinomas are presented in Tables 5-1, 5-2, and 5-3. Various investigators (12,33,41a,44,48,54), using some or even most of the criteria listed in these tables, however, have arrived at different conclusions about the frequencies of the three types of association of these tumors. Part of the confusion in the literature is attributable to the choice of cases being analyzed (for example, only those tumors confined to the ovary and uterus versus all the cases, including those with extragenital spread) and part is attributable to the

125

Table 5-1

ENDOMETRIOID TUMORS OF OVARY AND ENDOMETRIUM

Endometrial Primary Ovarian Secondary

1. Histologic similarity of the tumors
2. Large endometrial tumor - small ovarian tumor(s)
3. Atypical endometrial hyperplasia additionally present
4. Deep myometrial invasion
   a. Direct extension into adnexa
   b. Vascular space invasion in myometrium
5. Spread elsewhere in typical pattern of endometrial carcinoma
6. Ovarian tumors bilateral and/or multinodular
7. Hilar location, vascular space invasion, surface implants, or combination in ovary
8. Ovarian endometriosis absent
9. Aneuploidy with similar DNA indices or diploidy of both tumors*
10. Similar molecular genetic or karyotypic abnormalities in both tumors

*The possibility of tumor heterogeneity must be taken into account in the evaluation of the ploidy findings.

Table 5-2

ENDOMETRIOID TUMORS OF OVARY AND ENDOMETRIUM

Ovarian Primary Endometrial Secondary

1. Histologic similarity of the tumors
2. Large ovarian tumor - small endometrial tumor
3. Ovarian endometriosis present
4. Location in ovarian parenchyma
5. Direct extension from ovary predominantly into outer wall of uterus
6. Spread elsewhere in typical pattern of ovarian carcinoma
7. Ovarian tumor unilateral (80 to 90 percent of cases) and forming single mass
8. No atypical hyperplasia in endometrium
9. Aneuploidy with similar DNA indices or diploidy of both tumors*
10. Similar molecular genetic or karyotypic abnormalities in both tumors

*The possibility of tumor heterogeneity must be taken into account in the evaluation of the ploidy findings.

Table 5-3

ENDOMETRIOID TUMORS OF OVARY AND ENDOMETRIUM

Independent Primary Tumors

1. Histologic dissimilarity of the tumors
2. No or only superficial myometrial invasion of endometrial tumor
3. No vascular space invasion of endometrial tumor
4. Atypical endometrial hyperplasia additionally present
5. Absence of other evidence of spread of endometrial tumor
6. Ovarian tumor unilateral (80 to 90 percent of cases)
7. Ovarian tumor located in parenchyma
8. No vascular space invasion, surface implants, or predominant hilar location in ovary
9. Absence of other evidence of spread of ovarian tumor
10. Ovarian endometriosis present
11. Different ploidy or DNA indices, if aneuploid, of the tumors*
12. Dissimilar molecular genetic or karyotypic abnormalities in the tumors

*The possibility of tumor heterogeneity must be taken into account in the evaluation of the ploidy findings.

small size of the various series. The very good prognosis in those cases in which the tumor is confined to both organs (54), however, provides strong evidence that at least in that situation, the neoplasms are independent primary tumors in most cases. When endometrioid carcinomas are confined to the ovary and uterus, the major determinant of prognosis appears to be the depth of invasion of the myometrium (54). If strong evidence favoring any one of the three interpretations of the relation of the two tumors does not exist, the primary site of the tumor should be determined by its initial clinical manifestations according to the staging rules of the International Federation of Gynecology and Obstetrics (FIGO), a scientifically unsatisfying but practical solution for recording purposes.

A final, relatively common problem in the differential diagnosis of endometrioid adenocarcinoma is its distinction from extragenital metastatic carcinomas, particularly those arising in the intestine. This problem is discussed on page 341.

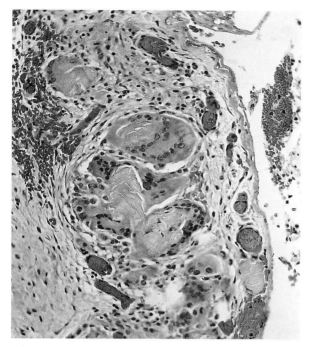

Figure 5-39
FOREIGN BODY GIANT CELL REACTION ON
PERITONEUM ASSOCIATED WITH
ENDOMETRIOID ADENOCARCINOMA WITH
SQUAMOUS DIFFERENTATION OF OVARY

Thin flakes of keratin are surrounded by foreign body giant cells. (Fig. 3 from Kim KR, Scully RE. Peritoneal keratin granulomas with carcinoma of endometrium and ovary and atypical polypoid adenomyoma of endometrium. A clinicopathological analysis of 22 cases. Am J Surg Pathol 1990;14:925–32.)

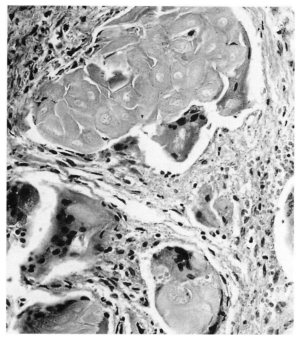

Figure 5-40
FOREIGN BODY GIANT CELL REACTION TO
GHOSTS OF SQUAMOUS CELLS ON
PERITONEUM ASSOCIATED WITH
ENDOMETRIOID ADENOCARCINOMA WITH
SQUAMOUS DIFFERENTIATION OF OVARY

(Fig. 4 from Kim KR, Scully RE. Peritoneal keratin granulomas with carcinoma of endometrium and ovary and atypical polypoid adenomyoma of endometrium. A clinicopathological analysis of 22 cases. Am J Surg Pathol 1990;14:925–32.)

Spread and Metastasis. Endometrioid carcinomas spread in a manner similar to that of ovarian carcinomas in general but their stage distribution differs from that of serous carcinomas. Thirty-one percent of the tumors are stage I; 20 percent, stage II; 38 percent, stage III; and 11 percent, stage IV (31). Peritoneal lesions associated with endometrioid adenocarcinomas with squamous differentiation, as well as endometrial carcinomas of the same histologic type, include, in addition to tumor implants, foreign body granulomas surrounding keratin (fig. 5-39), ghosts of mature squamous cells (fig. 5-40), or both (20). Although the finding of these granulomas should prompt a careful search for viable tumor cells within them or elsewhere on the peritoneum, their presence in the absence of viable-appearing tumor cells does not seem to affect the prognosis adversely. This conclusion, however, is based on only a small number of cases in which the peritoneal lesions had not been treated (20).

Treatment and Prognosis. The treatment of endometrioid carcinomas is similar to that of ovarian epithelial cancers in general (page 39). According to the FIGO annual report the 5-year survival rate of patients with stage I carcinoma is 78 percent; stage II, 63 percent; stage III, 24 percent; and stage IV, 6 percent (31). Kline and coworkers (23) found that the grade of endometrioid carcinoma was of prognostic significance in that patients with grade 1 and 2 tumors had a higher survival rate than those with grade 3 tumors, but there was no difference in the survival of patients with grade 1 and grade 2 tumors. Carey et al. (3), in contrast, found a significant difference in the survival of patients with grade 1 and those with grade 2 tumors, but not of those

127

with grade 2 and those with grade 3 tumors. The WHO method of grading endometrioid carcinomas of the endometrium (40), amplified by Zaino and Kurman (53), deserves a trial for grading endometrioid carcinomas of the ovary in view of its successful use for the former tumors.

TUMORS WITH A SARCOMATOUS COMPONENT

Malignant Mesodermal Mixed Tumors (Carcinosarcomas)

Definition. These tumors are composed of carcinoma of various mullerian types and sarcoma-like tissue, which may be homologous (characterized by tissue types native to the ovary) or heterologous (containing foreign tissue, such as cartilage, skeletal muscle, and osteoid). Although these neoplasms often contain nonendometrioid epithelial or stromal elements they are classified as endometrioid because of their close similarity to their more common counterparts in the endometrium.

General Features. These tumors account for well under 1 percent of all ovarian cancers, with over 250 cases reported in the literature (65,66, 68,72,76,79). They occur in the sixth to eighth decades in three quarters of the cases, and are rare below the age of 40 years. The recent application of immunohistochemical techniques to these neoplasms has renewed interest in their nature. Since their sarcoma-like components can be stained for epithelial antigens, such as various cytokeratins and epithelial membrane antigen, in a high percentage of the cases, a number of investigators have suggested that at least some of these tumors may be metaplastic carcinomas rather than true carcinosarcomas (58,62,64,65, 71,75). This interpretation is supported by the finding of similar immunostaining for p53 in the carcinomatous and sarcoma-like components of 17 uterine malignant mullerian mixed tumors (74) and clonality studies (80). If tumors of all stages are included, ovarian malignant mesodermal mixed tumors are bilateral in about one third of the cases.

Gross Findings. The tumor is typically large, may be predominantly solid or cystic, and commonly contains areas of necrosis and hemorrhage (fig. 5-41). Rarely, it arises within an endometriotic cyst (61,73,77).

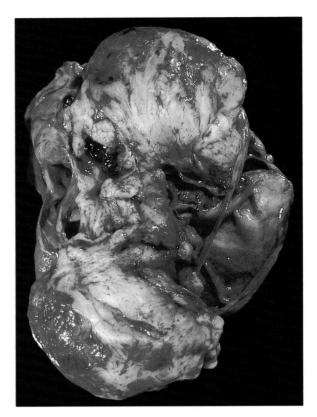

Figure 5-41
MALIGNANT MESODERMAL
MIXED TUMOR OF OVARY
The sectioned surface is composed of solid tissue with areas of necrosis and hemorrhage.

Microscopic Findings. The obviously epithelial component of the malignant mesodermal mixed tumor is most commonly serous, endometrioid, or undifferentiated carcinoma; occasionally, squamous cell or clear cell carcinoma is present, and rarely, mucinous carcinoma (figs. 5-42–5-47). In the homologous form of the tumor, the sarcoma-like component has the appearance of fibrosarcoma, malignant fibrous histiocytoma, a sarcoma with myxoid change, or high-grade endometrial stromal sarcoma (fig. 5-42). The heterologous tumor most commonly contains malignant-appearing cartilage, skeletal muscle, or both (figs. 5-43–5-46), and occasionally malignant-appearing osteoid, bone, or adipose tissue. An unusual but nonspecific feature of malignant mesodermal mixed tumors, which has been reported in half to all the cases, is the presence of hyaline bodies that are periodic acid–Schiff

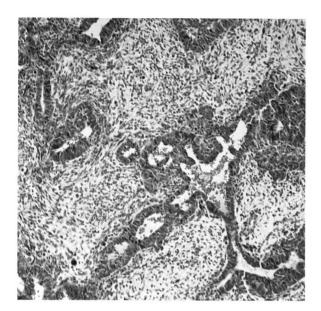

Figure 5-42
MALIGNANT MESODERMAL
MIXED TUMOR, HOMOLOGOUS
Glands and solid aggregates of carcinoma cells are separated by a fibrosarcomatous component.

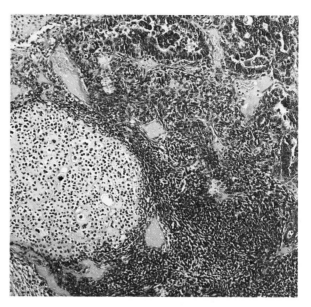

Figure 5-43
MALIGNANT MESODERMAL
MIXED TUMOR, HETEROLOGOUS
Areas of undifferentiated and serous carcinoma form irregular glands; malignant-appearing cartilage is present.

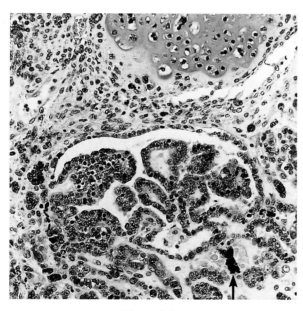

Figure 5-44
MALIGNANT MESODERMAL MIXED
TUMOR, HETEROLOGOUS
Serous papillary adenocarcinoma, malignant cartilage, and undifferentiated sarcoma are evident. A cell with a bizarre nucleus contains intracytoplasmic hyaline bodies (arrow). (Fig. 38 from Serov SF, Scully RE, Sobin LH. Histological typing of ovarian tumours. International Histological Classification of Tumours No. 9. Geneva: World Health Organization, 1973.)

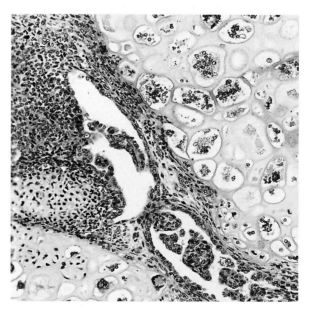

Figure 5-45
MALIGNANT MESODERMAL MIXED
TUMOR, HETEROLOGOUS
The cartilage contains bizarre, hyperchromatic nuclei. (Fig. 39 from Serov SF, Scully RE, Sobin LH. Histological typing of ovarian tumours. International Histological Classification of Tumours No. 9. Geneva: World Health Organization, 1973.)

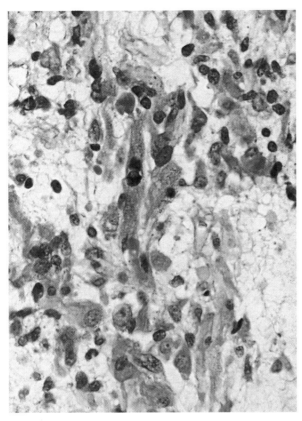

Figure 5-46
MALIGNANT MESODERMAL
MIXED TUMOR, HETEROLOGOUS
Rhabdomyosarcomatous differentiation and hyaline bodies are evident.

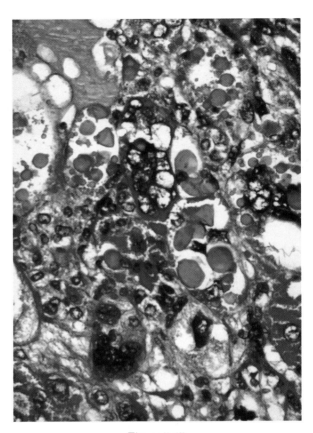

Figure 5-47
MALIGNANT MESODERMAL
MIXED TUMOR
Cells with bizarre nuclei contain numerous hyaline bodies.

(PAS) positive and diastase resistant (fig. 5-47). These structures are more common within the cells of the sarcomatous-appearing component but are also found within the obviously epithelial cells (56,67). Electron microscopic examination reveals a blending of the epithelial and stromal components of the tumor, with areas suggesting a transition between them (64).

Despite the designation of the tumor as mesodermal, nonmesodermal types of tissue have been identified in occasional cases, either in uterine or ovarian tumors of this type or in both. Glial and neuronal differentiation has been reported in both sites (69,70) and staining for chromogranin, neuron-specific enolase, and synaptophysin, alone or in combination, has been described in one sixth of the cases (71). We found islands of well-differentiated hepatic-type cells

in one ovarian specimen. Finally, trophoblastic differentiation (57) and increased levels of alpha-fetoprotein in the serum (59) have been reported in association with these tumors.

Differential Diagnosis. Malignant mesodermal mixed tumors are confused most often with immature teratomas (page 267). The different age incidence of the two tumors is generally the first clue to the differential diagnosis, with immature teratomas occurring predominantly in children and young women and not after the menopause, when most malignant mesodermal mixed tumors occur. Microscopic examination also reveals numerous differences. Immature teratomas typically contain elements derived from all three germ layers, and neuroectodermal tissue is almost always the predominant malignant component; neuroectodermal tissue is rare in malignant mesodermal mixed tumors, and when present, is typically a minor component. The malignant epithelial component of an immature teratoma characteristically appears embryonal and does not resemble a mullerian type of carcinoma, as it does in the malignant mesodermal mixed tumor. Finally, the cartilage in an immature teratoma has an immature or mature appearance with uniform nuclei in contrast to the highly atypical-appearing cartilage characteristic of a malignant mesodermal mixed tumor. Immunohistochemical staining for neuroendocrine cells, which are almost always demonstrable in immature teratomas and are much less common in malignant mesodermal mixed tumors, is another differential feature (60).

Other tumors that enter the differential diagnosis less frequently are moderately and poorly differentiated Sertoli-Leydig cell tumors, with or without heterologous elements, and endometrioid stromal sarcomas containing sex cord–like elements. Typically, better differentiated, more readily diagnosable areas are found focally in less differentiated Sertoli-Leydig cell tumors, which almost always occur in young women and are commonly virilizing. Also, the latter tumors rarely have epithelial components resembling mullerian-type carcinomas except for the heterologous form, which contains mucinous epithelium that usually appears benign or borderline, and the retiform type, which occurs in a much younger age group (average age, 15 years) and almost always contains more diagnostic areas. In a difficult case, staining for epithelial membrane antigen is useful because it is almost always demonstrable in malignant mesodermal mixed tumors, but only rarely and then in only a few Sertoli cells in Sertoli-Leydig cell tumors (55,63). Endometrioid stromal sarcomas with sex cord–like differentiation are better differentiated than malignant mesodermal mixed tumors, and the sex cord–like elements have a greater resemblance to the sex cord components of sex cord–stromal tumors than to the mullerian epithelial components of malignant mesodermal mixed tumors.

Finally, malignant mesodermal mixed tumors must be distinguished from carcinomas that contain an unusually cellular stroma with mitotic activity and sarcomatoid carcinomas. We diagnose malignant mesodermal mixed tumor when the stromal component has features that if seen in

pure form would warrant a diagnosis of sarcoma. In some cases it may be difficult to distinguish between a cellular stroma and a malignant stromal component, and such cases, as well as rare cases in which an ovarian primary tumor appears to be a pure carcinoma but metastasizes as a malignant mesodermal mixed tumor, suggest the existence of a spectrum of tumors ranging from pure carcinomas with a cellular stroma to malignant mesodermal mixed tumors. We diagnose sarcomatoid carcinoma when the sarcoma-like elements blend with obvious carcinomatous elements throughout the tumor in contrast to the sharp demarcation between the two components that is seen, at least focally, in the malignant mesodermal mixed tumor. This distinction may be more apparent than real if the latter tumor is a metaplastic carcinoma and may have little or no significance as far as prognosis and therapy are concerned.

Spread, Metastasis, and Prognosis. Over 90 percent of these tumors have spread beyond the ovary at the time of diagnosis, with 60 percent, stage III and 10 percent, stage IV (72,76). The metastatic deposits most commonly contain both carcinomatous and sarcoma-like components but may be purely sarcomatoid or purely carcinomatous. The prognosis is very poor but an occasional patient survives more than 5 years after removal of the tumor and combination chemotherapy (78).

Adenosarcoma

Definition. This tumor is composed of glands lined by one or more forms of benign-appearing or atypical mullerian-type epithelium, and a predominant sarcomatous component, which may have an endometrial-stromal or cellular fibromatous appearance and occasionally contains heterologous elements.

General Features. Twelve of the 14 reported examples have occurred in patients in the fifth and sixth decades (81,83–85). A history of radiation therapy for endometriosis was obtained in one case (81). Occasionally, a separate primary adenosarcoma arises in the uterus or in extraovarian endometriosis.

Gross Findings. The tumor was unilateral in the reported cases. It may be predominantly solid or cystic, with the solid tissue usually firm but occasionally soft, depending on its cellularity (fig. 5-48).

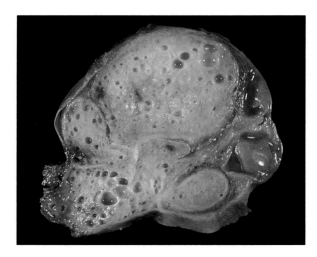

Figure 5-48
ADENOSARCOMA
The tumor is predominantly solid, and contains scattered small cysts.

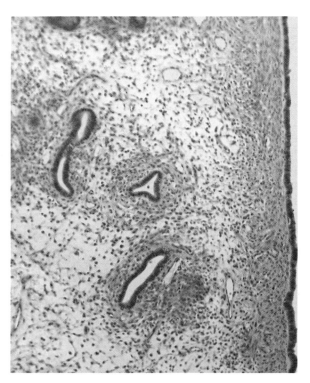

Figure 5-49
ADENOSARCOMA
Several glands are cuffed by stromal cells; most of the stromal component is edematous and hypocellular.

Microscopic Findings. The stromal component of the tumor may have the appearance of a cellular fibroma, low-grade fibrosarcoma, or low-grade endometrial stromal sarcoma, and typically is most cellular adjacent to the glands, forming cuffs around them (figs. 5-49, 5-50). When the glands become cystic polypoid projections of stroma into the lumens are often present (fig. 5-51). The stroma, which is typically cellular (fig. 5-51), may be hypocellular and densely fibrous or edematous in some areas, particularly away from the glands. The mitotic rate of the stromal cells ranges from 2 to over 40 per 10 high-power fields (fig. 5-52); varying degrees of stromal nuclear atypia may be present. The glandular epithelium is of various mullerian types, such as endometrioid, serous, mucinous, or clear cell. Heterologous elements are occasionally present in the stromal component. The epithelium may exhibit varying degrees of nuclear atypia, occasionally fulfilling the criteria for carcinoma in situ.

Differential Diagnosis. Adenosarcomas must be differentiated from adenofibromas and endometriosis that forms endometrial polyp–like masses (polypoid endometriosis) (86). The latter lesions are not characterized by the intracystic polypoid projections of cellular stroma, periglandular cuffing, mitotic activity, and nuclear atypia of typical adenosarcomas. Because of the paucity of reported cases the criteria for distinguishing between adenosarcomas and these benign lesions in difficult cases are not well established. On the basis of our experience with uterine adenosarcomas (82), however, we diagnose ovarian adenosarcoma if the stroma is unusually cellular, if there is more than minimal stromal-nuclear atypia, or if the mitotic count is 2 or greater per 10 high-power fields.

Spread and Metastasis. Adenosarcomas have spread beyond the ovary into the pelvis, abdomen, or both in about half of the cases (84). The treatment is primarily surgical although radiation therapy and multiagent chemotherapy have been used successfully in some cases (83).

Endometrioid Stromal Sarcoma

Definition. This tumor is characterized by an invasive proliferation of cells that resemble the stromal cells of a normal proliferative endometrium.

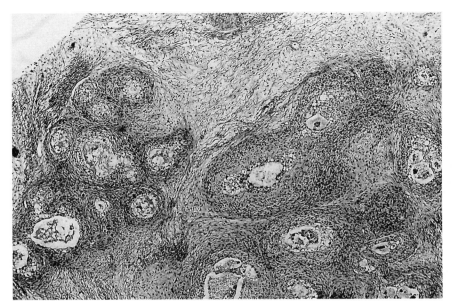

Figure 5-50
ADENOSARCOMA
There is striking periepithelial cuffing by sarcoma cells. The epithelial element in this tumor had the appearance of clear cell carcinoma in situ.

Figure 5-51
ADENOSARCOMA
The glands are of irregular shape with polypoid extensions of highly cellular stroma into the lumens. (Fig. 1 from Clement PB, Scully RE. Extrauterine mesodermal (müllerian) adenosarcoma. A clinicopathologic analysis of five cases. Am J Clin Pathol 1978; 69:276–83.)

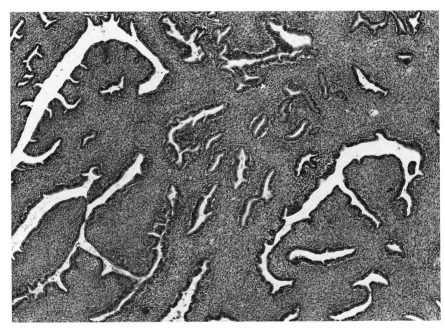

General Features. Approximately 45 cases of endometrioid stromal sarcoma involving the ovary have been reported (87–91). At least 40 percent of them have been contiguous with areas of endometriosis (87,90) and approximately 30 percent have been accompanied by a similar tumor in the uterus (91). The latter association raises the question whether some of the ovarian tumors were metastatic from the uterus (92) (page 361). Slightly over half the tumors have been diagnosed in women in the fifth and sixth decades, with an age range of 11 to 76 years.

Gross Findings. Seventy percent of the tumors are unilateral. Most of them are solid, but a substantial number are both solid and cystic, and occasional tumors are predominantly cystic.

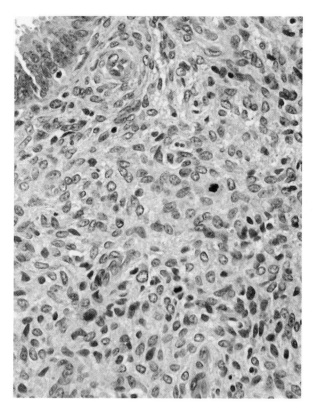

Figure 5-52
ADENOSARCOMA
Mitotic figures are present in the highly cellular stroma of the tumor depicted in figure 5-51.

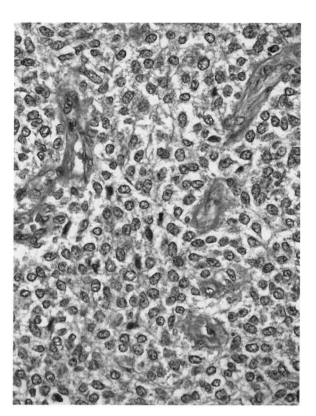

Figure 5-53
ENDOMETRIOID STROMAL SARCOMA
This well-differentiated tumor is composed of cells with small rounded nuclei. Numerous arterioles resembling the spiral arteries of the late secretory endometrium are a characteristic feature.

The solid areas are tan or yellow-white, often containing areas of necrosis or hemorrhage. The cysts range up to 15 cm in diameter, and most of them contain bloody fluid.

Microscopic Findings. Microscopic examination typically reveals a diffuse proliferation of small cells with scanty cytoplasm and round to oval nuclei, resembling endometrial stromal cells to varying degrees. A characteristic feature is the presence of numerous small arteries resembling the spiral arteries of the normal late secretory endometrium (fig. 5-53). Foam cells laden with lipid, presumably of endometrioid stromal cell origin, may be distributed throughout the tumor, singly and in small groups. The tumor may be intersected by fibrous bands, and hyaline plaques may be scattered throughout it.

A common feature of the ovarian endometrioid stromal sarcoma, which is only rarely shared by the uterine tumor of the same type, is a transi-tion to tissue indistinguishable from an ovarian fibroma (fig. 5-54). Like uterine endometrial stromal sarcomas, the ovarian tumors contain, in up to one third of the cases, cords and nests of cells and small tubules resembling those seen in sex cord–stromal tumors of the ovary (figs. 5-55, 5-56) (91). Less often, these tumors contain occasional benign-appearing endometrioid glands (88). Mitotic activity ranges from less than 1 to over 30 figures per 10 high-power fields. Some investigators (91) have divided endometrioid stromal sarcomas into low-grade and high-grade forms, depending on whether the mitotic count is less or greater than 10 per 10 high-power fields. Reticulin staining discloses individual investment of the tumor cells by fibrils (fig. 5-57); staining for lipid may reveal large numbers of fine droplets in the tumor cells as well as in the scattered foam cells

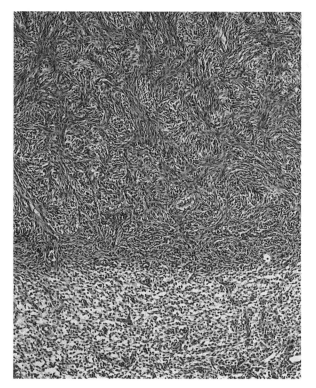

Figure 5-54
ENDOMETRIOID STROMAL SARCOMA
The tumor appears typical in the lower third of the figure and has the appearance of a fibroma in the upper two thirds. (Fig. 6 from Young RH, Prat J, Scully RE. Endometrioid stromal sarcomas of the ovary. A clinicopathological analysis of twenty-three cases. Cancer 1984;53:1143–55.)

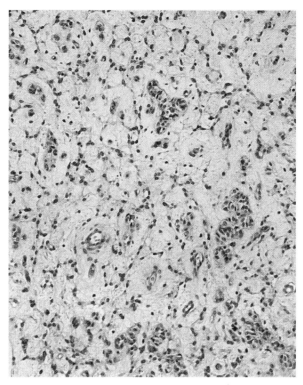

Figure 5-55
ENDOMETRIOID STROMAL SARCOMA WITH
SEX CORD–LIKE DIFFERENTIATION
The tumor is hypocellular with more edema than usual. Small clusters of epithelial-like cells suggesting sex cord elements are scattered within the tumor.

in some of the cases. A transition between the tumor and endometriosis is often seen.

Differential Diagnosis. Endometrioid stromal sarcomas may be confused with other small cell tumors of the ovary (Table 5-4), particularly the diffuse adult granulosa cell tumor. The lack of endocrine manifestations, the more frequent bilaterality, the presence of many small arteries throughout the tumor, the individual investment of tumor cells by reticulin fibrils, the tongue-like pattern of infiltration, particularly outside the ovary (fig. 5-58), and a lack of staining for α-inhibin (54a) are helpful in identifying the tumor as a stromal sarcoma. The foam cells that may be present are distinguishable from Leydig or lutein cells by their content of fine lipid vacuoles and their usually eccentric nuclei, which lack prominent nucleoli. The sex cord–like elements within a tumor of this type, which are usually a

minor component, differ from granulosa cell aggregates in a granulosa cell tumor by generally lacking the pale, often grooved nuclei of granulosa cells and from the Sertoli cell components of a Sertoli-Leydig cell tumor by lacking their distinctive patterns (page 206). The differentiation of the endometrioid stroma sarcoma with sex cord–like differentiation from the malignant mesodermal mixed tumor has been discussed on page 131.

The endometrioid stromal sarcoma has occasionally been confused with stromal hyperplasia or an ovarian fibroma or thecoma. Stromal hyperplasia is rarely associated with significant ovarian enlargement and lacks the marked cellularity, arterial content, and resemblance to endometrial stroma that are characteristic of endometrioid stromal sarcoma. Evidence of estrogenic manifestations and the lipid-rich cytoplasm and α-inhibin

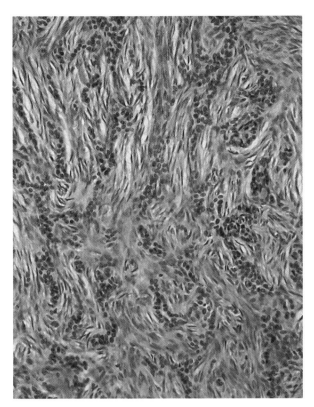

Figure 5-56
ENDOMETRIOID STROMAL SARCOMA
WITH SEX CORD–LIKE DIFFERENTIATION

Thin trabeculae composed of epithelial-like cells lie within a fibromatous endometrioid stromal component. (Fig. 9 from Young RH, Prat J, Scully RE. Endometrioid stromal sarcomas of the ovary. A clinicopathological analysis of twenty-three cases. Cancer 1984;53:1143–55.)

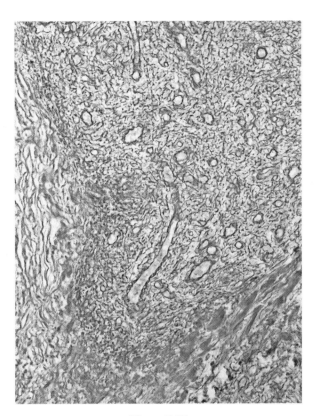

Figure 5-57
ENDOMETRIOID STROMAL SARCOMA,
RETICULIN STAIN
Fibrils envelop individual tumor cells.

staining of the tumor cells of a thecoma are lacking in the endometrioid stromal sarcoma (54a). Although fibromatous areas may be present in an endometrioid stromal sarcoma, the more cellular areas mimicking normal endometrial stroma with spiral arteries are absent in a fibroma.

The most difficult problem in differential diagnosis exists in cases in which an endometrioid stromal sarcoma of the ovary is associated with a similar tumor in the uterus; the latter has been diagnosed from 30 years before to 6 years after the discovery of the ovarian tumor (91). One has to apply general principles of pathology, particularly evaluating features that are helpful in general in differentiating primary and metastatic tumors of the ovary (see chapter 18) to determine whether this combination of neoplasms reflects

metastasis from one organ to the other or independent primary neoplasia. The most telling argument for an ovarian origin in such cases is continuity with endometriosis. The length of the interval between the discovery of the ovarian and the uterine tumors has to be considered in determining the primary or metastatic nature of the ovarian tumor, but with the realization that low-grade endometrial stromal sarcoma is well known for its indolent behavior and frequent late recurrence. The relative sizes of the uterine and ovarian tumors, their extent, and the presence or absence of vascular space invasion are helpful in determining whether they are independent primary tumors or reflect interorgan metastasis. Needless to say, it is important to review the uterine pathology of any patient with an endometrioid stromal tumor of the ovary who has had a prior hysterectomy; if a hysterectomy has not been performed, it may be impossible to

Table 5-4

TUMORS THAT MAY APPEAR IN OVARY AS SMALL ROUND CELL TUMORS

Primary Tumors
   Small cell carcinoma, hypercalcemic type
   Small cell carcinoma, pulmonary type
   Undifferentiated carcinoma
   Adult granulosa cell tumor
   Sertoli-Leydig cell tumor of intermediate and poor
      differentiation
   Endometrioid stromal sarcoma
   Malignant melanoma
   Small cell primitive neuroectodermal tumors
   Embryonal rhabdomyosarcoma

Metastatic Tumors
   Lymphoma; leukemia
   Small cell carcinomas, pulmonary type
   Endometrial stromal sarcoma
   Merkel cell tumor
   Malignant melanoma
   Desmoplastic small round cell tumor with
      divergent differentiation
   Alveolar and embryonal rhabdomyosarcoma
   Ewing's sarcoma
   Neuroblastoma
   Others, rarely or not yet reported

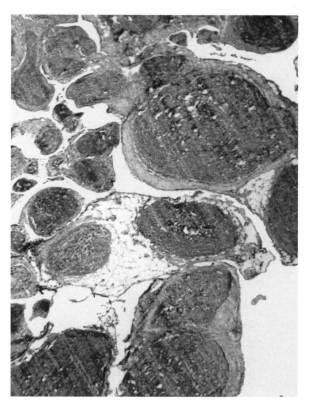

Figure 5-58
ENDOMETRIOID STROMAL SARCOMA,
METASTATIC TO OMENTUM
The tumor has grown in cellular nodules and tongues.

exclude the simultaneous presence of a uterine sarcoma. Chang et al. (88) regard as certainly primary only those cases in which the tumor is confined to the ovary, and the uterus has been shown to be free of tumor on pathologic examination; we, however, accept additionally continuity with ovarian endometriosis as evidence of an ovarian origin.

Spread and Metastasis. Approximately 75 percent of endometrioid stromal sarcomas have spread beyond the ovary at the time of exploration, either to the pelvis or the upper abdomen or both, and a rare tumor has already spread distantly, most commonly to the lung.

Treatment and Prognosis. The primary treatment of endometrioid stromal sarcoma is surgical removal of the neoplasm. Optimally, a hysterectomy and bilateral salpingo-oophorectomy should be performed because of the frequency of both bilaterality and uterine involvement, which may not be obvious either preoperatively or at the time of operation. There is suggestive evidence that, like uterine tumors of the same type, the ovarian tumors, especially if they are low grade, may respond to progesterone administration. Radiation therapy may be effective for the treatment of local disease; the role of chemotherapy remains unsettled. Follow-up studies indicate that low-grade endometrioid stromal sarcoma is often curable for limited periods but may be fatal after 10 or more postoperative years; long-term follow-up of a significant number of patients, however, is not available to evaluate the ultimate prognosis. High-grade tumors in a small series of cases appeared to be associated with a rapid course and a poor prognosis (91).

REFERENCES

Endometrioid Tumors in General and Epithelial Tumors

1. Aguirre P, Thor AD, Scully RE. Ovarian endometrioid carcinomas resembling sex cord-stromal tumors. An immunohistochemical study. Int J Gynecol Pathol 1989;8:364–73.

2. Bell DA, Scully RE. Atypical and borderline endometrioid adenofibromas of the ovary. A report of 27 cases. Am J Surg Pathol 1985;9:205–14.

3. Carey MS, Dembo AJ, Simm JE, Fyler AW, Treger T, Bush RS. Testing the validity of a prognostic classification in patients with surgically optimal ovarian carcinoma: a 15-year review. Int J Gynecol Cancer 1993;3:24–35.

4. Clement PB, Young RH, Scully RE. Endometrioid-like variant of ovarian yolk-sac tumor: a clinicopathological analysis of eight cases. Am J Surg Pathol 1987;11:767–78.

5. Costa MJ, Morris R, DeRose P, et al. Utility of immunohistochemistry in distinguishing ovarian Sertoli-stromal cell tumors from carcinosarcomas. Hum Pathol 1992;23:787–97.

6. Czernobilsky B. Endometrioid neoplasia of the ovary: a reappraisal. Int J Gynecol Pathol 1982;1:203–10.

7. Czernobilsky B, Silverman BB, Mikuta JJ. Endometrioid carcinoma of the ovary. A clinicopathologic study of 75 cases. Cancer 1970;26:1141–52.

8. Daly MB. The epidemiology of ovarian cancer. In: Ozols RF, ed. Ovarian cancer. Hematology/oncology clinics of North America. Philadelphia: WB Saunders, 1992;6:729–38.

9. Dardi LE, Miller AW, Gould VE. Sertoli-Leydig cell tumor with endometrioid differentiation. Case report and discussion of histogenesis. Diagn Gynecol Obstet 1982;4:227–34.

10. Daya D, Young RH, Scully RE. Endometrioid carcinoma of the fallopian tube resembling an adnexal tumor of probable wolffian origin. A report of six cases. Int J Gynecol Pathol 1992;11:122–30.

11. DePriest PD, Banks ER, Powell DE, et al. Endometrioid carcinoma of the ovary and endometriosis: the association in postmenopausal women. Gynecol Oncol 1992;47:71–5.

11a. Eichhorn JH, Lawrence WD, Young RH, Scully RE. Ovarian neuroendocrine carcinomas of non-small-cell type associated with surface epithelial adenocarcinomas. A study of five cases and review of the literature. Int J Gynecol Pathol 1996;15:303–14.

11b. Eichhorn JH, Scully RE. Endometrioid ciliated-cell tumors of the ovary: a report of five cases. Int J Gynecol Pathol 1996;15:248–56.

11c. Eichhorn JH, Young RH, Scully RE. Primary ovarian small cell carcinoma of pulmonary type. A clinicopathologic, immunohistologic, and flow cytometric analysis of 11 cases. Am J Surg Pathol 1992;16:926–38.

12. Eifel P, Hendrickson M, Ross J, Ballon S, Martinez A, Kempson R. Simultaneous presentation of carcinoma involving the ovary and the uterine corpus. Cancer 1982;50:163–70.

13. Fu YS, Stock RJ, Reagan JW, Storaasli JP, Wentz WB. Significance of squamous component in endometrioid carcinoma of the ovary. Cancer 1979;44:614–21.

13a. Fukunaga M, Nomura K, Ishikawa E, Ushigome S. Ovarian atypical endometriosis: its close association with malignant epithelial tumors. Histopathology 1997;30:249–55.

14. Gadducci A, Ferdeghini M, Prontera C, et al. The concomitant determination of different tumor markers in patients with epithelial ovarian cancer and benign ovarian masses: relevance of differential diagnosis. Gynecol Oncol 1992;44:147–54.

15. Heaps JM, Nieberg RK, Berek JS. Malignant neoplasms arising in endometriosis. Obstet Gynecol 1990;75:1023–8.

16. Hendrickson MR, Kempson RL. Ciliated carcinomas—a variant of endometrial adenocarcinoma: a report of 10 cases. Int J Gynecol Pathol 1983;2:1–12.

17. Hughesdon PE. Benign endometrioid tumours of the ovary and the müllerian concept of ovarian epithelial tumours. Histopathology 1984;8:977–90.

18. Katsube Y, Berg JW, Silverberg SG. Epidemiologic pathology of ovarian tumors: a histopathologic review of primary ovarian neoplasms diagnosed in the Denver standard metropolitan statistical area, 1 July 31—December 1969 and 1 July 31—December 1979. Int J Gynecol Pathol 1982;1:3–16.

19. Kempson RL, Hendrickson MR. Miscellaneous types of surface epithelial neoplasms. The well-differentiated end of the morphologic spectrum of endometrioid, clear cell, and Brenner tumors and mixed epithelial tumors of low malignant potential of mullerian type. State of the art reviews: pathology. Philadelphia, Hanley & Belfus, 1993;1:335–65.

20. Kim KR, Scully RE. Peritoneal keratin granulomas with carcinomas of endometrium and ovary and atypical polypoid adenomyoma of endometrium. A clinicopathological analysis of 22 cases. Am J Surg Pathol 1990;14:925–32.

21. Kleinman GM, Young RH, Scully RE. Primary neuroectodermal tumors of the ovary. A report of 25 cases. Am J Surg Pathol 1993;17:764–78.

22. Klemi PJ, Grönroos M. Endometrioid carcinoma of the ovary. A clinicopathologic, histochemical and electron microscopic study. Obstet Gynecol 1979;53:572–9.

23. Kline RC, Wharton JT, Atkinson EN, Burke TW, Gershenson DM, Edwards CL. Endometrioid carcinoma of the ovary: retrospective review of 145 cases. Gynecol Oncol 1990;39:337–46.

24. Koonings PP, Campbell K, Mishell DR Jr, Grimes DA. Relative frequency of primary ovarian neoplasms: a 10-year review. Obstet Gynecol 1989;74:921–6.

25. Leake J, Woolas RP, Daniel J, Oram DH, Brown CL. Immunohistochemical and serological expression of CA 125: a clinicopathological study of 40 malignant ovarian epithelial tumours. Histopathology 1994;24:57–64.

26. Liu WM, Chen CJ, Kan YY, Chao KC, Yuan CC, Ng HT. Simultaneous endometrioid carcinoma of the uterine corpus and ovary. Clin Med J (Taipei) 1989;44:38–44.

27. Moll R, Pitz S, Levy R, Weikel W, Franke WW, Czernobilsky B. Complexity of expression of intermediate filament proteins, including glial filament protein, in endometrial and ovarian adenocarcinomas. Hum Pathol 1991;22:989–1001.

28. Mostoufizadeh M, Scully RE. Malignant tumors arising in endometriosis. Clin Obstet Gynecol 1980;23:951–63.

29. Nilbert M, Pejovic T, Mandahl N, Iosif S, Willén H, Mitelman F. Monoclonal origin of endometriotic cysts. Int J Gynecol Cancer 1995;5:61–3.

29a. Nogales FF, Bergeron C, Carvia RE, Alvaro T, Fulwood HR. Ovarian endometrioid tumors with yolk sac tumor component, an unusual form of ovarian neoplasm. Analysis of six cases. Am J Surg Pathol 1996;10:1056–66.

30. Norris HJ. Proliferative endometrioid tumors and endometrioid tumors of low malignant potential of the ovary. Int J Gynecol Pathol 1993;12:134–40.

31. Pettersson F. Annual report of the results of treatment in gynecological cancer. Stockholm, International Federation of Gynecology and Obstetrics, 1991.

32. Pitman MB, Young RH, Clement PB, Dickersin GR, Scully RE. Oxyphilic endometrioid carcinoma of the ovary and endometrium: a report of nine cases. Int J Gynecol Pathol 1994;13:290–301.

33. Prat J, Matias-Guiu X, Barreto J. Simultaneous carcinoma involving the endometrium and the ovary. A clinicopathologic, immunohistochemical, and DNA flow cytometric study of 18 cases. Cancer 1991;68:2455–9.

34. Roth LM, Czernobilsky B, Langley FA. Ovarian endometrioid adenofibromatous and cystadenofibromatous tumors: benign, proliferating, and malignant. Cancer 1981;48:1838–45.

35. Roth LM, Liban E, Czernobilsky B. Ovarian endometrioid tumors mimicking Sertoli and Sertoli-Leydig cell tumors. Sertoliform variant of endometrioid carcinoma. Cancer 1982;50:1322–31.

36. Russell P. The pathological assessment of ovarian neoplasms: I: introduction to the common 'epithelial' tumours and analysis of benign 'epithelial' tumours. Pathology 1979;11:5–26.

37. Russell P, Bannatyne P. Surgical pathology of the ovaries. Edinburgh: Churchill Livingstone, 1989.

38. Rutgers JL, Young RH, Scully RE. Ovarian yolk sac tumor arising from an endometrioid carcinoma. Hum Pathol 1987;18:1296–9.

39. Scully RE, Bell DA, Abu-Jawdeh GM. Update on early ovarian cancer and cancer developing in benign ovarian tumors. In: Mason P, Sharp F, Blackett T, Berek J, eds. Ovarian cancer, biological and therapeutic challenges. London: Chapman and Hall, 1994:139–44.

40. Scully RE, Bonfiglio TA, Kurman RJ, Silverberg SG, Wilkinson EJ. World Health Organization histological classification of tumours. Histological typing of female genital tract tumours, 2nd ed. Berlin: Springer-Verlag. 1994.

41. Seidman JD. Prognostic importance of hyperplasia and atypia in endometriosis. Int J Gynecol Pathol 1996;15:1–9.

41a. Shenson DL, Gallion HH, Powell DE, Pieretti M. Loss of heterozygosity and genomic instability in synchronous endometrioid tumors of the ovary and endometrium. Cancer 1995;76:650–7.

42. Snyder RR, Norris HJ, Tavassoli F. Endometrioid proliferative and low malignant potential tumors of the ovary. A clinicopathologic study of 46 cases. Am J Surg Pathol 1988;12:661–71.

43. Stalsberg H, Blom PE, Bostad LH, Westgaard G. Ovarian tumours and endometriosis in Norway General Hospital material. In: Stalsberg H, ed. An international survey of distributions of histologic types of tumours of the testis and ovary. UICC technical report series. Geneva: UICC, 1983;75:307–12.

44. Symonds DA, Johnson DP, Wheeless CR Jr. Feulgen cytometry in simultaneous endometrial and ovarian carcinoma. Cancer 1988;61:2511–6.

45. Tavassoli FA, Andrade R, Merino M. Retiform wolffian adenoma. In: Fenoglio-Preiser CM, Wolffe M, Rilke F, eds. Progress in surgical pathology, vol. XI. New York: Field and Wood Medical Publishers, 1990:121–36.

46. Tornos C, Silva EG, Ordonez NG, Gershenson DM, Young RH, Scully RE. Endometrioid carcinoma of the ovary with a prominent spindle-cell component, a source of diagnostic confusion. A report of 14 cases. Am J Surg Pathol 1995;19:1343–53.

47. Ueda G, Yamasaki M, Inoue M, et al. Argyrophil cells in the endometrioid carcinoma of the ovary. Cancer 1984;54:1569–73.

48. Ulbright TM, Roth LM. Metastatic and independent cancers of the endometrium and ovary: a clinicopathologic study of 34 cases. Hum Pathol 1985;16:28–34.

49. Young RH, Prat J, Scully RE. Ovarian endometrioid carcinomas resembling sex-cord stromal tumors. A clinicopathological analysis of 13 cases. Am J Surg Pathol 1982;6:513–22.

50. Young RH, Scully RE. Ovarian Sertoli cell tumors. A report of ten cases. Int J Gynecol Pathol 1984;2:349–63.

51. Young RH, Scully RE. Ovarian Sertoli-Leydig cell tumors. A clinicopathological analysis of 207 cases. Am J Surg Pathol 1985;9:543–69.

52. Young RH, Scully RE. Ovarian tumors of probable wolffian origin. A report of 11 cases. Am J Surg Pathol 1983;7:125–35.

53. Zaino RJ, Kurman RJ, Diana KL, Morrow CP. The utility of the revised International Federation of Gynecology and Obstetrics histologic grading of endometrial adenocarcinoma using a defined nuclear grading system. A Gynecologic Oncology Group study. Cancer 1995;75:81–6.

54. Zaino RJ, Unger ER, Whitney C. Synchronous carcinomas of the uterine corpus and ovary. Gynecol Oncol 1984;19:329–35.

54a. Zheng W, Sung CJ, Hanna I, et al. α and β subunits of inhibin/activin as sex cord-stromal differentiation markers. Int J Gynecol Pathol 1997;16:263–71.

Malignant Mesodermal Mixed Tumor

55. Aguirre P, Thor AD, Scully RE. Ovarian endometrioid carcinomas resembling sex cord-stromal tumors. An immunohistochemical study. Int J Gynecol Pathol 1989;8:364–73.

56. Al-Nafussi AI, Hughes DE, Williams AR. Hyaline globules in ovarian tumours. Histopathology 1993;23:563–6.

57. Barua R, Richmond D. Trophoblastic differentiation in a malignant mixed mesodermal tumor of the ovary. Hum Pathol 1988;19:1235–6.

58. Bitterman P, Chun B, Kurman RJ. The significance of epithelial differentiation in mixed mesodermal tumors of the uterus. A clinicopathologic and immunohistochemical study. Am J Surg Pathol 1990:14:317–28.

59. Blumenfeld Z, Kerner H, Thaler I, Deutsch M, Beck D. Increased alpha-fetoprotein levels in mixed mesodermal tumor of the ovary. Gynecol Obstet Invest 1984;17:169–73.

60. Calame JJ, Schaberg A. Solid teratomas and mixed müllerian tumors of the ovary: a clinical, histological, and immunocytochemical comparative study. Gynecol Oncol 1989;33:212–21.

61. Cooper P. Mixed mesodermal tumor and clear cell carcinoma arising in ovarian endometriosis. Cancer 1978;42:2827–31.
62. Costa MJ, Khan R, Judd R. Carcinosarcoma (malignant mixed müllerian [mesodermal] tumor) of the uterus and ovary. Correlation of clinical, pathologic, and immunohistochemical features in 29 cases. Arch Pathol Lab Med 1991;115:583–90.
63. Costa MJ, Morris RJ, Wilson R, Judd R. Utility of immunohistochemistry in distinguishing ovarian Sertoli-stromal cell tumors from carcinosarcomas. Hum Pathol 1992;23:787–97.
64. DeBrito PA, Silverberg SG, Orenstein JM. Carcinosarcoma (malignant mixed müllerian [mesodermal] tumor) of the female genital tract: immunohistochemical and ultrastructural analysis of 28 cases. Hum Pathol 1993;24:132–42.
65. Dellers EA, Valente PT, Edmonds PR, Balsara G. Extrauterine mixed mesodermal tumors. An immunohistochemical study. Arch Pathol Lab Med 1991;115:918–20.
66. Dictor M. Malignant mixed mesodermal tumor of the ovary: a report of 22 cases. Obstet Gynecol 1985;65:720–4.
67. Dictor M. Ovarian malignant mixed mesodermal tumor: the occurrence of hyaline droplets containing α-1-antitrypsin. Hum Pathol 1982;13:930–3.
68. Dinh TV, Slavin RE, Bhagavan BS, Hannigan EV, Tiamson EM, Yandell RB. Mixed mesodermal tumors of the ovary: a clinicopathologic study of 14 cases. Obstet Gynecol 1988;72:409–12.
69. Ehrmann RL, Weidner N, Welch WR, Gleiberman I. Malignant mixed müllerian tumor of the ovary with prominent neuroectodermal differentiation (teratoid carcinosarcoma). Int J Gynecol Pathol 1990;9:272–82.
70. Fetissof F, Arbeille B, Lansac J, Lhuintre Y. Tumeur mixte mésodermique maligne de l'ovaire avec contingent neuro-ectodermique. Ann Pathol 1989;9:204–8.
71. George E, Manivel JC, Dehner LP, Wick MR. Malignant mixed müllerian tumors: an immunohistochemical study of 47 cases, with histogenetic considerations and clinical correlation. Hum Pathol 1991;22:215–23.
72. Hanjani P, Petersen RO, Lipton SE, Nolte SA. Malignant mixed mesodermal tumors and carcinosarcoma of the ovary: report of eight cases and review of literature. Obstet Gynecol Surv 1983;38:537–45.
73. Marchevsky AM, Kaneko M. Bilateral ovarian endometriosis associated with carcinosarcoma of the right ovary and endometrioid carcinoma of the left ovary. Am J Clin Pathol 1978;70:709–12.
74. Mayall F, Rutty K, Campbell F, Goddard H. p53 immunostaining suggests that uterine carcinosarcomas are monoclonal. Histopathology 1994;24:211–4.
75. Meis JM, Lawrence WD. The immunohistochemical profile of malignant mixed müllerian tumor. Overlap with endometrial adenocarcinoma. Am J Clin Pathol 1990;94:1–7.
76. Morrow CP, d'Ablaing G, Brady LW, Blessing JA, Hreshchyshyn MM. A clinical and pathologic study of 30 cases of malignant mixed mullerian epithelial and mesenchymal ovarian tumors: a Gynecologic Oncology Group study. Gynecol Oncol 1984;18:278–92.
77. Mostoufizadeh M, Scully RE. Malignant tumors arising in endometriosis. Clin Obstet Gynecol 1980;23:951–63.
78. Prendiville J, Murphy D, Renninson J, Buckley H, Crowther D. Carcinosarcoma of the ovary treated over a 10-year period at the Christie Hospital. Int J Gynecol Cancer 1994;4:200–5.
79. Terada KY, Johnson TL, Hopkins M, Roberts JA. Clinicopathologic features of ovarian mixed mesodermal tumors and carcinosarcomas. Gynecol Oncol 1989;32:228–32.
80. Thompson L, Chang B, Barsky SH. Monoclonal origins of malignant mixed tumors (carcinosarcomas). Evidence for a divergent histogenesis. Am J Surg Pathol 1996;20:277–85.

Adenosarcoma

81. Clement PB, Scully RE. Extrauterine mesodermal (müllerian) adenosarcoma: a clinicopathologic analysis of five cases. Am J Clin Pathol 1978;69:276–83.
82. Clement PB, Scully RE. Mullerian adenosarcoma of the uterus: a clinicopathological analysis of 100 cases with a review of the literature. Hum Pathol 1990;21:363–81.
83. Czernobilsky B, Gillespie JJ, Roth LM. Adenosarcoma of the ovary. A light- and electron-microscopic study with review of the literature. Diag Gynecol Obstet 1982;4:25–36.
84. Dellers EA, Valente PT, Edmonds PR, Balsara G. Extrauterine mixed mesodermal tumor. An immunohistochemical study. Arch Pathol Lab Med 1991;115:918–20.
84a. Fukunaga M, Nomura K, Endo Y, Ushigome A, Aizawa S. Ovarian adenosarcoma. Histopathology 1997;30:283–7.
85. Kao GF, Norris HJ. Benign and low grade variants of mixed mesodermal tumor (adenosarcoma) of the ovary and adnexal region. Cancer 1978;42:1314–24.
86. Mostoufizadeh M, Scully RE. Malignant tumors arising in endometriosis. Clin Obstet Gynecol 1980;23:951–63.

Endometrioid Stromal Sarcoma

87. Baiocchi G, Kavanagh JJ, Wharton JT. Endometrioid stromal sarcomas arising from ovarian and extraovarian endometriosis: report of two cases and review of the literature. Gynecol Oncol 1990;36:147–51.
88. Chang KL, Crabtree GS, Lim-Tan SK, Kempson RL, Hendrickson MR. Primary extrauterine endometrial stromal neoplasms: a clinicopathologic study of 20 cases and a review of the literature. Int J Gynecol Pathol 1993;12:282–96.
89. Shakfeh SM, Woodruff JD. Primary ovarian sarcomas: report of 46 cases and review of the literature. Obstet Gynecol Surv 1987;42:331–49.
90. Shiraki M, Otis CN, Powell JL. Endometrial stromal sarcoma arising from ovarian and extraovarian endometriosis—report of two cases and review of the literature. Surg Pathol 1991;4:333–43.
91. Young RH, Prat J, Scully RE. Endometrioid stromal sarcomas of the ovary. A clinicopathologic analysis of 23 cases. Cancer 1984;53:1143–55.
92. Young RH, Scully RE. Sarcomas metastatic to the ovary: a report of 21 cases. Int J Gynecol Pathol 1990;9:231–52.

6
CLEAR CELL TUMORS

Definition. Clear cell tumors have an epithelial component that contains one or more cell types, most commonly clear cells and hobnail cells, and less frequently cuboidal, flat, oxyphilic, or mucin-containing signet-ring cells.

General Features. Benign clear cell tumors are rare, and borderline forms account for less than 1 percent of ovarian borderline tumors (8). Clear cell carcinomas, however, account for 6 percent of epithelial-stromal cancers (18). Most clear cell carcinomas (87 percent) are diagnosed during the fifth through seventh decades, and 10 percent in the fourth decade (1,2,7,11,14,17,25,28). The clinical manifestations are mostly similar to those of other epithelial cancers. Clear cell carcinomas, however, have the highest association among all epithelial-stromal cancers with ovarian and pelvic endometriosis and with paraendocrine hypercalcemia (page 379) (see Table 20-1) (29).

Although clear cell carcinomas were initially called "mesonephromas" and subsequently "mesonephric carcinomas" and "mesonephroid carcinomas," their mullerian nature is now generally accepted in view of their association with endometriosis in the same ovary in 5 to 38 (average, 24) percent of the cases (4,7,13), their admixture with endometrioid carcinoma in 20 to 25 percent of the cases (fig. 6-1) (4,6,21), their occurrence in the endometrium, and their origin from vaginal adenosis of mullerian type in the vagina of girls and young women exposed prenatally to diethylstilbestrol (23). The mullerian epithelial cell types that the clear and hobnail cells of clear cell tumors resemble most closely, both on light microscopic and electron microscopic examination (6,24), are similar-appearing cells that often line endometrial glands during pregnancy (Arias-Stella change).

Gross Findings. Clear cell adenofibromas that are benign or borderline have a nonspecific adenofibromatous appearance. Occasionally, the glands are dilated, giving the sectioned surface of the tumor a sponge-like appearance (parvilocular cystoma) (fig. 6-2) (20). Clear cell carcinomas may be predominantly solid but are more often predominantly cystic, appearing as unilocular or sometimes multilocular cysts containing one or more white, yellow, or pale brown polypoid masses protruding into the lumens. The cyst lumens may contain serous or mucinous fluid; in cases in which the tumor has arisen in an endometriotic cyst, the fluid may be chocolate colored, with patchy brown discoloration of the cyst lining (fig. 6-3). The external surface of the tumor is often shaggy due to adhesions, which in some cases are related to associated endometriosis. Benign and borderline clear cell tumors are almost invariably unilateral; clear cell carcinomas are bilateral in only 2 percent of stage I cases (18).

Microscopic Findings. As in the case of endometrioid tumors, there is controversy regarding the criteria for the differential diagnosis of benign, borderline, and malignant clear cell adenofibromas (3,9,19). We restrict the diagnosis of clear cell adenofibroma to cases in which the

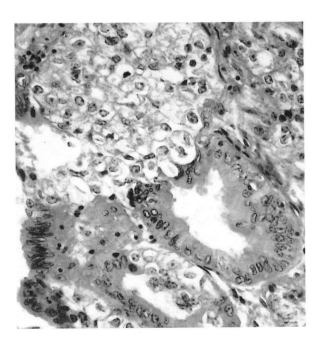

Figure 6-1
CLEAR CELL AND ENDOMETRIOID
ADENOCARCINOMA, MIXED
(Fig. 14 from Scully RE, Barlow JF. "Mesonephroma" of ovary. Tumor of müllerian nature related to the endometrioid carcinoma. Cancer 1967;20:1405–17.)

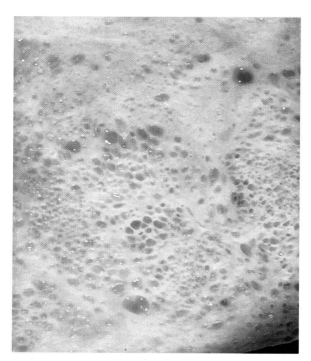

Figure 6-2
CLEAR CELL ADENOFIBROMA
OF BORDERLINE MALIGNANCY
The sectioned surface is parvilocular.

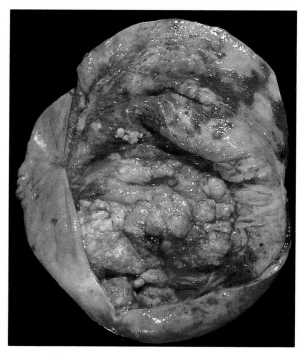

Figure 6-3
POLYPOID CLEAR CELL CARCINOMA
ARISING IN ENDOMETRIOTIC CYST
The cyst contained chocolate-colored fluid and its inner lining has areas of brown discoloration. (Fig. 3 from Scully RE, Barlow JF. "Mesonephroma" of ovary. Tumor of müllerian nature related to the endometrioid carcinoma. Cancer 1967;20:1405–17.)

epithelium appears benign; when it is atypical or carcinomatous without invasion, we designate the tumor borderline (fig. 6-4) and specify the appearance of the epithelial cells. We also diagnose microinvasion or larger areas of invasion if present, as described for endometrioid tumors (fig. 6-5) (page 112).

Clear cell carcinomas have a variety of patterns and cell types that are often admixed. The most common patterns are papillary (fig. 6-6) and tubulocystic (figs. 6-7, 6-8); a predominantly solid pattern (fig. 6-9) is less frequent. The papillae are often complex. The tubules and cysts frequently contain mucin, but intracellular mucin is not a feature of the lining cells. Rarely, the tumor has a reticular pattern, simulating a yolk sac tumor.

The most common cell types are the clear cell (fig. 6-9) and the hobnail cell (fig. 6-10). Clear cells may be arranged in solid nests or masses, or line cysts, tubules, and papillae; hobnail cells invariably line lumens and their papillae. The clear cells are typically rounded or polyhedral and have eccentric nuclei, generally without prominent nucle-

oli (fig. 6-9). The hobnail cells contain bulbous, usually dark nuclei that protrude into lumens beyond the apparent cytoplasmic limits of the cells (fig. 6-10). Psammoma bodies are occasionally present. Less common cell types are flat or cuboidal cells (fig. 6-8), oxyphilic cells with abundant eosinophilic cytoplasm (fig. 6-11), and signet-ring cells containing mucin, typically in the form of inspissated eosinophilic material in the center of a vacuole (figs. 6-12, 6-13). The flat cells, which may contain slightly bulging nuclei, line small cysts and often have a deceptively benign appearance (fig. 6-8, left). Occasionally, the cysts contain colloid-like material, imparting a struma-like appearance to the tumor. When the flat cell is the predominant or only cell type in a nonadenofibromatous tumor one should sample the tumor carefully to find areas diagnostic of carcinoma (fig. 6-8, right). Oxyphilic cells are sometimes prominent and in occasional

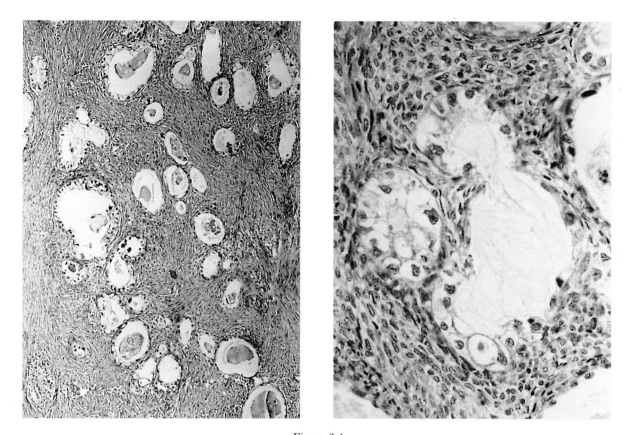

Figure 6-4
CLEAR CELL ADENOFIBROMA OF BORDERLINE MALIGNANCY
Left: The glands are lined by clear cells with hyperchromatic nuclei and lie in an abundant fibromatous stroma.
Right: The glands are lined by clear cells containing moderately atypical nuclei; thin mucin is present in the lumens.

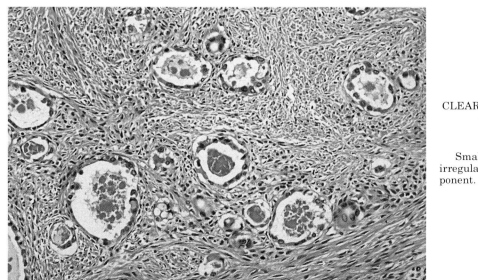

Figure 6-5
CLEAR CELL ADENOFIBROMA
OF BORDERLINE
MALIGNANCY,
MICROINVASIVE

Small clusters of tumor cells have irregularly invaded the stromal component.

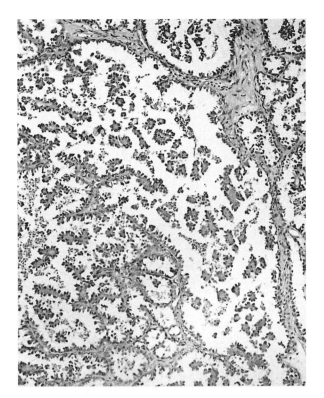

Figure 6-6
CLEAR CELL ADENOCARCINOMA
The tumor has a papillary pattern.

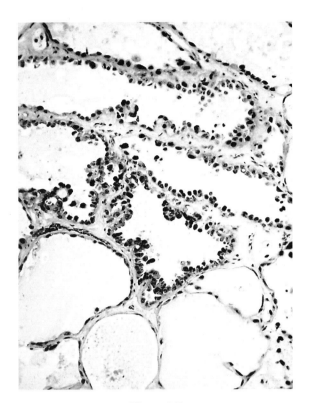

Figure 6-7
CLEAR CELL ADENOCARCINOMA
Hobnail and flat cells are evident. (Fig. 10 from Scully RE, Barlow JF. "Mesonephroma" of ovary. Tumor of müllerian nature related to the endometrioid carcinoma. Cancer 1967;20:1405–17.)

cases are the predominant cell type of the tumor. These cells may line glands but more often grow in nests and masses (figs. 6-11). Signet-ring cells, although commonly present, are usually encountered in small foci, but occasionally these cells form a prominent component of the tumor, and rarely, are the only cell type. In poorly differentiated areas of clear cell carcinoma, the cells lose their distinctive features, appearing as undifferentiated epithelial cells (fig. 6-14).

Two architectural features sometimes helpful in the recognition of clear cell carcinomas are multiple, complex papillae and densely hyaline accumulations of basement membrane material expanding the cores of the papillae (fig. 6-15). Benign and borderline adenofibromatous components are often present in clear cell carcinomas; indeed, tumors that appear to be clear cell adenofibromas on preliminary examination must be sampled carefully to exclude areas of carcinoma (fig. 6-16). A rare clear cell carcinoma contains an extensive infiltrate of round cells, a

large number of which are plasma cells; lymphocytes and polymorphonuclear leukocytes may also be present in the infiltrate (fig. 6-17). We have seen two cases of clear cell carcinoma admixed with rhabdomyosarcoma.

Special staining reveals abundant glycogen within the clear cells, which may also contain lipid. Mucin is typically located in the lumens and in the apex of the cytoplasm of the lining cells but is abundant within the cytoplasm of the signet-ring cells. Ultrastructural examination of clear cell carcinomas reveals short, irregular, blunt microvilli on the surfaces of the luminal cells, and glycogen and stacks of rough endoplasmic reticulin within the cytoplasm (24).

Differential Diagnosis. The distinctions between clear cell carcinoma and serous carcinoma and the secretory variant of endometrioid carcinoma are discussed on pages 73 and 123. Clear cell carcinomas are often confused with primitive

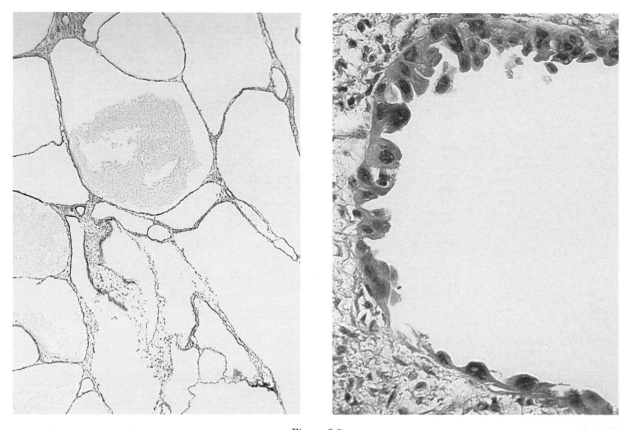

Figure 6-8
CLEAR CELL ADENOCARCINOMA
Left: The tumor has a cystic pattern, with flat cells lining almost all the cysts.
Right: A cyst in the tumor is lined by moderately atypical hobnail cells. The tumor recurred with a higher grade 4 years postoperatively.

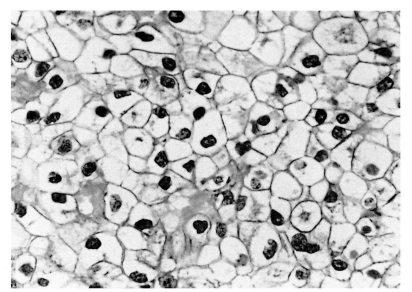

Figure 6-9
CLEAR CELL CARCINOMA
The tumor has a solid pattern. The cells are polyhedral and have eccentric, hyperchromatic nuclei without conspicuous nucleoli.

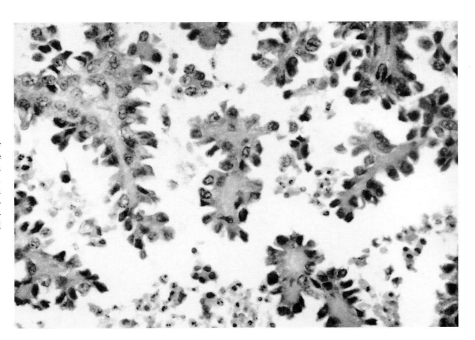

Figure 6-10
CLEAR CELL
ADENOCARCINOMA
The papillae are lined by hobnail cells and have hyalinized cores. (Fig. 42 from Serov SF, Scully RE, Sobin LH. Histological typing of ovarian tumours. International Histological Classification of Tumours No. 9. Geneva: World Health Organization, 1973.)

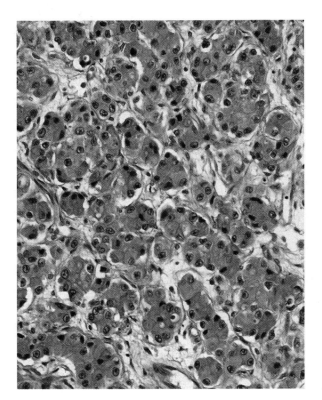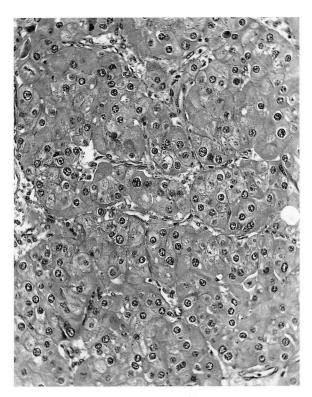

Figure 6-11
CLEAR CELL CARCINOMA, OXYPHILIC TYPE
Left: The tumor cells contain abundant eosinophilic cytoplasm and are arranged in small, closely packed groups.
Right: The tumor cells have abundant cytoplasm and form solid aggregates.

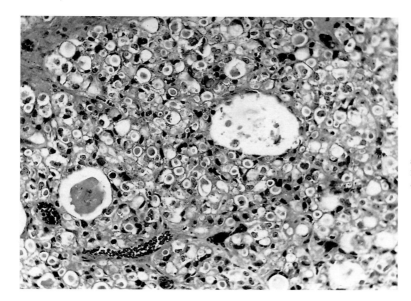

Figure 6-12
CLEAR CELL ADENOCARCINOMA
Most of the tumor cells contain inspissated secretion that was eosinophilic and mucicarmine positive, creating a targetoid appearance.

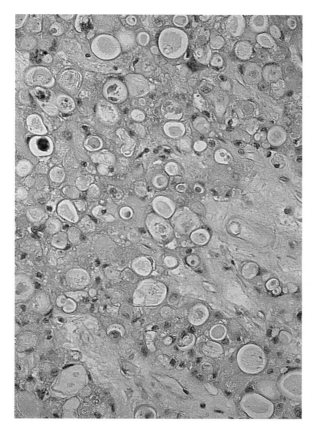

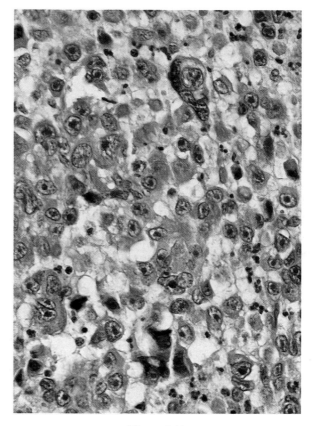

Figure 6-13
CLEAR CELL ADENOCARCINOMA
The tumor cells are vacuolated and some contain inspissated secretion, which was stained by mucicarmine.

Figure 6-14
CLEAR CELL CARCINOMA,
POORLY DIFFERENTIATED
The clear cell features of the cytoplasm are absent.

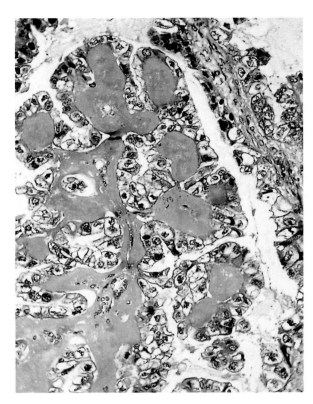

Figure 6-15
CLEAR CELL ADENOCARCINOMA
A complex glomeruloid papilla is lined by clear cells and has an extensively hyalinized core.

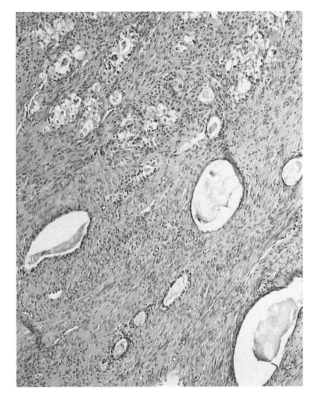

Figure 6-16
CLEAR CELL ADENOCARCINOMA
WITH ADENOFIBROMA COMPONENT

germ cell tumors, particularly dysgerminomas and yolk sac tumors. The difference in age incidence of patients with clear cell carcinoma and primitive germ cell tumors is a helpful clinical clue to the diagnosis. The pure, diffuse clear cell carcinoma may be confused with a dysgerminoma. The clear cells in the former, however, are typically polyhedral and have eccentric, hyperchromatic nuclei, usually without prominent nucleoli (see fig. 6-9). Dysgerminoma cells are characteristically rounded and flattened along their periphery, have nuclei that are more central, and contain one to four prominent discrete nucleoli. Lymphocytes are almost always sprinkled throughout a dysgerminoma whereas in the clear cell carcinoma with round cell infiltration plasma cells are a prominent component. Immunohistochemically, placental-like alkaline phosphatase can be demonstrated in both dysgerminomas and clear cell carcinomas, but much less often in the latter; in

contrast, keratin is almost always stainable in clear cell carcinoma, but only occasionally in dysgerminoma. Epithelial membrane antigen is one of the best differential immunohistochemical markers, being positive in clear cell carcinomas and negative in dysgerminomas (26,27).

Yolk sac tumors typically have a reticular pattern, which is an unusual feature in clear cell carcinomas. When papillae are present in yolk sac tumors they are almost always single and contain a central blood vessel (Schiller-Duval bodies) in contrast to the multiple complex papillae of clear cell carcinomas, which commonly have hyalinized cores (fig. 6-15). Hyaline bodies are a typical feature of yolk sac tumors but have been described in 25 percent of clear cell carcinomas as well (fig. 6-18) (12) and are not helpful in the differential diagnosis. Immunohistochemical stains for alpha-fetoprotein and Leu-M1 may aid in the differential diagnosis of these two

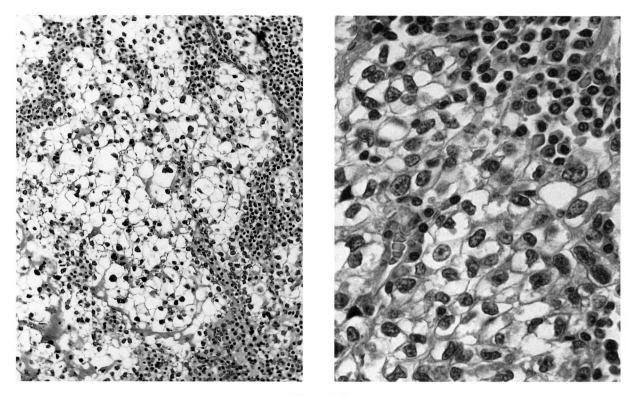

Figure 6-17
CLEAR CELL CARCINOMA WITH EXTENSIVE ROUND CELL INFILTRATION
Left: The polyhedral shape of the cells and their eccentric nuclei help to distinguish this tumor from a dysgerminoma. (Fig. 47 from Young RH, Clement PB, Scully RE. Pathology of the ovary. In: Sternberg SS, ed. Diagnostic surgical pathology, Vol 2, 1st ed. New York: Raven Press, 1989:1682.)
Right: Many of the round cells are plasma cells (top right).

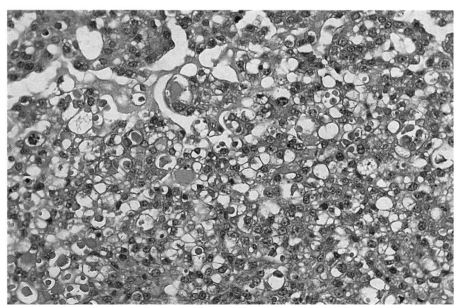

Figure 6-18
CLEAR CELL
CARCINOMA
Numerous intracytoplas-
mic hyaline bodies are visible.

tumors (31). Alpha-fetoprotein is demonstrable in almost all yolk sac tumors but was found in only 1 of 9 ovarian clear cell carcinomas (and only 3 of 17 clear cell carcinomas of the female genital tract); Leu-M1, in contrast, was stainable in 89 percent of ovarian clear cell carcinomas and only 28 percent (2 of 7) of yolk sac tumors.

Rarely, the follicles of the juvenile granulosa cell tumor are lined by cells with a hobnail shape. The typically young age of the patient, the usually associated estrogenic manifestations, and the presence of other more typical patterns of the tumor enable one to distinguish it from a clear cell carcinoma. Occasionally, cysts within an ovarian tumor of probable wolffian origin are lined by hobnail cells, but other more characteristic patterns of that tumor are almost always present as well. When signet-ring–type cells are abundant, the question of a Krukenberg tumor may arise. The latter tumor is commonly discovered in a patient known to have a primary mucinous tumor elsewhere, and is bilateral in 80 percent of the cases (22). Microscopic examination typically reveals a uniform distribution of signet cells and small mucinous glands in a cellular fibromatous stroma, features that are lacking in clear cell carcinoma.

Differentiation of primary clear cell carcinoma from metastatic renal cell carcinoma is discussed on page 353. Distinction from metastatic clear cell carcinomas that are primary in extrarenal sites, including the colon (page 344), is based on the usual criteria for differentiating primary and metastatic ovarian cancers (page 335) as well as the many distinctive features of primary clear cell carcinoma.

Oxyphilic clear cell carcinoma (30) is usually identified by the additional presence of other patterns of clear cell carcinoma. When the tumor occurs in pure form it may be impossible to distinguish by examination of routinely stained slides from hepatoid carcinoma, an oxyphilic carcinoma that resembles hepatocellular carcinoma and is immunoreactive for alpha-fetoprotein. Among the wide variety of other oxyphilic tumors of the ovary, both primary and metastatic, those that we have encountered in our practice and in the literature are listed in Table 6-1; other unlisted types may exist, especially in the metastatic category. The distinctive features of all the tumors listed in the table are described in the discussions of them elsewhere in the text.

Table 6-1

TUMORS THAT MAY APPEAR IN OVARY AS OXYPHILIC TUMORS

Primary Carcinomas
  Clear cell
  Hepatoid
  Endometrioid
  Anaplastic (with mucinous tumor)
  Small cell, hypercalcemic type, large cell variant

Metastatic Tumors
  Melanoma
  Hepatocellular carcinoma
  Carcinoma of breast
  Large cell carcinoma of lung
  Carcinoid tumor
  Others

Germ Cell Tumors
  Hepatoid yolk sac tumor
  Oxyphilic struma ovarii
  Oxyphilic pituitary-type tumor in dermoid cyst
  Malignant melanoma
  Apocrine carcinoma in dermoid cyst

Sex Cord–Stromal Tumors
  Luteinized granulosa cell tumor, juvenile and adult[†]
  Luteinized thecoma[†]
  Oxyphilic Sertoli cell tumor[†]

Steroid Cell Tumors and Pregnancy Luteoma[*†]

Paraganglioma

Malignant Mesothelioma

Soft Tissue Tumors
  Epithelioid smooth muscle tumor
  Others

---

[*] A tumor-like lesion.
[†] α-inhibin positive immunohistochemically.

Spread and Metastasis. Forty-three percent of clear cell carcinomas are stage I; 19 percent, stage II; 29 percent, stage III; and 9 percent, stage IV (18).

Treatment and Prognosis. The treatment of clear cell tumors is similar to that of surface epithelial-stromal tumors in general (page 39). Clear cell borderline tumors, including those with microinvasion of the stroma, almost always have a benign course. In one case (3), however, a tumor in the latter category that was incompletely resected continued to grow in the pelvis and was fatal. The 5-year survival rate for patients with stage I carcinomas is 69 percent; for stage II, 55 percent; for stage III, 14 percent; and for stage IV, 4 percent. These survival rates are poorer than those for epithelial cancers of other cell types, and are closer to those of undifferentiated carcinoma. There is no consensus in the literature about the value of pattern, cell type, mitotic index, or grade as a prognostic indicator (5,7,10,13,15,16).

REFERENCES

1. Anderson MC, Langley FA. Mesonephroid tumours of the ovary. J Clin Pathol 1970;23:210–8.
2. Aure JC, Hoeg K, Kolstad P. Mesonephroid tumors of the ovary. Clinical and histopathologic studies. Obstet Gynecol 1971;37:860–7.
3. Bell DA, Scully RE. Benign and borderline clear cell adenofibromas of the ovary. Cancer 1985;56:2922–31.
4. Brescia RJ, Dubin N, Demopoulos RI. Endometrioid and clear cell carcinoma of the ovary. Factors affecting survival. Int J Gynecol Pathol 1989;8:132–8.
5. Crozier MA, Copeland LJ, Silva EG, Gershenson DM, Stringer CA. Clear cell carcinoma of the ovary: a study of 59 cases. Gynecol Oncol 1989;35:199–203.
6. Czernobilsky B, Silverman BB, Enterline HT. Clear-cell carcinoma of the ovary. A clinicopathologic analysis of pure and mixed forms and comparison with endometrioid carcinoma. Cancer 1970;25:762–72.
7. Imachi M, Tsukamoto N, Shimamoto T, Hirakawa T, Uehira K, Nakano H. Clear cell carcinoma of the ovary: a clinicopathologic analysis of 34 cases. Int J Gynecol Cancer 1991;1:113–9.
8. Kaern J, Tropé CG, Kristensen GB, Abeler VM, Pettersen EO. DNA ploidy: the most important prognostic factor in patients with borderline tumors of the ovary. Int J Gynecol Cancer 1993;3:349–58.
9. Kao GF, Norris HJ. Unusual cystadenofibromas: endometrioid, mucinous, and clear cell types. Obstet Gynecol 1979;54:729–36.
10. Kennedy AW, Biscotti CV, Hart WR, Webster KD. Ovarian clear cell adenocarcinoma. Gynecol Oncol 1989;32:342–9.
11. Klemi PJ, Grönroos M. Mesonephroid carcinoma of the ovary. A clinicopathologic, histochemical, and electron microscopic study. Obstet Gynecol 1979;53:472–9.
12. Klemi PJ, Meurman L, Grönroos M, Talerman A. Clear cell (mesonephroid) tumors of the ovary with characteristics resembling endodermal sinus tumor. Int J Gynecol Pathol 1982;1:95–100.
13. Montag AG, Jenison EL, Griffiths CT, Welch WR, Lavin PT, Knapp RC. Ovarian clear cell carcinoma. A clinicopathologic analysis of 44 cases. Int J Gynecol Pathol 1989;8:85–96.
14. Nakashima N, Nagasaka T, Fukata S, et al. Study of ovarian tumors treated at Nagoya University Hospital, 1965–1988. Gynecol Oncol 1990;37:103–11.
15. Norris HJ, Robinowitz M. Ovarian adenocarcinoma of mesonephric type. Cancer 1971;28:1074–81.
16. O'Brien ME, Schofield JB, Tan S, Fryatt I, Fisher C, Wiltshaw E. Clear cell epithelial ovarian cancer (mesonephroid): bad prognosis only in early stages. Gynecol Oncol 1993;49:250–4.
17. Ohkawa K, Amasaki H, Terashima Y, Aizawa S, Ishikawa E. Clear cell carcinoma of the ovary: light and electron microscopic studies. Cancer 1977;40:3019–29.
18. Pettersson F. Annual report of the results of treatment in gynecological cancer. Stockholm, International Federation of Gynecology and Obstetrics, 1991.
19. Roth LM, Langley FA, Fox H, Wheeler JE, Czernobilsky B. Ovarian clear cell adenofibromatous tumors. Benign, of low malignant potential, and associated with invasive clear cell carcinoma. Cancer 1984;53:1156–63.
20. Schiller W. Parvilocular cystomas of the ovary. Arch Pathol 1943;35:391–413.
21. Scully RE, Barlow JF. "Mesonephroma" of ovary. Tumor of müllerian nature related to the endometrioid carcinoma. Cancer 1967;20:1405–16.
22. Scully RE, Richardson GS. Luteinization of the stroma of metastatic cancer involving the ovary and its endocrine significance. Cancer 1961;14:827–40.
23. Scully RE, Welch WR. Pathology of the female genital tract after prenatal exposure to diethylstilbestrol. In: Herbst AL, Bern HA, eds. Developmental effects of diethylstilbestrol (DES) in pregnancy. New York: Thieme-Stratton, 1981:26-45.
24. Silverberg SG. Ultrastructure and histogenesis of clear cell carcinoma of the ovary. Am J Obstet Gynecol 1973;115:394–400.
25. Tateno H, Sasano N. Ovarian tumours in Sendai, Japan. General hospital material. In: Stalsberg E, ed. UICC technical report series, vol 75. An international survey of distribution of histologic types of tumours of the testis and ovary. Geneva: UICC, 1983;291–6.
26. Viale G, Gambacorta M, Dell'Orto P, Coggi G. Coexpression of cytokeratins and vimentin in common epithelial tumors of the ovary: an immunocytochemical study of eighty-three cases. Virchows Arch [A] 1988;413:91–101.
27. Wick MR, Swanson PE, Manivel JC. Placental-like alkaline phosphatase reactivity in human tumors: an immunohistochemical study of 520 cases. Hum Pathol 1987;18:946–54.
28. Yoonessi M, Weldon D, Satchidand SK, Crickard K. Clear cell ovarian adenocarcinoma. J Surg Oncol 1984;27:289–97.
29. Young RH, Oliva E, Scully RE. Small cell carcinoma of the ovary, hypercalcemic type. A clinicopathological analysis of 150 cases. Am J Surg Pathol. 1994;18:1102–16.
30. Young RH, Scully RE. Oxyphilic clear cell carcinoma of the ovary. A report of nine cases. Am J Surg Pathol 1987;11:661–7.
31. Zirker TA, Silva EG, Morris M, Ordonez NG. Immunohistochemical differentiation of clear-cell carcinoma of the female genital tract and endodermal sinus tumor with the use of alpha-fetoprotein and Leu-M1. Am J Clin Pathol 1989;91:511–4.

7

TRANSITIONAL AND SQUAMOUS CELL TUMORS

TRANSITIONAL CELL TUMORS

Definition. Transitional cell tumors have an epithelial component made up predominantly of cells resembling urothelial cells. In benign Brenner tumors nests of transitional cells are distributed within a generally predominant fibromatous component. Borderline and malignant Brenner tumors have a background of benign Brenner neoplasia, which is lacking in the tumor designated transitional cell carcinoma.

General Features. Transitional cell tumors, most of which are benign, account for 1 to 2 percent of all ovarian tumors; the benign forms account for 4 to 5 percent of benign tumors in the surface epithelial–stromal category (11,12,15, 24,25). Approximately 95 percent of Brenner tumors are diagnosed in women between the ages of 30 and 70 years, with most presenting in women between 40 and 60 years of age (6,7,22, 27,29). In two series (9,14), the latter of which was composed of consultation cases, borderline and malignant Brenner tumors accounted for 3 and 5 percent, and 5 and 5 percent, respectively, of all Brenner tumors. Over half of the borderline tumors and over two thirds of the malignant tumors were diagnosed in women between the ages of 50 and 70 years (9,14,17,18). Three quarters of transitional cell carcinomas occur in women between 50 and 70 years of age (3). According to Silva et al. (21) pure transitional cell carcinomas account for 1 percent of carcinomas in the surface epithelial–stromal category; in another 5 percent of the cases transitional cell carcinoma is the predominant element; and in still another 3 percent, it is a minor component of a mixed tumor.

Most transitional cell tumors are considered to be of surface epithelial and stromal origin in view of: 1) the common presence of mucinous epithelium in Brenner tumors and the frequent association of these tumors with mucinous cystic tumors; 2) the occasional content of serous ciliated epithelium in Brenner tumors and their rare association with serous cystadenomas; 3) the occasional finding of a communication between Brenner tumor epithelial nests and surface epithelium that has undergone transitional cell metaplasia or of an association of the tumor with transitional cell nests in the superficial ovarian cortex (2,27); and 4) the close histologic, immunohistochemical, and ultrastructural resemblance between the epithelial nests of Brenner tumors and Walthard nests, which arise from mesothelium (16,20).

The occasional association of Brenner tumors with a dermoid cyst and their rare association with struma ovarii or carcinoid tumor (6a,27), on the other hand, suggest the possibility of a germ cell origin in some cases. Finally, the rare occurrence of a microscopic Brenner tumor in the ovarian hilus in relation to the rete ovarii supports an origin from rete epithelium, which may be of coelomic-epithelial or mesonephric origin (7,23,27).

Brenner tumors are occasionally associated with endocrine manifestations of estrogenic or less often androgenic type, apparently as a result of steroid hormone secretion by the stromal component of the tumor (see chapter 19).

Gross Findings. Benign Brenner tumors are typically small (fig. 7-1) and have no clinical manifestations; slightly over half are less than 2 cm in diameter and approximately one third are detectable only on microscopic examination (6,7,22,27). Ten percent of the tumors are over 10 cm, and rare examples are 20 cm or greater in diameter (7,22). Seven to 8 percent of Brenner tumors are bilateral (6,7,22,27,29). Gross examination reveals a sharply circumscribed, firm, nodular tumor that may have a smooth or slightly bosselated external surface. The sectioned surfaces are usually white but may be pale yellow (fig. 7-2); small cysts are often visible to the naked eye or with the use of a hand lens. The tumor tissue may have a gritty consistency caused by flecks of calcific material, and rarely, is extensively calcified. Large cysts lined by transitional epithelium are occasionally present and may predominate (fig. 7-3). In about one quarter of the cases another type of tumor is present in the same ovary, usually in contact with the Brenner tumor, and contributes to its gross appearance (6,7,22,27). Two thirds of the associated

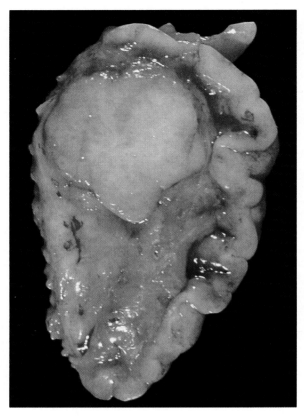

Figure 7-1
BRENNER TUMOR
The tumor is sharply demarcated; its sectioned surface has a thecoma-like yellow hue. (Fig. 53 from Young RH, Clement PB, Scully RE. Pathology of the ovary. In: Sternberg SS, ed. Diagnostic surgical pathology, Vol 2, 1st ed. New York: Raven Press, 1989:1685.)

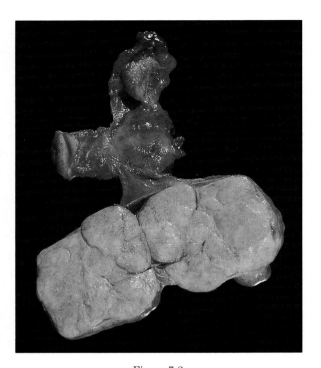

Figure 7-2
BRENNER TUMOR
The sectioned surfaces are lobulated and have a fibroma-like appearance.

tumors are mucinous cystic tumors, which are almost always benign; the remainder are mostly serous cystadenomas and dermoid cysts.

Brenner tumors of borderline malignancy typically have both solid and cystic components, with the former similar to those of the benign Brenner tumor and the latter usually containing papillary or polypoid masses (fig. 7-4). Almost all borderline Brenner tumors are unilateral (9,14,18,28).

Malignant Brenner tumors typically have both solid and cystic components, with the cysts containing papillary or polypoid masses or solid nodules in their walls (figs. 7-5, 7-6). Twelve percent of malignant Brenner tumors are bilateral (4). Transitional cell carcinomas grossly resemble other carcinomas of epithelial-stromal type, but differ from malignant Brenner tumors by lacking

gritty areas caused by calcification, which are evident in half the cases of malignant Brenner tumor (3). Transitional cell carcinomas are bilateral in approximately 15 percent of the cases (3).

Microscopic Findings. *Benign Brenner Tumor.* The typical benign Brenner tumor (figs. 7-7–7-11) is characterized by the presence of round or oval nests and, occasionally, trabeculae composed of transitional cells. These cells contain pale cytoplasm and oval nuclei; the nuclei often have conspicuous grooves, giving them a coffee-bean shape (fig. 7-8). The nests may be solid or have a central cavity filled with dense eosinophilic material (fig. 7-9); the cavity may be lined by mucinous (fig. 7-10), ciliated-serous (fig. 7-11), or indifferent glandular epithelium. When mucinous or ciliated-serous cells are present, the term "metaplastic Brenner tumor" has been used by some investigators (18). Pure mucinous glands and cysts may also be present in Brenner tumors. Criteria for the diagnosis of a mixed Brenner and mucinous tumor are presented on page 165. The Brenner epithelial nests are scattered throughout

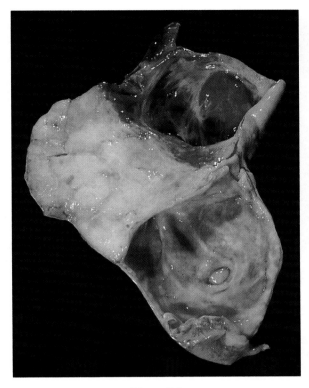

Figure 7-3
BRENNER TUMOR
Sectioning has revealed a solid fibroma-like component as well as two cysts, which were lined by transitional epithelium.

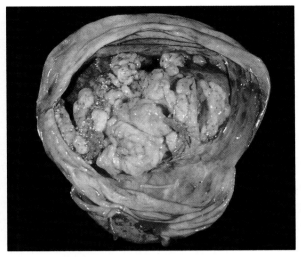

Figure 7-4
BRENNER TUMOR OF BORDERLINE MALIGNANCY
A polypoid mass protrudes into the lumen of the opened cyst. (Fig. 54 from Young RH, Clement PB, Scully RE. Pathology of the ovary. In: Sternberg SS, ed. Diagnostic surgical pathology, Vol 2, 1st ed. New York: Raven Press, 1989:1685.)

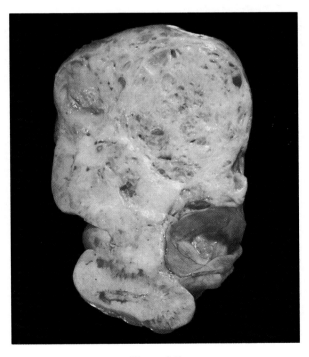

Figure 7-5
MALIGNANT BRENNER TUMOR
The sectioned surface contains soft tan areas with small cysts as well as firm white areas. (Fig. 6 from Halligrimsson J, Scully RE. Borderline and malignant Brenner tumours of the ovary. A report of 15 cases. Acta Pathol Microbiol Scand [A] Suppl 1972;233:56–66.)

a stromal component that resembles an ovarian fibroma (fig. 7-7) but rarely, has features more typical of thecoma, with plump cells that may contain abundant lipid-rich cytoplasm or with nests of lutein cells. Spicules of calcification are present in the stroma in approximately one third of the cases, typically in the form of slender plaques adjacent to the epithelial nests. Rarely, squamous differentiation is present centrally within the Brenner nests.

The ultrastructural features of Brenner tumors resemble those of transitional cell tumors of the urinary tract. Immunohistochemically, however, the urothelial tumors are almost always positive for cytokeratin-20, and the ovarian tumors, almost always negative (22a). Neuroendocrine granules are stainable in one third of Brenner tumors (1). These granules are frequently positive immunohisto-chemically for serotonin, but unlike the argyrophil granules in other ovarian epithelial tumors, are rarely positive for peptide hormones (1).

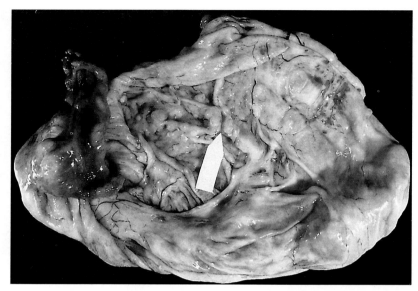

Figure 7-6
MALIGNANT
BRENNER TUMOR
The marker points to one of many solid nodules visible in the wall of the opened cyst. The nodules were composed of invasive transitional cell carcinoma (see figure 7-15). (Fig. 7 from Hallgrimsson J, Scully RE. Borderline malignant Brenner tumours of the ovary. A report of 15 cases. Acta Pathol Microbiol Scand [A] Suppl 1972;233:56–66.)

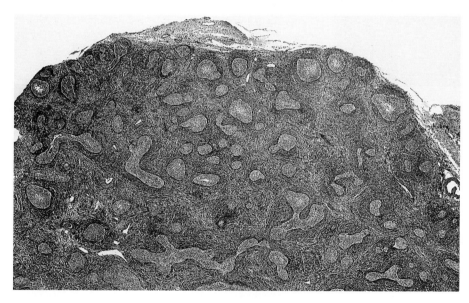

Figure 7-7
BRENNER TUMOR
Irregularly rounded solid nests of transitional cells are separated by a predominant fibromatous stromal component.

Borderline Brenner Tumor. The criteria for the diagnosis of borderline and frankly malignant Brenner tumors and the designations used for these neoplasms are controversial. The criteria used by various authorities are listed in Table 7-1. We favor the World Health Organization (WHO) approach, which requires obvious invasion for the diagnosis of malignancy (page 52), but we also specify whether the noninvasive cells of the borderline Brenner tumor are only atypical (equivalent to grade 1 transitional cell carcinoma of the urinary tract) (figs. 7-12, 7-13) or carcinomatous

(equivalent to grade 2 or 3), and if the latter, we designate the grade (fig. 7-14).

Malignant Brenner Tumor. Obviously invasive components of malignant Brenner tumors are made up exclusively or predominantly of malignant-appearing transitional cells or squamous cells and may contain mucinous cells as well (figs. 7-15–7-17). The invasive elements are typically grade 2 or higher but occasionally take the form of crowded, irregularly shaped islands of transitional cells of grade 1 malignancy (17). The rare mucinous adenocarcinoma associated with a

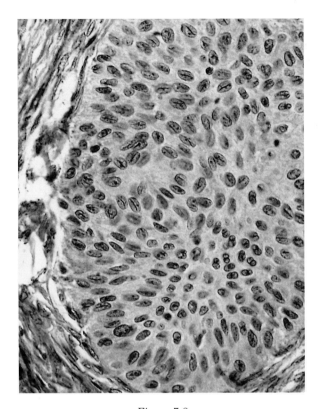

Figure 7-8
BRENNER TUMOR
Many of the nuclei in the solid epithelial nest are grooved, resembling coffee beans.

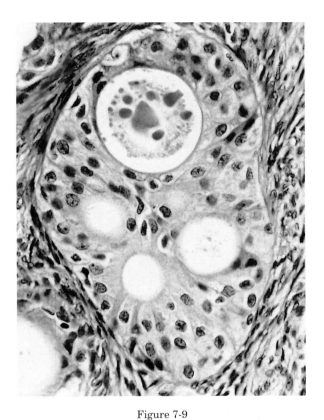

Figure 7-9
BRENNER TUMOR
The epithelial nest has several lumens, one of which contains hyaline material that was eosinophilic. (Fig. 47 from Serov SF, Scully RE, Sobin LH. Histological typing of ovarian tumours. International Histological Classification of Tumours No. 9. Geneva: World Health Organization, 1973.)

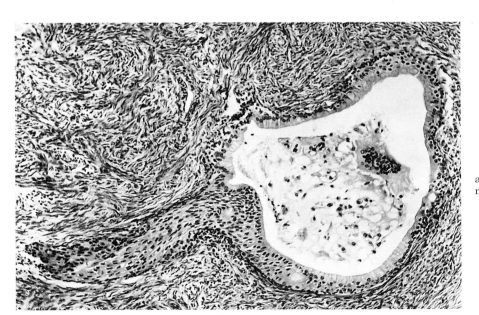

Figure 7-10
BRENNER TUMOR
The epithelial nest contains a cavity that is lined predominantly by mucinous epithelium.

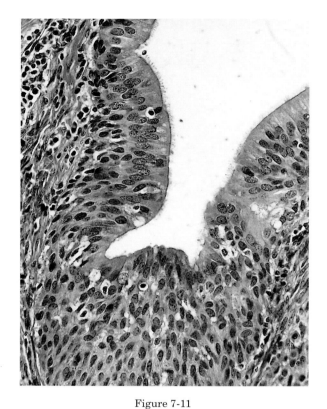

Figure 7-11
BRENNER TUMOR
The epithelial nest contains a lumen lined by ciliated epithelium.

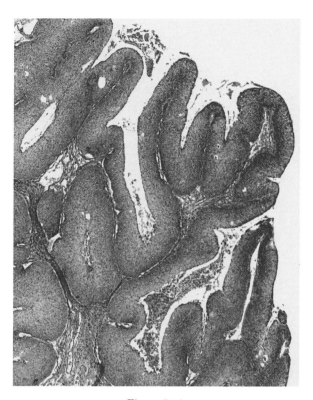

Figure 7-12
BRENNER TUMOR OF BORDERLINE MALIGNANCY
Papillae lined by transitional cells protrude into the lumen. (Fig. 49 from Serov SF, Scully RE, Sobin LH. Histological typing of ovarian tumours. International Histological Classification of Tumours No. 9. Geneva: World Health Organization, 1973.)

Table 7-1

CRITERIA FOR SUBCLASSIFICATION OF BRENNER TUMORS ACCORDING TO LITERATURE

Microscopic Features	WHO	Fascicle Authors	Colgan & Norris (5) Roth et al. (17,18)	Trebeck et al. (26)*
Benign epithelium	Benign	Benign	Benign	Benign
No stromal invasion				
Atypical epithelium				
Grade 1	Borderline	Borderline	Proliferative	Proliferative
Grade 2	Borderline	Borderline[†]	Proliferative	Proliferative
Grade 3	Borderline	Borderline[†]	Borderline	Malignant
Stromal invasion	Malignant	Malignant	Malignant	Malignant

*These authors suggest separation of proliferative and "noninvasive" malignant Brenner tumors on the basis of diploid and aneuploid findings, respectively, on flow cytometry, although a subsequent case of invasive malignant Brenner tumor was shown to be diploid (13).
[†]With intraepithelial carcinoma.

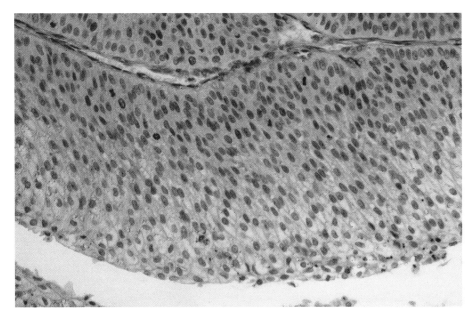

Figure 7-13
BRENNER TUMOR
OF BORDERLINE
MALIGNANCY
The lining of the papilla is composed of well-differentiated transitional cells with mitotic figures in the basal portion of the epithelium.

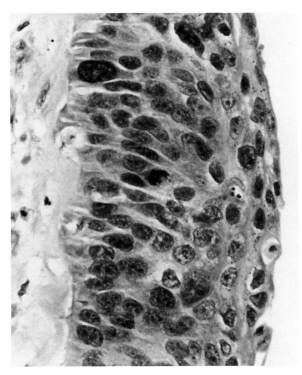

Figure 7-14
BRENNER TUMOR OF BORDERLINE MALIGNANCY
WITH INTRAEPITHELIAL CARCINOMA
The lining of the cyst is high-grade transitional cell carcinoma. (Fig. 5 from Hallgrimsson J, Scully RE. Borderline and malignant Brenner tumours of the ovary. A report of 15 cases. Acta Pathol Microbiol Scand [A] Suppl 1972;233:56–66.)

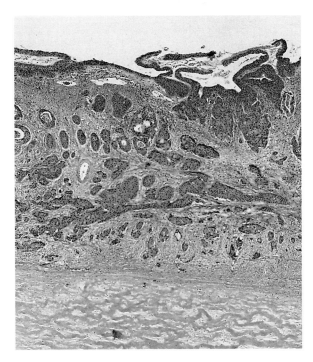

Figure 7-15
MALIGNANT BRENNER TUMOR
The cyst is lined by malignant transitional cells, which irregularly invade the wall of the cyst. (Same tumor as illustrated in figure 7-6.) (Fig. 8 from Hallgrimsson J, Scully RE. Borderline and malignant Brenner tumours of the ovary. A report of 15 cases. Acta Pathol Microbiol Scand [A] Suppl 1972;233:56–66.)

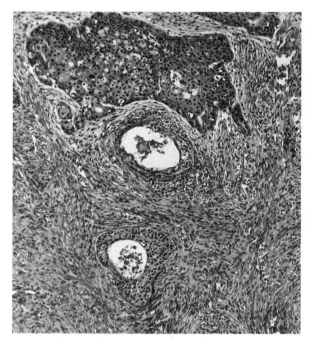

Figure 7-16
MALIGNANT BRENNER TUMOR
A large irregular nest of malignant transitional cells with jagged margins lies above two benign Brenner nests with central cavities.

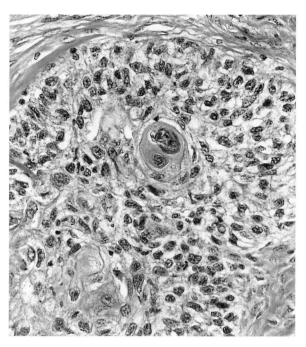

Figure 7-17
MALIGNANT BRENNER TUMOR
Early squamous differentiation in the form of an abortive pearl is present within a nest of transitional cells with high-grade nuclei. (Fig. 9 from Hallgrimsson J, Scully RE. Borderline and malignant Brenner tumours of the ovary. A report of 15 cases. Acta Pathol Microbiol Scand [A] Suppl 1972;233:56–66.)

benign Brenner tumor should be designated as such rather than as a malignant Brenner tumor.

Transitional Cell Carcinoma. Transitional cell carcinoma, not otherwise specified, which by definition, lacks benign and borderline Brenner elements, is characterized by an intracystic papillary pattern, designated "papillary type" by Roth et al. (19,19a); an arrangement of nests of epithelial cells separated by fibrous stroma, designated "malignant Brenner-like type" by those authors; or both patterns (fig. 7-18). The cells have the characteristics of malignant transitional cells, which in most cases are grade 2 or 3 (8,21). In over half the cases, in addition to transitional cells, small pools of mucin, which may be surrounded by glandular epithelium, are present (fig. 7-19). In most of the cases the tumor is impure, being admixed with other types of surface epithelial carcinoma, most commonly of serous type (8,21).

Differential Diagnosis. The benign Brenner tumor is rarely confused with neoplasms of other types. Its distinction from endometrioid adenofibroma with squamous differentiation is

discussed on page 123. The epithelial elements of Brenner tumors differ in their appearance from those of insular granulosa cell tumors and insular carcinoid tumors, which may create a problem when they contain an abundant fibromatous stroma (page 293). Brenner tumors of borderline malignancy, malignant Brenner tumors, and transitional cell carcinomas can be mimicked closely by very rare metastatic transitional cell carcinomas of urothelial origin. The often difficult distinction between these tumors is discussed on page 356. Transitional cell carcinomas are distinguished from undifferentiated carcinomas by their frequent content of thick papillae with smooth luminal borders in contrast to the pseudopapillae secondary to tumor cell necrosis that may be present in undifferentiated carcinomas. Also, in nonpapillary areas of transitional cell carcinoma a nesting pattern of tumor cells is more common than in undifferentiated carcinomas (8,21). Mucin pools are also more

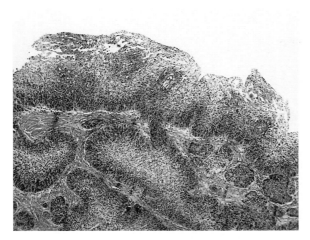

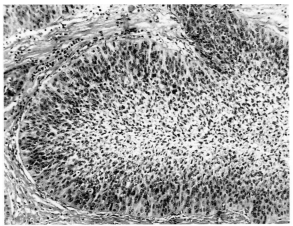

Figure 7-18
TRANSITIONAL CELL CARCINOMA
Top: Transitional cells line a cyst and extend into the underlying stroma as irregularly rounded nests and trabeculae.
Bottom: High-power view showing moderately differentiated transitional cells.

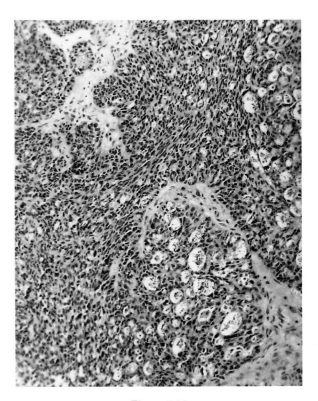

Figure 7-19
TRANSITIONAL CELL CARCINOMA, GRADE 3
The irregular mass of transitional cells contains many small pools filled with mucin.

frequent in transitional cell than in undifferentiated carcinomas. The most important criterion, however, is the presence of moderate to abundant cytoplasm, and in well-differentiated tumors, distinctive nuclei that have the appearance of urothelial cell nuclei. Finally, a rare granulosa cell tumor of either the juvenile or adult type has a papillary-cystic pattern similar to that of a borderline Brenner tumor or a transitional cell carcinoma. The age of the patient, the usually associated endocrine manifestations of the tumor, and the presence in most cases of other more typical patterns of granulosa cell tumor enable one to make the correct diagnosis.

Spread and Metastasis. No Brenner tumor in the borderline category, whether designated atypical, proliferative, borderline, or malignant without demonstrable invasion (i.e. borderline with intraepithelial carcinoma) has as yet been documented to spread beyond the ovary. Nevertheless, only small numbers of patients with these tumors have had long-term follow-up. Malignant Brenner tumors present at a stage higher than I in approximately 20 percent of the cases; in contrast, over two thirds of transitional cell carcinomas have spread to the abdomen or beyond at the time of diagnosis (3).

Treatment and Prognosis. In view of the lack of evidence of spread of borderline Brenner tumors they can be treated by conservative surgery when they occur in young women. Malignant Brenner tumors are managed like other epithelial cancers; they have an excellent prognosis when confined to the ovary (3). Patients with transitional cell carcinomas have a poorer prognosis than those with malignant Brenner tumors, stage for stage, with an overall 5-year survival rate of 35 percent (3). Silva et al. (21), however, have pointed out that when the metastases of ovarian carcinoma are composed solely or predominantly of transitional cell carcinoma the patients respond far better to chemotherapy and have a higher 5-year survival rate than do patients with other forms of epithelial ovarian cancer considered as a group (56 versus 7 percent) (21). Hollingsworth et al. (10), in contrast, found no chemoresponse or survival advantage for patients with advanced stage transitional cell carcinoma.

SQUAMOUS CELL TUMORS

Epidermoid cysts and some squamous cell carcinomas are included in the epithelial-stromal category even though an origin from surface epithelium has not been established conclusively in all the cases.

Epidermoid Cyst

Approximately 20 examples of epidermoid cyst lined by keratinizing squamous epithelium and lacking skin appendages have been reported (32,42). All of them were unilateral and were located within the ovarian medulla except for a single cyst in the hilus. They ranged in diameter from 0.2 to 4.6 cm and were filled with yellow-white creamy material. Origins from surface epithelial inclusion glands and the rete ovarii have been proposed. One group of authors found nests resembling Walthard nests and the epithelial components of a Brenner tumor in the walls of all three cysts that they described (fig. 7-20), suggesting a relation to the latter tumor (42). Another group mentioned, but did not document, the presence of hair or a cartilaginous nodule accompanying two cysts associated with Walthard nests, suggesting a teratomatous nature of epidermoid cysts in some cases (32).

Squamous Cell Carcinoma

Squamous cell carcinomas of the ovary arise most commonly from the lining of a dermoid cyst (19 cases), less often in endometriosis (12 cases) (31,33,34,36,37,41) or a Brenner tumor (38), and in one cited but undocumented case, in a mucinous cystadenoma with squamous differentiation (30). Only the last three forms of squamous cell

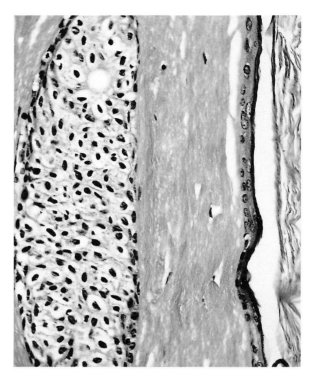

Figure 7-20
EPIDERMOID CYST
The cyst contains keratinized material. A solid nest of transitional cells simulating a Walthard nest lies in the wall of the cyst (left). (Fig. 3 from Young RH, Prat J, Scully RE. Epidermoid cyst of the ovary. A report of three cases with comments on histogenesis. Am J Clin Pathol 1980;73:272–6.).

carcinoma can be classified confidently in the surface epithelial–stromal category. The literature also contains 24 cases of pure squamous cell carcinoma of the ovary with few or no clues to their origin (37). In 10 of these cases carcinoma in situ of the cervix was also diagnosed, either previously or synchronously (33a), raising the question of metastasis from an undiscovered focus of invasive cervical cancer instead of an ovarian origin (fig. 7-21). Five of the 10 ovarian squamous cell carcinomas associated with carcinoma in situ of the cervix were purely or almost purely cystic, three without obvious invasion, one with minimal invasion, and one with deeper invasion of the adjacent ovarian stroma; in the other five cases solid invasive components were present as well as cysts lined by tumor. In two cases the additional presence of benign squamous epithelium in an ovarian cyst lined partly by malignant epithelium supported the diagnosis of a

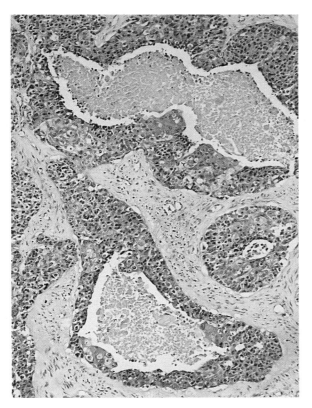

Figure 7-21
SQUAMOUS CELL CARCINOMA
Islands of malignant squamous cells are centrally necrotic.

primary ovarian carcinoma (35,39), possibly arising in an epidermoid cyst. In another case, the patient was alive and free of tumor 5 years after the removal of the uterus and adnexa (40) providing evidence against spread of tumor from the cervix to the ovary.

Primary squamous cell carcinomas of the ovary must be distinguished from endometrioid adenocarcinomas with extensive squamous differentiation and from secondary squamous cell tumors originating in the uterine cervix and possibly other sites. The finding of closely associated benign squamous epithelium, endometriosis, or a Brenner tumor provides strong evidence for an origin in the ovary.

Patients with squamous cell carcinoma belonging definitely or probably in the surface epithelial–stromal category have ranged in age from 27 to 90 years, with a mean age of 53 years (37).

Too few cases have been reported to establish the prognosis associated with primary squamous cell carcinomas that originate in endometriosis or are pure, but after a follow-up period of at least 1 year, all 10 patients with a tumor in the former group died of their disease (33,34,36, 37,41), and only 7 of 19 patients in the latter category were alive without evidence of disease 1 to 5 years postoperatively (37).

REFERENCES

Transitional Cell Tumors

1. Aguirre P, Scully RE, Wolfe HJ, DeLellis RA. Argyrophil cells in Brenner tumors: histochemical and immunohistochemical analysis. Int J Gynecol Pathol 1986;5:223–34.
2. Arey LB. The origin and form of the Brenner tumor. Am J Obstet Gynecol 1961;81:743–51.
3. Austin RM, Norris HJ. Malignant Brenner tumor and transitional cell carcinoma of the ovary: a comparison. Int J Gynecol Pathol 1987;6:29–39.
4. Chen KT. Bilateral malignant Brenner tumor of the ovary. J Surg Oncol 1984;26:194–7.
5. Colgan TJ, Norris HJ. Ovarian epithelial tumours of low malignant potential: a review. Int J Gynecol Pathol 1983;1:367–82.
6. Ehrlich CE, Roth LM. The Brenner tumor. A clinicopathologic study of 57 cases. Cancer 1971;27:332–42.
6a. Elemenoglou A, Zizi-Serbetzoglou A, Trihia H, Vasilakaki T, Bournia E. Mixed ovarian neoplasm composed of struma ovarii and Brenner tumor. Eur J Gynaec Oncol 1994;15:138–41.
7. Fox H, Agrawal K, Langley FA. The Brenner tumour of the ovary. A clinicopathological study of 54 cases. J Obstet Gynaecol Brit Cmwlth 1972;79:661–5.
8. Gersell DJ. Primary ovarian transitional cell carcinoma. Diagnostic and prognostic considerations [Editorial]. Am J Clin Pathol 1990;93:586–8.
9. Hallgrímsson J, Scully RE. Borderline and malignant Brenner tumours of the ovary. A report of 15 cases. Acta Path Microbiol Scand [A] 1972;80(Supp. 233):56–66.
10. Hollingsworth HC, Steinberg SM, Silverberg SG, Merino MJ. Advanced stage transitional cell carcinoma of the ovary. Hum Pathol 1996;27:1267–72.
11. Katsube Y, Berg JW, Silverberg SG. Epidemiologic pathology of ovarian tumors: a histopathologic review of primary ovarian neoplasms diagnosed in the Denver standard metropolitan statistical area, 1 July–31 December 1969 and 1 July–31 December 1979. Int J Gynecol Pathol 1982;1:3–16.

12. Koonings PP, Campbell K, Mishell DR Jr, Grimes DA. Relative frequency of primary ovarian neoplasms: a 10-year review. Obstet Gynecol 1989;74:921–6.

13. Martin AR, Cotylo PK, Kennedy JC, Fineberg NS, Roth LM. Flow cytometric DNA analysis of ovarian Brenner tumors and transitional cell carcinomas. Int J Gynecol Pathol 1992;11:188–96.

14. Miles PA, Norris HJ. Proliferative and malignant Brenner tumors of the ovary. Cancer 1972;30:174–86.

15. Nakashima N, Nagasaka T, Fukata S, et al. Study of ovarian tumors treated at Nagoya University Hospital, 1965–1988. Gynecol Oncol 1990;37:103–11.

16. Roth LM. The Brenner tumor and the Walthard cell nest. An electron microscopic study. Lab Invest 1974;31:15–23.

17. Roth LM, Czernobilsky B. Ovarian Brenner tumors. II. Malignant. Cancer 1985;56:592–601.

18. Roth LM, Dallenbach-Hellweg G, Czernobilsky B. Ovarian Brenner tumors. I. Metaplastic, proliferating, and of low malignant potential. Cancer 1985;56:582–91.

19. Roth LM, Gersell DJ, Ulbright TM. Ovarian Brenner tumors and transitional cell carcinoma: recent developments. Int J Gynecol Pathol 1993;12:128–33.

19a. Roth LM, Gersell DJ, Ulbright TM. Transitional cell carcinoma and other transitional cell tumors of the ovary. In: Fechner RE, Rosen PP, eds. Anatomic Pathology, Vol. 1. Chicago: ASCP Press, 1996:179–91.

20. Santini D, Gelli MC, Mazzoleni G, et al. Brenner tumor of the ovary: a correlative histologic, histochemical, immunohistochemical, and ultrastructural investigation. Hum Pathol 1989;20:787–95.

21. Silva EG, Robey-Cafferty SS, Smith TL, Gershenson DM. Ovarian carcinomas with transitional cell carcinoma pattern. Am J Clin Pathol 1990;93:457–65.

22. Silverberg SG. Brenner tumor of the ovary. A clinicopathologic study of 60 tumors in 54 women. Cancer 1971;28:588–96.

22a. Soslow RA, Rouse RV, Hendrickson MR, Silva EG, Longacre TA. Transitional cell neoplasms of the ovary and urinary bladder: a comparative immunohistochemical analysis. Int J Gynecol Pathol 1996;15:257–65.

23. Stohr G. The relationship of Brenner tumor to the rete ovarii. Am J Obstet Gynecol 1956;72:389–99.

24. Tateno H, Sasano N. Ovarian tumours in Sendai, Japan. General hospital material. In: Stalsberg H, ed. UICC technical report series, Vol 75. An international survey of distribution of histologic types of tumours of the testis and ovary. Geneva: UICC, 1983;291–6.

25. Tiltman AJ, Sweerts M. Ovarian neoplasms in the Western Cape. S Afr Med J 1982;61:343–5.

26. Trebeck CE, Friedlander ML, Russell P, Baird RI. Brenner tumors of the ovary: a study of the histology, immunochemistry, and cellular DNA content in benign, borderline, and malignant ovarian tumors. Pathology 1987;19:241–6.

27. Waxman M. Pure and mixed Brenner tumors of the ovary: clinicopathologic and histogenetic observations. Cancer 1979;43:1830–9.

28. Woodruff JD, Dietrich D, Genadry R, Parmley TH. Proliferative and malignant Brenner tumors. Review of 47 cases. Am J Obstet Gynecol 1981;141:118–25.

29. Yoonessi M, Abell MR. Brenner tumors of the ovary. Obstet Gynecol 1979;54:90–6.

Squamous Cell Tumors

30. Black WC, Benitez RE. Nonteratomatous squamous cell carcinoma in situ of the ovary. Obstet Gynecol 1964;24:865–8.

31. Chen KT. Squamous cell carcinoma of the ovary [Letter]. Arch Pathol Lab Med. 1988;112:114–5.

32. Fan LD, Zang HY, Zhang XS. Ovarian epidermoid cyst: report of eight cases. Int J Gynecol Pathol 1996;15:69–71.

33. Lele SB, Piver MS, Barlow JJ, Tsukada Y. Squamous cell carcinoma arising in ovarian endometriosis. Gynecol Oncol 1978;6:290–3.

33a. Mai KT, Yazdi M, Bertrand MA, Le Saux N, Cathcart L. Bilateral primary ovarian squamous cell carcinoma associated with human papilloma virus infection and vulvar and cervical intraepithelial neoplasia. Am J Surg Pathol 1996;20:767–72.

34. McCullough K, Froats ER, Falk HC. Epidermoid carcinoma arising in an endometrial cyst of the ovary. Arch Pathol Lab Med 1946;41:335–7.

35. McGrady BJ, Sloan JM, Lamki H, Fox H. Bilateral ovarian cysts with squamous intraepithelial neoplasia. Int J Gynecol Pathol 1993;12:350–4.

36. Naresh KN, Ahuja VK, Rao CR, Mukherjee G, Bhargava MK. Squamous cell carcinoma arising in endometriosis of the ovary. J Clin Pathol 1991;44:958–9.

37. Pins MR, Young RH, Daly WJ, Scully RE. Primary squamous cell carcinoma of the ovary. A report of 37 cases. Am J Surg Pathol 1996;20:823–33.

38. Roth LM, Czernobilsky B. Ovarian Brenner tumors. II. Malignant. Cancer 1985;56:592–601.

39. Shingleton HM, Middleton FF, Gore H. Squamous cell carcinoma of the ovary. Am J Obstet Gynecol 1974;120:556–60.

40. Sworn MJ, Jones H, Letchworth AT, Herrington CS, McGee JO. Squamous intraepithelial neoplasia in an ovarian cyst, cervical intraepithelial neoplasia and human papillomavirus. Hum Pathol 1995;26:344–7.

41. Tetu B, Silva EG, Gershenson DM. Squamous cell carcinoma of the ovary. Arch Pathol Lab Med 1987;111:864–6.

42. Young RH, Prat J, Scully RE. Epidermoid cyst of the ovary. A report of three cases with comments on histogenesis. Am J Clin Pathol 1980;73:272–6.

8
MIXED EPITHELIAL TUMORS AND UNDIFFERENTIATED CARCINOMA

MIXED EPITHELIAL TUMORS

Since most of the tumors in the surface epithelial–stromal category have a similar origin, it is not surprising that admixtures of the various subtypes often occur. To avoid diagnosis of an unwieldy number of mixed tumors, the World Health Organization (WHO) limits their identification to those neoplasms in which different tumor types are recognizable on gross examination, and those in which one or more components other than the predominant component account for at least 10 percent of the tumor on microscopic examination. Almost all combinations of mixed epithelial neoplasia have been encountered. Among those that have received particular emphasis in the literature are Brenner tumor with a mucinous cystic component, an endocervical-like mucinous cystic tumor of borderline malignancy containing other epithelial cell types (fig. 8-1) (12), an endometrioid carcinoma admixed with a clear cell carcinoma (see fig. 6-1) (4,7,13), a transitional cell carcinoma with another type of carcinoma (14), and an endometrioid carcinoma with a serous or undifferentiated component (fig. 8-2) (16). In cases of Brenner and mucinous neoplasia, specific criteria for the diagnosis of a mixed epithelial tumor are essential for diagnostic uniformity. According to our criteria, if both the mucinous and Brenner components (Brenner tumor and pure mucinous tumor) are detectable on gross examination or if the minor component (Brenner tumor or pure mucinous tumor) accounts for at least 10 percent of the neoplasm, the diagnosis is mixed mucinous and Brenner tumor. Mucinous epithelium within Brenner epithelial nests is not sufficient to warrant a diagnosis of a mixed epithelial tumor. The presence of additional cell types in endocervical-like mucinous borderline tumors does not appear to affect the prognosis (12). Since endometrioid carcinomas and clear cell carcinomas are associated with a roughly similar prognosis (2,7), the combination of the two tumor types would not be expected to have a significant effect on survival.

The controversial improvement in prognosis associated with a predominance of transitional cell carcinoma in mixed epithelial-stromal cancers has been discussed on page 162. The addition of a serous or undifferentiated carcinoma component to a stage III or IV endometrioid carcinoma has been reported to reduce the 5- and 10-year survival rates from 63 to 8 percent and 45 to 0 percent, respectively (16). The International Federation of Gynecology and Obstetrics (FIGO) annual report has no survival figures for patients with mixed epithelial borderline tumors and carcinomas; according to its classification

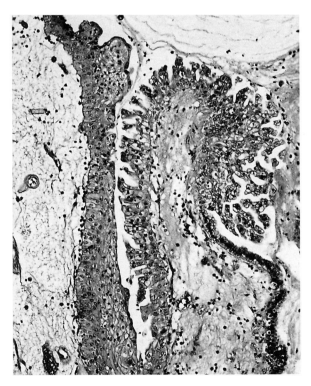

Figure 8-1
CYSTIC TUMOR OF BORDERLINE MALIGNANCY
OF MIXED EPITHELIAL TYPES
Part of the cyst is lined by proliferating endocervical-like mucinous cells forming cellular papillae and part is lined by squamous epithelium. The intracellular mucin is not clearly visible at this magnification.

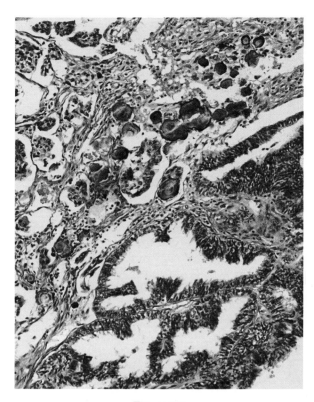

Figure 8-2
MIXED EPITHELIAL TUMOR
The tumor consists of serous papillary carcinoma (above) and endometrioid adenocarcinoma (below).

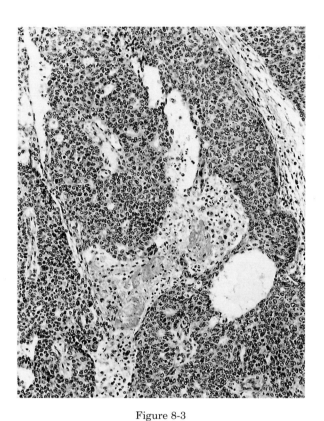

Figure 8-3
UNDIFFERENTIATED CARCINOMA
The tumor cells are growing in masses with a central area of necrosis.

criteria these tumors are designated according to the predominant cell type (11), an approach that makes it impossible to ascertain the significance of an additional minor component of another cell type.

UNDIFFERENTIATED CARCINOMA

Definition. According to the WHO, an undifferentiated carcinoma is one that shows no differentiation or contains only rare, minor areas of differentiation (figs. 8-3, 8-4). Silva et al. (15), however, defined undifferentiated carcinoma as one in which over half the tumor lacks differentiation. If the WHO criteria are used, 5 percent or less of ovarian cancers of epithelial type belong in the undifferentiated category.

General Features. According to FIGO (11) undifferentiated carcinomas account for 14 percent of epithelial cancers of the ovary. Nineteen percent of stage IA and IB tumors are bilateral.

Twelve percent of undifferentiated carcinomas are confined to the ovary; 11 percent are stage II; 51 percent, stage III; and 26 percent, stage IV. The respective 5-year survival rates are 68 percent, 40 percent, 17 percent, and 6.3 percent (11).

Pathologic Features. Undifferentiated carcinomas have no distinctive gross features that distinguish them from other high-grade ovarian carcinomas. Microscopic examination reveals a uniform or almost uniform population of cells with high-grade nuclear features and typically scanty cytoplasm. The tumor may have a sarcomatoid appearance. Rare minor foci of differentiation into glands, mucin-filled cells, and psammoma bodies may be present. Such differentiation is nonspecific, occurring with varying degrees of frequency in many subtypes in the epithelial-stromal cell category (9).

Rare undifferentiated carcinomas are of small cell type. Some of these tumors resemble carcinomas of the lung and have neuroendocrine features (5,6)

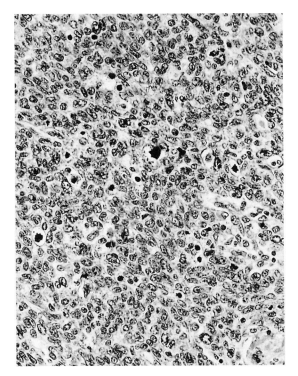

Figure 8-4
UNDIFFERENTIATED CARCINOMA
The tumor cells have atypical nuclei with mitotic figures and scanty cytoplasm.

(page 320). More often, they are small cell carcinomas of the hypercalcemic type, a tumor of unknown lineage (page 316).

Rarely, undifferentiated carcinomas exhibit focal transformation into choriocarcinoma, with the typical microscopic features of that tumor and the production of chorionic gonadotropin (10).

Immunohistochemical staining of undifferentiated carcinoma is positive for epithelial membrane antigen (EMA) and cytokeratins, negative for vimentin, and only occasionally positive for CA125 (8).

Differential Diagnosis. Undifferentiated carcinomas are most often confused with transitional cell carcinomas (page 160) and diffuse adult granulosa cell tumors. The nuclear hyperchromatism and frequent pleomorphism, the atypical mitotic activity, and the rarity of associated endocrine manifestations in cases of undifferentiated carcinoma contrast with the typically pale, often grooved nuclei, the absence of atypical mitotic activity, and the common association with endocrine manifestations of the granulosa cell tumor. Also, the stages of the two tumors and their clinical courses differ markedly. In difficult cases, staining of undifferentiated carcinomas for EMA and lack of staining for vimentin and α-inhibin in contrast to the results in granulosa cell tumors are helpful in the differential diagnosis (1,3,8,15).

Undifferentiated carcinomas must also be distinguished from poorly differentiated sarcomas, carcinosarcomas (page 128), and lymphomas by the usual criteria for identifying these tumors. Undifferentiated carcinomas arising elsewhere rarely metastasize to the ovary. Diagnosis of these tumors is based on the criteria for distinguishing ovarian primary from metastatic tumors in general (page 335).

REFERENCES

1. Aguirre P, Thor AD, Scully RE. Ovarian endometrioid carcinomas resembling sex cord-stromal tumors. An immunohistochemical study. Int J Gynecol Pathol 1989;8:364–73.
2. Brescia RJ, Dubin N, Demopoulos RI. Endometrioid and clear cell carcinoma of the ovary. Int J Gynecol Pathol 1989;8:132–8.
3. Costa MJ, DeRose PB, Roth LM, Brescia RJ, Zaloudek CJ, Cohen C. Immunohistochemical phenotype of ovarian granulosa cell tumors: absence of epithelial membrane antigen has diagnostic value. Hum Pathol 1994;25:60–6.
4. Czernobilsky B, Silverman BB, Enterline HT. Clear-cell carcinoma of the ovary. A clinicopathologic analysis of pure and mixed forms and comparison with endometrioid carcinoma. Cancer 1970;25:762–72.
5. Eichhorn JH, Lawrence WD, Young RH, Scully RE. Ovarian neuroendocrine carcinomas of non-small cell type associated with surface epithelial adenocarcinomas. A study of five cases and a review of the literature. Int J Gynecol Pathol 1996;15:303–14.
6. Eichhorn JH, Young RH, Scully RE. Primary ovarian small cell carcinoma of pulmonary type. A clinicopathologic, immunohistologic, and flow cytometric analysis of 11 cases. Am J Surg Pathol 1992;16:926–38.

7. Kurman RJ, Craig JM. Endometrioid and clear cell carcinoma of the ovary. Cancer 1972;29:1653–64.

8. Kuwashima Y, Uehara T, Kishi K, Shiromizu K, Matsuzawa M, Takayama S. Immunohistochemical characterization of undifferentiated carcinomas of the ovary. J Cancer Res Clin Oncol 1994;120:672–7.

9. O'Donnell M, Al-Nafussi AI. Intracytoplasmic lumina and mucinous inclusions in ovarian carcinomas. Histopathology 1995;26:181–4.

10. Oliva E, Andrada E, Pezzica E, Prat J. Ovarian carcinomas with choriocarcinomatous differentiation. Cancer 1993;72:2441–6.

11. Pettersson F. Annual report of the results of treatment in gynecological cancer. Stockholm, International Federation of Gynecology and Obstetrics, 1991.

12. Rutgers JL, Scully RE. Ovarian mixed-epithelial papillary cystadenoms of borderline malignancy of mullerian type. A clinicopathologic analysis. Cancer 1988;61:546–54.

13. Scully RE, Barlow JF. "Mesonephroma" of ovary. Tumor of mullerian nature related to the endometrioid carcinoma. Cancer 1967;20:1405–16.

14. Silva EG, Robey-Cafferty SS, Smith TL, Gershenson DM. Ovarian carcinomas with transitional cell carcinoma pattern. Am J Clin Pathol 1990;93:457–65.

15. Silva EG, Tornos C, Bailey MA, Morris M. Undifferentiated carcinoma of the ovary. Arch Pathol Lab Med 1991;115:377–81.

16. Tornos C, Silva EG, Khorana SM, Burke TW. High-stage endometrioid carcinoma of the ovary. Prognostic significance of pure versus mixed histologic types. Am J Surg Pathol 1994;18:687–93.

9
SEX CORD–STROMAL TUMORS, GRANULOSA CELL TUMORS

SEX CORD–STROMAL TUMORS

This category of neoplasms, which accounts for approximately 8 percent of all primary ovarian tumors, comprises all neoplasms that contain granulosa cells, theca cells, and their luteinized derivatives, as well as Sertoli cells, Leydig cells, and fibroblasts of stromal origin, singly or in various combinations and in varying degrees of differentiation (1,2). In the developing testis the sex cords are clearly distinguishable by the 7th week of embryonic life as slender columns of primitive Sertoli cells, but similar cords, at least in the sense of thin columns, are not encountered in the developing ovary; instead, packets of small pregranulosa cells enveloping germ cells become evident later in embryonic life. For that reason, the term "sex cords" has been criticized as inacurrate to describe the progenitors of granulosa cells. Nevertheless, the long-established usage of this designation by embryologists and the lack of a better term justify its retention. The term "sex cord–stromal tumors," which has been adopted by the World Health Organization (WHO), has the advantage of acknowledging the presence in neoplasms in this general category of derivatives of either or both the sex cords and the stroma. The components derived from the sex cords (granulosa and Sertoli cells) are typically arranged in epithelial configurations, whereas those derived from the stroma have the appearance of gonadal stroma or its specialized derivatives: theca, lutein, and Leydig cells.

Most sex cord–stromal tumors are composed of ovarian cell types (granulosa-stromal cell tumors) but some (Sertoli-stromal cell tumors) contain only cells of testicular type; occasionally, cells and patterns of growth characteristic of both gonads coexist (gynandroblastomas). When the neoplastic cells are immature, when their appearance is intermediate between those of testicular and ovarian cell types, or when the architectural patterns of the tumor are not specific for either the testis or the ovary, it may be impossible to determine whether the tumor belongs in the granulosa-stromal or Sertoli-stromal cell category; in such cases the term "sex cord–stromal tumor, unclassified" is used. In a 25-year period at one large institution (1) the distribution of the various sex cord–stromal tumors, excluding consultation material, was as follows: tumors in the thecoma-fibroma group (87 percent), granulosa cell tumors (12 percent), Sertoli-Leydig cell tumors (0.05 percent), and unclassified (0.05 percent). The granulosa cell tumor accounts for most clinically malignant tumors in the sex cord–stromal category.

GRANULOSA CELL TUMORS

These are tumors in which granulosa cells account for at least 10 percent of a granulosa-stromal cell tumor. Two main histopathologic subtypes exist: adult and juvenile. The adult form typically has microfollicles, cells with scanty cytoplasm and pale nuclei, and occurs mainly in middle-aged and older women; the juvenile form typically has large follicles, cells with moderate to abundant cytoplasm and darker nuclei, and occurs mainly in children and younger women.

Adult Granulosa Cell Tumor

General Features. Adult granulosa cell tumors account for 1 to 2 percent of all ovarian tumors and 95 percent of all granulosa cell tumors (4,6,9,10,12,14,21,28,36,37,42). They occur more often in menopausal and postmenopausal than premenopausal women, with a peak age incidence between 50 and 55 years, but they may be seen at any age. They are the most common ovarian tumors with estrogenic manifestations but the proportion that secrete hormones is difficult to establish because a specimen of endometrium for evaluation of the presence or absence of an estrogenic effect is often unavailable. When the tumor is functioning, the typical endometrial effect is cystic hyperplasia, usually exhibiting some degree of precancerous atypia (17). Carcinoma of the endometrium, which is almost always well differentiated, occurs in slightly less than 5 percent of the cases, and twice as often in postmenopausal as in premenopausal patients (17).

An endocrine presentation of an adult granulosa cell tumor is almost always related to hyperestrinism and varies according to the age of the patient. Postmenopausal women typically have uterine bleeding. Women in the reproductive age group usually experience irregular, excessive uterine bleeding but amenorrhea, which may last for months to years, often precedes the bleeding or may be the only endocrine manifestation, sometimes being mistaken for menopausal amenorrhea. In the rare cases in which the adult granulosa cell tumor appears before puberty the endocrine presentation is isosexual pseudoprecocity. Occasional adult granulosa cell tumors are accompanied by an endometrial change suggestive of progesterone production by the tumor (a decidual reaction of the stroma or secretory activity of the glands). In some cases this phenomenon is associated with varying degrees of luteinization of the granulosa cells (40). Rarely, androgenic changes, usually virilization but occasionally only a recent onset of hirsutism, accompany adult granulosa cell tumors (26,29). A disproportionate number of androgenic granulosa cell tumors have been unilocular or multilocular thin-walled cystic tumors. In addition to endocrine manifestations most women with adult granulosa cell tumors have signs and symptoms related to a mass, usually in the form of abdominal pain or swelling; approximately 10 percent present with acute abdominal symptoms due to rupture of the neoplasm with hemoperitoneum.

In two large studies, 78 and 91 percent of granulosa cell tumors were stage I (4–6,37), most of the remainder were stage II, and no more than 5 percent, stage III. A mass is usually palpable, at least on pelvic examination; in up to 12 percent of the cases the tumor cannot be detected on physical examination (12), but is almost always large enough to be visible on ultrasound examination.

Gross Findings. The tumors are unilateral in over 95 percent of the cases (4–6,14,36,37). They usually have an intact external surface but 10 to 15 percent are ruptured. The size varies from microscopic to huge masses that distend the abdomen; the average diameter is approximately 12 cm. The sectioned surfaces have several highly distinctive appearances. They may be predominantly cystic, with numerous compartments that are typically filled with fluid or clotted blood (fig. 9-1) and separated by solid tissue, which varies

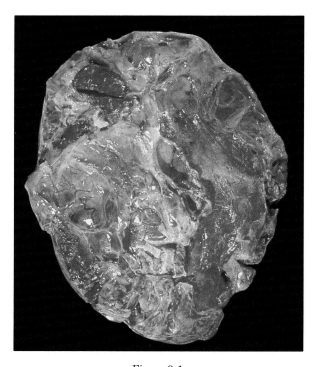

Figure 9-1
ADULT GRANULOSA CELL TUMOR
The sectioned surface is solid and cystic, with a number of the cysts containing clotted blood.

from yellow to white depending on the proportion of lipid-containing cells, and from soft to firm depending on the relative prominence of granulosa cell and stromal elements. Some tumors are composed entirely of solid, white to yellow tissue (fig. 9-2), which often contains areas of hemorrhage and occasionally areas of necrosis. Uncommonly, the tumor forms a thin-walled multilocular (fig. 9-3) or unilocular cyst that contains watery fluid and has a smooth lining, resembling a serous cystadenoma (26,28).

Microscopic Findings. Microscopic examination typically reveals granulosa cells growing in a wide variety of patterns, which are frequently admixed. A common low-power pattern, which predominated in one series (23), is diffuse (sarcomatoid) (fig. 9-4); high-power examination often shows an epithelial pattern of the tumor cells within the diffuse areas. Trabecular (fig. 9-5) and insular (fig. 9-6) arrangements of granulosa cells separated by a fibrothecomatous stroma are also frequent. The best differentiated pattern is follicular, and the most common follicular pattern is

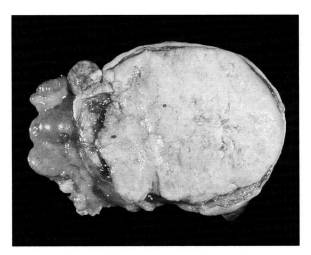

Figure 9-2
ADULT GRANULOSA CELL TUMOR
The sectioned surface is uniformly solid and yellow.

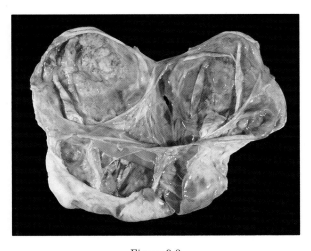

Figure 9-3
ADULT GRANULOSA CELL TUMOR
The tumor is composed of several locules with predominantly smooth linings. (Fig. 2 from Young RH, Scully RE. Ovarian sex cord–stromal tumors: problems in differential diagnosis. Pathol Ann 1988;23(Pt 1):237–96.)

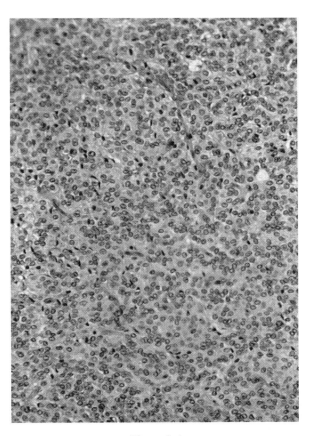

Figure 9-4
ADULT GRANULOSA CELL TUMOR,
DIFFUSE PATTERN
The small cells have scanty cytoplasm.

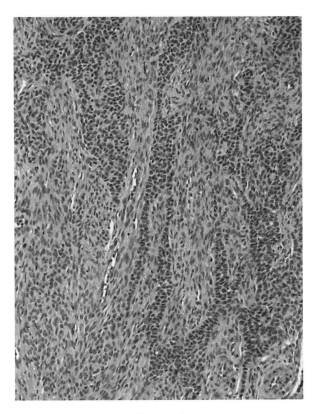

Figure 9-5
ADULT GRANULOSA CELL TUMOR,
TRABECULAR PATTERN
The granulosa cells are growing in trabeculae and cords separated by cellular fibromatous tissue.

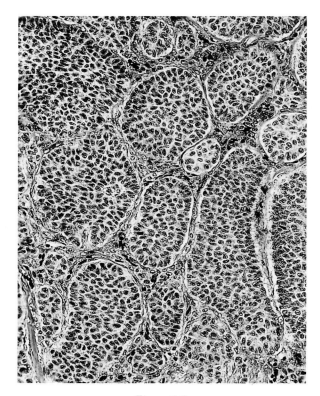

Figure 9-6
ADULT GRANULOSA CELL TUMOR,
INSULAR PATTERN
The granulosa cells are growing in well delineated nests.

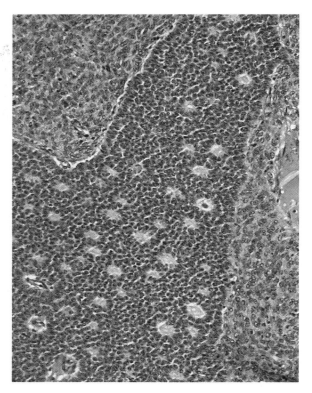

Figure 9-7
ADULT GRANULOSA CELL TUMOR,
MICROFOLLICULAR PATTERN
A large, discrete island of granulosa cells contains numerous Call-Exner bodies and is surrounded by a diffuse pattern of granulosa cells.

microfollicular, characterized by the presence of numerous small cavities simulating the Call-Exner bodies of a graafian follicle (figs. 9-7, 9-8). These cavities may contain eosinophilic fluid, one or a few degenerating nuclei, hyalinized basement membrane material, or rarely, basophilic fluid. The cavities are separated typically by well-differentiated granulosa cells that contain scanty cytoplasm and pale, angular or oval, often grooved nuclei arranged haphazardly in relation to one another and to the microfollicles. Less common is a macrofollicular pattern, characterized by cysts lined by well-differentiated granulosa cells, beneath which theca cells are usually present; this pattern rarely predominates (fig. 9-9). Other patterns of granulosa cell tumor are watered-silk (moiré-silk) (fig. 9-10) and gyriform (fig. 9-11), characterized by undulating parallel rows and zigzag cords of granulosa cells, respectively. Finally, rare neoplasms are composed of spindle-shaped granulosa cells or contain hollow or solid

tubules; the latter may be uniformly cellular or have peripheral nuclei and a central accumulation of cytoplasm. The tubular patterns are indistinguishable from those of well-differentiated Sertoli cell tumors, but their presence in a granulosa cell tumor is ignored diagnostically unless they account for 10 percent or more of the tumor; in such cases, a diagnosis of gynandroblastoma is warranted. The cells lining large cysts may have a number of the above patterns; aggregates of granulosa cells or a layer of theca cells may be present in the cyst wall (fig. 9-12). The lining cells may be denuded focally in cystic tumors. The above typical patterns may be obscured to varying extents during the last trimester of pregnancy because of prominent edema and in some cases, extensive luteinization (39).

Although the cells in most adult granulosa cell tumors have only scanty to small amounts of cytoplasm, a component of cells with moderate

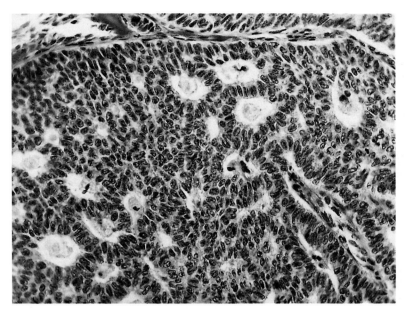

Figure 9-8
ADULT GRANULOSA CELL TUMOR,
MICROFOLLICULAR PATTERN
Call-Exner bodies containing fluid and pyknotic nuclei are surrounded by cells with oval and angular nuclei and scanty cytoplasm.

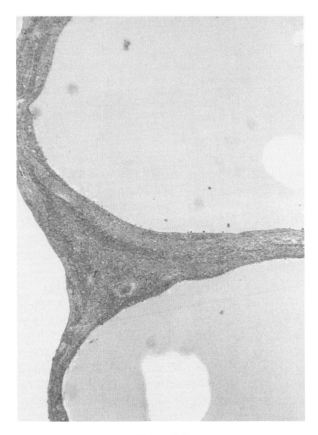

Figure 9-9
ADULT GRANULOSA CELL TUMOR,
MACROFOLLICULAR PATTERN
Large fluid-filled follicles resemble follicle cysts.

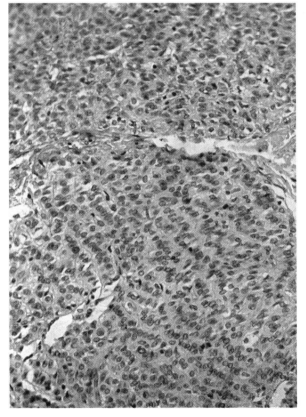

Figure 9-10
ADULT GRANULOSA CELL TUMOR,
WATERED-SILK (MOIRÉ-SILK) PATTERN
The tumor cells are arranged in parallel wavy rows.

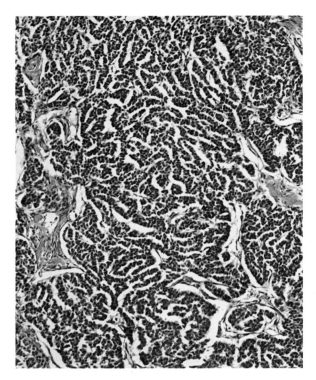

Figure 9-11
ADULT GRANULOSA CELL TUMOR,
GYRIFORM PATTERN
There is a zigzag arrangement of cords of granulosa cells.

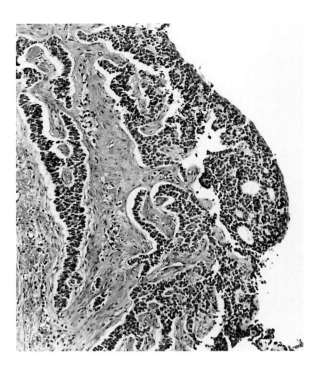

Figure 9-12
ADULT GRANULOSA CELL TUMOR, CYSTIC
Granulosa cells not only line the cyst but are present in irregular aggregates in its wall. (Fig. 5 from Nakashima N, Young RH, Scully RE. Androgenic granulosa cell tumors of the ovary. A clinicopathological analysis of 17 cases and review of the literature. Arch Pathol Lab Med 1984;108:786–91.)

to abundant eosinophilic cytoplasm (luteinized cells) is seen occasionally. In approximately 2 percent of the cases most of the tumor cells are luteinized (figs. 9-13, 9-14) (40).

Although the diagnosis of a granulosa cell tumor is usually strongly suggested on the basis of its low-power microscopic architecture, it must be confirmed by identifying typically pale, relatively uniform nuclei, at least some of which often contain grooves (figs. 9-15, 9-16). The prominence of the grooves varies from case to case; even when they are not prominent the nuclei are almost always pale and uniform (fig. 9-16). An exception to the characteristic nuclear features occurs in approximately 2 percent of granulosa cell tumors, which contain cells with bizarre, enlarged, hyperchromatic nuclei, including multinucleated forms (fig. 9-17) (41). Such cells are typically focal but may be numerous and divert attention from more characteristic areas. Nucleoli are occasionally prominent, particularly in luteinized granulosa cells (fig. 9-14) (40).

The mitotic rate in granulosa cell tumors varies (fig. 9-16). In one series of cases, 49 percent of the tumors had less than 1 mitotic figure per 10 high-power fields, 27 percent had 1 to 2, 15 percent had 3 to 5, and 9 percent had 6 or more (37). If numerous mitotic figures and especially if abnormal forms are present, the diagnosis of granulosa cell tumor should be made with caution.

The stromal component of granulosa cell tumors varies in prominence but in most cases at least a minor amount is present; occasionally, it predominates. It may be fibromatous (fig. 9-5) or fibrous but more typically contains a component of cells resembling theca externa cells, theca interna cells, or lutein cells (fig. 9-18). In some tumors, particularly those with a diffuse pattern, differentiation of granulosa and theca cells with routine staining may be difficult or impossible. In such cases a reticulin stain may be helpful. In a granulosa cell tumor, as in a graafian follicle, the fibrils typically invest theca cells or fibroblasts in

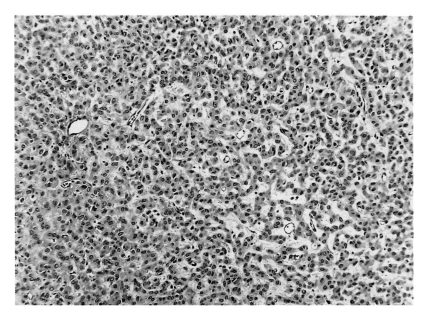

Figure 9-13
ADULT GRANULOSA CELL
TUMOR, LUTEINIZED
The cells contain moderate amounts
of cytoplasm, which was eosinophilic.

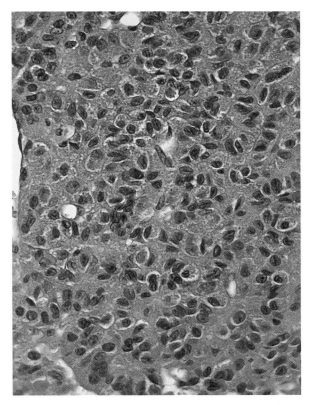

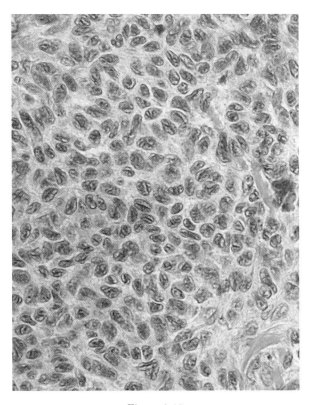

Figure 9-14
ADULT GRANULOSA CELL TUMOR, LUTEINIZED
The tumor cells contain abundant eosinophilic cytoplasm and mostly pale, oval and angular nuclei in a disorderly arrangement. A few nuclei have prominent nucleoli.

Figure 9-15
ADULT GRANULOSA CELL TUMOR
The cells have scanty cytoplasm and pale, oval and angular nuclei, many of which are grooved. (Fig. 3-2 from Young RH, Scully RE. Ovarian sex cord-stromal and steroid cell tumors. In: Roth LM, Czernobilsky B, eds. Tumors and tumor-like conditions of the ovary. New York: Churchill-Livingstone, 1985:43–73.)

175

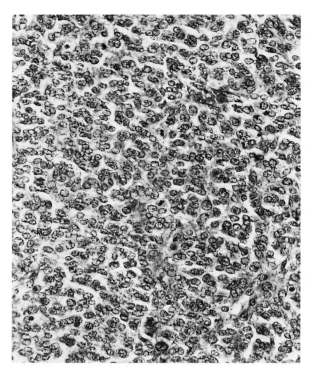

Figure 9-16
ADULT GRANULOSA CELL TUMOR
Nuclear grooves are not as conspicuous as in figure 9-15 but the nuclei are uniform and pale.

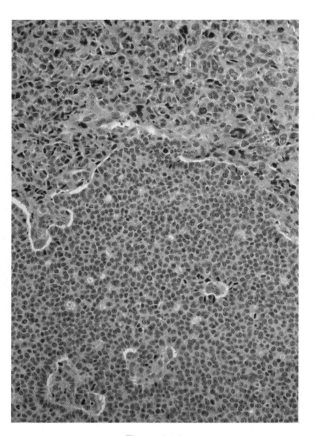

Figure 9-17
ADULT GRANULOSA CELL TUMOR
Many cells have enlarged, hyperchromatic, bizarre nuclei (top).

the stromal component individually or in very small groups; in contrast, the granulosa cell portion of the tumor contains few fibrils, most of which are perivascular (fig. 9-19). In occasional cases the reticulin stain is not useful because of an intermediate pattern of fibril distribution. Distinction between a granulosa cell tumor and a cellular fibroma or thecoma is important because of the greater malignant potential of the granulosa cell tumor. The occurrence of hemorrhage in many granulosa cell tumors often results in fibrosis with deposition of blood pigment.

Rarely, a granulosa cell tumor undergoes sarcomatous transformation (38) or has features similar to those of a poorly differentiated carcinoma containing highly atypical cells. One well-differentiated granulosa cell tumor containing scattered small islands of cells with the morphologic and immunocytochemical properties of mature hepatic cells has been reported (27) and we have seen four similar cases. Another granulosa cell tumor was situated in the wall of a mucinous cystic tumor (32).

Several special stains that are typically positive in steroid hormone-producing cells, particularly stains for intracellular lipid and immunostains for enzymes involved in steroid hormone biosynthesis from cholesterol (8a,33), as well as ultrastructural observations (15), suggest that the theca cell component of granulosa cell tumors produces androgens that are aromatized to estrogens by the granulosa cell component. Since the granulosa cells of the corpus luteum are capable of steroid hormone production, however, luteinized granulosa cells within granulosa cell tumors may be capable of synthesizing steroid hormones without the participation of theca cells.

The most important immunohistochemical findings in adult granulosa cell tumors, which can be decisive in the diagnosis of problem cases, are: α-inhibin (+), vimentin (+), cytokeratin (may be +, typically with punctate staining), cytokeratin-7 (–), and epithelial membrane antigen (–) (3,7,8,13,

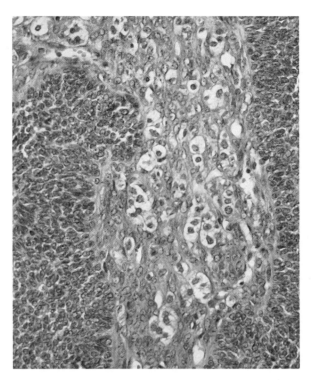

Figure 9-18
ADULT GRANULOSA CELL TUMOR
The stroma between the darkly staining aggregates of granulosa cells contains theca cells with pale vacuolated cytoplasm.

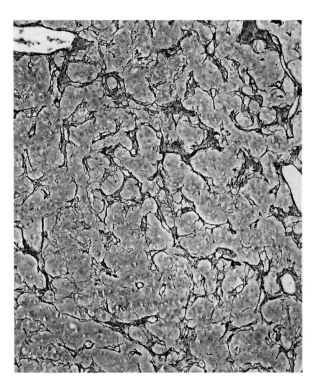

Figure 9-19
ADULT GRANULOSA CELL TUMOR
A reticulin stain shows fibrils surrounding nests and larger aggregates of granulosa cells. (Compare with figure 10-6.) (Fig. 19.14 from Young RH, Scully RE. Sex cord-stromal tumors, steroid cell tumors and other ovarian tumors with endocrine and paraendocrine and paraneoplastic manifestations. In: Kurman RJ, ed. Blaustein's pathology of the female genital tract, 4th ed. New York: Springer-Verlag, 1994:791.)

16a,24,25,30,31,32a,42). The granulosa cell component is often positive for S-100 protein (8) and smooth muscle actin (8), and the stromal component may be focally positive for desmin (30).

Differential Diagnosis. The misinterpretation of an undifferentiated carcinoma as a diffuse adult granulosa cell tumor is common; the differential diagnosis has been discussed on page 167. The small cell carcinoma of hypercalcemic type (page 316) may also be misdiagnosed as an adult granulosa cell tumor because of the presence of small cells with scanty cytoplasm and follicle-like structures in most of the cases. In addition to the presence of hypercalcemia in two thirds of patients with small cell carcinoma (absent in those with adult granulosa cell tumors) and the lack of estrogenic manifestations, the most helpful distinguishing histologic features of the small cell carcinoma are the more hyperchromatic nuclei, the much higher mitotic rate, and the lack of other characteristic patterns of the adult granulosa cell tumor. The distinction of a diffuse

adult granulosa cell tumor from an endometrioid stromal sarcoma (primary or metastatic from the uterus) is discussed on page 135. Other small cell tumors that may be in the differential diagnosis are included in Table 5-4.

Adult granulosa cell tumors with a diffuse pattern may be difficult to distinguish from pure stromal tumors, particularly highly cellular fibromas and thecomas. Reticulin stains may be helpful in this differential diagnosis (page 174).

Occasionally, the distinction of a unilocular or multilocular macrofollicular adult granulosa cell tumor from single or multiple follicle cysts of large size is difficult, particularly if the patient is pregnant or in the puerperium. The large, solitary, luteinized follicle cyst of pregnancy and the puerperium (page 426) is indistinguishable grossly from a unilocular cystic adult granulosa cell tumor. The large luteinized cells of the former, some of which contain large bizarre nuclei, differ from those of a unilocular adult granulosa cell tumor, which usually is lined by nonluteinized cells (fig. 9-12) and only rarely contains bizarre nuclei. Large solitary luteinized follicle cysts have rarely been seen in the absence of a current or very recent pregnancy.

Endometrioid carcinomas, usually those that are well or moderately well differentiated, are occasionally misdiagnosed as adult granulosa cell tumors when they have a focal diffuse, insular, trabecular, or microglandular pattern resembling on low-power examination similar patterns of granulosa cell tumors. The differential diagnosis is discussed on page 125.

The rare adult granulosa cell tumor in which most of the cells are luteinized may resemble a steroid cell tumor or another type of oxyphilic tumor of the ovary (see Table 6-1) (40). The focal presence of areas with the architectural and cytologic features of a nonluteinized granulosa cell tumor usually facilitates the diagnosis in these cases.

It is important also to distinguish the Call-Exner bodies of adult granulosa cell tumors from the acini of carcinoid tumors and from the hyaline deposits that are seen in gonadoblastomas and sex cord tumors with annular tubules (SCTATs). The acini of carcinoid tumors often contain dense eosinophilic secretion which is sometimes calcified; calcification is not a feature of the adult granulosa cell tumor. The nuclei of carcinoid tumors have coarse chromatin in contrast to the pale nuclei of adult granulosa cell tumors, and the cytoplasm is almost always positive for neuroendocrine markers unlike the cytoplasm of adult granulosa cell tumors. The hyaline deposits in gonadoblastomas and SCTATs are typically larger than Call-Exner bodies and can sometimes be observed to be continuous with hyaline thickening of the basement membrane along the periphery of the tumor cell nests; these deposits may undergo calcification. Also, gonadoblastomas contain germ cells, and SCTATs exhibit prominent, ring-shaped, simple and complex tubules. Occasionally, however, foci of SCTAT may be present in adult granulosa cell tumors and vice versa. The differentiation from gonadoblastoma and SCTAT is aided by distinctive clinical and gross features in many cases, for example, the background of intersex in cases of gonadoblastoma

(see chapter 16) and the very small size and multiplicity of the SCTATs associated with the Peutz-Jeghers syndrome (page 220).

The adult granulosa cell tumor may be confused also with metastatic malignant melanoma and metastatic breast carcinoma. Metastatic melanomas may contain cells with scanty cytoplasm that grow diffusely, imparting a low-power microscopic appearance similar to that of an adult granulosa cell tumor. Patterns of growth incompatible with a diagnosis of adult granulosa cell tumor and intracytoplasmic melanin pigment are usually found when a melanoma is thoroughly sampled; staining for α-inhibin and HMB-45 is helpful in problematic cases; adult granulosa cell tumors, however, may stain for S-100 protein (8). Metastatic breast carcinomas, particularly those of the lobular type, may have a diffuse pattern and uniform small cells with scanty cytoplasm, simulating an adult granulosa cell tumor. In cases in which the existence of a breast cancer is not suspected, the presence of focal patterns more suggestive of breast carcinoma than a granulosa cell tumor and the absence of the typical nuclear features of a granulosa cell tumor should alert the pathologist to the correct diagnosis. Special staining for intracellular mucin and staining for α-inhibin, epithelial membrane antigen, and gross cystic disease fluid protein-15 should provide the answer in difficult cases (page 352).

Spread and Metastasis. Adult granulosa cell tumors of all patterns have a malignant potential, with a capacity to extend beyond the ovary or recur after apparently complete removal. Spread is largely within the pelvis and lower abdomen; distant metastases are rare, but have been reported in many sites. Although recurrences may appear within 5 years, they are commonly detected much later, occasionally three or more decades postoperatively. In one series the mean time from diagnosis to death was 10.5 years and the median time 7.5 years (6). In another series in which 30 tumors recurred, 15 did so within 5 years (36). Elevations of the serum inhibin level may be helpful in detecting recurrent disease (19,22).

Treatment. The optimal treatment of a granulosa cell tumor in menopausal or postmenopausal women is bilateral salpingo-oophorectomy with total hysterectomy. In younger women in whom the preservation of fertility is an important consideration, however, removal of only the involved ovary is justifiable if extraovarian spread is not evident and examination of the contralateral ovary shows no evidence of involvement. Recurrence is usually fatal, but reoperation, radiation therapy, chemotherapy, or a combination thereof, has been used with various degrees of success (16,34). The chemotherapy in most cases has been similar to that used in the treatment of malignant germ cell tumors (35).

Prognosis. The 10-year survival figures that have been recorded in the literature have varied widely from under 60 to over 90 percent (4–6,14, 23,36,37) and progressive declines in survival have been documented after longer follow-up periods. Patients with stage I granulosa cell tumors have a considerably better prognosis than those with higher stage tumors, as shown by an 86 percent versus a 49 percent survival rate at 10 years in one large series (37) and a 96 percent versus a 26 percent survival rate in another (6). Rupture also adversely affects the outlook, with an 86 percent 25-year survival for patients with intact stage I tumors in contrast to only 60 percent for those with ruptured tumors of the same stage (6).

The size of granulosa cell tumors has also been analyzed in relation to prognosis. In one series all the patients with tumors 5 cm or less in diameter survived for 10 years, but only 57 percent of those with tumors 6 to 15 cm in diameter and 53 percent of those with even larger tumors survived for that period of time (14). Other investigators reported a 73 percent survival rate for patients with tumors under 5 cm in diameter, 63 percent for those with tumors between 5 and 15 cm, and 34 percent for those with a still larger tumor (37). In another series, stage I tumors 5 cm or less in diameter were associated with a 100 percent 10-year survival rate in contrast to 92 percent for patients with larger stage I tumors (6). The last series is the only one in which the survival rate was corrected for stage, but the difference in prognosis in that series was not statistically significant.

Attempts to correlate the histologic pattern and the degrees of nuclear atypia and mitotic activity with prognosis have met with varying success. Kottmeier (21) reported a better prognosis if the tumor was well differentiated (with a follicular or "cylindromatous" pattern) than if it was more poorly differentiated ("sarcomatoid"). This difference was reflected in 5-year survival figures of 87 percent and 64 percent, respectively,

but was more striking in the figures for 10 years, which were 82 percent versus 29 percent. The latter figures emphasize that very long follow-up is necessary before survival data for any series of granulosa cell tumors become meaningful. Several investigators, in contrast, have not confirmed the prognostic importance of pattern alone in granulosa cell tumors (4–6,10,14,23,28,36,37,42).

The degree of nuclear atypia in granulosa cell tumors has also been correlated with prognosis. In one study, the 5-year survival rate for patients whose tumors were free of atypia was 92 percent compared to 80 percent for those with slight atypia and 30 percent for those with moderate atypia (37). In another study there was an 80 percent 25-year survival of patients with tumors of grade 1 nuclear atypia in contrast to only a 60 percent survival of those with grade 2 atypia (6). In both of these studies nuclear atypia was the most reliable prognostic finding in stage I cases; in higher stage cases nuclear atypia and mitotic rate were of similar significance. There is no current evidence that the rare granulosa cell tumors that contain cells with bizarre nuclei are associated with a worse prognosis than tumors lacking those cells, but follow-up information on the former is limited (41).

Correlation of the mitotic activity of granulosa cell tumors with prognosis has also been attempted. In one study, there was a 70 percent 10-year survival of patients whose tumors had 2 or fewer mitotic figures per 10 high-power fields compared to only a 37 percent survival of those with 3 or more (37). In another investigation (14), tumors with many mitotic figures were associated with a worse prognosis than those with few, but most of the tumors with high mitotic rates presented at a higher stage than those with low mitotic rates, and differences in mitotic rate did not have a statistically significant effect on the prognosis of stage I tumors. Miller et al. (25a), however, reported that mitotic activity and nuclear atypia were greater in cases of early than in cases of late recurrence (over 10 years).

Flow cytometric studies have produced contradictory results. Two groups of investigators found that aneuploidy was not predictive of an adverse outcome (11,18) whereas another group concluded that it was (20). However, in the latter investigation almost two thirds of the neoplasms were higher than stage I, and two of them had

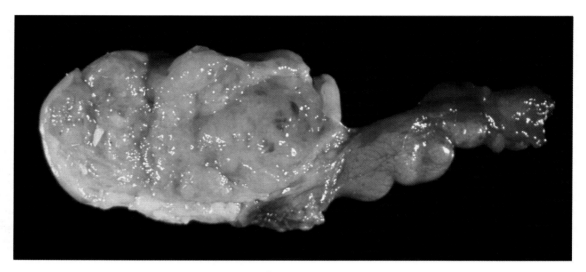

Figure 9-20
JUVENILE GRANULOSA CELL TUMOR
The sectioned surface is almost entirely solid and slightly lobulated, and is composed of yellow tissue.

mitotic rates of over 40 per 10 high-power fields; both findings cast doubt on the authors' diagnostic criteria for granulosa cell tumor.

Juvenile Granulosa Cell Tumor

General Features. Less than 5 percent of granulosa cell tumors are diagnosed before the age of normal puberty. Most of these tumors, as well as many granulosa cell tumors in young adults, differ histologically from adult granulosa cell tumors. The designation "juvenile" has been selected for such tumors because 97 percent of them occur in the first three decades (50). Approximately 80 percent of juvenile granulosa cell tumors (JGCTs) occurring in prepubertal children result in isosexual pseudoprecocity (43,46,49, 50,51). Typically this is heralded by breast development, followed by the appearance of pubic and axillary hair, stimulation and enlargement of the external and internal secondary sex organs, irregular uterine bleeding, and a whitish vaginal discharge, believed to originate in the stimulated endocervical glands; somatic and skeletal development are typically accelerated as well. Androgenic manifestations such as clitoromegaly occasionally occur. When the JGCT occurs after puberty, the patient usually presents with abdominal pain or swelling, sometimes associated with menstrual irregularities or amenorrhea. Approximately 6 percent of all the patients present with acute abdominal symptoms due to rupture of the tumor and hemoperitoneum (50). Eight patients have had Ollier's disease (enchondromatosis), and three additional patients, Maffucci's syndrome (enchondromatosis and hemangiomatosis) (48,50) (page 388).

The tumor is ruptured at operation in approximately 10 percent of the cases, and ascites is present in a similar percentage (50). Extraovarian spread is found in only 2 percent of the patients and is usually confined to the pelvis. A mass is almost always detectable clinically but on rare occasions is impalpable preoperatively on pelvic or bimanual rectal examination (44).

Gross Findings. The JGCT is bilateral in only about 2 percent of the cases. The diameter of the tumor has ranged from 3 to 32 cm, with an average of 12.5 cm (50). The gross features are similar to those of the adult granulosa cell tumor (figs. 9-20–9-22), with the single most common appearance as a solid and cystic neoplasm, in which the cysts may contain hemorrhagic fluid. Both uniformly or predominantly solid (fig. 9-20) and uniformly or predominantly cystic masses (fig. 9-21) are also encountered; the latter may be multilocular or unilocular. The solid tissue is typically yellow-tan or gray, and occasionally exhibits extensive necrosis, hemorrhage, or both (fig. 9-22).

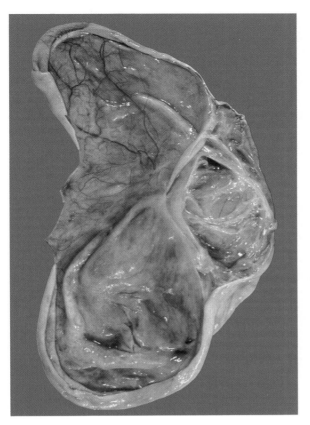

Figure 9-21
JUVENILE GRANULOSA CELL TUMOR
The sectioned surface shows several large locules with smooth linings.

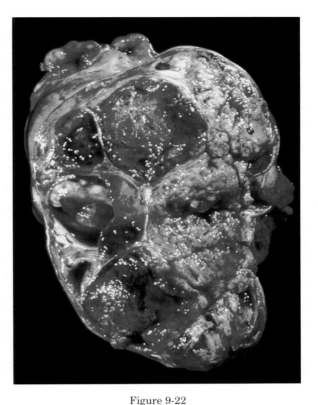

Figure 9-22
JUVENILE GRANULOSA CELL TUMOR
The sectioned surface is solid and cystic with extensive hemorrhage and areas of necrosis.

Microscopic Findings. Microscopic examination typically reveals a solid cellular neoplasm, with focal follicle formation (figs. 9-23, 9-24), but the tumor may be uniformly solid or contain numerous follicles. The solid areas may be diffuse or separated into nodules by fibrothecomatous septa (fig. 9-25); the nodules may become hyalinized, resembling somewhat corpora albicantia. Occasionally the granulosa cells lie in clusters in a fibrous stroma or are scattered irregularly on a background of basophilic fluid. In the solid foci the granulosa cells usually predominate but often there is an admixture of theca cells and in some areas the latter may predominate. Occasionally, the granulosa cells and theca cells are admixed in a haphazard fashion. In such cases reticulin stains may aid in their differentiation (page 174). A final rare pattern is papillary (fig. 9-26). Foci resembling typical thecoma with hyaline bands, and areas of sclerosis and calcification, are encountered rarely, but are usually small.

The follicles usually vary in size and shape (fig. 9-24) but may be round to oval (fig. 9-23). Their lumens contain eosinophilic or basophilic secretion (fig. 9-23), which can be stained by mucicarmine in approximately two thirds of the cases (fig. 9-27). Granulosa cells of varying layers of thickness line the follicles and are occasionally surrounded by mantles of theca cells (fig. 9-28). More often, however, the cells lining the follicles blend into the intervening diffusely cellular areas. Rarely, the lining cells have a hobnail contour (fig. 9-30).

The two characteristic cytologic features of the neoplastic granulosa cells that distinguish them from those of the adult granulosa cell tumor are their generally rounded, euchromatic or hyperchromatic nuclei, which almost always lack

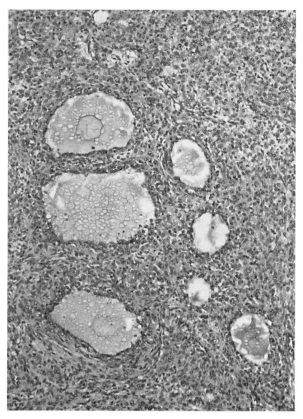

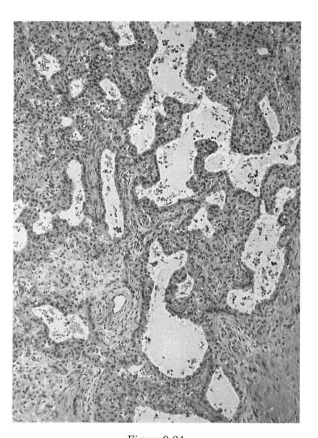

Figure 9-23
JUVENILE GRANULOSA CELL TUMOR
A solid pattern of cells is punctured by oval to round follicles differing in size and containing basophilic fluid.

Figure 9-24
JUVENILE GRANULOSA CELL TUMOR
There is marked variation in size and shape of the follicles.

Figure 9-25
JUVENILE GRANULOSA
CELL TUMOR
The granulosa cells are growing in solid nodules.

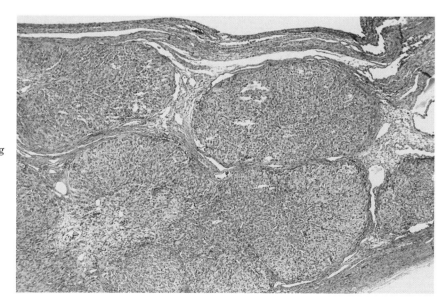

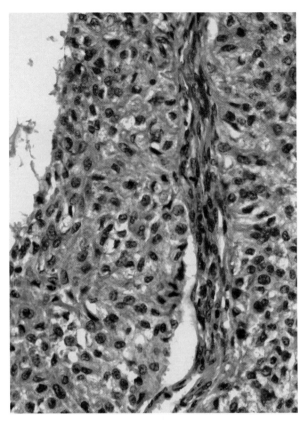

Figure 9-26
JUVENILE GRANULOSA CELL TUMOR
A papilla is lined by cells with pale to eosinophilic cytoplasm and slightly atypical nuclei. There is a superficial resemblance to a transitional cell neoplasm (see figure 7-13).

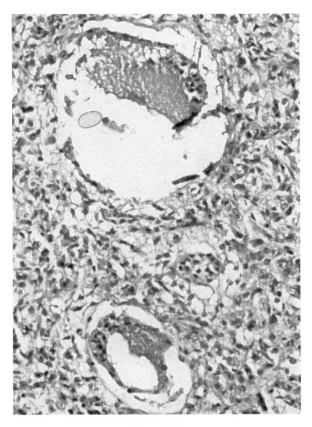

Figure 9-27
JUVENILE GRANULOSA CELL TUMOR
The fluid within two follicles is mucicarminophilic.

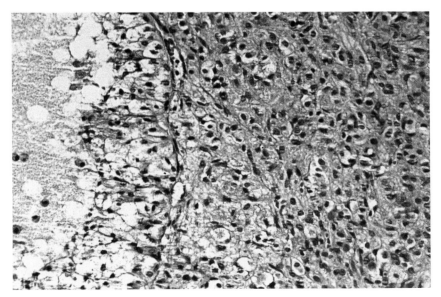

Figure 9-28
JUVENILE GRANULOSA
CELL TUMOR
The cells lining the follicle have abundant vacuolated cytoplasm. Adjacent theca cells contain abundant eosinophilic, focally vacuolated cytoplasm.

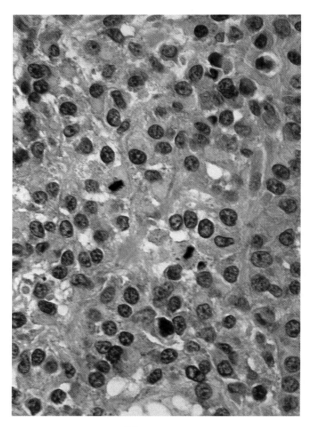

Figure 9-29
JUVENILE GRANULOSA CELL TUMOR
The tumor cells have abundant eosinophilic cytoplasm and round, slightly hyperchromatic nuclei. Two mitotic figures are seen near the center.

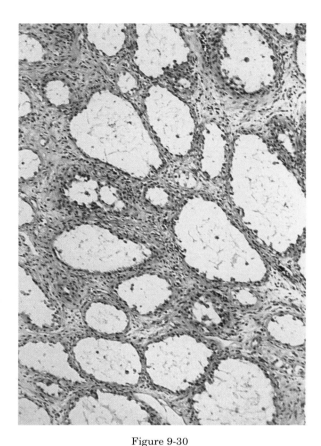

Figure 9-30
JUVENILE GRANULOSA CELL TUMOR
Many follicles are lined by cells with atypical "hobnail" nuclei simulating a tubulocystic clear cell carcinoma.

grooves, and their usual abundant content of eosinophilic or vacuolated (luteinized) cytoplasm (figs. 9-28, 9-29). The theca cell component of the tumor often contains moderate to large amounts of intracytoplasmic lipid. The theca cells are more often spindle shaped than the granulosa cells, and like the latter, usually have hyperchromatic nuclei. Nuclear atypia varies from minimal (fig. 9-30) to severe (fig. 9-31). Severe nuclear atypia has been observed in about 13 percent of the cases (50). Mitotic activity ranges from slight to marked (43a,50). Rare JGCTs are admixed with intermediate Sertoli-Leydig cell tumors (page 219). The JGCT is α-inhibin positive and epithelial membrane antigen negative.

Differential Diagnosis. The follicles of the JGCT are almost always more irregular in size and shape than those of an adult granulosa cell

tumor and its cells are typically more extensively luteinized, with nuclei that are typically round and more chromatic, and lack nuclear grooves. The mucicarminophilic, often basophilic follicular content of the JGCT is rare in the adult tumor, and Call-Exner bodies are almost never present in the JGCT.

The JGCT may be misinterpreted as a malignant germ cell tumor, usually a yolk sac tumor or embryonal carcinoma, especially if the nuclear atypia is marked. Paradoxically, the nuclear atypia of some JGCTs exceeds that seen in these biologically more aggressive primitive germ cell tumors. The nuclei of the JGCT are usually not as malignant-appearing as those of either germ cell tumor, however. Also, the follicular pattern of the JGCT is not a feature of primitive germ cell tumors, although the vesicles of the polyvesicular

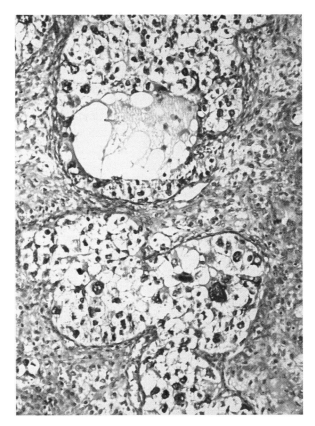

Figure 9-31
JUVENILE GRANULOSA CELL TUMOR
Large, bizarre nuclei and a single follicle are present.

vitelline yolk sac tumor may resemble superficially the follicles of a JGCT. The typical patterns of embryonal carcinomas and yolk sac tumors, as well as the immunohistochemical demonstration of chorionic gonadotropin in the former and alpha-fetoprotein in the latter tumor, and negative results for α-inhibin in both tumors can be decisive in difficult cases.

The JGCT is sometimes misinterpreted as a thecoma because of the occasional absence or rarity of follicles, the typically abundant cytoplasm of the neoplastic cells, and the occasional predominance of theca cells. Thorough sampling to demonstrate follicles and the use of reticulin stains to establish the granulosa cell nature of at least 10 percent of the tumor cells are important diagnostically. Also, thecomas only occasionally occur before 30 years of age and only exceptionally exhibit more than slight mitotic activity or nuclear atypia. Diffusely luteinized areas within a JGCT may suggest the diagnosis of a steroid cell tumor but other areas within the specimen should reveal diagnostic features. The pregnancy luteoma occasionally contains rounded follicle-like spaces and may suggest a luteinized JGCT, but again its pattern and cytologic features are uniform throughout the lesion. In contrast to the JGCT, the pregnancy luteoma is multiple in one half and bilateral in one third of the cases.

The surface epithelial–stromal tumors with which a JGCT may be confused are clear cell, undifferentiated, and transitional cell carcinomas. The tubulocystic variant of clear cell carcinoma is suggested rarely when follicles in a JGCT are lined by cells with a hobnail shape (fig. 9-30); JGCTs with high-grade nuclear atypia (fig. 9-31) may suggest an undifferentiated carcinoma. Transitional cell carcinoma is mimicked in rare cases in which a cystic JGCT contains papillae lined by uniform granulosa cells with moderate amounts of cytoplasm (fig. 9-26). All these carcinomas are very rare in the age group in which JGCTs almost always occur, and have immunohistochemical profiles that differ from those of granulosa cell tumors (page 176).

The JGCT may be confused with a small cell carcinoma of hypercalcemic type because both neoplasms contain follicles and both are found in young patients (page 316). Clinically, the two tumors typically differ because the former is usually associated with estrogenic manifestations and the latter, with paraendocrine hypercalcemia. From a histologic viewpoint, the typical small cell carcinoma is composed of cells with scanty cytoplasm, in marked contrast to the JGCT, in which the tumor cells typically have moderate to large amounts of cytoplasm. The follicles of small cell carcinoma rarely contain the mucicarminophilic basophilic secretion seen in many JGCTs. Although the JGCT often has many mitotic figures, they are generally much fewer than in the small cell carcinoma. Particular difficulty may be encountered in cases of the large cell variant of small cell carcinoma, in which the tumor cells have abundant eosinophilic cytoplasm. In most such cases, the more common small cell type of neoplasia is present, at least focally. If it is absent, the tumor tends to be uniform in appearance throughout without the typical variations in pattern seen in JGCTs. Also, a thecal component is absent in both the large cell and small cell forms of small cell carcinoma and the large cells sometimes have a distinctive dense, globular condensation of their cytoplasm, a feature seen only rarely in the JGCT. Also, small cell carcinomas are negative for α-inhibin and occasionally positive for epithelial membrane antigen in contrast to JGCTs.

The metastatic tumor that is mostly likely to be confused with a JGCT is malignant melanoma because it may contain follicle-like spaces and cells with abundant eosinophilic cytoplasm (page 354). Metastatic melanoma is rare in the first two decades, during which approximately 80 percent of JGCTs are encountered. The clinical history is helpful in many cases, but even if a history of a primary melanoma is absent or it has regressed, the possibility of metastatic melanoma should still be considered, particularly when the patient is over 20 years of age. The likelihood of metastatic melanoma is higher if the ovarian tumor is bilateral. Immunohistochemical staining for HMB-45 and α-inhibin is almost always helpful in difficult cases.

Treatment and Prognosis. In view of the rarity of bilateral ovarian involvement and the excellent prognosis of stage I JGCTs, removal of the involved ovary is almost always curative. Little experience has accumulated on the roles of chemotherapy and radiation therapy in the management of persistent or recurrent tumor, but examples of their efficacy in achieving long-term, disease-free survival have been recorded (43a,46a,50). Although the JGCT usually appears less well-differentiated than the adult type, follow-up data indicate a higher survival rate. In contrast to the adult granulosa cell tumor, which often recurs late, almost all the recurrences of the juvenile tumor appear within 3 postoperative years (43,46,49,50, 51). In one series of JGCTs, the feature of greatest prognostic significance was the stage of the tumor (50). Only 2 of the 80 stage I tumors for which follow-up information was available were clinically malignant. All 3 stage II tumors were fatal. Although both the mitotic rate and the degree of nuclear atypia correlated with the prognosis when tumors of all stages were considered, no such correlation was evident when only stage I tumors were evaluated. Two studies of the DNA content in small series of cases of JGCT showed that neither the DNA ploidy or the S-phase fraction was predictive of the outcome (45,47).

REFERENCES

Sex Cord–Stromal Tumors

1. Gee DC, Russell P. The pathological assessment of ovarian neoplasms. IV. The sex cord stromal tumors. Pathology 1981;13:235–55.

2. Young RH, Scully RE. Ovarian sex cord-stromal tumors: problems in differential diagnosis. Path Ann 1988;23 (pt I):237–96.

Adult Granulosa Cell Tumors

3. Benjamin E, Law S, Bobrow LG. Intermediate filaments cytokeratin and vimentin in ovarian sex cord-stromal tumors with correlative studies in adult and fetal ovaries. J Pathol 1987;152:253–63.

4. Bjorkholm E. Granulosa cell tumors: a comparison of survival in patients and matched controls. Am J Obstet Gynecol 1980;138:329–31.

5. Bjorkholm E, Pettersson F. Granulosa-cell and theca-cell tumors. The clinical picture and long term outcome for the Radiumhemmet series. Acta Obstet Gynecol Scand 1980;59:361–65.

6. Bjorkholm E, Silversward C. Prognostic factors in granulosa cell tumors. Gynecol Oncol 1981;11:261–74.

7. Chadha S, van der Kwast TH. Immunohistochemistry of ovarian granulosa cell tumors. The value of tissue specific proteins and tumor markers. Virchows Arch [A] 1989;414:439–45.

8. Costa MJ, DeRose PB, Roth LM, Brescia RJ, Zaloudek C, Cohen C. Immunohistochemical phenotype of ovarian granulosa cell tumors: absence of epithelial membrane antigen has diagnostic value. Hum Pathol 1994;25:60–6.

8a. Costa MJ, Morris R, Sasano H. Sex steroid biosynthesis enzymes in ovarian sex-cord stromal tumors. Int J Gynecol Pathol 1994;13:109–19.

9. Diddle AW. Granulosa- and theca-cell ovarian tumors: prognosis. Cancer 1951;15:215–28.

10. Evans AT, Gaffey TA, Malkasian GD Jr, Annegers JF. Clinicopathologic review of 118 granulosa and 82 theca cell tumors. Obstet Gynecol 1980;55:231–37.

11. Evans MP, Webb MJ, Gaffey TA, Katzmann JA, Suman VJ, Hu TC. DNA ploidy of ovarian granulosa cell tumors. Lack of correlation between DNA index or proliferative index and outcome in 10 patients. Cancer 1995;75:2295–8.

12. Fathalla MF. The occurrence of granulosa and theca tumors in clinically normal ovaries. A study of 25 cases. J Obstet Gynaecol Brit Cmwlth 1967;74:278–82.

13. Flemming P, Wellmann A, Maschek H, Lang H, Georgii A. Monoclonal antibodies against inhibin represent key markers of adult granulosa cell tumors of the ovary even in their metastases. A report of three cases with late metastasis, being previously misinterpreted as hemangiopericytoma. Am J Surg Pathol 1995;19:927–33.

14. Fox H, Agrawal K, Langley FA. A clinicopathological study of 92 cases of granulosa cell tumor of the ovary with special reference to the factors influencing prognosis. Cancer 1975;35:231–41.

15. Genton CY. Some observations on the fine structure of human granulosa cell tumors. Virchows Arch [A] 1980;387:353–69.

16. Gershenson DM, Copeland LJ, Kavanagh JJ, Stringer CA, Saul PB, Wharton JT. Treatment of metastatic stromal tumors of the ovary with cisplatin, doxorubicin, and cyclophosphamide. Obstet Gynecol 1987;5:765–9.

16a. Guerrieri C, Frånlund B, Malström H, Boeryd B. Ovarian endometrioid carcinomas simulating sex cord-stromal tumors: a study employing inhibin and cytokeratin 7. Int J Gynecol Pathol 1998;17:266–71.

17. Gusberg SB, Kardon P. Proliferative endometrial response to theca-granulosa cell tumors. Am J Obstet Gynecol 1967;111:633–43.

18. Hitchcock CL, Norris HJ, Khalifa MA, Wargotz ES. Flow cytometric analysis of granulosa tumors. Cancer 1989;64:2127–32.

19. Jobling T, Mamers P, Healy DL, et al. A prospective study of inhibin in granulosa cell tumors of the ovary. Gynecol Oncol 1994;55:285–9.

20. Klemi PJ, Joensuu H, Salmi T. Prognostic value of flow cytometric DNA content analysis in granulosa cell tumor of the ovary. Cancer 1990;65:1189–93.

21. Kottmeier HL. Carcinoma of the female genitalia. The Abraham Flexner Lectures, series no 11. Baltimore: Williams & Wilkins, 1953.

22. Lappöhn RE, Burger HG, Bouma J, Bangah M, Krans M, De Bruijn HW. Inhibin as a marker for granulosa-cell tumors. N Engl J Med 1989;321:790–3.

23. Malmström H, Högberg T, Björn R, Simonsen E. Granulosa cell tumors of the ovary: prognostic factors and outcome. Gynecol Oncol 1994;52:50–5.

24. Miettinen M, Lehto VP, Virtanen I. Expression of intermediate filaments in normal ovaries and ovarian epithelial, sex cord-stromal, and germinal tumors. Int J Gynecol Pathol 1983;2:64–71.

25. Miettinen M, Wahlstrom T, Virtanen I. Talerman A, Astengo-Osuna C. Cellular differentiation in ovarian sex-cord-stromal and germ-cell tumors studied with antibodies to intermediate-filament proteins. Am J Surg Pathol 1985;9:640–51.

25a. Miller BE, Barron BA, Wan JY, Delmore JE, Silva EG, Gershenson DM. Prognostic factors in adult granulosa cell tumor of the ovary. Cancer 1997;79:1951–5.

26. Nakashima N, Young RH, Scully RE. Androgenic granulosa cell tumors of the ovary. A clinicopathological analysis of seventeen cases and review of the literature. Arch Path Lab Med 1984;108:786–91

27. Nogales FF, Concha A, Plata C, Ruiz-Avila I. Granulosa cell tumor of the ovary with diffuse true hepatic differentiation simulating stromal luteinization. Am J Surg Pathol 1993;17:85–90.

28. Norris HJ, Taylor HB. Prognosis of granulosa-theca tumors of the ovary. Cancer 1968;21:255–63.

29. Norris HJ, Taylor HB. Virilization associated with cystic granulosa tumors. Obstet Gynecol 1969;34:629–35.

30. Otis CN, Powell JL, Barbuto D, Carcangiu ML. Intermediate filamentous proteins in adult granulosa cell tumors. An immunohistochemical study of 25 cases. Am J Surg Pathol 1992;16:962–68.

31. Park SH, Kim I. Histogenetic consideration of ovarian sex cord-stromal tumors analyzed by expression pattern of cytokeratins, vimentin, and laminin. Correlation studies with human gonads. Path Res Pract 1994;190:449–56.

32. Price A, Russell P, Elliott P, Bannatyne P. Composite mucinous and granulosa-cell tumor of ovary: case report of a unique neoplasm. Int J Gynecol Pathol 1990;9:372–8.

32a. Rishi M, Howard LN, Bratthauer GL, Tavassoli FA. Use of monoclonal antibody against human inhibin as a marker for sex cord-stromal tumors of the ovary. Am J Surg Pathol 1997;21:583–9.

33. Sasano H, Okamoto M, Mason JI, et al. Immunohistochemical studies of steroidogenic enzymes (aromatase, 17-alpha-hydroxylase and cholesterol side-chain cleavage cytochromes P-450) in sex cord-stromal tumors of the ovary. Hum Pathol 1989;20:452–7.

34. Schwartz PE, Smith JP. Treatment of ovarian stromal tumors. Am J Obstet Gynecol 1976;125:402–11.

35. Segal R, DePetrillo AD, Thomas G. Clinical review of adult granulosa cell tumors of the ovary. Gynecol Oncol 1995;56:338–44.

36. Sjostedt S, Wahlen T. Prognosis of granulosa cell tumors. Acta Obstet Gynecol Scand 1961;40:1–26.

37. Stenwig JT, Hazekamp JT, Beecham JB. Granulosa cell tumors of the ovary. A clinicopathological study of 118 cases with long-term follow-up. Gynec Oncol 1979;7:136–52.

38. Susil BJ. Sumithran E. Sarcomatous change in granulosa cell tumor. Hum Pathol 1987;18:397–9.

39. Young RH, Dudley AG, Scully RE. Granulosa cell, Sertoli-Leydig cell and unclassified sex cord-stromal tumors associated with pregnancy: a clinicopathological analysis of thirty-six cases. Gynecol Oncol 1984;18:181–205.

40. Young RH, Oliva E, Scully RE. Luteinized adult granulosa cell tumors of the ovary: a report of four cases. Int J Gynecol Pathol 1994;13:302–10.

41. Young RH, Scully RE. Ovarian sex cord-stromal tumors with bizarre nuclei: a clinicopathologic analysis of seventeen cases. Int J Gynecol Pathol 1983;1:325–35.

42. Zheng W, Sung CJ, Hanna I, et al. α and β subunits of inhibin/activin as sex cord-stromal differentiation markers. Int J Gynecol Pathol 1997;16:236–71.

Juvenile Granulosa Cell Tumors

43. Biscotti CV, Hart WR. Juvenile granulosa cell tumors of the ovary. Arch Pathol Lab Med 1989;113:40–6.

43a. Calaminus G, Wessalowski R, Harms D, Gobel U. Juvenile granulosa cell tumors of the ovary in children and adolescents: results from 33 patients registered in a prospective cooperative study. Gynecol Oncol 1997;65:447–52.

44. Case Records of the Massachusetts General Hospital Case 21-1983. N Engl J Med 1983;308:1279–84.

45. Jacoby AF, Young RH, Colvin RB, et al. DNA content in juvenile granulosa cell tumors of the ovary: a study of early- and advanced-stage disease. Gynecol Oncol 1992;46:97–103.

46. Lack EE, Perez-Atayde AR, Murthy AS, et al. Granulosa theca cell tumors in premenarchal girls. A clinical and pathologic study of ten cases. Cancer 1981;48:1846–54.

46a. Powell JL, Otis CN. Management of advanced juvenile granulosa cell tumor of the ovary. Gynecol Oncol 1997;64:282–4.

47. Swanson SA, Norris HJ, Kelsten ML, Wheeler J. DNA content of juvenile granulosa tumors determined by flow cytometry. Int J Gynecol Pathol 1990;9:101–9.

48. Tanaka Y, Sasaki Y, Nishihira H, Izawa T, Nishi T. Ovarian juvenile granulosa cell tumor associated with Maffucci's syndrome. Am J Clin Pathol 1992;97:523–7.

49. Vassal G, Flamant F, Caillaud JM, et al. Juvenile granulosa cell tumor of the ovary in children: a clinical study of 15 cases. J Clin Oncol 1988;6:990–5.

50. Young RH, Dickersin GR, Scully RE. Juvenile granulosa cell tumor of the ovary. A clinicopathologic analysis of 125 cases. Am J Surg Pathol 1984;8:575–96.

51. Zaloudek C, Norris HJ. Granulosa tumors of the ovary in children. A clinical and pathologic study of 32 cases. Am J Surg Pathol 1982;6:503–12.

10
STROMAL TUMORS

THECOMA

Definition. This is a stromal tumor composed of lipid-containing cells that resemble theca interna cells, with less than 10 percent granulosa cells. The *typical thecoma* is composed of sheets of theca-like cells; a variable fibromatous component is usually present as well (1,2,4,12). The *luteinized thecoma* has the basic appearance of a fibroma or a typical thecoma but also contains lutein cells. These cells are polyhedral or rounded cells with abundant eosinophilic to lipid-rich cytoplasm and central, round nuclei, which typically contain single prominent nucleoli (5,10,18).

General Features. Typical thecomas are approximately one third as common as granulosa cell tumors. They are usually estrogenic, occur in patients of an older average age than granulosa cell tumors, and are rare prior to puberty and uncommon before the age of 30 years. In one large series, 84 percent of the patients were postmenopausal, with a mean age of 59 years; only 10 percent were under 30 years of age (2). In the same series 60 percent of the postmenopausal women presented with uterine bleeding and 21 percent had endometrial carcinoma. Rarely, thecomas have been associated with other uterine tumors such as mullerian mixed tumors and endometrial stromal sarcomas, suggesting a possible role of estrogen production in the genesis of those tumors (9).

In one large series of luteinized thecomas, half of them were estrogenic, 39 percent were nonfunctioning, and 11 percent were androgenic (18). Masculinization is rarely, if ever, seen in association with typical thecomas, presumably because they contain enough aromatase to transform androgens to estrogens. Luteinized thecomas occur in younger patients than typical thecomas. Although they are most common in postmenopausal women, 30 percent occur in patients under 30 years of age (18). When, on rare occasions, crystals of Reinke are identified in the lutein-like cells of what otherwise would be considered a luteinized thecoma, the term "stromal Leydig cell tumor" is appropriate (8,11,13,18). This tumor is virilizing in approximately half of the cases. Rare luteinized

thecomas with distinctive features are associated with sclerosing peritonitis (3) (page 192).

Gross Findings. Thecomas are unilateral in 97 percent of the cases. They range in size from small, impalpable tumors to large, solid masses; most are 5 to 10 cm in diameter. Sectioning typically discloses a solid yellow mass (fig. 10-1), but in some cases the tumor is white with only focal tinges of yellow; cystic change and areas of hemorrhage and necrosis occur occasionally. Foci of calcification may be present; extensively calcified thecomas tend to occur in young women (15).

Microscopic Findings. Microscopic examination reveals masses of cells, most of which are

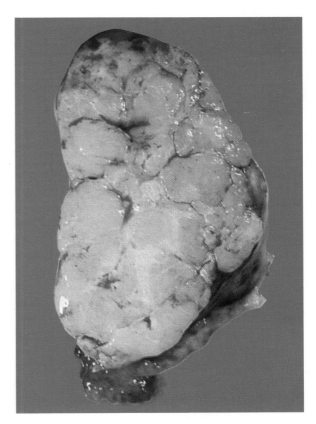

Figure 10-1
THECOMA

The sectioned surface is lobulated and yellow. (Fig. 31 from Young RH, Scully RE. Ovarian sex cord–stromal tumors: problems in differential diagnosis. Pathol Ann 1988;23(Pt 1):237–96.)

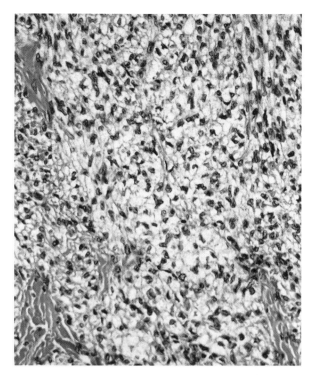

Figure 10-2
THECOMA
The tumor cells are vacuolated. (Fig. 9 from Young RH, Scully RE. Ovarian sex cord stromal tumors. Recent advances and current status. Clin Obstet Gynecol 1984;11:93–134.)

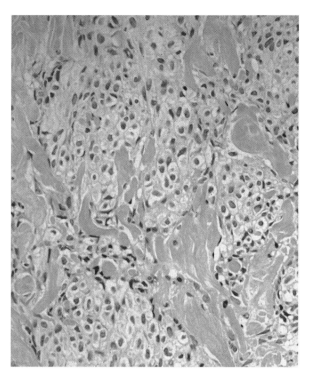

Figure 10-3
THECOMA
The tumor cells have abundant pale, dense cytoplasm. Hyaline plaques are conspicuous.

ill-defined and oval or rounded. The cytoplasm is usually abundant and vacuolated (fig. 10-2) or pale and dense (fig. 10-3); it usually contains moderate to large amounts of lipid (fig. 10-4). The nuclei vary from round to spindle shaped and typically exhibit little or no atypia; mitotic figures are absent or infrequent. Rarely, large bizarre nuclei with a degenerative appearance are seen (16). Hyaline plaques are often conspicuous (fig. 10-3). The stroma may exhibit calcification (fig. 10-5). In thecomas, in contrast to granulosa cell tumors, reticulin fibrils typically surround individual tumor cells (fig. 10-6). In luteinized thecomas, lutein cells are present as single cells, in nests (fig. 10-7), or rarely, in large nodules. Stromal Leydig cell tumors have an identical appearance except that some of the lutein-like cells contain crystals of Reinke (fig. 10-8).

Most of the tumors reported as "malignant thecomas," are better interpreted as endocrinologically inactive fibrosarcomas or diffuse granulosa cell tumors (14), but rare, mitotically active, typical and luteinized thecomas with nuclear abnormalities metastasize (14,18). Thecomas, like fibromas, are often aneuploid (7), but this finding should not lead to a diagnosis of malignant thecoma.

Differential Diagnosis. The dividing line between thecomas and fibromas is imprecise. Because of the overlap between them some authors use the designation "fibrothecoma." We place tumors in the fibroma category unless they contain the typical cytoplasm-rich cells of the thecoma or show more than minimal staining for α-inhibin. Cellular thecomas are occasionally misinterpreted as granulosa cell tumors; this differential diagnosis is discussed on page 174.

Rarely, thecomas contain scattered minor cellular aggregates of sex cord type, including nests of indifferent cells, nests of cells resembling granulosa cells, or tubules lined by cells resembling Sertoli cells. The overall appearance and behavior of these tumors is closer to those of a

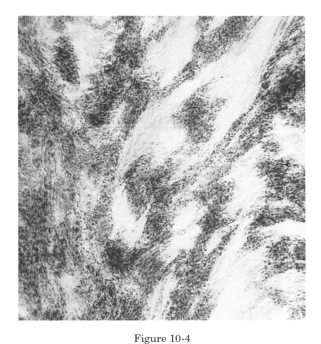

Figure 10-4
THECOMA
The tumor cells contain abundant intracytoplasmic lipid demonstrated by an oil red-O stain.

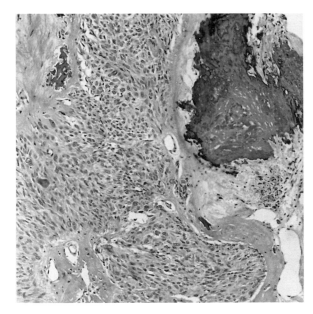

Figure 10-5
THECOMA
There are several foci of stromal calcification.

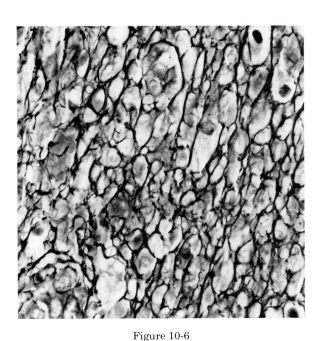

Figure 10-6
THECOMA
Reticulin stain highlights an investment of individual cells by fibrils. (Compare with figure 9-19.) (Fig. 65 from Serov SF, Scully RE, Sobin LH. Histological typing of ovarian tumours. International Histological Classification of Tumours No. 9. Geneva: World Health Organization, 1973.)

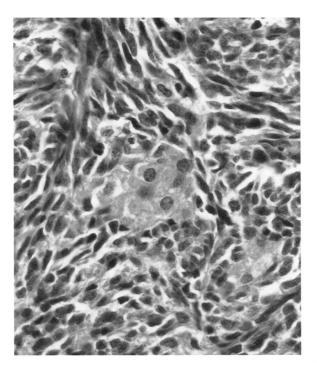

Figure 10-7
LUTEINIZED THECOMA
A cluster of luteinized cells is present within fibromatous tissue.

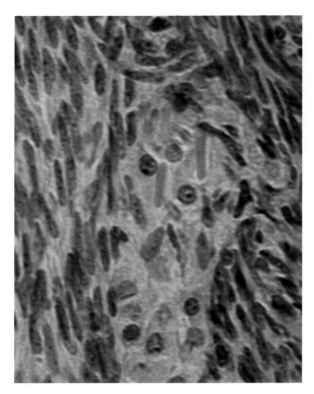

Figure 10-8
STROMAL–LEYDIG CELL TUMOR
Crystals of Reinke are present within lutein-like cells.

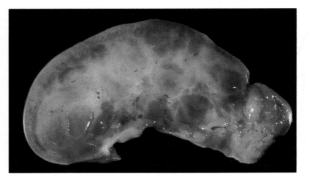

Figure 10-9
LUTEINIZED THECOMA IN PATIENT
WITH SCLEROSING PERITONITIS
The sectioned surface is tan-white with small cysts.
(Courtesy of Jun Miyauchi, MD, Tokyo, Japan.)

thecoma than a granulosa cell or Sertoli-stromal cell tumor; the designation "thecoma with minor sex cord elements" (17) is used when the latter account for less than 10 percent of the composition of the tumor.

When a thecoma is extensively luteinized, its appearance may suggest a steroid cell tumor. Indeed, Hughesdon (5) proposed that the steroid cell tumor is a fully luteinized thecoma. Since the typical luteinized thecoma and steroid cell tumor differ greatly in their clinical and pathologic features and are almost always easily differentiated, they should be classified separately. We diagnose steroid cell tumor when an underlying fibromatous or thecomatous component is present in less than 10 percent of the specimen. Luteinized thecomas must also be distinguished from stromal hyperthecosis. The latter is almost always bilateral in contrast to the luteinized thecoma, which is rarely bilateral except for the variant associated with sclerosing peritonitis (see below). Microscopic examination of stromal hyperthecosis

reveals lutein cells on a background of small stromal cells with minimal collagen production; in luteinized thecomas, in contrast, the background consists of large collagen-producing spindle cells or plump theca cells.

The diffuse luteinization of thecomas that may occur in pregnant patients can lead to confusion with pregnancy luteomas. The latter, however, are multiple in half the cases, contain little or no lipid, and do not have a background of fibroma or typical thecoma.

Luteinized Thecoma with Sclerosing Peritonitis

Fifteen unusual ovarian lesions associated enigmatically with sclerosing peritonitis have been reported (3,6), most of them interpreted as variants of luteinized thecomas. Like luteinized thecomas of the usual type, these tumors occurred in patients younger than those with typical thecomas; 10 of the 15 patients were under 30 and only 2 over 50 years of age. The patients usually present with abdominal swelling, occasionally with ascites and symptoms of bowel obstruction. In most cases both ovaries are involved, with appearances ranging from large masses up to 31 cm in diameter to normal-sized or slightly enlarged ovaries, which may have a prominent nodular surface. The sectioned surfaces may have edematous areas with cyst formation (fig. 10-9). Microscopic examination shows a dense proliferation of spindle cells with focal differentiation into lutein cells (fig. 10-10), which are typically smaller than those in the usual

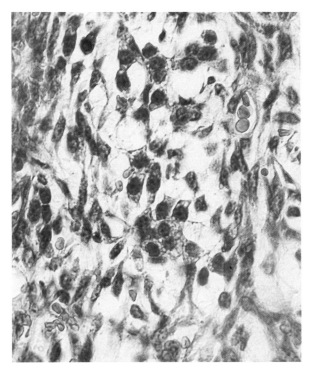

Figure 10-10
LUTEINIZED THECOMA IN PATIENT
WITH SCLEROSING PERITONITIS
Nests of pale lutein cells are present on a background of spindle cells. (Fig. 7 from Clement PB, Young RH, Hanna W, Scully RE. Sclerosing peritonitis associated with luteinized thecomas of the ovary. A clinicopathological analysis of six cases. Am J Surg Pathol 1994;18:1–13.)

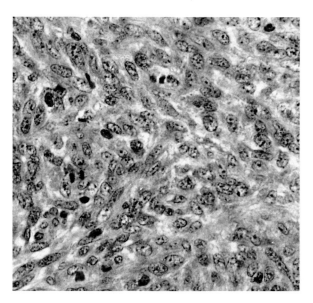

Figure 10-11
LUTEINIZED THECOMA IN PATIENT
WITH SCLEROSING PERITONITIS
Spindle cells with plump nuclei exhibit prominent mitotic activity. (Fig. 6 from Clement PB, Young RH, Hanna W, Scully RE. Sclerosing peritonitis associated with luteinized thecomas of the ovary. A clinicopathological analysis of six cases. Am J Surg Pathol 1994;18:1–13.)

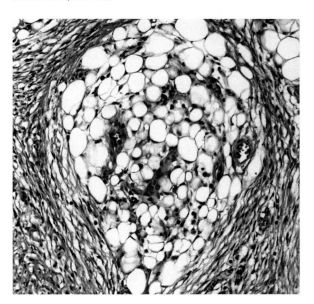

Figure 10-12
SCLEROSING PERITONITIS IN PATIENT
WITH LUTEINIZED THECOMA
A cellular fibroblastic proliferation surrounds lobules of omental fat. (Fig. 9 from Clement PB, Young RH, Hanna W, Scully RE. Sclerosing peritonitis associated with luteinized thecomas of the ovary. A clinicopathological analysis of six cases. Am J Surg Pathol 1994;18:1–13.)

luteinized thecoma. Although mitotic figures are absent or rare in some cases, many tumors have brisk mitotic activity, up to 47 per 10 high-power fields, predominantly in the spindle cells (fig. 10-11). In some cases there is striking edema with microcyst formation; rarely, nests of cells of sex cord type are present within the tumors. The peritoneal process consists of a variably cellular proliferation of fibroblasts and myofibroblasts separated by collagen, fibrin, and occasional inflammatory cells (fig. 10-12). Despite the high mitotic rate in many cases, spread of tumor cells beyond the ovary has not been reported. In several cases, however, intermittent episodes of small bowel obstruction occurred after the ovarian tumors were excised, and three patients have died of complications of their peritoneal disease.

The differential diagnosis of this variant of luteinized thecoma includes stromal hyperthecosis,

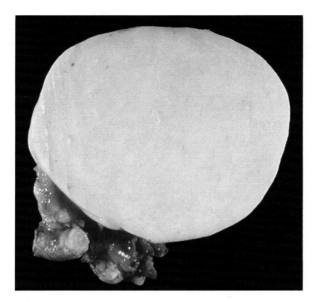

Figure 10-13
FIBROMA
The sectioned surface is chalky white and appears flat.

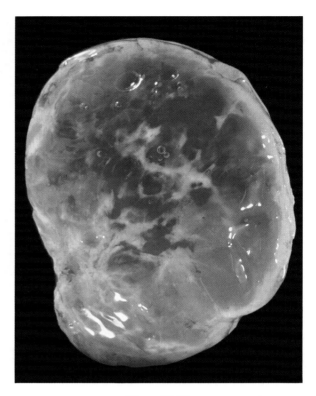

Figure 10-14
FIBROMA
The sectioned surface is edematous and focally hemorrhagic.

massive edema, and fibromatosis. Stromal hyperthecosis, however, is not accompanied by ascites, does not cause marked ovarian enlargement, and lacks mitotic activity. Massive edema and fibromatosis, in contrast to this variant of luteinized thecoma, are hypocellular and associated with either diffuse marked edema or diffuse collagen deposition. Edematous cellular fibromas and sclerosing stromal tumors are typically unilateral, are unassociated with peritonitis, and lack the striking mitotic activity seen in some luteinized thecomas with sclerosing peritonitis.

FIBROMA AND CELLULAR FIBROMA

Definition. These tumors are composed entirely or almost entirely of spindle, oval, or round cells forming variable amounts of collagen.

General Features. Fibromas account for 4 percent of all ovarian tumors. They occur at all ages, but are most frequent during middle age, with an average patient age of 48 years; fewer than 10 percent of fibromas are encountered in patients under the age of 30 years (20), and they are rare in children (19). The fibroma is only exceptionally associated with evidence of steroid hormone production but is occasionally accompanied by two unusual clinical syndromes: Meigs'

syndrome (page 389) (23) and the nevoid basal cell carcinoma syndrome (Gorlin's syndrome) (page 387). The former, which complicates about 1 percent of ovarian fibromas, is defined as ascites and pleural effusion accompanying a fibrous ovarian tumor, usually a fibroma, and disappearing after the removal of the tumor. Ascites alone is associated with 10 to 15 percent of ovarian fibromas over 10 cm in diameter (25).

Gross Findings. Fibromas are bilateral in about 8 percent of the cases (20). They range in size from microscopic to very large, with an average diameter of 6 cm (20). Sectioning typically reveals hard, flat, chalky-white surfaces (fig. 10-13). Areas of edema, occasionally with cyst formation, are relatively common, and some tumors are predominantly edematous (fig. 10-14) or cystic. Hemorrhage is occasionally seen, usually in tumors that prove to be cellular on microscopic examination. Focal or diffuse calcification is observed in fewer than 10 percent of the cases, but, this feature, along with bilateral involvement, is

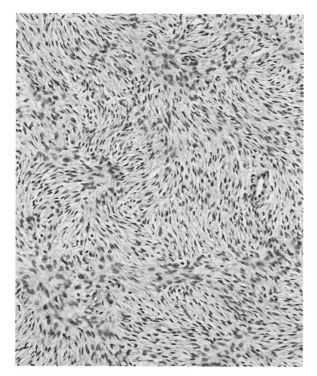

Figure 10-15
FIBROMA
The cells are arranged in a storiform pattern.

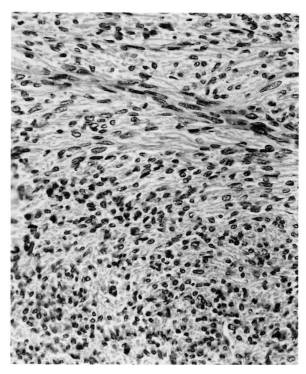

Figure 10-16
FIBROMA
The cells have small spindle-shaped and round nuclei lacking atypia or mitotic activity. (Fig. 67 from Serov SF, Scully RE, Sobin LH. Histological typing of ovarian tumours. International Histological Classification of Tumours No. 9. Geneva: World Health Organization, 1973.)

almost always present in patients with the nevoid basal cell carcinoma syndrome.

Microscopic Findings. Microscopic examination reveals intersecting bundles of spindle cells producing collagen; a storiform pattern is often seen (figs. 10-15, 10-16). Hyaline bands are not uncommon. Many tumors show varying degrees of intercellular edema (fig. 10-17), which may have a myxoid appearance. The cytoplasm of the neoplastic cells may contain small quantities of lipid. Occasionally, it contains eosinophilic hyaline droplets (fig. 10-18). Most fibromas are only moderately cellular, exhibit no nuclear atypia, and have only rare mitotic figures. Approximately 10 percent of fibromas are densely cellular (closely approaching or attaining the cellularity of a diffuse granulosa cell tumor) and merit the designation "cellular fibroma" (fig. 10-19) (24); mitotic figures are found in increased numbers in these tumors, which have an average mitotic count of 3 or fewer per 10 high-power fields. An occasional fibroma contains a minor component

of sex cord elements (fig. 10-20) (17). One fibroma was associated with Leydig cell hyperplasia in the adjacent stroma (21).

Differential Diagnosis. Fibromas must be distinguished from thecomas (page 190) as well as several non-neoplastic ovarian processes, specifically massive edema, fibromatosis, and stromal hyperplasia. The first two disorders are usually unilateral but may be bilateral. Massive edema is characterized by a proliferation of ovarian stromal cells with marked intercellular edema, and fibromatosis by the production of abundant dense collagen. Unlike fibromas, which almost always displace follicles, corpora lutea, and corpora albicantia, massive edema and fibromatosis encompass these structures. Stromal hyperplasia, in contrast to the ovarian fibroma, is almost always bilateral and is characterized by a multinodular or diffuse proliferation of closely packed, small stromal cells with minimal collagen formation.

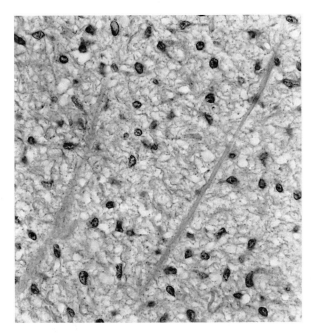

Figure 10-17
FIBROMA
There is prominent intercellular edema. (Fig. 68 from Serov SF, Scully RE, Sobin LH. Histological typing of ovarian tumours. International Histological Classification of Tumours No. 9. Geneva: World Health Organization, 1973.)

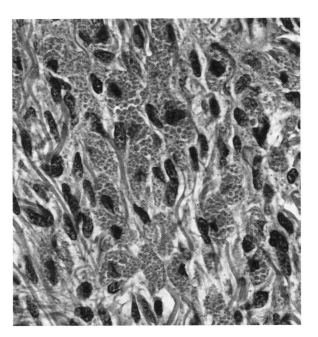

Figure 10-18
FIBROMA
Numerous small hyaline droplets are present.

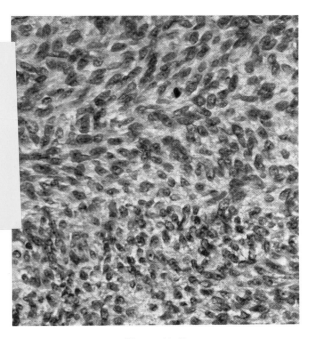

Figure 10-19
CELLULAR FIBROMA
The tumor is cellular but devoid of significant atypia. A mitotic figure is evident.

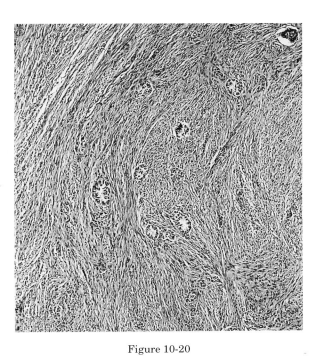

Figure 10-20
FIBROMA WITH MINOR SEX CORD ELEMENTS
Sertoliform tubules are scattered within a fibromatous tumor. (Fig. 4 from Young RH, Scully RE. Ovarian stromal tumors with minor sex cord elements. A report of seven cases. Int J Gynecol Pathol 1983;2:227–34.)

Distinction of a fibroma from a primary endometrioid or metastatic endometrial stromal sarcoma and from a Krukenberg tumor is discussed on pages 135 and 339, respectively.

Prognosis. Ovarian fibromas are almost always benign. Cellular forms with an average of 3 or fewer mitotic figures per 10 high-power fields and no more than minimal nuclear atypia have a low malignant potential, however, occasionally recurring in the pelvis or upper abdomen, particularly if they are adherent or ruptured (24). One fibroma that presumably lacked any unusual features was associated with peritoneal implants (22).

FIBROSARCOMA

Only pure fibrosarcomas are considered here; those that are components of more complex neoplasms are discussed elsewhere. In our experience pure fibrosarcomas are among the most common forms of ovarian sarcoma. They may be seen at any age but are found most often in older women (26–30). They are usually unilateral and large. Sectioning typically shows solid tissue, which commonly has areas of hemorrhage and necrosis. Occasionally, when a fibrosarcoma occupies only a portion of a fibromatous tumor its presence may not be suspected on gross examination.

Microscopic examination shows a densely cellular neoplasm with moderate to severe nuclear atypia and an average mitotic count of 4 or more per 10 high-power fields (fig. 10-21). Abnormal mitotic figures and areas of necrosis and hemorrhage are common.

Primary and metastatic endometrioid stromal sarcomas, which are typically composed of small cells with round nuclei and scanty cytoplasm, may be confused with fibrosarcomas if the characteristic arterioles of the former tumors are overlooked.

The ovarian fibrosarcomas that have been reported have been associated with a malignant course.

SCLEROSING STROMAL TUMOR

Definition. This tumor is characterized by cellular pseudolobules that are composed of fibroblasts and rounded vacuolated cells and are separated by edematous or dense, much less cellular collagenous tissue.

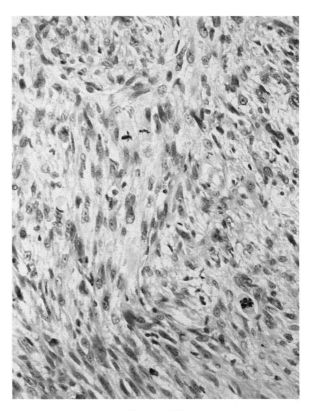

Figure 10-21
FIBROSARCOMA
There is moderate cytologic atypia with mitotic figures, including atypical forms.

General Features. This tumor differs clinically from fibromas and thecomas by being most common in the first three decades, during which over 80 percent of the cases occur; the average patient age is 27 years (46). In contrast to the thecoma, the sclerosing stromal tumor has been associated with evidence of estrogen secretion only rarely; androgenic manifestations have been present in two cases during pregnancy (31,36). All sclerosing stromal tumors encountered to date have been benign (31–47).

Gross Findings. The tumors are typically unilateral, discrete, and sharply demarcated. The sectioned surface is basically solid and white but often shows areas of edema and cyst formation, as well as yellow foci (figs. 10-22, 10-23). A rare tumor forms a unilocular cyst (46).

Microscopic Findings. Microscopic examination discloses a pseudolobular pattern (figs. 10-24, 10-25) in which cellular nodules are separated

197

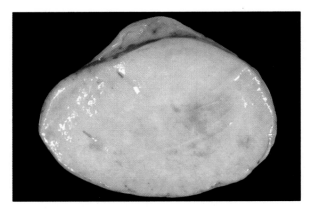

Figure 10-22
SCLEROSING STROMAL TUMOR
The sectioned surface of the tumor is white and edematous centrally, and yellow at the periphery. (Fig. 1 from Chalvardjian A, Scully RE. Sclerosing stromal tumors of the ovary. Cancer 1973;31:664–70.)

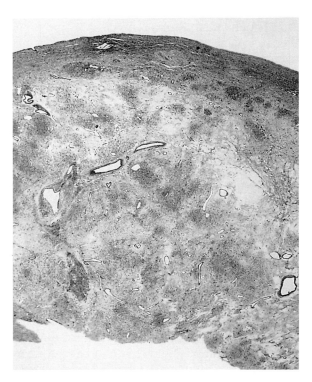

Figure 10-24
SCLEROSING STROMAL TUMOR
Cellular pseudolobules are separated by edematous hypocellular fibrous tissue. (Fig. 74 from Young RH, Clement PB, Scully RE. Pathology of the ovary. In: Sternberg SS, ed. Diagnostic surgical pathology, Vol 2, 2nd ed. New York: Raven Press, 1994:2235.)

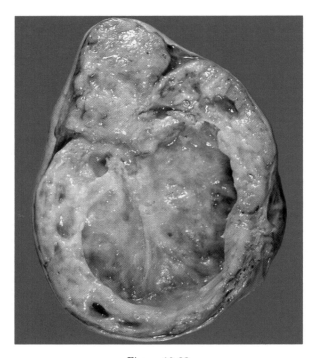

Figure 10-23
SCLEROSING STROMAL TUMOR
The sectioned surface contains a number of cysts.

by poorly cellular areas of densely collagenous or edematous connective tissue. Prominent thin-walled vessels are commonly present within the nodules (fig. 10-26), which may also exhibit varying degrees of sclerosis. The vessels may be di-

lated and resemble those of a hemangiopericytoma (fig. 10-27). The cellular component of the nodules consists of a disorganized admixture of fibroblasts and rounded, vacuolated cells (fig. 10-26). The latter cells appear to be degenerating lutein cells with shrunken nuclei, which occasionally are eccentric and resemble signet-ring cells (fig. 10-28). In the rare functioning tumors the lutein cells more closely resemble those of a luteinized thecoma; occasionally, lutein cells with abundant eosinophilic cytoplasm are also prominent in nonfunctioning tumors.

Differential Diagnosis. This neoplasm has a much more heterogeneous appearance than either a fibroma or a thecoma. It is most closely related to the luteinized thecoma but its distinctive pseudolobular pattern, its intimate admixture of fibroblasts and inactive-appearing lutein cells, and its ectatic blood vessels are not found in the latter tumor. Occasionally, the signet-ring–like cells in

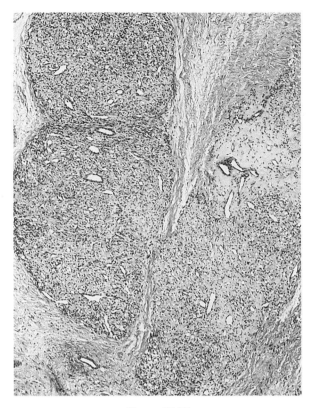

Figure 10-25
SCLEROSING STROMAL TUMOR
Cellular pseudolobules are separated by fibrous stroma.

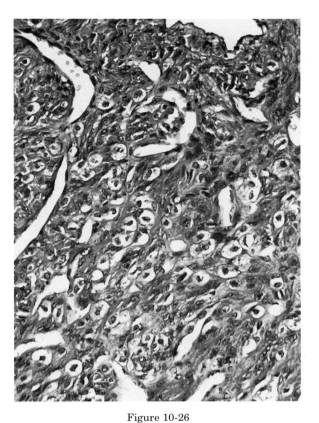

Figure 10-26
SCLEROSING STROMAL TUMOR
The collagen-producing spindle cells are admixed with rounded vacuolated cells.

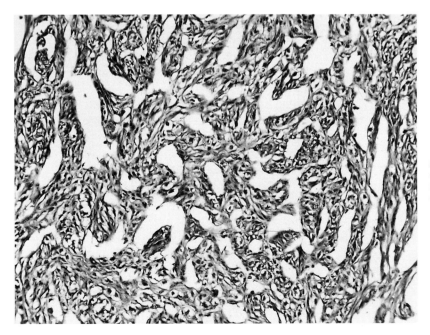

Figure 10-27
SCLEROSING
STROMAL TUMOR
A pseudolobule is richly vascularized, simulating a hemangiopericytoma. (Fig. 5 from Chalvardjian A, Scully RE. Sclerosing stromal tumors of the ovary. Cancer 1973;31:664–70.)

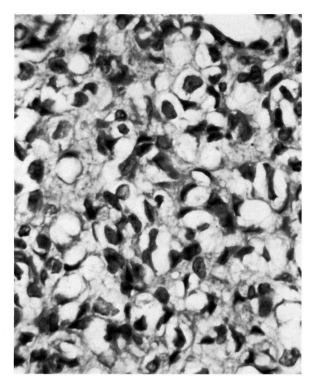

Figure 10-28
SCLEROSING STROMAL TUMOR
Many vacuolated cells have eccentric nuclei, simulating signet-ring cells.

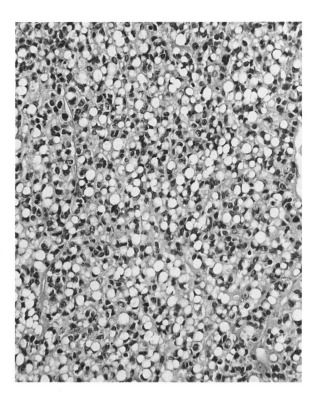

Figure 10-29
SIGNET-RING STROMAL TUMOR
There is a diffuse growth of cells with eccentric nuclei and clear cytoplasm.

a sclerosing stromal tumor suggest a Krukenberg tumor but their cytoplasm contains lipid rather than mucin. The ectatic vessels in the cellular pseudolobules sometimes suggest a hemangiopericytoma, but the latter lacks the other distinctive features of the sclerosing stromal tumor.

SIGNET-RING STROMAL TUMOR

Definition. This is a cellular stromal tumor containing signet-ring–like cells that do not contain mucin or lipid.

General Features. Only five examples of this neoplasm have been described (48–50). All of them have occurred in adults and have been nonfunctioning.

Pathology. Two of the five tumors were both solid and cystic; the others were uniformly solid. Microscopic examination reveals spindle cells that merge almost imperceptibly with rounded cells containing eccentric nuclei and single large vacuoles, resembling signet-ring cells (fig. 10-29). The signet-ring cell component may be diffuse or may occupy only a portion of an otherwise typical fibroma. Stains for mucin and lipid are negative. Ultrastructural examination has suggested that the vacuoles may have several origins. In some cases they appear to result from generalized edema of the cytoplasmic matrix, in other cases from swelling of mitochondria, and in still others from cytoplasmic pseudoinclusions of edematous extracellular matrix (48).

Differential Diagnosis. This tumor must be distinguished from other neoplasms with signet-ring–like cells, especially the Krukenberg tumor. Mucin stains facilitate this differential diagnosis. The signet-ring stromal tumor lacks the pseudolobulation and lipid-rich cells of a sclerosing stromal tumor.

REFERENCES

Thecoma

1. Banner EA, Dockerty MB. Theca cell tumors of the ovary. A clinical and pathological study of twenty-three cases (including thirteen new cases) with a review. Surg Gynecol Obstet 1945;81:234–42.
2. Bjorkholm E, Silfversward C. Theca-cell tumors. Clinical features and prognosis. Acta Radiol Oncol 1980;19:241–4.
3. Clement PB, Young RH, Hanna W, Scully RE. Sclerosing peritonitis associated with luteinized thecomas of the ovary. A clinicopathological analysis of six cases. Am J Surg Pathol. 1994;18:1–13.
4. Geist SH, Gaines JA. Theca cell tumors. Am J Obstet Gynecol 1938;35:39–51.
5. Hughesdon PE. Lipid cell thecomas of the ovary. Histopathology 1983;7:681–92.
6. Khan EM, Pandey R. Sarcoma-like ovarian nodules associated with retractile mesenteritis and retroperitoneal fibrosis. Histopathology 1994;24:276–8.
7. Lage JM, Weinberg DS, Huettner PC, Mark SD. Flow cytometric analysis of nuclear DNA content in ovarian tumors. Association of ploidy with tumor type, histologic grade, and clinical stage. Cancer 1992;69:2668–75.
8. Paoletti M, Pridjian G, Okagaki T, Talerman A. A stromal Leydig cell tumor of the ovary occurring in a pregnant 15-year-old girl. Ultrastructural findings. Cancer 1987;60:2806–10.
9. Press MF, Scully RE. Endometrial "sarcoma" complicating ovarian thecoma, polycystic ovarian disease and estrogen therapy. Gynecol Oncol 1985;21:135–54.
10. Roth LM, Sternberg WH. Partly luteinized theca cell tumor of the ovary. Cancer 1983;51:1697–704.
11. Scully RE. An unusual ovarian tumor containing Leydig cells but associated with endometrial hyperplasia, in a postmenopausal woman. J Clin Endocrinol Metab 1953;13:1254–63.
12. Sternberg WH, Gaskill CJ. Theca-cell tumors with a report of twelve new cases and observations on the possible etiologic role of ovarian stromal hyperplasia. Am J Obstet Gynecol 1950;59:575–87.
13. Sternberg WH, Roth LM. Ovarian stromal tumors containing Leydig cells. 1. Stromal-Leydig cell tumor and non-neoplastic transformation of ovarian stroma to Leydig cells. Cancer 1973;32:940–51.
14. Waxman M, Vuletin JC, Urcuyo R, Belling CG. Ovarian low-grade stromal sarcoma with thecomatous features. A critical reappraisal of the so-called "malignant thecoma." Cancer 1979;44:2206–17.
15. Young RH, Clement PB, Scully RE. Calcified thecomas in young women. A report of four cases. Int J Gynecol Pathol 1988;7:343–50.
16. Young RH, Scully RE. Ovarian sex-cord-stromal tumors with bizarre nuclei. a clinicopathologic analysis of seventeen cases. Int J Gynecol Pathol 1983;1:325-35.
17. Young RH, Scully RE. Ovarian stromal tumors with minor sex cord elements: a report of seven cases. Int J Gynecol Pathol 1983;2:227–34.
18. Zhang J, Young RH, Arseneau J, Scully RE. Ovarian stromal tumors containing lutein or Leydig cells (luteinized thecomas and stromal Leydig cell tumors). A clinicopathological analysis of fifty cases. Int J Gynecol Pathol 1982;1:270–85.

Fibroma

19. Bower JF, Erickson ER. Bilateral ovarian fibromas in a 5-year-old. Am J Obstet Gynecol 1967;99:880–2.
20. Dockerty MB, Masson JC. Ovarian fibromas: a clinical and pathologic study of two hundred and eighty-three cases. Am J Obstet Gynecol 1944;47:741–52.
21. Konishi I, Fujii S, Ishikawa Y, Suzuki A, Okamura H, Mori T. Ovarian fibroma with Leydig cell hyperplasia of the adjacent stroma: a light and electron microscopic study. Int J Gynecol Pathol 1986;5:170–8.
22. Lyday RO. Fibroma of the ovary with abdominal implants. Am J Surg 1952;84:737–8.
23. Meigs JV. Fibroma of the ovary with ascites and hydrothorax. Meigs' syndrome. Am J Obstet Gynecol 1954;67:962–87.
24. Prat J, Scully RE. Cellular fibromas and fibrosarcomas of the ovary: a comparative clinicopathologic analysis of seventeen cases. Cancer 1981;47:2663–70.
25. Samanth KK, Black WC. Benign ovarian stromal tumors associated with free peritoneal fluid. Am J Obstet Gynecol 1970;107:538–45.
25a. Young RH, Scully RE. Ovarian stromal tumors with minor sex cord elements: a report of seven cases. Int J Gynecol Pathol 1983;2:227–34.

Fibrosarcoma

26. Anderson B, Turner DA, Benda J. Ovarian sarcoma. Gynecol Oncol 1987;26:183–92.
27. Azoury RS, Woodruff JD. Primary ovarian sarcomas. Report of 43 cases from the Emil Novak Ovarian Tumor Registry. Obstet Gynecol 1971;37:920–41.
28. Christman JE, Ballon SC. Ovarian fibrosarcoma associated with Maffucci's syndrome. Gynecol Oncol 1990;37:290–1.
29. Kraemer BB, Silva EG, Sneige N. Fibrosarcoma of ovary. A new component in the nevoid basal-cell carcinoma syndrome. Am J Surg Pathol 1984;8:231–6.
30. Miles PA, Kiley KC, Mena H. Giant fibrosarcoma of the ovary. Int J Gynecol Pathol 1985;4:83–7.

Sclerosing Stromal Tumor

31. Cashell AW, Cohen ML. Masculinizing sclerosing stromal tumor of the ovary during pregnancy. Gynecol Oncol 1991;43:281–5.
32. Chalvardjian A, Scully RE. Sclerosing stromal tumors of the ovary. Cancer 1973;31:664–70.
33. Damjanov I, Drobnjak P, Grizelj V, Longhino N. Sclerosing stromal tumor of the ovary. A hormonal and ultrastructural analysis. Obstet Gynecol 1975;45:675–9.
34. Gee DC, Russell P. Sclerosing stromal tumours of the ovary. Histopathology 1979;3:367–76.
35. Hsu C, Ma L, Mak L. Sclerosing stromal tumor of the ovary: case report and review of the literature. Int J Gynecol Pathol 1983;2:192–200.
36. Ismail SM, Walker SM. Bilateral virilizing sclerosing stromal tumours of the ovary in a pregnant woman with Gorlin's syndrome: implications for pathogenesis of ovarian stromal neoplasms. Histopathology 1990;17:159–63.
37. Katsube Y, Iwaoki Y, Silverberg SG, Fujiwara A. Sclerosing stromal tumor of the ovary associated with endometrial adenocarcinoma. A case report. Gynecol Oncol 1988;29:392–8.
38. Martinelli G, Govoni E, Pileri S, Grigioni FW, Doglioni C, Pelusi G. Sclerosing stromal tumor of the ovary. A hormonal, histochemical and ultrastructural study. Virchows Arch [A] 1983;402:155–61.
39. Quinn MA, Oster AO, Fortune D, Hudson B. Sclerosing stromal tumor of the ovary. Case report with endocrine studies. Br J Obstet Gynaecol 1981;88:555–8.
40. Saitoh A, Tsutsumi Y, Osamura RY, Watanabe K. Sclerosing stromal tumor of the ovary. Immunohistochemical and electron-microscopic demonstration of smooth-muscle differentiation. Arch Pathol Lab Med 1989;113:372–6.
41. Suit PF, Hart WR. Sclerosing stromal tumor of the ovary. An ultrastructural study and review of the literature to evaluate hormonal function. Cleve Clin J Med 1988;55:189–94.
42. Tang M, Liu T. Ovarian sclerosing stromal tumors. Clinicopathologic study of 10 cases. Chinese Med J 1982;95:186–90.
43. Tenti P, Carnevali L, Zampatti C, Franchi M. Sclerosing stromal tumour of the ovary. Ultrastructural study. Eur J Gynaec Oncol 1988;9:464–9.
44. Tiltman AJ. Sclerosing stromal tumor of the ovary: demonstration of ligandin in three cases. Int J Gynecol Pathol 1985;4:362–9.
45. Tsukamoto N, Nakamura M, Ishikawa H. Sclerosing stromal tumor of the ovary. Gynecol Oncol 1976;4:335–9.
46. Young RH, Scully RE. Ovarian sex cord-stromal tumors: recent progress. Int J Gynecol Pathol 1982;1:101–23.
47. Yuen BH, Robertson I, Clement PB, Mincey EK. Sclerosing stromal tumor of the ovary. Obstet Gynecol 1982;60:252–6.

Signet-Ring Stromal Tumor

48. Dickersin GR, Young RH, Scully RE. Signet-ring stromal and related tumors of the ovary. Ultrastruct Pathol 1995;19:401–19.
49. Ramzy I. Signet-ring stromal tumor of ovary. Histochemical, light, and electron microscopic study. Cancer 1976;38:l66–72.
50. Suarez A, Palacios J, Burgos E, Gamallo C. Signet-ring stromal tumor of the ovary: a histochemical and ultrastructural study. Virchows Arch [A] 1993;422:333–6.

❖❖❖

11

SERTOLI–STROMAL CELL TUMORS
MIXED AND UNCLASSIFIED SEX CORD–STROMAL TUMORS

SERTOLI–STROMAL CELL TUMORS

"Sertoli-stromal cell tumors" is a generic term for tumors composed of Sertoli cells, cells resembling rete epithelial cells, and Leydig cells, either in pure form or as mixtures of any of these cell types.

Sertoli Cell Tumor

Definition. This tumor is characterized by hollow or solid tubules separated by a stroma that contains only rare or no Leydig cells. Tumors with a predominant component of annular tubules, considered by some authors (7) to be Sertoli cell tumors, are designated separately as sex cord tumors with annular tubules by the World Health Organization (WHO).

General Features. These tumors account for approximately 4 percent of Sertoli-stromal cell tumors (7–9,11). They may be seen at any age, with an average age of 30 years (11). They are usually nonfunctioning but may be estrogenic or occasionally androgenic. Seven tumors, most or all of which appear to have been of the lipid-rich type, have resulted in isosexual pseudoprecocity. Four of these tumors, two of them from sisters (6) and two others of the uncommon oxyphil cell type (4), were from patients with the Peutz-Jeghers syndrome. One Sertoli cell tumor was associated with high levels of serum progesterone and estrogen (10), and a few tumors were associated with renin production (page 382) (2,3,5). One Sertoli cell tumor was malignant, with distant metastases (11).

Gross Findings. All the Sertoli cell tumors reported to date have been unilateral and stage I. They average 9 cm in diameter and typically form lobulated, solid, yellow (fig. 11-1) or brown masses (11).

Microscopic Findings. Microscopic examination shows a variable component of tubules, which may be round or elongated, hollow or solid, or have a combination of these features (figs. 11-2–11-5). The tubules often grow in lobules separated by a typically fibrous stroma, which may be hyalinized and sometimes replaces the tubules in portions of the neoplasm. The hollow tubules are lined by cuboidal cells with moderate (fig. 11-3) to abundant cytoplasm, which may be dense and eosinophilic or pale and vacuolated. The solid tubules may contain closely packed cells with small nuclei and scanty cytoplasm (fig. 11-4) or large cells, which may be oxyphilic (fig. 11-5) or have abundant cytoplasmic lipid (lipid-rich Sertoli cell tumor) (fig. 11-2). In all forms of Sertoli cell tumor the tubular pattern may merge with a diffuse arrangement of the neoplastic cells. A few Leydig cells may be present. There is usually little, if any, nuclear atypia or mitotic activity but rare tumors have significant degrees of each; the one fatal tumor was poorly differentiated focally (11). Immunohistochemical staining of Sertoli cell tumors has typically shown reactivity for cytokeratins, and in one study two of five tumors were positive for vimentin (1). A negative immunohistochemical reaction for epithelial membrane antigen and a positive reaction for α-inhibin are helpful in confirming the diagnosis of Sertoli cell tumor (page 125) (4a,11a).

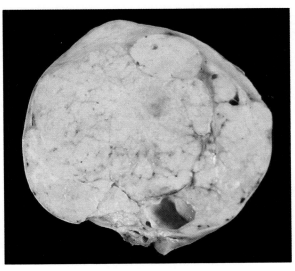

Figure 11-1
SERTOLI CELL TUMOR
The sectioned surface is yellow and lobulated.

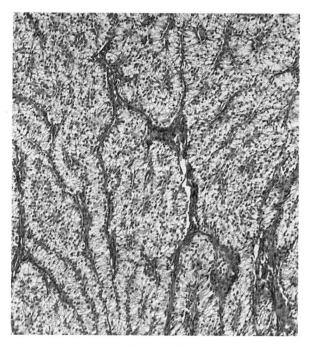

Figure 11-2
LIPID-RICH SERTOLI CELL TUMOR
Anastomosing solid tubules contain cells with abundant pale cytoplasm that contained lipid.

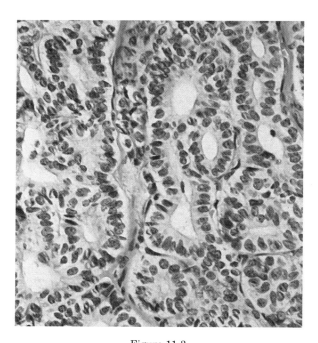

Figure 11-3
SERTOLI CELL TUMOR
Hollow tubules are lined by cuboidal cells with bland cytologic features.

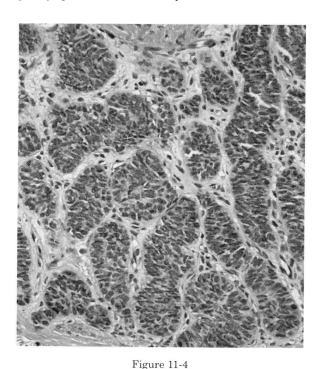

Figure 11-4
SERTOLI CELL TUMOR
Solid tubules resemble those of the prepubertal testis except for their greater cellularity.

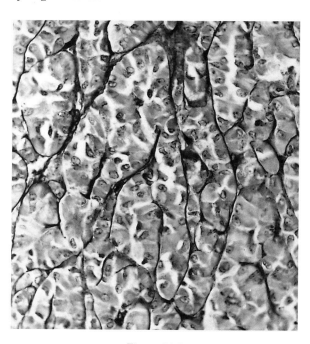

Figure 11-5
SERTOLI CELL TUMOR, OXYPHILIC CELL TYPE
The tumor cells have abundant cytoplasm that was eosinophilic. (Fig. 3 from Ferry JA, Young RH, Engel S, Scully RE. Oxyphilic Sertoli cell tumor of the ovary. A report of three cases, two in patients with the Peutz-Jeghers syndrome. Int J Gynecol Pathol 1994;13:259–66.)

Sertoli–Leydig Cell Tumors

Definition. These tumors are composed of Sertoli cells and cells of stromal derivation, including Leydig cells, in variable proportions and variable degrees of differentiation. There may be a prominent component of cells resembling rete epithelial cells growing in patterns similar to those of the rete testis. Sertoli-Leydig cell tumors have been divided by WHO into four major subtypes, three of which have variants that contain heterologous elements such as mucinous epithelium, carcinoid, cartilage, and skeletal muscle (Table 2-1).

General Features. These tumors account for less than 0.5 percent of all ovarian tumors (20,21, 25,31,35). The average patient age is 25 years; 75 percent of the patients are 30 years of age or younger and only 10 percent are over 50 years of age (31). The well-differentiated tumors occur at an average age of 35 years (34) and retiform tumors at an average age of 15 years (31,32).

Although the most striking mode of presentation of Sertoli-Leydig cell tumors is virilization, it occurs in only about one third of the cases (31). In such cases a patient who has been having normal periods typically experiences oligomenorrhea, followed within a few months by amenorrhea. There is a concomitant loss of female secondary sex characteristics, with atrophy of the breasts and disappearance of normal bodily contours. Progressive masculinization is heralded by acne, with hirsutism, temporal balding, deepening of the voice, and enlargement of the clitoris following in its wake. The androgen secretion by the tumor may also result in erythrocytosis. Although two early studies had reported an increased frequency of virilization in association with poorly differentiated tumors (20,21), there was no significant difference in its frequency among the various subtypes in the largest reported series except that it was lower in association with retiform tumors and variants containing heterologous elements (31).

Plasma levels of testosterone, androstenedione, and other androgens, alone or in combination, may be elevated. The urinary 17-ketosteroid values are usually normal or only slightly raised although occasionally, a high level has been recorded. These findings are in contrast to those associated with virilizing adrenal tumors, which may be accompanied by high urinary levels of 17-ketosteroids. The values for plasma androgens and urinary 17-ketosteroids are not reliable, however, in the differentiation of ovarian and adrenal virilizing tumors since the latter are often associated with elevated testosterone and normal urinary 17-ketosteroid levels. Also, tests involving attempted stimulation by tropic hormones and suppression by gonadal and adrenocortical steroids have not proved decisive in differentiating these tumors. Approximately 20 Sertoli-Leydig cell tumors associated with elevated serum levels of alpha-fetoprotein have been reported (17), but values as high as those accompanying yolk sac tumors are rare (29).

Approximately 50 percent of patients with Sertoli-Leydig cell tumors have no endocrine manifestations, and usually complain of abdominal swelling or pain. Occasional tumors have been associated with estrogenic manifestations, including menometrorrhagia in women in the reproductive age group and postmenopausal bleeding in older women (31). Other unusual clinical aspects of these tumors are their rare association with sarcoma botryoides of the cervix, occasional association with thyroid disease, and rare familial occurrence (page 388) (31).

Gross Findings. Over 98 percent of Sertoli-Leydig cell tumors are unilateral. The tumors are stage Ia in about 80 percent of the cases; rupture or involvement of the external surface of the ovary occurs in 12 percent of the cases and ascites in 4 percent. Only 2 to 3 percent of the tumors have spread beyond the ovary at presentation, usually within the pelvis and occasionally into the upper abdomen (31).

These tumors vary as greatly in their gross appearance as granulosa cell tumors but less often contain cysts filled with blood and rarely form unilocular thin-walled cysts (figs. 11-6–11-10). They vary from microscopic lesions to huge masses, but most are between 5 and 20 (average, 13.5) cm in diameter (31). They are often solid, lobulated, yellow masses (fig. 11-6). Poorly differentiated tumors, including those with mesenchymal heterologous elements (fig. 11-9) (23), tend to be larger than well-differentiated tumors and contain areas of hemorrhage and necrosis more frequently. Tumors with heterologous (fig. 11-8) or retiform (fig. 11-10) components are more often cystic than other forms but rarely, tumors without

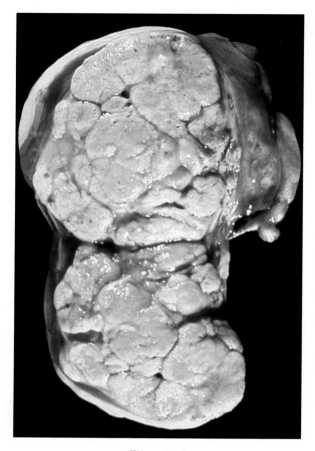

Figure 11-6
SERTOLI-LEYDIG CELL TUMOR
The sectioned surface is lobulated and bright yellow.

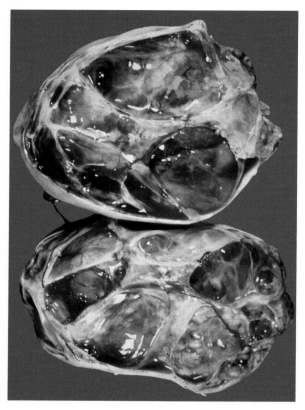

Figure 11-7
SERTOLI-LEYDIG CELL TUMOR
The sectioned surface contains numerous cysts. This tumor did not have a retiform component or heterologous mucinous elements.

either of these components are predominantly cystic (fig. 11-7). The cysts in the retiform tumors may contain numerous papillae and polypoid excrescences, which vary from small to large and edematous, simulating serous papillary cystic tumors or a hydatidiform mole (fig. 11-10) (32). Tumors with a large heterologous mucinous component (fig. 11-8) may be mistaken for mucinous cystic tumors on gross examination.

Microscopic Findings. Well differentiated Sertoli-Leydig cell tumors are characterized by a predominantly tubular pattern (figs. 11-11, 11-12) (34). On low-power examination fibrous bands are often conspicuous, separating lobules composed of hollow, or less often, solid, tubules and Leydig cells; in some tumors tubules of both types are present. The hollow tubules are typically round to oval and small (fig. 11-11), but may

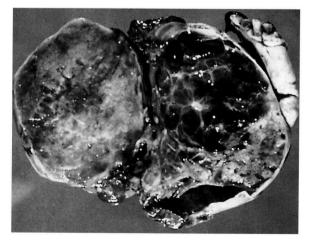

Figure 11-8
SERTOLI-LEYDIG CELL TUMOR
WITH HETEROLOGOUS ELEMENTS
The right half of the sectioned surface is composed of thin-walled cysts that were filled with mucin.

206

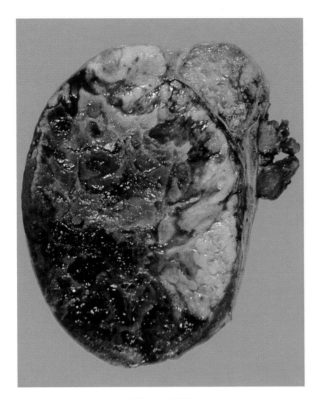

Figure 11-9
SERTOLI-LEYDIG CELL TUMOR,
POORLY DIFFERENTIATED, WITH
MESENCHYMAL HETEROLOGOUS ELEMENTS
The sectioned surface shows extensive hemorrhage and
necrosis.

be slightly irregular or cystically dilated; rarely,
they simulate endometrial glands (fig. 11-12) (16).
The lumens are usually devoid of conspicuous
secretion but in some cases eosinophilic fluid,
which is occasionally mucicarminophilic, is present. The solid tubules are typically elongated but
may be round or oval, and may resemble prepubertal or atrophic testicular tubules. The tubules
contain cells with moderate to large amounts of
cytoplasm that may be dense or vacuolated and
lipid-rich; the cells lining hollow tubules are typically cuboidal or columnar. The nuclei are round
or oblong without prominent nucleoli; nuclear atypia is usually absent or minimal and mitotic figures are rare. The stromal component consists of
bands of mature fibrous tissue in which variable
but usually conspicuous numbers of Leydig cells
are present (fig. 11-11); they contain variable
amounts of lipid and occasionally abundant

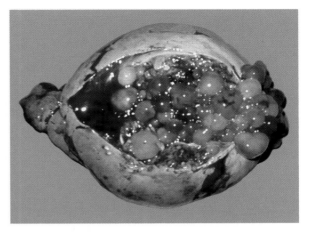

Figure 11-10
SERTOLI-LEYDIG CELL TUMOR, RETIFORM
Numerous polypoid, vesicle-like structures occupy the
lumen of a cyst. (Fig. 1 from Young RH, Scully RE. Ovarian
Sertoli-Leydig cell tumors with a retiform pattern: a prob-
lem in histopathologic diagnosis. A report of 25 cases. Am J
Surg Pathol 1983;7:755–71.)

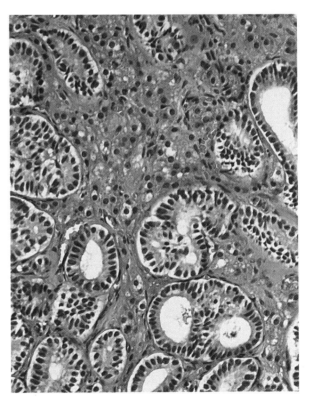

Figure 11-11
SERTOLI-LEYDIG CELL TUMOR,
WELL DIFFERENTIATED
Well differentiated tubules are separated by Leydig cells
with abundant eosinophilic cytoplasm.

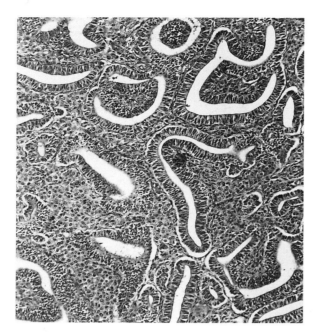

Figure 11-12
SERTOLI-LEYDIG CELL TUMOR,
WELL DIFFERENTIATED

The tubules are irregular in shape and lined by stratified epithelium, resembling endometrial glands. Numerous Leydig cells are present in the intervening stroma. (Fig. 6 from Young RH, Scully RE. Well differentiated ovarian Sertoli-Leydig cell tumors. A clinicopathological analysis of 23 cases. Int J Gynecol Pathol 1984;3:77–90.)

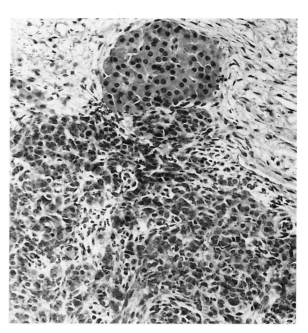

Figure 11-13
SERTOLI-LEYDIG CELL TUMOR
OF INTERMEDIATE DIFFERENTIATION

Irregular clusters and cords of darkly staining Sertoli cells are associated with a nodule of Leydig cells (top). (Fig. 46 from Young RH, Scully RE. Ovarian sex cord–stromal tumors: problems in differential diagnosis. Pathol Ann 1988;23(Pt 1):237–96.)

lipochrome pigment. Rare crystals of Reinke can be found in approximately 20 percent of the cases (34).

Sertoli-Leydig cell tumors of intermediate and poor differentiation form a continuum characterized by a variety of patterns and combinations of cell types (figs. 11-13–11-26). There may be intermediate differentiation in some areas and poor differentiation in others; less commonly, tumors of intermediate differentiation contain well-differentiated foci. Either the Sertoli cells, Leydig cells, or both exhibit variable degrees of immaturity.

In tumors of intermediate differentiation, immature Sertoli cells with small, round, oval, or angular nuclei are arranged typically in ill-defined masses, often creating a lobulated appearance on low-power examination. Within the masses the Sertoli cells may be arranged diffusely or in aggregates (fig. 11-14). Solid and hollow tubules; nests; thin, usually short, cords (figs. 11-15, 11-16) resembling the sex cords of the embryonic testis;

and occasionally, broad columns of Sertoli cells may be present (fig. 11-18). Small or large cysts may be conspicuous (fig. 11-19), sometimes containing eosinophilic secretion and creating a thyroid-like appearance (fig. 11-20). Follicle-like spaces are encountered occasionally. Rarely, hobnail-like cells line cysts. The Sertoli cells, Leydig cells, or both exceptionally have bizarre nuclei similar to those seen in other sex cord--stromal tumors (33). The Sertoli cell aggregates are separated by a stromal component that ranges from fibromatous to densely cellular to edematous, and typically contains clusters of well differentiated Leydig cells (figs. 11-12–11-14, 11-16, 11-17, 11-21). Edematous fibrous tissue may also separate individual tumor cells. Edema is particularly conspicuous in tumors from pregnant patients (fig. 11-24), often obscuring typical patterns. Occasionally, part or all of the stromal component is made up of immature, cellular mesenchymal tissue. The Sertoli and Leydig cells, singly or together, may contain variable and sometimes large amounts of

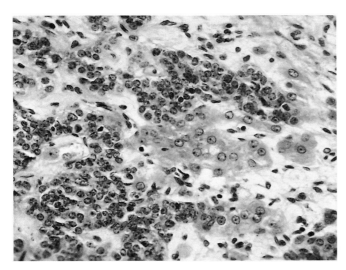

Figure 11-14
SERTOLI-LEYDIG CELL TUMOR
OF INTERMEDIATE DIFFERENTIATION
Anastomosing aggregates of darkly staining Sertoli cells are separated by clusters of Leydig cells. The latter have abundant cytoplasm, which was eosinophilic, and nuclei with prominent nucleoli.

Figure 11-15
SERTOLI-LEYDIG CELL TUMOR OF
INTERMEDIATE DIFFERENTIATION
Numerous thin cords of immature Sertoli cells are evident.

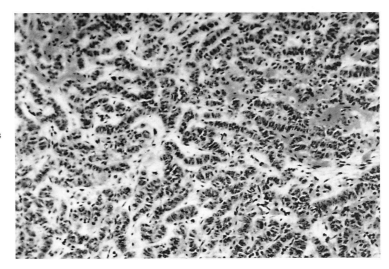

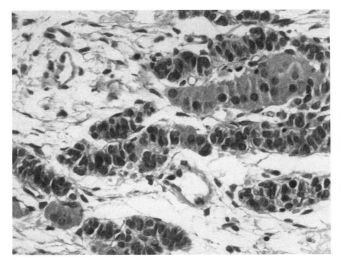

Figure 11-16
SERTOLI-LEYDIG CELL TUMOR
OF INTERMEDIATE
DIFFERENTIATION
Thin cords of darkly staining Sertoli cells lie in an edematous stroma containing nests of Leydig cells with abundant eosinophilic cytoplasm. (Fig. 79 from Young RH, Clement PB, Scully RE. Pathology of the ovary. In: Sternberg SS, ed. Diagnostic surgical pathology, Vol 2, 2nd ed. New York: Raven Press, 1994:2238.)

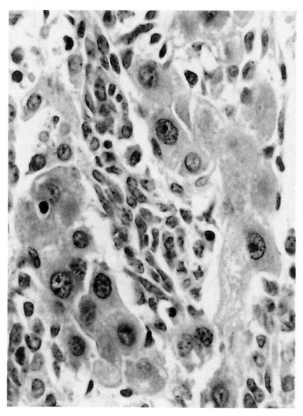

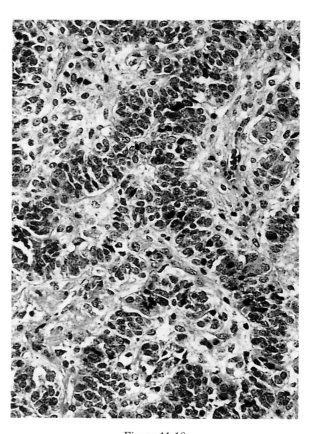

Figure 11-17
SERTOLI-LEYDIG CELL TUMOR
OF INTERMEDIATE DIFFERENTATION
Several clusters of Leydig cells with abundant cytoplasm, which was eosinophilic, separate aggregates of smaller Sertoli cells with scanty cytoplasm.

Figure 11-18
SERTOLI-LEYDIG CELL TUMOR OF
INTERMEDIATE DIFFERENTIATION
Long, thick ribbons of Sertoli cells are conspicuous. This tumor had a retiform pattern in other areas.

Figure 11-19
SERTOLI-LEYDIG CELL
TUMOR OF INTERMEDIATE
DIFFERENTIATION
A solid pattern merges with a microcystic pattern.

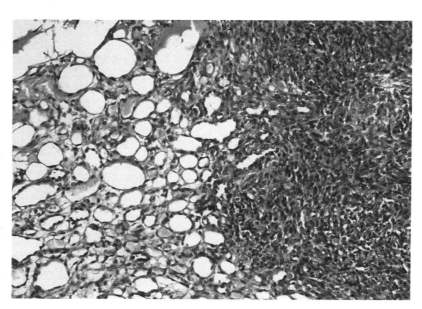

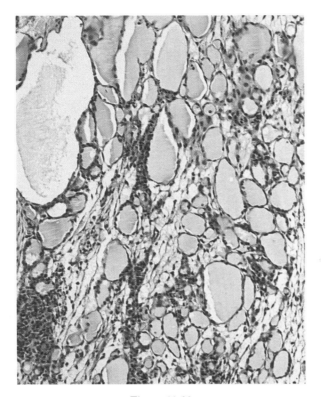

Figure 11-20
SERTOLI-LEYDIG CELL TUMOR
OF INTERMEDIATE DIFFERENTATION
Cysts contain eosinophilic secretion and superficially resemble thyroid follicles.

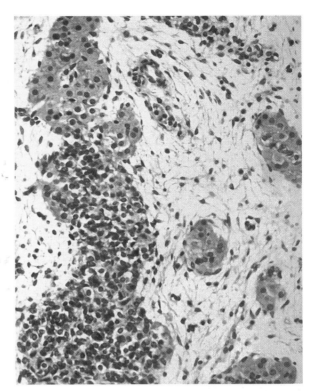

Figure 11-21
SERTOLI-LEYDIG CELL TUMOR OF
INTERMEDIATE DIFFERENTATION
Edematous stroma separates aggregates of Sertoli cells and nodules of Leydig cells.

lipid in the form of small or large droplets (fig. 11-23). Often, the most clear-cut differentiation into Sertoli cell aggregates and Leydig cell clusters is at the periphery of cellular lobules (figs. 11-13, 11-21). Leydig cell aggregates tend to be particularly large when the patient is pregnant. Rarely, crystals of Reinke can be identified in a few Leydig cells (fig. 11-22).

Poorly differentiated Sertoli-Leydig cell tumors were originally classified as sarcomatoid because, aside from the presence of specifically diagnostic elements, they often resemble fibrosarcomas (fig. 11-25); however, they may also be composed of poorly differentiated Sertoli cells growing in a diffuse pattern (fig. 11-26). Poorly differentiated tumors either lack the lobulation or orderly arrangement of Sertoli and stromal elements seen in most tumors of intermediate differentiation or exhibit those features in only minor foci. Additionally, they typically have a mitotic rate of over 10 per

10 high-power fields in contrast to tumors of intermediate differentiation, which in one series had an average of 5.5 mitotic figures per 10 high-power fields (31).

Fifteen percent of Sertoli-Leydig cell tumors have a retiform component, which has a pattern simulating, to variable degrees, that of the rete testis. A retiform pattern predominates in approximately half of these cases and is the exclusive or almost exclusive component in about 15 percent of them (2 percent of all Sertoli-Leydig cell tumors) (26,27,32). A retiform pattern has not yet been reported in association with well-differentiated Sertoli-Leydig cell tumors. Microscopic examination reveals a network of irregularly branching, elongated, narrow, often slit-like tubules and cysts (figs. 11-27, 11-28), into which papillae or polypoid structures may project (figs. 11-29, 11-30). The tubules and cysts may contain eosinophilic secretion and are lined by epithelial cells

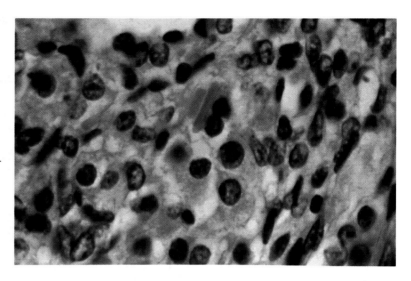

Figure 11-22
SERTOLI-LEYDIG CELL TUMOR
OF INTERMEDIATE
DIFFERENTIATION
Rod-shaped crystals of Reinke are present in the center.

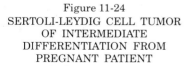

Figure 11-23
SERTOLI-LEYDIG CELL
TUMOR OF INTERMEDIATE
DIFFERENTIATION
There is prominent (lipid) vacuolization of Leydig cells.

Figure 11-24
SERTOLI-LEYDIG CELL TUMOR
OF INTERMEDIATE
DIFFERENTIATION FROM
PREGNANT PATIENT
Prominent intercellular edema has resulted in a reticular pattern, which may lead to the misdiagnosis of a yolk sac tumor.

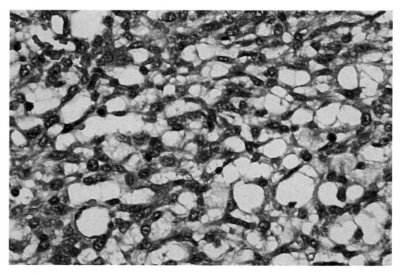

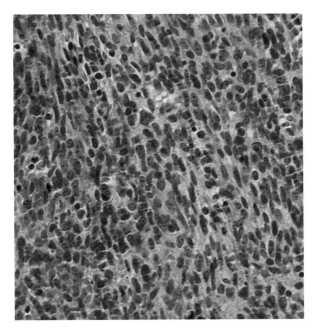

Figure 11-25
SERTOLI-LEYDIG CELL TUMOR,
POORLY DIFFERENTIATED
The tumor cells are spindle shaped; the appearance resembles that of a sarcoma.

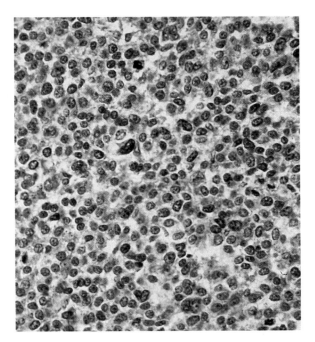

Figure 11-26
SERTOLI-LEYDIG CELL TUMOR,
POORLY DIFFERENTIATED
There is a diffuse growth of Sertoli cells with conspicuous nuclear atypia and mitotic activity. Features diagnostic of Sertoli cells were present elsewhere in the tumor.

that exhibit varying degrees of stratification and nuclear atypia (fig. 11-28). There are three types of papillae and polyps: most commonly, they are small and rounded or blunt, often containing hyalinized cores (fig. 11-30); less often, they are large and bulbous, with edematous cores (fig. 11-29) or delicate and branching and lined by stratified cells, simulating the papillae of a borderline or invasive serous tumor (fig. 11-28); prominent cellular budding may heighten this resemblance. A common finding in the retiform Sertoli-Leydig cell tumor is the presence of columns or ribbons of immature Sertoli cells (fig. 11-18). The stroma within a retiform area may be hyalinized or edematous, or moderately or densely cellular and immature.

Heterologous elements occur in approximately 20 percent of Sertoli-Leydig cell tumors, most of which are otherwise of intermediate differentiation, but some of which are poorly differentiated or retiform (23,24,28,30). Most commonly, glands and cysts lined by moderately to well differentiated gastric-type or intestinal-type mucinous epithelium are seen (figs. 11-31–11-33) (12,30); the

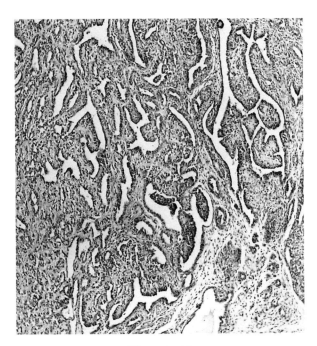

Figure 11-27
SERTOLI-LEYDIG CELL TUMOR, RETIFORM
Elongated, branching tubules are conspicuous.

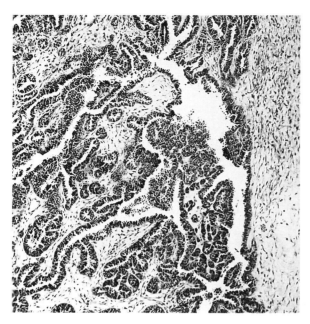

Figure 11-28
SERTOLI-LEYDIG CELL TUMOR, RETIFORM
Elongated, branching tubules with papillae and a stratified cellular lining impart a resemblance to a malignant serous papillary tumor (see figure 3-12).

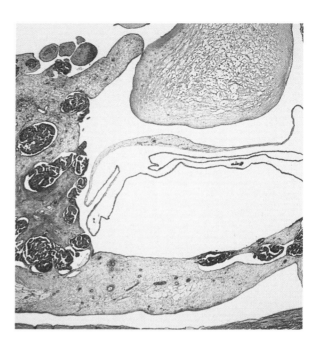

Figure 11-29
SERTOLI-LEYDIG CELL TUMOR, RETIFORM
One large edematous polypoid structure and several smaller cellular papillae with a glomeruloid pattern are evident.

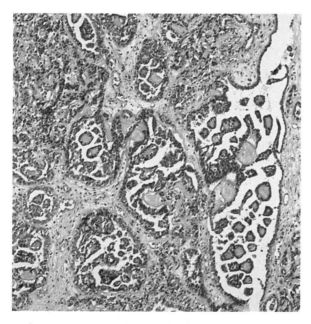

Figure 11-30
SERTOLI-LEYDIG CELL TUMOR, RETIFORM
The papillae are small, and many have hyalinized cores, simulating those of a clear cell adenocarcinoma. (Fig. 7 from Young RH, Scully RE. Ovarian Sertoli-Leydig cell tumors with a retiform pattern: a problem in histopathologic diagnosis. A report of 25 cases. Am J Surg Pathol 1983;7:755–71.)

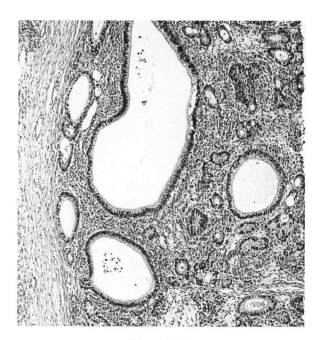

Figure 11-31
SERTOLI-LEYDIG CELL TUMOR
WITH HETEROLOGOUS ELEMENTS
Mucinous glands and cysts are separated by cellular tissue containing cords of Sertoli cells.

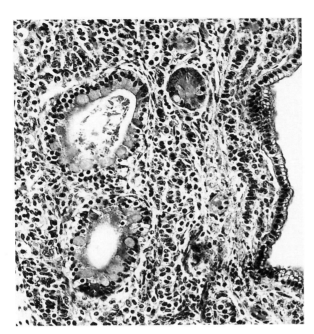

Figure 11-32
SERTOLI-LEYDIG CELL TUMOR
WITH HETEROLOGOUS ELEMENTS
Ribbons and poorly defined aggregates of immature Sertoli cells lie in the tissue between the mucinous glands and cyst. Goblet cells are visible in the epithelium lining two glands. (Fig. 4 from Young RH, Prat J, Scully RE. Ovarian Sertoli-Leydig cell tumors with heterologous elements (i). Gastrointestinal epithelium and carcinoid. A clinicopathologic analysis of 36 cases. Cancer 1982;50:2448–56.)

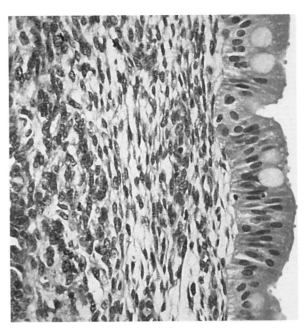

Figure 11-33
SERTOLI-LEYDIG CELL TUMOR
WITH HETEROLOGOUS ELEMENTS
Goblet cells are present in the epithelium lining a mucinous cyst.

latter may include goblet cells (fig. 11-33), argentaffin cells, and rarely, Paneth cells. The mucinous epithelium may appear benign or have the features of borderline malignancy or even low-grade adenocarcinoma (fig. 11-34). Mucin extravasation into the stroma is often present (fig. 11-35) and may elicit a prominent giant cell reaction, including epulis-like giant cells. Occasionally, tumors with mucinous elements contain scattered foci of insular (figs. 11-36, 11-37) or goblet cell carcinoid, which are usually of microscopic size (30) but rarely form a grossly visible mass. Stromal heterologous elements, encountered in 5 percent of all Sertoli-Leydig cell tumors (23), include islands of cartilage arising on a sarcomatous background (fig. 11-38), areas of embryonal rhabdomyosarcoma, or both (fig. 11-39). One heterologous tumor contained cells resembling hepatocytes (29) and in another case, neuroblastoma was present in a recurrent Sertoli-Leydig cell tumor (23).

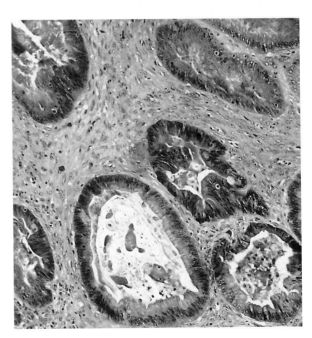

Figure 11-34
SERTOLI-LEYDIG CELL TUMOR WITH
HETEROLOGOUS ELEMENTS
The mucinous component is focally low-grade adenocarcinoma. Sertoli and Leydig cells are absent in this area.

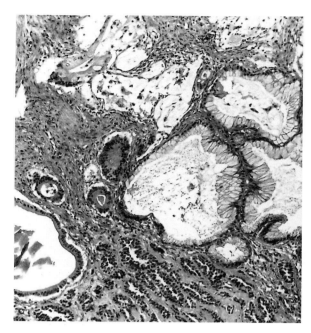

Figure 11-35
SERTOLI-LEYDIG CELL TUMOR
WITH HETEROLOGOUS ELEMENTS
AND RETIFORM COMPONENT
Mucin extravasation into the stroma is present (top).

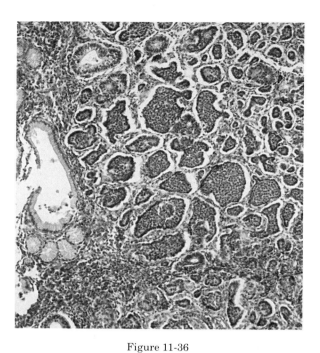

Figure 11-36
SERTOLI-LEYDIG CELL TUMOR
WITH HETEROLOGOUS ELEMENTS
Numerous nests of carcinoid tumor occupy most of the field;
mucinous elements are present at the left.

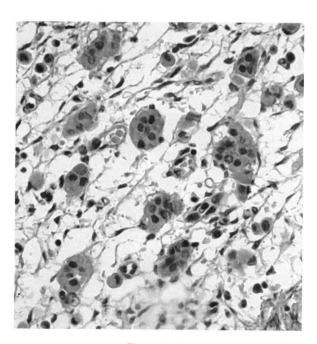

Figure 11-37
SERTOLI-LEYDIG CELL TUMOR
WITH HETEROLOGOUS ELEMENTS
Many small clusters of carcinoid tumor are present. A
Grimelius stain revealed argyrophil cells in the clusters.

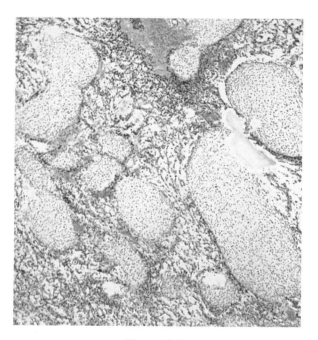

Figure 11-38
SERTOLI-LEYDIG CELL TUMOR
WITH HETEROLOGOUS ELEMENTS
Numerous islands of fetal-type cartilage are present
within cellular mesenchyme.

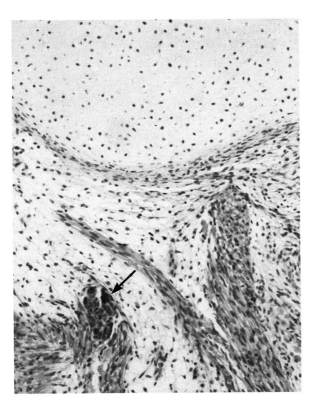

Figure 11-39
SERTOLI-LEYDIG CELL TUMOR WITH
HETEROLOGOUS ELEMENTS
An island of fetal-type cartilage is present at the top and
bands of rhabdomyoblasts at the bottom. A small, darkly
staining cluster of immature Sertoli cells is visible (arrow).

In the cases of Sertoli-Leydig cell tumor associated with elevated alpha-fetoprotein levels in the serum, immunohistochemical staining demonstrated this antigen in a variety of cell types: Sertoli cells, Leydig cells, and the mucinous cells and hepatocyte-like cells of heterologous tumors (17). Other immunohistochemical findings are discussed below (13–15,19,22,35a).

Differential Diagnosis. Sertoli cell tumors and Sertoli-Leydig cell hamartomas can replace the abdominal testis of a woman with the androgen-insensitivity syndrome and simulate ovarian Sertoli-stromal cell tumors. Both the testicular lesions and the syndrome in which they develop have distinctive diagnostic features (page 401).

Alpha-inhibin is stainable immunohistochemically in most Sertoli-Leydig cell tumors, more uniformly and intensely in Leydig than Sertoli cell components. A positive result is very helpful in differentiating these tumors from those dis-

cussed below, all of which are negative or at most, minimally positive for this antigen (35a).

The sometimes difficult differential diagnosis of a distinctive form of endometrioid carcinoma and a Sertoli-stromal cell tumor has been discussed on page 125. Sertoli-stromal cell tumors may also be simulated, although rarely, by endometrioid stromal sarcomas with sex cord–like differentiation (page 134).

The tubular Krukenberg tumor (page 336) may mimic a Sertoli-stromal cell tumor, especially if intracellular mucin is not a prominent feature on routine staining and luteinization of the stroma is present; further confusion arises in the occasional cases in which the Krukenberg tumor is associated with virilization, particularly during pregnancy. Tubular Krukenberg tumors are frequently bilateral, and contain atypical cells, including signet-ring cells filled with mucin, easily demonstrable by special stains.

Carcinoid tumors of the trabecular type may be confused with Sertoli-Leydig cell tumors of intermediate differentiation. The ribbons of the former, however, are much longer and more uniformly distributed than the sex cord–like formations of the latter. Rare carcinoid tumors with a solid tubular pattern can be difficult to distinguish from well-differentiated Sertoli-stromal cell tumors. Examination of the stroma of these tumors may be helpful in the differential diagnosis; it is typically less cellular and more fibromatous in carcinoid tumors than in Sertoli-stromal cell tumors and does not contain Leydig cells, although steroid-type cells are occasionally conspicuous at the tumor periphery (see chapter 19). The most specific diagnostic criterion is the presence of argyrophil granules in almost all carcinoid tumors and of argentaffin granules in many of them. In contrast, only glands and cysts lined by gastrointestinal-type epithelium and carcinoid tumorlets within heterologous Sertoli-Leydig cell tumors contain such granules (30). Finally, primary carcinoid tumors are associated with teratomatous elements in 70 percent of the cases, and metastatic carcinoids are most commonly bilateral and usually associated with a known primary tumor and metastases elsewhere.

Rare examples of struma ovarii have a solid tubular pattern almost indistinguishable on routine staining from that of a Sertoli cell tumor (page 287). Identification of more typical patterns of struma elsewhere and immunohistochemical staining for thyroglobulin facilitate the differential diagnosis. The reverse problem, simulation of struma by a Sertoli-Leydig cell tumor, also occurs rarely when the latter contains cysts distended with eosinophilic secretion (fig. 11-20). The presence of areas of typical Sertoli-Leydig cell neoplasia, however, is almost always diagnostic.

Solid and hollow tubules in ovarian wolffian tumors (page 325) may be indistinguishable from those in Sertoli-stromal cell tumors but the wolffian tumors lack Leydig cells, are rarely associated with endocrine manifestations, and virtually always have other distinctive patterns that establish the diagnosis.

A rare tumor that may be confused with Sertoli-stromal cell tumors is the ependymoma (page 300), which may contain ribbons of epithelial cells and even slit-like spaces and polypoid structures simulating those seen in retiform Sertoli-Leydig cell tumors. Adequate sampling of each tumor usually shows diagnostic features, and immunostaining for glial fibrillary acidic protein should confirm the diagnosis of ependymoma.

When diagnostic sex cord elements are few, poorly differentiated Sertoli-Leydig cell tumors may be misinterpreted as sarcomas or undifferentiated tumors of other types. The diagnosis of poorly differentiated Sertoli-Leydig cell tumor should be evaluated by thorough sampling, particularly in young women with androgenic manifestations.

Heterologous Sertoli-Leydig cell tumors can be mistaken for teratomas (24), but gonadal teratomas have not been reported to contain gonadal cell types and the former tumors have never been reported to contain ectodermal elements except in a single example with neuroblastoma. In most heterologous tumors the Sertoli-Leydig cell component is easily identified but in some cases in which it is overlooked (fig. 11-34), an erroneous diagnosis of a pure mucinous cystic tumor may be made (page 97).

The retiform Sertoli-Leydig cell tumor may be misinterpreted as a yolk sac tumor because of the youth of the patient and the presence of papillae within cystic spaces. Androgenic manifestations accompany about one quarter of retiform Sertoli-Leydig cell tumors (32) in contrast to their rare association with yolk sac tumors that have a functioning stroma (see chapter 19). Retiform tumors typically exhibit a complex pattern of papillae in contrast to the single papillae lined by poorly differ-

entiated cells in yolk sac tumors. The presence of other distinctive patterns of either tumor and immunohistochemical staining for alpha-fetoprotein in the yolk sac tumor almost always facilitate the diagnosis, although less extensive staining is occasionally observed in a Sertoli-Leydig cell tumor. Similar findings are helpful in the diagnosis of Sertoli-Leydig cell tumors in pregnancy, during which marked edema may result in a pattern simulating the reticular pattern of a yolk sac tumor (fig. 11-24). Retiform Sertoli-Leydig cell tumors may also be confused with serous borderline tumors and carcinomas and with the exceptionally rare Wilms tumor of the ovary (page 331).

Sarcomatoid areas in retiform or heterologous Sertoli-Leydig cell tumors containing skeletal muscle or cartilage, may lead to a misdiagnosis of malignant mesodermal mixed tumor. However, the latter usually occurs in patients older than those with Sertoli-Leydig cell tumor. This differential diagnosis is discussed on page 131.

Treatment and Prognosis. The treatment depends on the age of the patient, the stage of the tumor, the presence or absence of rupture, and the degree of differentiation. In young women the low frequency of bilaterality justifies a unilateral salpingo-oophorectomy if the tumor is confined to one ovary. More aggressive surgical therapy and chemotherapy are indicated for tumors higher than stage I. Adjuvant therapy may be advisable for stage I tumors that are poorly differentiated or contain mesenchymal heterologous elements, and for tumors of intermediate differentiation that have ruptured. Experience with the therapy of persistent or recurrent Sertoli-Leydig cell tumors is relatively limited. Radiation therapy, combination chemotherapy of the types effective against primitive germ cell tumors, or both, have been beneficial in occasional reported cases (18).

After the removal of a virilizing Sertoli-Leydig cell tumor, normal menses characteristically resume in about 4 weeks. The excessive hair usually diminishes to some extent. Clitoromegaly and deepening of the voice are less apt to regress. The prognosis in cases of Sertoli-Leydig cell tumor is closely related to its subtype and stage. In one large series, none of the well-differentiated tumors, 11 percent of those of intermediate differentiation, 59 percent of the poorly differentiated tumors, and 19 percent of those with heterologous elements were clinically malignant (31). In the clinically malignant heterologous tumors, the Sertoli-Leydig component of the tumor was typically poorly differentiated and the heterologous elements usually included skeletal muscle, cartilage, or both. The presence of a retiform pattern has an adverse effect on prognosis; in one series, 25 percent of stage I tumors with a retiform component were malignant in contrast to only 10 percent of those with no retiform component (32). Rupture also adversely affects the outcome of patients with stage I Sertoli-Leydig tumors (31); 30 percent of the tumors of intermediate differentiation that had ruptured were clinically malignant in contrast to only 7 percent of those that had not; parallel figures for the poorly differentiated tumors were 86 and 45 percent. The rare tumors that present at a stage higher than I are almost always fatal.

In contrast to granulosa cell tumors, which often recur many years after primary therapy, recurrences of Sertoli-Leydig cell tumors are typically early. In one series, 66 percent of the clinically malignant tumors recurred within 1 year and only 7 percent after 5 years (31) The recurrent tumor is usually confined to the pelvis and abdomen but metastases to the lung, liver, skin, and supraclavicular lymph nodes have been reported. The recurrent tumor often is less differentiated than the primary tumor and may resemble a soft tissue sarcoma. The history is almost always helpful in establishing the correct interpretation in such a situation.

GYNANDROBLASTOMA

According to WHO, this term should be used only if well differentiated ovarian and testicular-type cells are clearly recognizable within the neoplasm (fig. 11-40) (36–38). This conclusion was reached because components that suggest, but do not establish ovarian or testicular differentiation are not specifically diagnosable in a reproducible fashion. Also, since small foci of ovarian cell types are often encountered in well-sampled, otherwise typical Sertoli-stromal cell tumors, and testicular cell types in occasional granulosa-stromal cell tumors, the diagnosis of gynandroblastoma should be restricted to the very rare tumors that contain more than minor components of both forms of neoplasia. Accord-

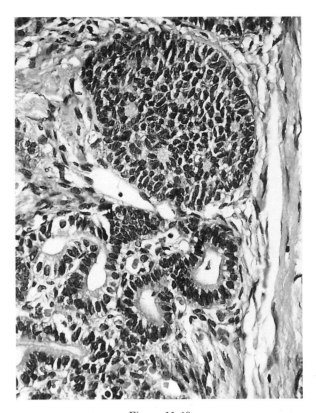

Figure 11-40
GYNANDROBLASTOMA
A focus of microfollicular adult granulosa cell tumor (above) is associated with several hollow tubules (below).

ing to our criteria, the well differentiated minor component should account for at least 10 percent of a mixed tumor to warrant a diagnosis of gynandroblastoma. When combinations such as Sertoli-Leydig cell tumor and juvenile granulosa cell tumor occur (37a), we prefer to diagnose both components, estimating the quantity of each. Gynandroblastomas usually occur in young adults but may be seen at any age. They may have androgenic or estrogenic manifestations. Almost all are stage I and clinically benign.

SEX CORD TUMOR
WITH ANNULAR TUBULES

Definition. This tumor is characterized by the presence of simple and complex ring-shaped tubules, often exhibiting focal differentiation into typical Sertoli cell tumor, granulosa cell tumor, or both.

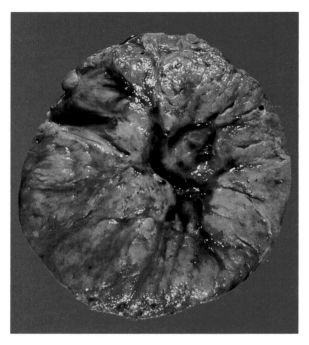

Figure 11-41
SEX CORD TUMOR WITH ANNULAR TUBULES
The large tumor has a yellow-orange sectioned surface (from a patient without the Peutz-Jeghers syndrome).

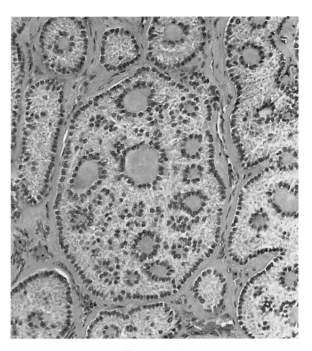

Figure 11-42
SEX CORD TUMOR WITH ANNULAR TUBULES
A few simple and several complex annular tubules are present (from a patient without the Peutz-Jeghers syndrome).

General Features. Sex cord tumors with annular tubules (SCTATs) vary in their clinical manifestations, depending on whether or not the patient has the Peutz-Jeghers syndrome (PJS) (gastrointestinal hamartomatous polyposis, mucocutaneous pigmentation, occasionally adenoma malignum of the uterine cervix, and carcinoma of the gastrointestinal tract, pancreas, or breast) (page 387) (45,49,51). In the one third of the patients who have PJS the lesions are incidental findings at operation for another indication or at autopsy (47,49,51). In those patients without the syndrome, the tumors almost always form palpable masses (39–44,46,48,51). Forty percent of the patients without the syndrome, and occasional patients with the syndrome, have had estrogenic manifestations. Progesterone secretion, which may result in decidual change of the endometrium, has been reported in a number of patients without the syndrome (42,50). The lesions in patients with PJS have been found at an average age of 27 years and those in patients without PJS at 34 years (51).

Gross Findings. In patients without PJS the tumors are almost always unilateral and are typically moderately large, predominantly solid, and frequently yellow (fig. 11-41). In patients with the syndrome the tumors are bilateral in at least two thirds of the cases. They are usually not recognized grossly but yellow nodules up to 3 cm in diameter have been observed in some cases.

Microscopic Findings. In cases both with and without the PJS, simple or complex annular tubules characterize the tumor either entirely or predominantly (fig. 11-42). The simple tubules are ring shaped, with the nuclei oriented peripherally and around a central hyaline body composed of basement membrane material; an intervening anuclear cytoplasmic zone forms the major component of the ring (fig. 11-42). The more numerous complex tubules are rounded structures made up of intercommunicating rings revolving around multiple hyaline bodies (fig. 11-42). In patients with the syndrome, multiple tumorlets varying from single tubules to clusters of them are scattered within the ovarian stroma

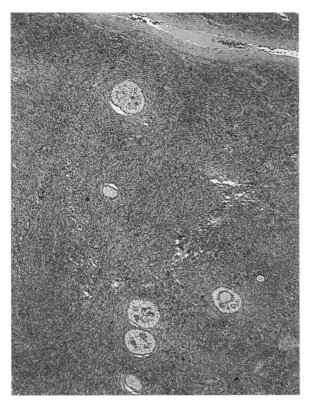

Figure 11-43
SEX CORD TUMOR WITH ANNULAR TUBULES
Scattered annular tubules are present in the ovarian stroma (from a patient with the Peutz-Jeghers syndrome).

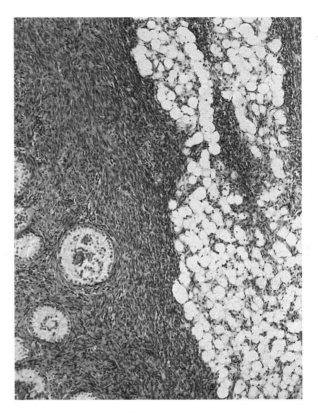

Figure 11-44
SEX CORD TUMOR WITH ANNULAR TUBULES
Islands of sex cord cells filled with large (lipid) vacuoles are adjacent to typical foci of sex cord tumor with annular tubules (from a patient with the Peutz-Jeghers syndrome).

(fig. 11-43). Islands of vacuolated sex cord cells loaded with lipid may also be present (fig. 11-44) as well as foci in which the tubular pattern is replaced by a diffuse growth of cells (fig. 11-45). Calcification of the tubules, which is occasionally extensive, is present in over half the cases with PJS (fig. 11-46). In large tumors unassociated with the syndrome, extensive hyalinization of the tubules and stroma may occur (fig. 11-47). Also, areas of microfollicular granulosa cell tumor (fig. 11-48), well-differentiated Sertoli cell tumor characterized by elongated solid tubules (fig 11-49), or both are often present. Ultrastructural examination has disclosed bundles of Charcot-Bottcher filaments in the cells of the annular tubules in occasional cases, consistent with Sertoli cell differentiation (40,50). The above findings have led some authorities (44,50) to consider SCTAT a subtype of Sertoli or granulosa cell tumor. In our opinion, the distinctive features of the tumor and its frequent association with the PJS warrant its classification as a specific form of sex cord–stromal tumor.

Treatment and Prognosis. The treatment of SCTAT is primarily surgical. At least one fifth of the tumors unassociated with PJS have been clinically malignant, with a characteristic spread via lymphatics. Recurrences are often late. In one remarkable case, multiple recurrences, mostly in regional and distant lymph nodes, including mediastinal and cervical lymph nodes, occurred over a period of 24 years, with each recurrent tumor removed surgically and followed by a long interval of remission (43). In that case the tumor produced large amounts of mullerian-inhibiting substance as well as progesterone and inhibin; the first two substances were useful serum tumor markers in monitoring the course of the

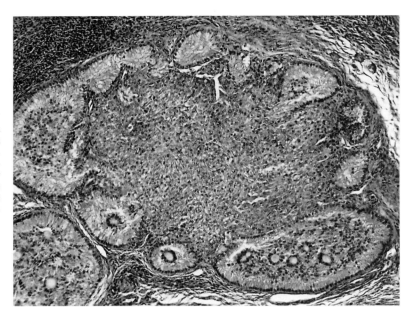

Figure 11-45
SEX CORD TUMOR
WITH ANNULAR TUBULES
Annular tubules surround a focus in which there is a diffuse growth of cells (from a patient with the Peutz-Jeghers syndrome). (Fig. 8 from Young RH, Welch WR, Dickersin GR, Scully RE. Ovarian sex cord tumor with annular tubules. Review of 74 cases including 27 with Peutz-Jeghers syndrome and 4 with adenoma malignum of the cervix. Cancer 1982;50:1384–402.)

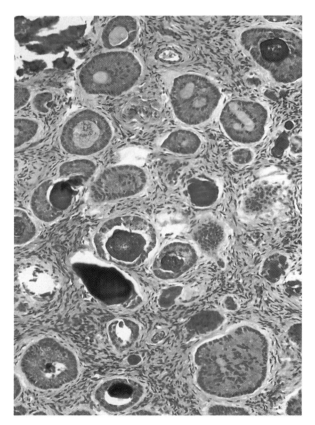

Figure 11-46
SEX CORD TUMOR
WITH ANNULAR TUBULES
There is calcification in several tubules (from a patient with the Peutz-Jeghers syndrome).

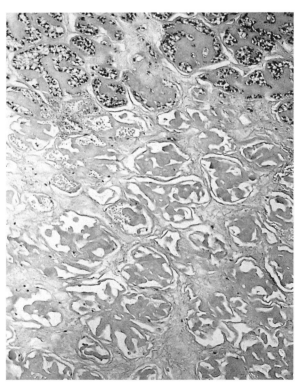

Figure 11-47
SEX CORD TUMOR WITH ANNULAR TUBULES
There is prominent hyalinization of the tubules and stroma (from a patient without the Peutz-Jeghers syndrome). (Fig. 16 from Young RH, Welch WR, Dickersin GR, Scully RE. Ovarian sex cord tumor with annular tubules. Review of 74 cases including 27 with Peutz-Jeghers syndrome and 4 with adenoma malignum of the cervix. Cancer 1982;50:1384–402.)

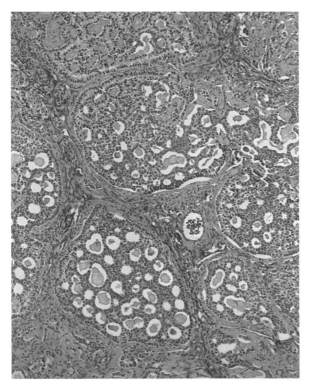

Figure 11-48
SEX CORD TUMOR WITH ANNULAR TUBULES
This area of the neoplasm has the features of a microfollicular granulosa cell tumor (from a patient without the Peutz-Jeghers syndrome).

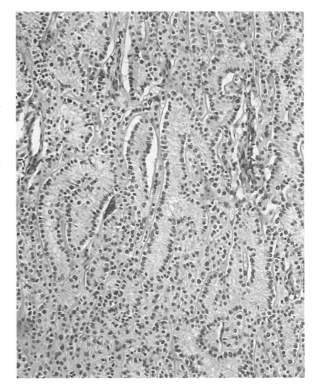

Figure 11-49
SEX CORD TUMOR WITH ANNULAR TUBULES
This area has the tubular architecture of a Sertoli cell tumor (from a patient without the Peutz-Jeghers syndrome).

patient. In another case mullerian-inhibiting substance and inhibin were useful tumor markers (46). All the tumorlets associated with PJS have been benign.

SEX CORD–STROMAL TUMORS, UNCLASSIFIED

These tumors, which account for 5 to 10 percent of those in the sex cord–stromal category (52), have patterns and cell types intermediate between or common to granulosa-stromal cell tumors and Sertoli-stromal cell tumors.

In one study, 17 percent of 36 sex cord–stromal tumors that were removed during pregnancy were placed in the unclassified group, and many of those that were classified as granulosa cell or Sertoli-stromal cell had large areas with an indifferent appearance (55). The features that led to difficulty in classification were the pres-

ence of prominent intercellular edema, increased luteinization in the granulosa cell tumors, and marked degrees of Leydig cell maturation in one third of the Sertoli-stromal cell tumors. All of these alterations, which were most common during the third trimester, tended to obscure the underlying tumor architecture.

Talerman et al. (53) described a group of sex cord–stromal tumors characterized by diffuse cellular fibrothecoma-like areas, granulosa cell–like areas, or both in combination with small areas of tubular differentiation in most of the cases. These authors interpreted such tumors, which differ in appearance from other Sertoli-stromal cell tumors, as "diffuse nonlobular androblastomas." Because of their predominant differentiation into cells of ovarian type we believe that many of these tumors can be classified as cellular fibromas or thecomas with minor sex cord elements (fig. 10-20) or as granulosa cell tumors with minor areas of

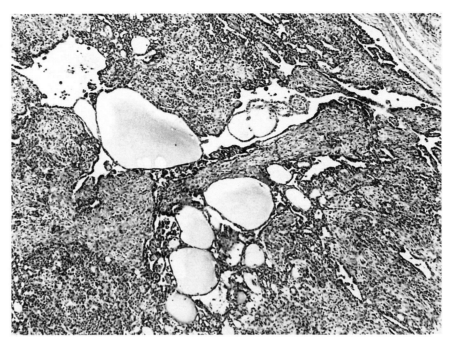

Figure 11-50
SEX CORD–STROMAL
TUMOR, UNCLASSIFIED
This tumor (from a patient with the Peutz-Jeghers syndrome) is characterized by retiform tubules with polyps, and cells with abundant cytoplasm, which was eosinophilic.

Sertoli cell differentiation. Other examples may not have distinctive enough features or the appropriate quantitative requirements for one or another of these diagnoses; we place such tumors in the unclassified sex cord–stromal category. Although the tumors were benign in all the reported cases, we have seen one example that recurred.

A rare type of sex cord–stromal tumor occurring in patients with the PJS and causing isosexual pseudoprecocity is characterized by a pattern that resembles that of the retiform Sertoli-Leydig cell tumor to some extent. This unique tumor, however, has sufficiently unusual features, including a proliferation of cells with abundant eosinophilic cytoplasm, some of which appear to be Sertoli cells and others, Leydig cells (54), to warrant separate categorization (fig. 11-50). Until the nature of the neoplastic cells is established we believe that this tumor belongs in the unclassified category.

Seidman (52) evaluated 32 cases of unclassified sex cord–stromal tumors, and concluded that their behavior is similar to that of granulosa cell and Sertoli-Leydig cell tumors.

REFERENCES

Sertoli Cell Tumors

1. Aguirre P, Thor AD, Scully RE. Ovarian small cell carcinoma. Histogenetic considerations based on immunohistochemical and other findings. Am J Clin Pathol 1989;92:140–9.
2. Aiba M, Hirayama A, Sakurada M, Naruse K, Ishikawa C, Aiba S. Spironolactone bodylike structure in renin-producing Sertoli cell tumor of the ovary. Surg Pathol 1990;3:143–9.
3. Ehrlich EN, Dominguez OV, Samuels LT, Lynch D, Oberhelman H, Warner NE. Aldosteronism and precocious puberty due to an ovarian androblastoma (Sertoli cell tumor). J Clin Endocrinol Metab 1963;23:358–67.
4. Ferry JA, Young RH, Engel G, Scully RE. Oxyphil Sertoli cell tumor of the ovary: a report of three cases, two in patients with the Peutz-Jeghers syndrome. Int J Gynecol Pathol 1994;13:259–66.

4a. Guerrieri C, Frånlund B, Melmstrom H, Boeryd B. Ovarian endometrioid carcinomas simulating sex cord-stromal tumors: a study employing inhibin and cytokeratin 7. Int J Gynecol Pathol 1998;17:266–71.

5. Korzets A, Nouriel H, Steiner Z, et al. Resistant hypertension associated with a renin-producing ovarian Sertoli cell tumor. Am J Clin Pathol 1986;85:242–7.

6. Solh HM, Azoury RS, Najjar SS. Peutz-Jeghers syndrome associated with precocious puberty. J Pediatr 1983;103:593–5.

7. Tavassoli FA, Norris HJ. Sertoli tumors of the ovary. A clinicopathologic study of 28 cases with ultrastructural observations. Cancer 1980;46:2281–97.

8. Teilum G. Classification of testicular and ovarian androblastoma and Sertoli cell tumors. A survey of comparative studies with consideration of histogenesis, endocrinology, and embryological theories. Cancer 1958;11:769–82.

9. Teilum G. Estrogen producing Sertoli cell tumors (androblastoma tubulare lipoides) of the human testis and ovary. Homologous ovarian and testicular tumors. III. J Clin Endocrinol 1949;9:301–18.

10. Tracy SL, Askin FB, Reddick RL, Jackson B, Kurman RJ. Progesterone secreting Sertoli cell tumor of the ovary. Gynecol Oncol 1985;22:85–96.

11. Young RH, Scully RE. Ovarian Sertoli cell tumors. A report of ten cases. Int J Gynecol Pathol 1984;2:349–63.

11a. Zheng W, Sung CJ, Harna I, et al. α and β subunits of inhibin/activin as sex cord-stromal differentiation markers. Int J Gynecol Pathol 1997;16:263–71.

Sertoli-Leydig Cell Tumors

12. Aguirre P, Scully RE, Delellis RA. Ovarian heterologous Sertoli-Leydig cell tumors with gastrointestinal-type epithelium. An immunohistochemical analysis. Arch Pathol Lab Med 1986;110:528–33.

13. Aguirre P, Thor AD, Scully RE. Ovarian endometrioid carcinomas resembling sex cord-stromal tumors: an immunohistochemical study. Int J Gynecol Pathol 1989;8:364–73.

13a. Aguirre P, Thor AD, Scully RE. Ovarian small cell carcinoma. Histogenetic considerations based on immunohistochemical and other findings. Am J Clin Pathol 1989;92:140–9.

14. Benjamin E, Law S, Bobrow LG. Intermediate filament cytokeratin and vimentin in ovarian sex cord-stromal tumors with correlative studies in adult and fetal ovaries. J Pathol 1987;52:253–63.

15. Costa MJ, Morris RJ, Wilson R, Judd R. Utility of immunohistochemistry in distinguishing ovarian Sertoli-stromal cell tumors from carcinosarcomas. Hum Pathol 1992;23:787–97.

16. Dardi LE, Miller AW, Gould VE. Sertoli-Leydig cell tumor with endometrioid differentiation. Case report and discussion of histogenesis. Diagn Gynecol Obstet 1982;4:227–34.

17. Gagnon S, Tetu B, Silva EG, McCaughey WT. Frequency of alpha-fetoprotein production by Sertoli-Leydig cell tumors of the ovary: an immunohistochemical study of eight cases. Mod Pathol 1989;2:63–7.

18. Gershenson DM, Copeland LJ, Kavanagh JJ, Stringer CA, Saul PB, Wharton JT. Treatment of metastatic stromal tumors of the ovary with cisplatin, doxorubicin, and cyclophosphamide. Obstet Gynecol 1987;70:765–9.

19. Miettinen M, Wahlstrom T, Virtanen I, Talerman A, Astengo-Osuna C. Cellular differentiation in ovarian sex-cord-stromal and germ-cell tumors studied with antibodies to intermediate-filament proteins. Am J Surg Pathol 1985;9:640–51.

20. Novak ER, Long JH. Arrhenoblastoma of the ovary. A review of the Ovarian Tumor Registry. Am J Obstet Gynecol 1965;92:1082–93.

21. O'Hern TM, Neubecker RD. Arrhenoblastoma. Obstet Gynecol 1962;l9:758–70.

22. Park SH, Kim I. Histogenetic consideration of ovarian sex cord-stromal tumors analyzed by expression pattern of cytokeratins, vimentin, and laminin. Correlation studies with human gonads. Path Res Pract 1994;190:449–56.

23. Prat J, Young RH, Scully RE. Ovarian Sertoli-Leydig cell tumors with heterologous elements. (ii) Cartilage and skeletal muscle: a clinicopathologic analysis of twelve cases. Cancer 1982;50:2465–75.

24. Reddick RL, Walton LA. Sertoli-Leydig cell tumor of the ovary with teratomatous differentiation: clinicopathologic considerations. Cancer 1982;50:1171–6.

25. Roth LM, Anderson MC, Govan AD, Langley FA, Gowing NF, Woodcock AS. Sertoli-Leydig cell tumors. A clinicopathologic study of 34 cases. Cancer 1981;48:187–97.

26. Roth LM, Slayton RE, Brady LW, Blessing JA, Johnson G. Retiform differentiation in ovarian Sertoli-Leydig cell tumors. A clinicopathologic study of six cases from a gynecologic oncology group study. Cancer 1985; 55:1093–8.

27. Talerman A. Ovarian Sertoli-Leydig cell tumor (androblastoma) with retiform pattern. A clinicopathologic study. Cancer 1987;60:3056–64.

28. Waxman M, Damjanov I, Alpert L, Sardinsky T. Composite mucinous ovarian neoplasms associated with Sertoli-Leydig and carcinoid tumors. Cancer 1981; 47:2044–52.

29. Young RH, Perez-Atayde AR, Scully RE. Ovarian Sertoli-Leydig cell tumor with retiform and heterologous components. Report of a case with hepatocytic differentiation and elevated serum alpha-fetoprotein. Am J Surg Pathol 1984;8:709–18.

30. Young RH, Prat J, Scully RE. Ovarian Sertoli-Leydig cell tumors with heterologous elements. (i) Gastrointestinal epithelium and carcinoid: a clinicopathologic analysis of thirty-six cases. Cancer 1982;50:2448–56.

31. Young RH, Scully RE. Ovarian Sertoli-Leydig cell tumors. A clinico-pathological analysis of 207 cases. Am J Surg Pathol 1985;9:543–69.

32. Young RH, Scully RE. Ovarian Sertoli-Leydig cell tumors with a retiform pattern: a problem in histopathologic diagnosis. A report of 25 cases. Am J Surg Pathol 1983;77:755–71.

33. Young RH, Scully RE. Ovarian sex cord stromal tumors with bizarre nuclei: a clinicopathological analysis of 17 cases. Int J Gynecol Pathol 1983;1:325–35.

34. Young RH, Scully RE. Well-differentiated ovarian Sertoli-Leydig cell tumors. A clinicopathological analysis of 23 cases. Int J Gynecol Pathol 1984;3:277–90.

35. Zaloudek C, Norris HJ. Sertoli-Leydig tumors of the ovary. A clinico-pathologic study of 64 intermediate and poorly differentiated neoplasms. Am J Surg Pathol 1984;8:405–18.

35a. Zheng W, Sung CJ, Harma I, et al. α and β subunits of inhibin/activin as sex cord-stromal differentiation markers. Int J Gynecol Pathol 1997;16:263–71.

Gynandroblastoma

36. Anderson MC, Rees DA. Gynandroblastoma of the ovary. Brit J Obstet Gynaecol 1975;82:68–73.

37. Chalvardjian A, Derzko C. Gynandroblastoma: its ultrastructure. Cancer 1982;50:710–21.

37a. McCluggage WG, Sloan JM, Murnaghan M, White R. Gynandroblastoma of ovary with juvenile granulosa cell component and heterologous intestinal type glands. Histopathology 1996;29:251–7.

38. Neubecker RD, Breen JL. Gynandroblastoma. A report of five cases with a discussion of the histogenesis and classification of ovarian tumors. Am J Clin Pathol 1962;38:60–9.

Sex Cord Tumor with Annular Tubules

39. Ahn GH, Chi JG, Lee SK. Ovarian sex cord tumor with annular tubules. Cancer 1986;57:1066-73.

40. Astengo-Osuna C. Ovarian sex-cord tumor with annular tubules. Case report with ultrastructural findings. Cancer 1984;54:1070–5.

41. Czernobilsky B, Gaedcke G, Dallenbach-Hellweg G. Endometrioid differentiation in ovarian sex cord tumor with annular tubules accompanied by gestagenic effect. Cancer 1985;55:738–44.

42. Dolan J, Al-Timimi AH, Richards SM, et al. Does ovarian sex cord tumor with annular tubules produce progesterone? J Clin Pathol 1986;39:29–35.

43. Gustafson ML, Lee MM, Scully RE, et al. Mullerian inhibiting substance as a marker for ovarian sex-cord tumor. N Engl J Med 1992;326:466–71.

44. Hart WR, Kumar N, Crissman JD. Ovarian neoplasms resembling sex cord tumors with annular tubules. Cancer 1980;45:2352–63.

45. McGowan L, Young RH, Scully RE. Peutz-Jeghers syndrome with "adenoma malignum" of the cervix. A report of two cases. Gynecol Oncol 1980;10:125–33.

46. Puls LE, Hamous J, Morrow MS, Schneyer A, MacLaughlin DT, Castracane VD. Recurrent ovarian sex cord tumor with annular tubules: tumor marker and chemotherapy experience. Gynecol Oncol 1994;54:396–401.

47. Scully RE. Sex cord tumor with annular tubules. A distinctive ovarian tumor of the Peutz-Jeghers syndrome. Cancer 1970;25:1107–21.

48. Shen K, Wu PC, Lang JH, Huang RL, Tang MT, Lian LJ. Ovarian sex cord tumor with annular tubules: a report of six cases. Gynecol Oncol 1993;48:180-4.

49. Srivatsa PJ, Keeney GL, Podratz KC. Disseminated cervical adenoma malignum and bilateral ovarian sex cord tumors with annular tubules associated with Peutz-Jeghers syndrome. Gynecol Oncol 1994;53:256–64.

50. Tavassoli FA, Norris HJ. Sertoli tumors of the ovary. A clinicopathologic study of 28 cases with ultrastructural observations. Cancer 1980;46:2281–97.

51. Young RH, Welch WR, Dickersin GR, Scully RE. Ovarian sex cord tumor with annular tubules: review of 74 cases including 27 with Peutz-Jeghers syndrome and 4 with adenoma malignum of the cervix. Cancer 1982;50:1384–402.

Sex Cord-Stromal Tumors, Unclassified

52. Seidman JD. Unclassified gonadal stromal tumors. A clinicopathologic study of 32 cases. Am J Surg Pathol 1996;20:699–706.

53. Talerman A, Hughesdon PE, Anderson MC. Diffuse nonlobular ovarian androblastoma usually associated with feminization. Int J Gynecol Pathol 1982;1:155–71.

54. Young RH, Dickersin GR, Scully RE. A distinctive ovarian sex cord-stromal tumor causing sexual precocity in the Peutz-Jeghers syndrome. Am J Surg Pathol 1983;7:233–43.

55. Young RH, Dudley AG, Scully RE. Granulosa cell, Sertoli-Leydig cell and unclassified sex cord-stromal tumors associated with pregnancy: a clinicopathological analysis of thirty-six cases. Gynecol Oncol 1984; 18:181–205.

❖❖❖

12
STEROID CELL TUMORS

The terms "lipid cell tumor" and "lipoid cell tumor" have been applied to ovarian neoplasms composed entirely of cells resembling typical steroid hormone–secreting cells, i.e., lutein cells, Leydig cells, and adrenal cortical cells (26). These terms are inaccurate as well as nonspecific, however, since up to 25 percent of tumors in this category contain little or no lipid. The term "steroid cell tumors" has been accepted by the World Health Organization (WHO) for these neoplasms, because it reflects both the morphologic features of the neoplastic cells and their propensity to secrete steroid hormones (1). These tumors, which account for only 0.1 percent of ovarian tumors, have been subdivided into two subtypes of known origin, the stromal luteoma and the Leydig cell tumor, and a third subtype whose cell lineage is uncertain, steroid cell tumor not otherwise specified (NOS). Some tumors in the last category are clinically malignant whereas those in the first two categories are benign.

STROMAL LUTEOMA

General Features. The stromal luteoma accounts for approximately 20 percent of steroid cell tumors (3). It is a small tumor that lies within the ovarian stroma and is therefore assumed to arise from it (4). Such an origin is supported by the capacity of the ovarian stroma to differentiate into lutein cells in cases of stromal hyperthecosis. Adrenal rest cells and Leydig cells, the other possible sources of tumors of this type, in contrast, have been identified within the ovarian stroma only exceptionally (5,6). The diagnosis of stromal luteoma is further supported in approximately 90 percent of the cases by the finding of stromal hyperthecosis elsewhere in the same ovary or in the contralateral ovary (3). In some cases of the latter disorder, the nests of lutein cells may form nodules (nodular hyperthecosis). The dividing line between a large hyperthecotic nodule and a stromal luteoma is arbitrary: we draw the line at 0.5 cm. In nodular hyperthecosis the nodules are typically multiple in contrast to the usually solitary stromal luteoma.

Eighty percent of stromal luteomas occur in postmenopausal women (3). The initial symptom in 60 percent of patients is abnormal vaginal bleeding, probably related to hyperestrinism, although whether the tumor secretes an estrogen directly or an androgen that is converted peripherally to an estrogen is unknown. Androgenic manifestations are present in only 12 percent of the cases (3). This profile of hormonal function is in contrast to that associated with other categories of steroid cell tumor, which are usually androgenic and only occasionally estrogenic. Underlying stromal hyperthecosis may contribute to the clinical picture in some patients with stromal luteoma, particularly those in whom there is a long history of a hormonal disturbance. At least one stromal luteoma was associated with the hyperandrogenism-insulin resistance-acanthosis nigricans syndrome (2), in which the ovaries are polycystic with stromal hyperthecosis (page 413). All the reported stromal luteomas have been benign.

Gross Findings. Stromal luteomas are almost always under 3 cm in diameter because if larger, confinement to the ovarian stroma, a requisite for the diagnosis, is no longer recognizable. With rare exceptions, stromal luteomas are unilateral. They are well circumscribed, solid, and usually gray-white or yellow (fig. 12-1), but one third have red or brown areas.

Microscopic Findings. Microscopic examination reveals a rounded nodule of cells of lutein type (fig. 12-2), which generally contain relatively little lipid; intracytoplasmic lipochrome pigment may be conspicuous. The nuclei are small and round with single prominent nucleoli; mitotic figures are generally rare. The cells may be arranged diffusely or in small nests or cords, and are completely or almost completely surrounded by ovarian stroma. One confusing feature, seen in about 20 percent of cases, is focal degeneration, with the formation of irregular spaces that may simulate glands or vessels (fig. 12-3). The spaces may contain lipid-laden cells and chronic inflammatory cells or may be separated by cells of those types as well as fibrotic tissue.

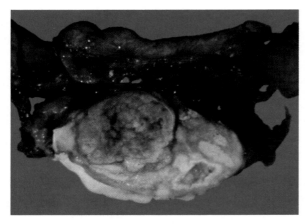

Figure 12-1
STROMAL LUTEOMA
The sectioned surface of the ovary contains a sharply demarcated, small, yellow tumor.

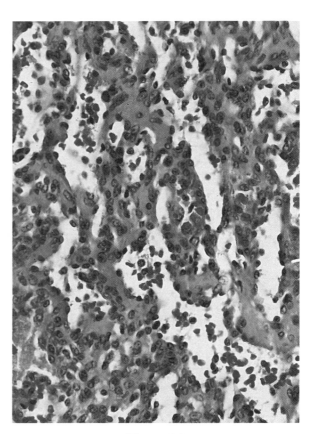

Figure 12-3
STROMAL LUTEOMA
Degenerative changes have produced irregular spaces containing red blood cells, suggesting the erroneous diagnosis of a vascular tumor.

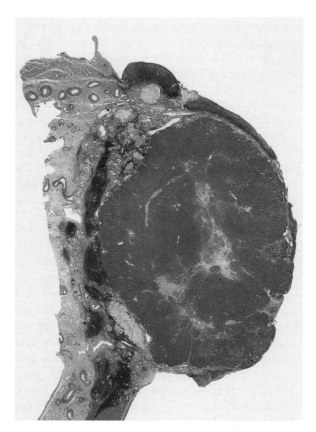

Figure 12-2
STROMAL LUTEOMA
The tumor occupies the ovarian parenchyma.

LEYDIG CELL TUMORS

General Features. The Leydig cell nature of a steroid cell tumor is established only by the identification of crystals of Reinke in the cytoplasm of the neoplastic cells on either light or electron microscopic examination (15). Since only 35 to 40 percent of testicular Leydig cell tumors contain these crystals on light microscopic examination, and Leydig cells cannot be differentiated from lutein cells or adrenal cortical cells in the absence of these inclusions, it is probable that a number of unclassified steroid cell tumors are Leydig cell tumors that cannot be specifically identified as such.

Ovarian Leydig cell tumors have been divided into two subtypes by Roth and Sternberg (12), the hilus cell tumor and the Leydig cell tumor,

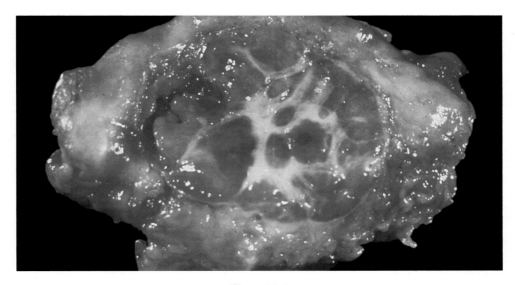

Figure 12-4
LEYDIG CELL TUMOR
A light brown mass lobulated by septa occupies the center of the sectioned surface of the ovary.

nonhilar type. The former arises from hilar Leydig cells and lies in the ovarian hilus separated from the medullary stroma. Leydig cell tumors of nonhilar type originate from ovarian stromal cells and lie within the ovarian stroma. Only four examples of the nonhilar type tumor have been reported and except for their location, the clinical and pathologic features do not differ from those of hilus cell tumors. An ovarian stromal cell derivation of these tumors is supported by the very rare finding of Leydig cells containing crystals in the steroid cell nests of ovaries that otherwise have the typical appearance of stromal hyperthecosis (17). Some Leydig cell tumors are centered at the junction of the hilus and medulla. In such cases it is impossible to be certain whether the tumor arose from medullary stroma or hilus cells.

Leydig cell tumors, which account for approximately 20 percent of steroid cell tumors, are detected at an average age of 58 years and cause hirsutism or virilization in three quarters of the cases (8,11,13,14,16); rarely, they are associated with estrogenic manifestations (10). The androgenic changes typically have a less abrupt onset and are milder than those associated with Sertoli-Leydig cell tumors, and sometimes have been present for many years. The urinary 17-ketosteroid levels are usually normal or only slightly elevated because the tumors produce predominantly the potent androgen, testosterone, which is not a 17-ketosteroid, instead of the weaker androgens, androstenedione and dehydroepiandrosterone, elevations of which are typically associated with high values of urinary 17-ketosteroids. Leydig cell tumors are occasionally palpable preoperatively. Almost all of those recorded in the literature have been benign; only one case of malignant Leydig cell tumor merits serious consideration, but the presence of crystals of Reinke in the neoplastic cells in that case was not convincingly documented in the illustrations (9).

Gross Findings. Leydig cell tumors are usually red-brown (fig. 12-4) to yellow but may be dark brown to black (fig. 12-5). They are typically centered in the hilus (fig. 12-5), are rarely large (mean diameter, 2.4 cm) (11), and are rarely bilateral (7).

Microscopic Findings. Microscopic examination typically reveals a circumscribed mass of steroid cells that are usually diffusely arranged. Occasionally, their nuclei cluster and are separated by nucleus-free eosinophilic zones (fig. 12-6); this pattern is highly suggestive of a Leydig cell tumor even in the absence of crystals of Reinke. In some tumors a prominent fibrous stroma imparts a nodular appearance (fig. 12-7). An unusual feature in one third of the cases is fibrinoid replacement of the walls of moderate-sized vessels,

229

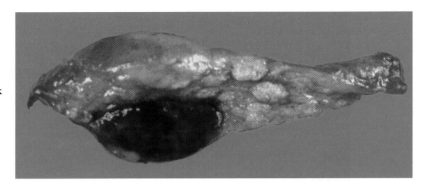

Figure 12-5
HILUS CELL TUMOR
A sharply circumscribed brown-black nodule is present in the ovarian hilus.

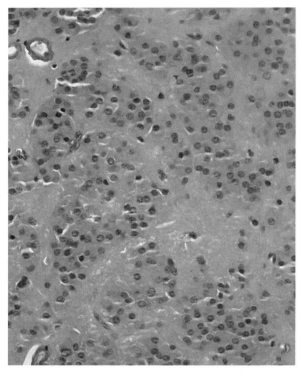

Figure 12-6
LEYDIG CELL TUMOR
Cellular areas are separated by anuclear eosinophilic areas. (Fig. 84 from Young RH, Clement PB, Scully RE. Pathology of the ovary. In: Sternberg SS, ed. Diagnostic surgical pathology, Vol 2, 2nd ed. New York: Raven Press, 1994:2242.)

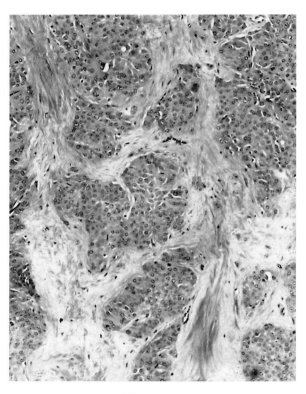

Figure 12-7
LEYDIG CELL TUMOR
A prominent fibrous stroma subdivides the tumor into cellular lobules.

unaccompanied by an inflammatory cell infiltration (fig. 12-8). Degenerative spaces similar to those seen in stromal luteomas may be present. The tumor cells typically contain abundant eosinophilic cytoplasm; some cells may have spongy cytoplasm, indicating the presence of lipid (fig. 12-9). Cytoplasmic lipochrome pigment is present in many cases; it is usually sparse but

may be abundant. The typically round nuclei are often hyperchromatic and contain single small nucleoli. There may be slight to moderate variation in nuclear size and shape, and occasionally the nuclei are bizarre (fig. 12-10) and multiple. Rare mitotic figures may be present.

Pseudoinclusions of cytoplasm into the nucleus may be seen. Elongated eosinophilic

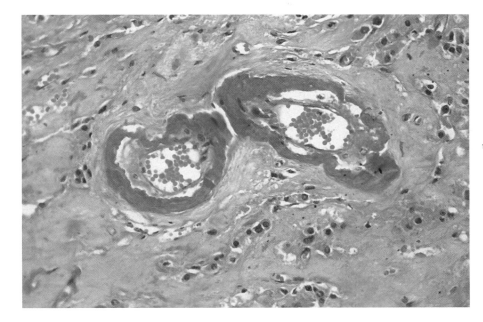

Figure 12-8
LEYDIG CELL TUMOR
Fibrinoid material occupies
the walls of two blood vessels.

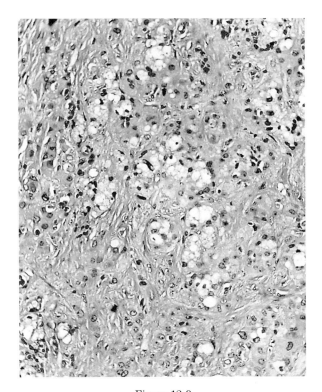

Figure 12-9
LEYDIG CELL TUMOR
Many of the tumor cells have abundant, pale, vacuolated
cytoplasm.

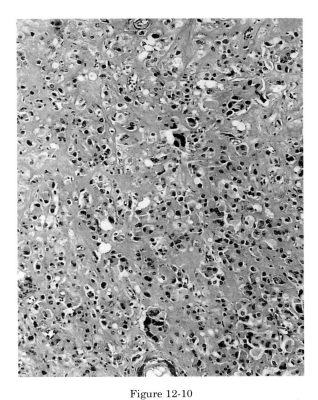

Figure 12-10
LEYDIG CELL TUMOR
Many of the nuclei have enlarged, hyperchromatic, bi-
zarre nuclei.

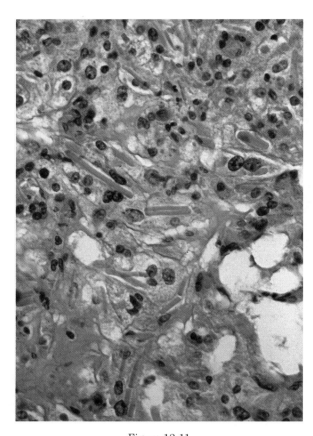

Figure 12-11
LEYDIG CELL TUMOR
Elongated eosinophilic crystals of Reinke are conspicuous in the cytoplasm of several tumor cells.

Reinke crystals of varying sizes are present in the cytoplasm or sometimes in the nucleus, but are often found only after prolonged search (fig. 12-11). The diagnosis of a Leydig cell tumor is favored if a crystal-free steroid cell tumor located in the hilus has a background of hilus cell hyperplasia, is associated with nonmedullated nerve fibers, exhibits fibrinoid necrosis of blood vessel walls, or shows nuclear clustering with intervening nucleus-free zones. On electron microscopic examination crystals of Reinke are typically rod shaped when cut longitudinally, and hexagonal in cross section. The interior of the crystal has a cross-hatched appearance. Intracytoplasmic eosinophilic spheres, which may be crystal precursors, are also typically present, but are not specific for Leydig cell tumors.

STEROID CELL TUMOR, NOT OTHERWISE SPECIFIED (NOS)

General Features. Tumors in this category, which account for approximately 60 percent of steroid cell tumors, are almost certainly large stromal luteomas or Leydig cell tumors, but because they lack crystals of Reinke and their topographic features have been obscured by their large size, they cannot be identified specifically as either type of tumor.

Steroid cell tumors NOS occur at any age but typically at a younger age (mean, 43 years) (22) than other types of steroid cell tumor, and in contrast to the latter, occasionally occur before puberty (19). These tumors are associated with androgenic changes, which may be of many years' duration (20), in half the cases; estrogenic changes, including rare examples of isosexual pseudoprecocity (18) in 10 percent of the cases; and occasionally progestagenic changes. Five reported tumors secreted cortisol and caused Cushing's syndrome (18,21,24,28), and a few others have been accompanied by elevated serum cortisol levels in the absence of clinical manifestations of Cushing's syndrome; one tumor secreted aldosterone (23). Rare examples have been associated with hypercalcemia, erythrocytosis, or ascites (22). Hormone studies performed in patients with androgenic changes, Cushing's syndrome, or both, typically show elevated urinary levels of 17-ketosteroids and 17-hydroxycorticosteroids as well as increased plasma levels of testosterone and androstenedione. The tumors that resulted in Cushing's syndrome were associated with elevated levels of free cortisol in the blood or urine (18,21,24,28). Only about 5 percent of the tumors are bilateral.

Gross Findings. The tumors are typically solid and well circumscribed, are occasionally lobulated, and have a mean diameter of 8.4 cm (22). The sectioned surfaces are typically yellow or orange if large amounts of intracytoplasmic lipid are present (fig. 12-12), red to brown if the cells are lipid-poor, or dark brown to black if large quantities of intracytoplasmic lipochrome pigment are present (fig. 12-13). Necrosis, hemorrhage, and cystic degeneration are occasionally observed (fig. 12-14).

Microscopic Findings. The cells are typically arranged diffusely (fig. 12-15), but occasionally grow in large aggregates, small nests

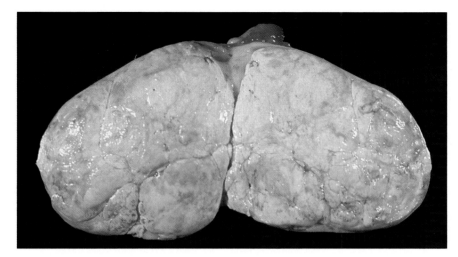

Figure 12-12
STEROID CELL TUMOR
NOT OTHERWISE
SPECIFIED
The sectioned surfaces are lobulated and yellow-orange.

Figure 12-13
STEROID CELL TUMOR
NOT OTHERWISE SPECIFIED
The tumor is well circumscribed and dark brown. (Fig. 2 from Hayes MC, Scully RE. Steroid tumors not otherwise specified (lipid cell tumors): a clinicopathological analysis of 63 cases. Am J Surg Pathol 1987;11:835–45.)

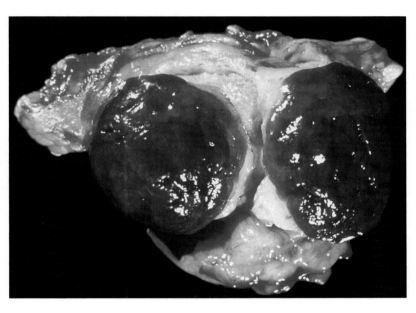

(fig. 12-16), irregular clusters, thin cords, or columns. The stroma is inconspicuous in most cases but is prominent in approximately 15 percent. A minor fibromatous component may be seen. Rarely, the stroma is edematous or myxoid, with tumor cells loosely dispersed within it, and exceptionally, it is calcified and may contain psammoma bodies. Necrosis and hemorrhage may be prominent, particularly in tumors with significant cytologic atypia.

The polygonal to rounded tumor cells have distinct cell borders, central nuclei, many of which contain prominent nucleoli (fig. 12-17), and moderate to abundant cytoplasm that varies

from eosinophilic and granular (lipid free or lipid poor) to spongy (lipid rich) (fig. 12-18); lipid was present in 75 percent of the tumors in one series (fig. 12-19) (22). Rarely, cells with large lipid vacuoles have a signet-ring cell appearance. Intracytoplasmic lipochrome pigment is found in 40 percent of the cases. In 60 percent of the cases in the largest published series (22), nuclear atypia was absent or minimal, and mitotic figures were fewer than 2 per 10 high-power fields. In the remaining cases, grade 1 to 3 nuclear atypia, usually associated with an increase in mitotic figures up to 15 per 10 high-power fields, was present (fig. 12-20).

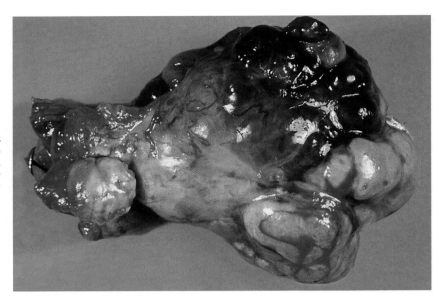

Figure 12-14
STEROID CELL TUMOR
NOT OTHERWISE SPECIFIED
The outer surface is partly bright yellow and partly red due to extensive hemorrhage. This neoplasm, which was associated with widespread intra-abdominal metastasis, was from a patient with Cushing's syndrome.

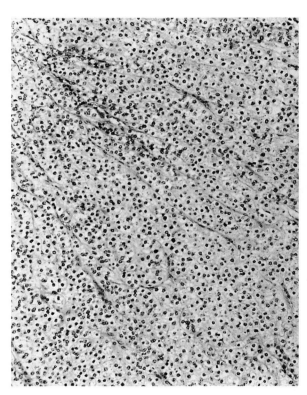

Figure 12-15
STEROID CELL TUMOR
NOT OTHERWISE SPECIFIED
The tumor has a diffuse pattern interrupted by delicate fibrovascular septa.

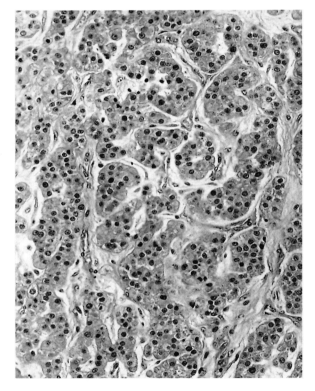

Figure 12-16
STEROID CELL TUMOR
NOT OTHERWISE SPECIFIED
The tumor cells are growing in discrete aggregates and have abundant cytoplasm, which was eosinophilic, and small, uniform nuclei. (Fig. 3 from Young RH, Scully RE. Ovarian steroid cell tumors associated with Cushing's syndrome. A report of three cases. Int J Gynecol Pathol 1987;6:40–8.)

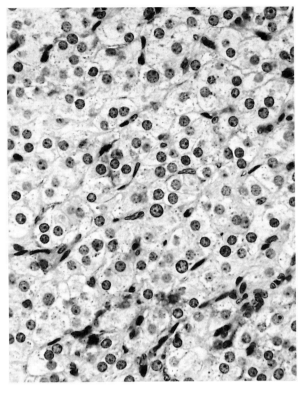

Figure 12-17
STEROID CELL TUMOR
NOT OTHERWISE SPECIFIED
   The tumor cells are round and have uniform nuclei. Nucleoli are prominent in some nuclei.

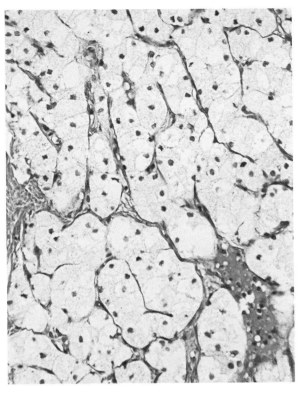

Figure 12-18
STEROID CELL TUMOR
NOT OTHERWISE SPECIFIED
   The tumor cells have abundant pale (lipid-rich) cytoplasm and small nuclei.

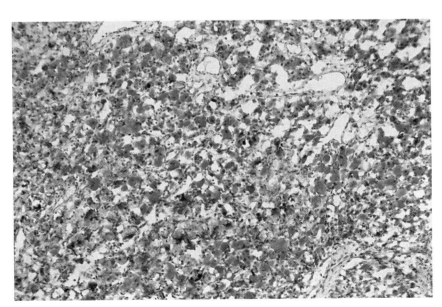

Figure 12-19
STEROID CELL TUMOR
NOT OTHERWISE SPECIFIED
   The tumor cells contain abundant lipid, demonstrated by an oil red-O stain.

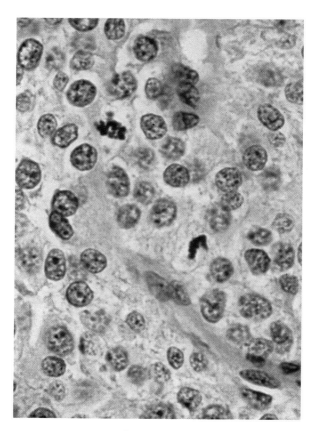

Figure 12-20
STEROID CELL TUMOR NOT OTHERWISE
SPECIFIED, CLINICALLY MALIGNANT
Two atypical mitotic figures are present.

Immunohistochemical staining is positive for α-inhibin, vimentin (75 percent); CAM 5.2 (46 percent) (globoid, paranuclear); AE1/AE3, CK1 (37 percent); epithelial membrane antigen (8 percent); and S-100 protein (7 percent). There is no staining for carcinoembryonic antigen, chromogranin A, alpha-fetoprotein, or HMB-45. These findings occasionally help in the differential diagnosis (25,26,29).

Differential Diagnosis. Stromal luteomas and Leydig cell tumors usually do not pose great diagnostic difficulty for the pathologist because of their characteristic locations and obvious composition of steroid-type cells, which contain crystals of Reinke in the Leydig cell tumor. The extensive space formation in occasional tumors in these categories, however, may simulate a vascular tumor or less often an adenocarcinoma. Awareness of this

degenerative phenomenon and its association with cellular debris, inflammatory cell infiltration, and fibrosis, as well as the finding of typical areas elsewhere in the specimen, particularly at the periphery, facilitate the diagnosis.

Steroid cell tumors in the NOS category vary more widely in appearance than the stromal luteoma and the Leydig cell tumor from both architectural and cytologic viewpoints, and accordingly, cause greater diagnostic difficulty. Many of the tumors in the differential diagnosis are listed in Table 6-1. The presence of characteristic nonluteinized cells in both luteinized granulosa cell tumors and thecomas, as well as the typical cytologic features and patterns of those neoplasms, and the finding of abundant reticulin in thecomas, help in their identification. Recognition of areas with a solid tubular pattern helps distinguish a usually estrogenic, lipid-rich Sertoli cell tumor with a predominant diffuse pattern from a typically androgenic steroid cell tumor. In contrast to steroid cell tumors, the clear cells of clear cell carcinomas and metastatic renal cell carcinomas have glycogen-rich cytoplasm and eccentric nuclei. Also, the presence of other patterns such as tubular, glandular, and papillary, inconsistent with a steroid cell tumor, generally facilitate the differential diagnosis. Oxyphilic clear cell carcinomas, oxyphilic endometrioid carcinomas, hepatoid yolk sac tumors, hepatoid carcinomas, and metastatic hepatocellular carcinoma are all characterized by neoplastic cells with abundant eosinophilic cytoplasm. The first two tumors generally exhibit epithelial patterns, may contain glandular lumens, and are almost always accompanied by more easily recognized patterns. The oxyphilic clear cell carcinoma almost invariably has a component of cells, such as hobnail cells, or patterns, such as tubulocystic, that are not seen in steroid cell tumors. The hepatoid tumors also have epithelial patterns, may contain glandular lumens, and are characterized by immunohistochemical staining for alpha-fetoprotein. We are not aware of any adrenocortical carcinomas that have presented as an ovarian tumor, but the possibility exists; radiologic and other studies might be necessary in such cases to achieve a diagnosis. Amelanotic primary and metastatic melanomas can simulate steroid cell tumors, and melanin granules may be confused with the lipochrome granules of a steroid cell tumor. Melanomas generally have more malignant nuclear features than steroid cell tumors. Special staining, including staining for S-100 protein and HMB-45, may be helpful in difficult cases. An association with other teratomatous elements, the presence of colloid, and immunohistochemical staining for thyroglobulin should distinguish an oxyphilic struma from a steroid cell tumor NOS. The exceptionally rare pituitary-type adenoma in the wall of a dermoid cyst (page 381) might be confused with a steroid cell tumor. Immunohistochemical staining for adrenocorticotropic hormone (ACTH) and other pituitary hormones may be helpful in such cases. Immunohistochemical staining for chromogranin should establish the diagnosis of the very rare primary paraganglioma of the ovary (page 330). Electron microscopic examination of most of the neoplasms that simulate steroid cell tumors should disclose strikingly different features and immunohistochemical staining of steroid cell tumors NOS for α-inhibin should exclude tumors in the differential diagnosis except for those in the sex cord–stromal category (25,29).

Pregnancy luteomas resemble lipid-poor or lipid-free steroid cell tumors grossly and microscopically, and like the latter, are often virilizing. In contrast, however, approximately half of pregnancy luteomas are multiple and approximately one third are bilateral. Mitotic figures may be numerous in pregnancy luteomas but nuclear atypia is absent; in contrast, a steroid cell tumor with brisk mitotic activity is more apt to exhibit significant nuclear atypia. It may be impossible, however, to distinguish a solitary pregnancy luteoma from a lipid-free or lipid-poor steroid cell tumor NOS occurring during pregnancy.

Treatment and Prognosis. The treatment of steroid cell tumors NOS is primarily surgical. Unilateral oophorectomy is indicated in stage Ia cases in young patients because of the low frequency of bilaterality. Chemotherapy has not been effective for high-stage tumors or those that have recurred. Extraovarian spread is present at the time of operation in 20 percent of the cases. In one of the two largest series in the literature, the proportion of tumors that were clinically malignant was 25 percent but the length of patient follow-up is not known (27). In the largest series, 43 percent of the tumors from patients followed for 3 or more years were clinically malignant (22); rare tumors recurred as many as 19 years postoperatively. Patients with clinically malignant tumors were on average 16 years older than those with "probably benign" tumors in one series (22); no malignant tumors have been reported in patients in the first two decades. Most of the patients with Cushing's disease have had extensive intra-abdominal spread of tumor (28).

The best pathologic correlates with malignant behavior in one series that included tumors of all stages were: a diameter of 7 cm or greater (78 percent malignant); 2 or more mitoses per 10 high-power fields (92 percent malignant); necrosis (86 percent malignant); hemorrhage (77 percent malignant); and grade 2 or 3 nuclear atypia (64 percent malignant) (22). Occasional tumors that appear cytologically benign, however, may be clinically malignant. The metastatic tumor is similar to the primary tumor in some cases but is more poorly differentiated in others.

REFERENCES

General Reference

1. Young RH, Scully RE. Sex cord-stromal, steroid cell and other ovarian tumors with endocrine, paraendocrine and paraneoplastic manifestations. In: Kurman RJ, ed. Blaustein's pathology of the female genital tract, 4th ed. New York: Springer-Verlag, 1994:783–847.

Stromal Luteoma

2. Givens JR, Kerber IJ, Wiser WL, Anderson RW, Coleman SA, Fish SA. Remission of acanthosis nigricans associated with polycystic ovarian disease and a stromal luteoma. J Clin Endocrinol Metab 1974;38:347–55.
3. Hayes MC, Scully RE. Stromal luteoma of the ovary: a clinicopathological analysis of 25 cases. Int J Gynecol Pathol 1987;6:313–21.
4. Scully RE. Stromal luteoma of the ovary. A distinctive type of lipoid-cell tumor. Cancer 1964;17:769–78.
5. Sternberg WH, Roth LM. Ovarian stromal tumors containing Leydig cells. I. Stromal-Leydig cell tumors and non-neoplastic transformation of ovarian stroma to Leydig cells. Cancer 1973;32:940–51.
6. Symonds DA, Driscoll SG. An adrenal cortical rest within the fetal ovary: report of a case. Am J Clin Pathol 1973;60:562–4.

Leydig Cell Tumors

7. Baramki TA, Leddy AL, Woodruff JD. Bilateral hilus cell tumors of the ovary. Obstet Gynecol 1983;62:128–31.
8. Boivin Y, Richart RM. Hilus cell tumors of the ovary. A review with a report of 3 new cases. Cancer 1965;18:231–40.
9. Echt CR, Hadd HE. Androgen excretion patterns in a patient with metastatic hilus cell tumor of the ovary. Am J Obstet Gynecol 1968;100:1055–61.
10. Ichinohasama R, Teshima S, Kishi K, et al. Leydig cell tumor of the ovary associated with endometrial carcinoma and containing 17 beta-hydroxysteroid dehydrogenase. Int J Gynecol Pathol 1989;8:64–71.
11. Paraskevas M, Scully RE. Hilus cell tumor of the ovary. A clinico-pathological analysis of 12 Reinke crystal-positive and 9 crystal-negative cases. Int J Gynecol Pathol 1989;8:299–310.
12. Roth LM, Sternberg WH. Ovarian stromal tumors containing Leydig cells. II. Pure Leydig cell tumor, non-hilar type. Cancer 1973;32:952–60.
13. Salm R. Ovarian hilus-cell tumours: their varying presentations. J Pathol 1974;113:117–27.
14. Salm R. Pure and mixed hilus cell tumours of ovary. Ann Roy Coll Surg Engl 1967;41:344–63.
15. Schnoy N. Ultrastructure of a virilizing ovarian Leydig-cell tumor. Hilar cell tumor. Virchows Arch [A] 1982;397:17–27.
16. Sternberg WH. The morphology, endocrine function, hyperplasia and tumors of the human ovarian hilus cells. Am J Pathol 1949;25:493–511.
17. Sternberg WH, Roth LM. Ovarian stromal tumors containing Leydig cells. I. Stromal-Leydig cell tumors and non-neoplastic transformation of ovarian stroma to Leydig cells. Cancer 1973;32:940–51.

Steroid Cell Tumors, Not Otherwise Specified

18. Adeyemi SD, Grange AO, Giwa-Osagie OF, et al. Adrenal rest tumour of the ovary associated with isosexual precocious pseudopuberty and cushingoid features. Eur J Pediatr 1986;145:236–8.
19. Campbell PE, Danks DM. Pseudoprecocity in an infant due to a luteoma of the ovary. Arch Dis Child 1963;38:519–23.
20. Davidson BJ, Waisman J, Judd HL. Long-standing virilism in a woman with hyperplasia and neoplasia of ovarian lipidic cells. Obstet Gynecol 1981;58:753–9.
21. Donovan JT, Otis CN, Powell JL, Cathcart HK. Cushing's syndrome secondary to malignant lipoid cell tumor of the ovary. Gynecol Oncol 1993;50:249–53.
22. Hayes MC, Scully RE. Ovarian steroid cell tumor (not otherwise specified): a clinicopathological analysis of 63 cases. Am J Surg Pathol 1987;11:835–45.
23. Kulkarni JN, Mistry RC, Kamat MR, Chinoy R, Lotlikar RG. Autonomous aldosterone-secreting ovarian tumor. Gynecol Oncol 1990;37:284–9.
24. Marieb HJ, Spangler S, Kashgarian M, Heiman A, Schwartz ML, Schwartz PE. Cushing's syndrome secondary to ectopic cortisol production by an ovarian carcinoma. J Clin Endocrinol Metab 1983; 57:737–40.
25. Rishi M, Howard LN, Bratthauer GL, Tavassoli FA. Use of monoclonal antibody against human inhibin as a marker for sex cord-stromal tumors of the ovary. Am J Surg Pathol 1997;21:583–9.
26. Seidman JD, Abbondanzo SL, Bratthauer GL. Lipid cell (steroid cell) tumor of the ovary: immunophenotype with analysis of potential pitfalls due to endogenous biotin-like activity. Int J Gynecol Pathol 1995;14:331–8.
27. Taylor HB, Norris HJ. Lipid cell tumors of the ovary. Cancer 1967;20:1953–62.
28. Young RH, Scully RE. Ovarian steroid cell tumors associated with Cushing's syndrome. A report of three cases. Int J Gynecol Pathol 1987;6:40–8.
29. Zheng W, Sung CJ, Hanna I, et al. α and β subunits of inhibin/activin as sex cord-stromal differential markers. Int J Gynecol Pathol 1997;16:263–71.

13

GERM CELL TUMORS:
GENERAL FEATURES AND PRIMITIVE FORMS

GENERAL FEATURES

Germ cell tumors account for approximately 30 percent of primary ovarian tumors (2); in one North American study, however, the figure was a surprisingly high 58 percent (3). Over 95 percent of these tumors are dermoid cysts (mature cystic teratomas) and most of the remaining germ cell tumors are malignant (2,3). Dermoid cysts account for 35 to 58 percent of benign ovarian neoplasms, and malignant germ cell tumors for 1 to 3 percent of all ovarian cancers in western countries. The latter figures, however, have been reported to be 9 to 14 percent in blacks (1,11) and approximately 20 percent in Japanese (7,9) populations in which surface epithelial cancers are lower in frequency. In patients under the age of 21 years, approximately 60 percent of ovarian tumors are of germ cell type, and as many as one third of germ cell tumors are malignant, accounting for two thirds of ovarian cancers in the first two decades (5,8). Shulman et al. (10) found that first-degree and second-degree relatives of patients with ovarian germ cell cancers do not have an increased risk for similar tumors. Mandel et al. (6), however, reported a familial clustering of germ cell tumors, and one member of the family had histiocytosis X.

Most malignant germ cell tumors occur in pure form, but in 10 percent of the cases two or more types are combined within the same specimen. It is essential, therefore, to examine carefully and sample judiciously each germ cell cancer. In general, examination of one microscopic section for every centimeter in diameter of the tumor is appropriate, with modification according to the degree of heterogeneity of the neoplastic tissue. The prognosis of patients with a mixed germ cell tumor generally reflects that of its most malignant element, but according to some investigators (4) a minor component of a highly malignant element affects the prognosis less adversely than a major component. The more common malignant germ cell tumors are composed of primitive or immature elements, and occur predominantly in the first three decades of life. Less frequent are malignant tumors of adult types, which almost always develop in dermoid cysts and are usually encountered in older women.

DYSGERMINOMA

Definition. This is a primitive germ cell tumor composed of large, rounded cells with typically clear cytoplasm that resemble primordial germ cells. The dysgerminoma is indistinguishable from the testicular seminoma and extragonadal germinomas.

General Features. Dysgerminomas are the most common of the malignant primitive germ cell tumors. They account for nearly half of the latter, for 1 percent of all ovarian cancers, for 5 to 10 percent of ovarian cancers in patients in the first two decades, and for 20 to 30 percent of ovarian cancers encountered during pregnancy. The proportion of dysgerminomas among all ovarian cancers is higher in Japan (5 to 13 percent) than in Western countries partly because of a much lower prevalence of other types of ovarian cancer in that country. Rare dysgerminomas arise in phenotypic females with gonadal dysgenesis, and in most such cases, they arise from gonadoblastomas (see chapters 16 and 21). Most commonly the patients have 46,XY pure gonadal dysgenesis or mixed gonadal dysgenesis, which is typically associated with 45,X/46,XY mosaicism. Seminomas masquerading as dysgerminomas also arise in the testes of phenotypic females with the androgen insensitivity syndrome (testicular feminization) and a 46,XY karyotype (page 401). Rare dysgerminomas have been associated with ataxia-telangiectasia (page 389).

Approximately 80 percent of dysgerminomas occur in patients in the second and third decades (24); the mean and median patient ages in most large series are the late teens or early 20s (15–17,29). Five percent occur before the age of 10 years; the tumors are rare in patients under 5 years and over 50 years of age. Most of the patients present with signs or symptoms related to an abdominal mass. In patients with an associated

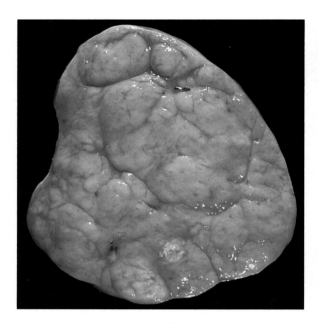

Figure 13-1
DYSGERMINOMA
The sectioned surface is solid, fleshy, and lobulated. (Fig. 86 from Young RH, Clement PB, Scully RE. Pathology of the ovary. In: Sternberg SS, ed. Diagnostic surgical pathology, Vol 2, 1st, ed. New York: Raven Press, 1989:1704.)

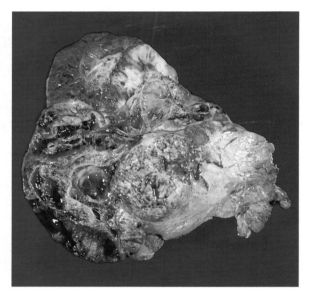

Figure 13-2
DYSGERMINOMA
The sectioned surface exhibits extensive hemorrhage and necrosis, and occasional cysts.

gonadoblastoma, an underlying abnormality in gonadal development may dominate the clinical presentation. Elevated serum levels of chorionic gonadotropin (hCG) occur in approximately 3 percent of patients with dysgerminomas (43), and usually result in hormonal manifestations, which are typically estrogenic (isosexual precocity, menstrual irregularities), but occasionally androgenic. The clinical picture may mimic that of an ectopic or intrauterine pregnancy or a hydatidiform mole (43).

Up to 95 percent of patients with dysgerminoma have an elevated serum level of lactic dehydrogenase (usually isoenzymes 1 and 2) at presentation, with the level varying with the size and stage of the tumor (18,22,25,36,39). Determination of this marker may also be useful in detecting recurrent tumor and monitoring response to therapy (36). Serum levels of alkaline phosphatase (18), neuron-specific enolase (26), and CA125 (12,25) have also been elevated in some patients. The serum alpha-fetoprotein (AFP) level is almost always normal; two of 17 apparently pure dysgerminomas, however, were associated with elevated levels of this marker (250 to 300 ng/ml) in one study (25).

About 65 percent of dysgerminomas are stage Ia (15,41). In higher stage tumors, the contralateral ovary, pelvic and para-aortic lymph nodes, peritoneum, or combinations thereof, are typically involved. Distant spread is occasionally evident at the time of presentation.

Gross Findings. Dysgerminomas are typically solid, with a median diameter of 15 cm. Their external surfaces are smooth or bosselated. The sectioned surfaces are typically soft, fleshy, and lobulated, and may be cream-colored, gray, pink, or tan (fig. 13-1). Areas of cystic degeneration, necrosis, and hemorrhage may be present (figs. 13-1, 13-2), and should be sampled microscopically to exclude other germ cell elements. Calcification suggests an underlying gonadoblastoma. The tumor is grossly bilateral in about 10 percent of the cases; in another 10 percent microscopic foci of tumor are present in a grossly normal-appearing contralateral ovary.

Microscopic Findings. The tumor is composed of uniform cells resembling primordial germ cells in diffuse, insular, trabecular, and cord-like patterns (figs. 13-3, 13-4). Rarely, the tumor cells line irregular or rounded gland-like spaces (fig. 13-5) or form solid tubular structures (fig. 13-6). In appropriately fixed specimens, the uniform,

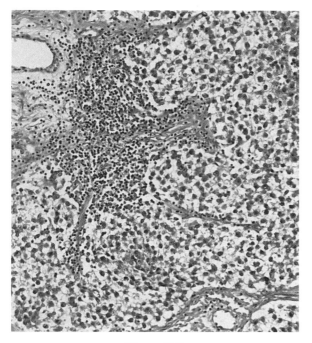

Figure 13-3
DYSGERMINOMA
The stroma contains numerous lymphocytes.

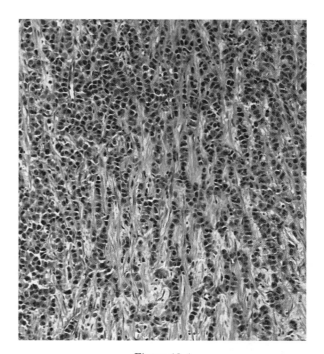

Figure 13-4
DYSGERMINOMA
The tumor cells are arranged in cords.

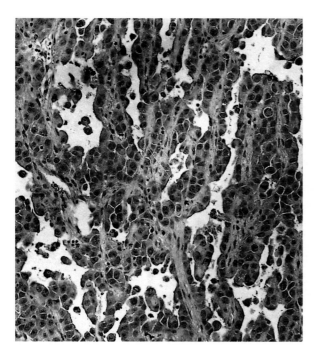

Figure 13-5
DYSGERMINOMA
Irregular spaces result in a pseudoglandular pattern.

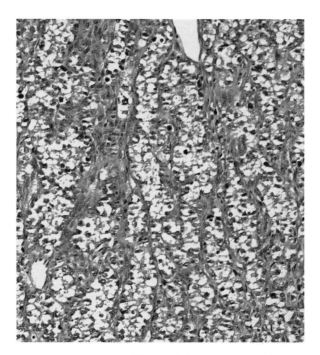

Figure 13-6
DYSGERMINOMA
A solid tubular pattern simulates that of a Sertoli cell tumor.

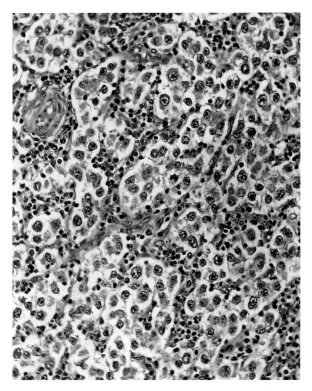

Figure 13-7
DYSGERMINOMA
The tumor cells have clear cytoplasm and large rounded nuclei with a prominent nucleolus. The stroma contains lymphocytes.

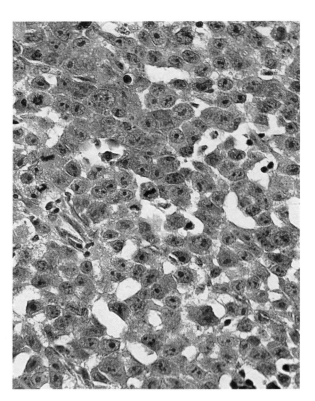

Figure 13-8
DYSGERMINOMA
The tumor cells have dense cytoplasm.

rounded tumor cells typically have clear cytoplasm, which is almost always glycogen-rich (fig. 13-7). Occasionally, however, the cytoplasm is dense and homogeneous (fig. 13-8). The tumor cells have discrete cell membranes, and a central, large, rounded or flattened nucleus, which contains coarsely clumped chromatin and one or several prominent nucleoli (fig. 13-7). Mitotic figures are usually numerous. The characteristic stroma consists of thin to broad fibrous bands that almost invariably contain mature lymphocytes (figs. 13-3, 13-7) which occasionally form lymphoid follicles. Most of the lymphoid cells are T lymphocytes (40). Areas of caseation-like necrosis of the neoplastic cells are frequent. Sarcoid-like granulomas are present in 20 percent of the cases, and rarely are sufficiently numerous to obscure the underlying tumor cells (fig. 13-9). A similar granulomatous response can be found in lymph nodes containing metastatic dysgerminoma.

Approximately 3 percent of dysgerminomas contain syncytiotrophoblastic giant cells (SGCs) (fig. 13-10), which are immunoreactive for hCG; the serum level of hCG is frequently elevated in such cases (43). The SGCs may be intimately associated with blood-filled sinusoids, but the characteristic biphasic growth pattern of choriocarcinoma, characterized by the additional presence of cytotrophoblast, is absent. Extensive sampling of tumors associated with hCG production is important to exclude foci of choriocarcinoma or embryonal carcinoma, the presence of which, in contrast to that of SGCs alone, warrants a diagnosis of mixed germ cell tumor. Rare pure dysgerminomas associated with an elevated hCG level contain no demonstrable SGCs.

Luteinized stromal cells, which may be admixed with the neoplastic cells or at the periphery of the tumor (37), are occasionally present, especially when the tumor is producing hCG; the luteinized stromal cells may be the source of the

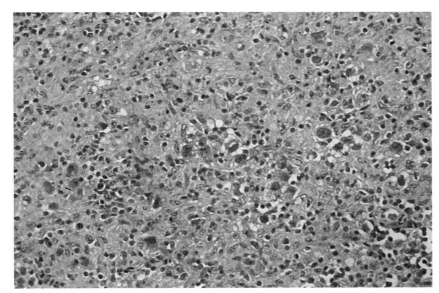

Figure 13-9
DYSGERMINOMA
A diffuse granulomatous reaction isolates scattered neoplastic cells.

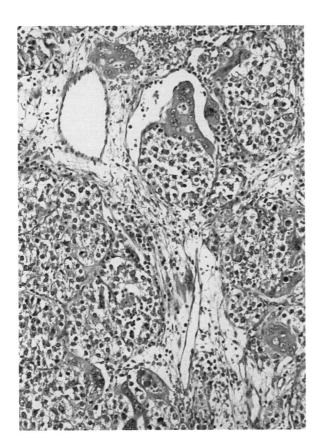

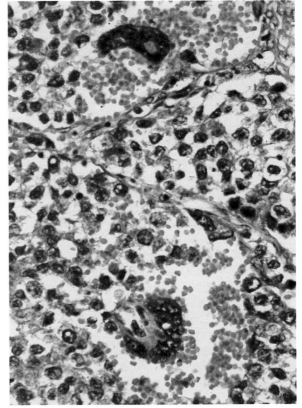

Figure 13-10
DYSGERMINOMA
Left and right: Syncytiotrophoblastic giant cells are admixed with the dysgerminoma cells. (Left figure is Fig. 91 from Young RH, Clement PB, Scully RE. Pathology of the ovary. In: Sternberg SS, ed. Diagnostic surgical pathology, Vol 2, 2nd, ed. New York: Raven Press, 1994:2245.)

excessive estrogens or androgens found in some cases (see chapter 19). The presence of focal calcification, which suggests that a gonadoblastoma may have been obliterated by the tumor, warrants additional sampling to identify residual gonadoblastoma.

Dysgerminoma cells are typically immunoreactive for placental-like alkaline phosphatase (14,30,33), vimentin (30,31), and in at least some cases, lactic dehydrogenase, neuron-specific enolase, Leu-7, cytokeratin, desmin, and glial fibrillary acidic protein (18–20,26,27,30,33). The tumor cells were invariably negative for epithelial membrane antigen and carcinoembryonic antigen in one study (33). Bailey et al. (13) have developed a monoclonal antibody (M2A, IgG2a) that they claim is specific for dysgerminomas (and seminomas). Dietl et al. (19) have shown frequent overexpression of p53 in dysgerminomas, and Tsuura et al. (42) have found c-kit localization in 92 percent of dysgerminomas (and seminomas). SGCs are typically immunoreactive for hCG (43) and cytokeratin. In the rare cases of hCG-secreting dysgerminomas in which SGCs are not identified, the cytoplasm of the dysgerminoma cells may be hCG positive (18,32).

Differential Diagnosis. Dysgerminomas should be distinguished from other malignant germ cell tumors in which a diffuse pattern may occur, specifically, yolk sac tumor with a solid pattern and embryonal carcinoma. The solid yolk sac tumor is distinguished by its greater nuclear variation, hyaline bodies, an absence or sparsity of lymphocytes in the stroma, immunoreactivity for AFP, and in almost all cases, other characteristic patterns that are absent in dysgerminomas. The rare embryonal carcinoma is composed typically of larger cells with larger nuclei that are more hyperchromatic and variable than those of the dysgerminoma. Moreover, embryonal carcinomas lack a lymphocytic stroma and almost always contain syncytiotrophoblastic giant cells (SGCs). Embryonal carcinomas are cytokeratin positive, whereas seminomas are only occasionally positive, and in such cases are typically only focally positive. Use of the BER-H2 antibody facilitates the distinction of testicular embryonal carcinomas from seminomas (21), but no comparative studies have been performed on the ovarian counterparts of these tumors. In one investigation, seven of eight testicular embryo-

nal carcinomas were positive with BER-H2, but 19 of 19 seminomas were negative (21).

The clear cell carcinoma with an exclusively diffuse pattern may resemble a dysgerminoma; this differential is discussed on page 148. Large cell lymphomas may simulate dysgerminomas both grossly and microscopically, and the frequent sprinkling of lymphocytes in the stroma of the latter enhances their microscopic similarity. The differing features of the nuclei of the two tumors, the almost invariable absence of glycogen in lymphomas, and a variety of distinctive immunohistochemical reactions (placental-like alkaline phosphatase positivity in dysgerminomas and leukocyte common antigen positivity in lymphomas) facilitate the differential diagnosis. Other cellular tumors with solid growth patterns of round cells, such as the granulosa cell tumor and primary or metastatic poorly differentiated carcinoma, are occasionally confused with dysgerminoma, but lack its distinctive microscopic features. Rare dysgerminomas with pseudoglandular and solid tubular patterns have been confused with Sertoli cell tumors, but the latter lack the distinctive nuclear features, the lymphocytic stroma, and the immunohistochemical findings of the dysgerminoma.

Treatment. In young patients with stage IA dysgerminoma in whom preservation of reproductive function is important, unilateral salpingo-oophorectomy with close clinical, radiologic, and serologic follow-up, is the treatment recommended by most investigators (23,24,28, 38,41). With this approach, chemotherapy is reserved for the treatment of recurrent disease, which occurs in approximately 20 percent of adequately staged patients. In young patients with higher stage disease, unilateral salpingo-oophorectomy followed by combination chemotherapy may be curative and spare contralateral ovarian function (38,41). In patients in whom preservation of fertility is not a factor, a hysterectomy with bilateral salpingo-oophorectomy, followed by chemotherapy is recommended for higher stage tumors (38,41). Radiation therapy is now generally reserved for the rare patients in whom chemotherapy fails. In cases in which conservative therapy is chosen, the contralateral ovary should be carefully evaluated. Bivalving or biopsy is recommended by some investigators, but each of these procedures is best avoided in a young woman with a normal-appearing ovary because it increases the risk of subsequent infertility. A small number of patients with minor involvement of the contralateral ovary have been successfully treated with unilateral salpingo-oophorectomy and chemotherapy, with preservation of fertility, suggesting that bilateral oophorectomy may not be essential in such cases (38).

Prognosis. Patients with dysgerminomas have an excellent prognosis; the most important and probably only prognostic factor is stage. The 5-year survival rate approaches 100 percent for patients with stage I tumor, and 80 to 90 percent for those with higher stage or recurrent tumor (15,17,24,29,41). A tumor diameter exceeding 10 cm has been considered an adverse prognostic factor in some (28), but not all studies (24), and a large tumor size without evidence of spread should not be a deterrent to conservative therapy in a young patient (41). Although the term "anaplastic dysgerminoma" has been applied to tumors with a high mitotic rate, there is no evidence that such tumors are associated with a worse prognosis, and use of this designation is not recommended. Two studies have found that most dysgerminomas are not diploid, and ploidy is not useful in predicting survival (34,35).

YOLK SAC TUMOR

Definition. The yolk sac tumor (also referred to as *endodermal sinus tumor)* is a primitive malignant germ cell tumor characterized by a variety of distinctive microscopic patterns, some of which recapitulate phases in the development of the normal yolk sac (66–71,79,82). Enteric and hepatic differentiation in some yolk sac tumors is consistent with origin of the primitive gut and its derivatives from the secondary yolk sac during embryogenesis (64,72,83).

General Features. In 1946, Teilum (81) recognized that one of the two types of ovarian tumor reported 7 years earlier by Schiller (76) under the designation "mesonephroma" was of germ cell origin. In 1959, Teilum (82) proposed the designation "endodermal sinus tumor" for this tumor because of the frequent presence of distinctive papillary structures resembling the yolk sac–derived endodermal sinuses of the rodent placenta. Subsequently, the microscopic spectrum of these neoplasms has expanded, jus-

tifying the more generic term, yolk sac tumor, for all the microscopic subtypes. Yolk sac tumors account for approximately 20 percent of primitive germ cell tumors, and are almost as common as dysgerminomas in the first two decades. A few yolk sac tumors have occurred in intimate association with an endometrioid or mucinous ovarian tumor (60,68a,73) indicating a somatic cell rather than germ cell origin in such cases.

Yolk sac tumors are most common in patients in the second and third decades; the median age is between 16 and 19 years (51,54,58,59). Approximately 10 percent of these tumors occur in the first decade (58,59). Although they are rare over the age of 40 years, exceptional examples have been reported in elderly women (57,60). Occasional yolk sac tumors have arisen in patients with gonadal dysgenesis (44,59,72). Patients usually present with abdominal pain, frequently of sudden onset, and a large abdominal or pelvic mass. Some women have been pregnant at presentation (49). Almost all the patients have an elevated serum level of AFP preoperatively, and this finding in a young female with an adnexal mass, although not specific, suggests the diagnosis of yolk sac tumor, especially if the level is greater than 1000 ng/ml (53,55). Nonspecific markers that may be found in the sera of patients with yolk sac tumors include CA125 and carcinoembryonic antigen, which were elevated in 100 percent and 10 percent of the patients, respectively, in one study (55). At laparotomy, there is evidence of spread of tumor to the peritoneum, retroperitoneal lymph nodes, or both, in 30 to 70 percent of the cases (51,54,58,59); the figure of 30 percent is from an older study (58) and probably reflects incomplete staging. Rare patients have distant metastases at presentation.

Gross Findings. The tumors are typically large, with a median diameter of 15 cm (58). The external surface is usually smooth and glistening although 25 percent have capsular tears due to preoperative or intraoperative rupture (58). The sectioned surfaces are typically solid and cystic and composed of soft, friable, yellow to gray tissue (fig. 13-11); rare tumors are entirely cystic (44). Extensive areas of hemorrhage and necrosis are common. A honeycomb appearance due to many small cysts may indicate the presence of a polyvesicular-vitelline component (fig. 13-12). Gross evidence of other germ cell elements, most

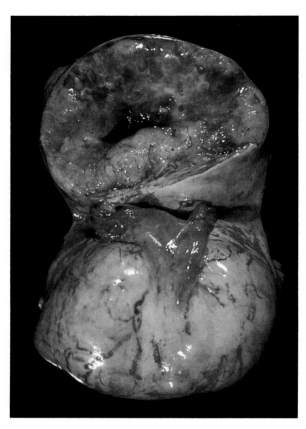

Figure 13-11
YOLK SAC TUMOR
The tumor has a predominantly solid and fleshy sectioned surface, with areas of necrosis, gelatinous degeneration, and cyst formation. (Fig. 15 from Scully RE. Recent progress in ovarian cancer. Human Pathol 1970;1:73–98.)

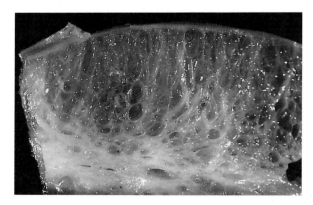

Figure 13-12
YOLK SAC TUMOR,
POLYVESICULAR-VITELLINE VARIANT
The sectioned surface has a honeycomb or microcystic appearance.

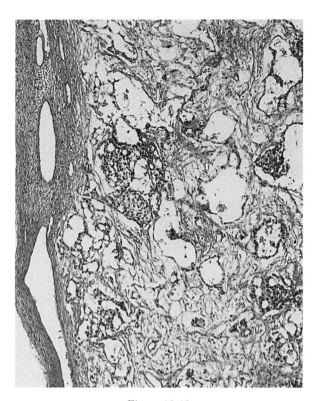

Figure 13-13
YOLK SAC TUMOR
A loose stroma separates reticular foci, solid nests, and small cysts.

commonly a dermoid cyst, is seen in 15 percent of the cases (58). Yolk sac tumors are virtually never bilateral unless the opposite ovary is involved as part of generalized peritoneal spread, but another tumor, almost always a dermoid cyst, is present in the contralateral ovary in 5 percent of the cases (58).

Microscopic Findings. Yolk sac tumors exhibit a wide variety of microscopic patterns (figs. 13-13–13-30), but most tumors have, at least focally, a reticular pattern. It is characterized by a loose meshwork of communicating spaces (figs. 13-13, 13-14, 13-16) lined by primitive tumor cells with cytoplasm that is typically clear, containing glycogen and occasionally, lipid. The hyperchromatic, irregular, large nuclei have prominent nucleoli; mitotic figures are usually numerous. Reticular areas frequently merge with microcystic or macrocystic areas.

The presence of Schiller-Duval bodies is a characteristic feature of yolk sac tumors. These

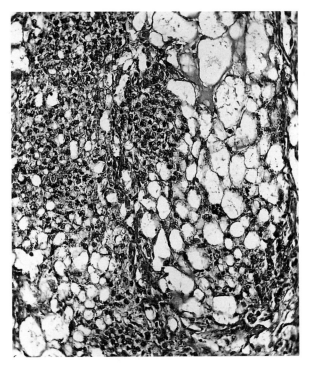

Figure 13-14
YOLK SAC TUMOR
Solid areas merge with areas showing a microcystic pattern. (Fig. 3 from Kurman RJ, Norris HJ. Endodermal sinus tumor of the ovary. A clinical and pathologic analysis of 71 cases. Cancer 1976;38:2404–19.)

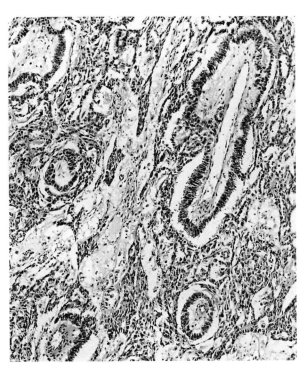

Figure 13-15
YOLK SAC TUMOR
Schiller-Duval bodies are seen in both cross and longitudinal sections. (Fig. 36 from Serov SF, Scully RE, Sobin LH. Histological typing of ovarian tumours. International Histological Classification of Tumours No. 9. Geneva: World Health Organization, 1973.)

structures are typically found within reticular areas. Although they have been reported in up to 75 percent of the cases (58), they are less common in our experience. They consist of single papillae that are rounded or elongated depending on the plane of section, with fibrovascular cores containing single vessels (figs. 13-15, 13-16). Primitive columnar cells cover the papillae, which occupy spaces lined by cuboidal, flat, or hobnail cells. Schiller-Duval bodies are usually sparsely distributed, but when numerous and closely packed create a distinctive papillary pattern (fig. 13-15). Variably sized, brightly eosinophilic, periodic acid–Schiff (PAS)-positive, diastase-resistant, intracellular hyaline bodies are present in most yolk sac tumors (fig. 13-17), and are most numerous in areas with a reticular or hepatoid pattern. Their immunohistochemical profile is discussed on page 254.

Three histologic variants of yolk sac tumor are recognized: polyvesicular-vitelline, hepatoid,

and glandular. When one or another of these patterns is prominent or occurs in pure form, a diagnosis of that specific variant is warranted. The polyvesicular-vitelline pattern is characterized by the presence of cysts lined by columnar, cuboidal, or flattened cells and usually separated by a dense spindle cell stroma (figs. 13-18, 13-19) (69). The vesicles may exhibit eccentric constrictions (fig. 13-19) simulating subdivision of the primary yolk sac vesicle to form a generally smaller component lined by taller epithelium, corresponding to the forerunner of the primitive gut in normal embryogenesis.

Minor foci of hepatoid differentiation are encountered in 16 to 48 percent of yolk sac tumors (64,72,83), but tumors with predominant hepatoid differentiation are rare (72,80). These tumors are characterized by the presence of large polygonal cells with prominent cell borders, abundant eosinophilic cytoplasm, and round central nuclei with prominent single nucleoli, growing in compact

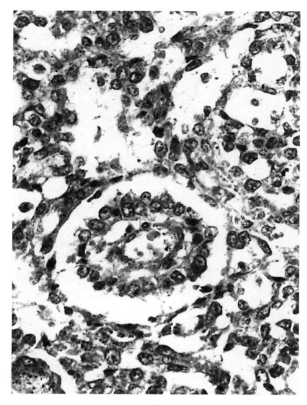

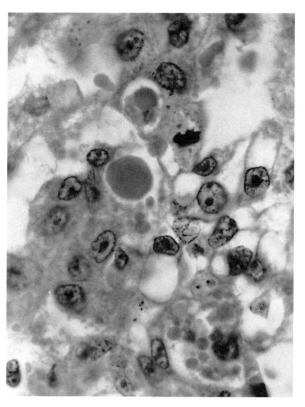

Figure 13-16
YOLK SAC TUMOR

A Schiller-Duval body containing a central blood vessel is surrounded by tumor with a reticular pattern. (Fig. 3 from Scully RE. Germ cell tumors of the ovary and fallopian tube. In: Meigs JV, Sturgis S, eds. Progress in gynecology, 1963;4:335–47.)

Figure 13-17
YOLK SAC TUMOR

Hyaline bodies, malignant nuclear features, and a mitotic figure are evident. (Fig. 93 from Serov SF, Scully RE, Sobin LH. Histological typing of ovarian tumours. International Histological Classification of Tumours No. 9. Geneva: World Health Organization, 1973.)

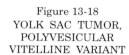

Figure 13-18
YOLK SAC TUMOR,
POLYVESICULAR
VITELLINE VARIANT

Large vesicles lie in a cellular stroma. (Fig. 91 from Serov SF, Scully RE, Sobin LH.Histological typing of ovarian tumours. International Histological Classification of Tumours No. 9. Geneva: World Health Organization, 1973.)

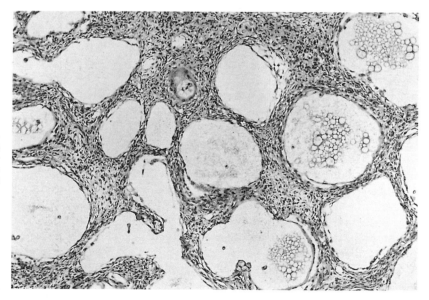

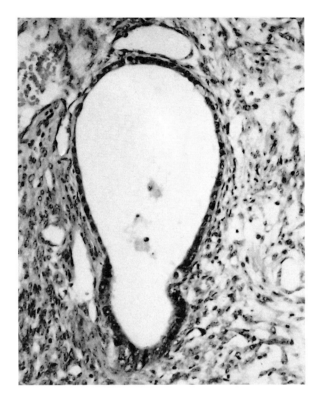

Figure 13-19
YOLK SAC TUMOR,
POLYVESICULAR-VITELLINE VARIANT
Secondary yolk sac vesicle lined by columnar epithelium (bottom) is continuous with primary yolk sac vesicle lined by flat epithelium (top). (Fig. 92 from Serov SF, Scully RE, Sobin LH. Histological typing of ovarian tumours. International Histological Classification of Tumours No. 9. Geneva: World Health Organization, 1973.)

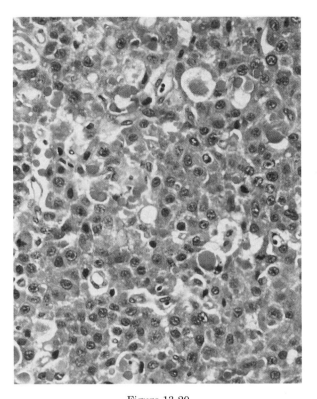

Figure 13-20
YOLK SAC TUMOR, HEPATOID VARIANT
The polygonal tumor cells have eosinophilic cytoplasm and contain hyaline bodies.

masses separated by thin fibrous bands, resembling hepatocellular carcinoma. Hyaline bodies are often numerous (fig. 13-20) (72); stainable bile has not been identified. In some cases, an admixed cribriform or glandular pattern of "intestinal" type (see below) is present.

Glands of endodermal derivation may be present in up to 54 percent of yolk sac tumors, usually sparsely distributed within reticular and polyvesicular-vitelline areas (51,58,83). The glands are lined by simple or pseudostratified columnar epithelium, which may contain subnuclear vacuoles or resemble more mature enteric epithelium, with argyrophil, goblet, and rarely, Paneth cells. Similar glands have been observed in normal human yolk sacs (68). Rare yolk sac tumors have a predominant glandular pattern, of which two types have been reported: the intestinal variant (45,56),

composed predominantly of large nests of primitive epithelial cells with a cribriform pattern (fig. 13-21) and the endometrioid-like variant in which glandular or villoglandular differentiation predominates, typically mimicking endometrioid adenocarcinoma (figs. 13-22–13-25) (44). The presence of subnuclear vacuoles, supranuclear vacuoles, or both, in the glands of some endometrioid-like tumors creates an appearance similar to that of a secretory endometrioid carcinoma (fig. 13-23), and nests of hepatoid cells within the gland lumens may mimic the squamous morules of an endometrioid carcinoma with squamous differentiation (fig. 13-25). One endometrioid yolk sac tumor had an additional component of mucinous adenocarcinoma with goblet cells and foci of carcinoid tumor (48). An abundant fibrous stroma in endometrioid-like yolk sac tumors may result in an adenofibromatous appearance, while in other cases a densely cellular stroma with mitotically active spindle cells may cause confusion with a

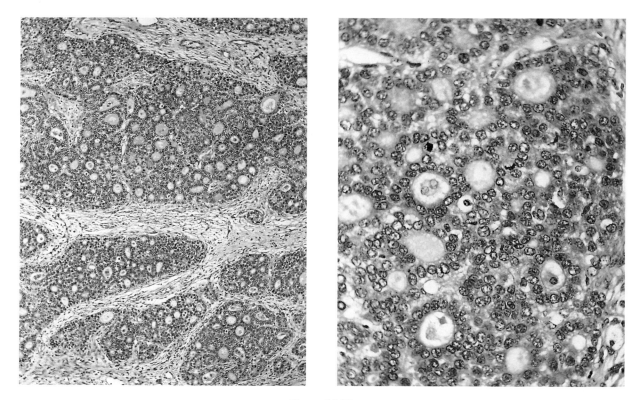

Figure 13-21
YOLK SAC TUMOR, GLANDULAR VARIANT, INTESTINAL TYPE
Left: A cribriform pattern is evident.
Right: A cribriform pattern and malignant-appearing nuclei with occasional mitotic figures are evident. (Figs. 17-6 and 17-7 respectively, from Young RH, Scully RE. Unusual patterns, subtypes, and differential diagnosis of gonadal yolk sac tumors. In: Nogales FF, ed. The human yolk sac and yolk sac tumors. Heidelberg: Springer-Verlag, 1993:309–42.)

Figure 13-22
YOLK SAC TUMOR,
ENDOMETRIOID-LIKE
GLANDULAR VARIANT
The tumor has a villoglandular pattern.

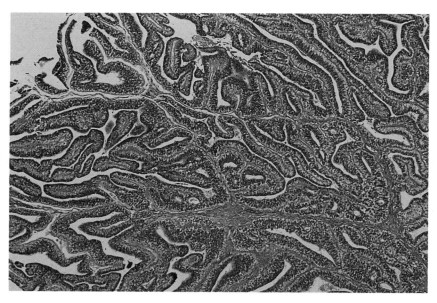

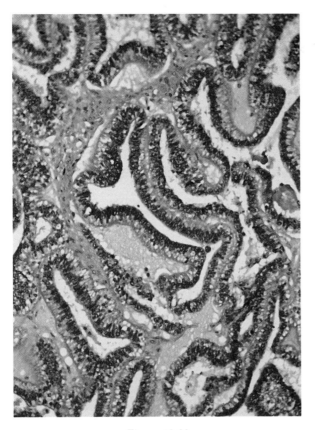

Figure 13-23
YOLK SAC TUMOR,
ENDOMETRIOID-LIKE GLANDULAR VARIANT
The glands are lined by stratified epithelium with sub-nuclear vacuoles.

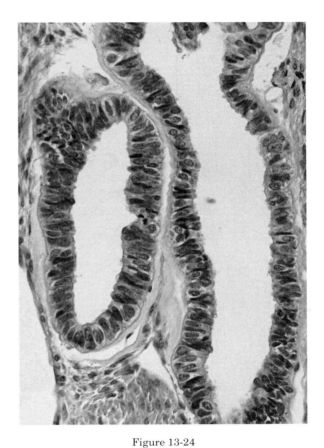

Figure 13-24
YOLK SAC TUMOR, ENDOMETRIOID-LIKE
GLANDULAR VARIANT
The endometrioid-like glands are lined by columnar cells with relatively bland nuclear features, simulating a grade 1 endometrioid adenocarcinoma.

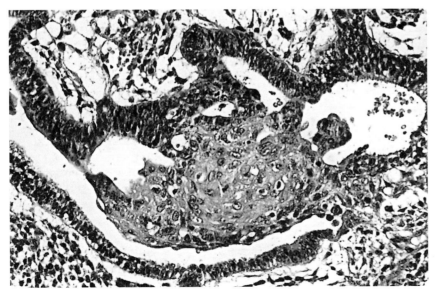

Figure 13-25
YOLK SAC TUMOR,
ENDOMETRIOID-LIKE
GLANDULAR VARIANT
A solid focus of cells representing hepatoid differentiation within a gland lumen resembles a squamous morule. (Fig. 17-14 from Young RH, Scully RE. Unusual patterns, subtypes, and differential diagnosis of gonadal yolk sac tumors. In: Nogales FF, ed. The human yolk sac and yolk sac tumors. Heidelberg: Springer-Verlag, 1993:309–42.)

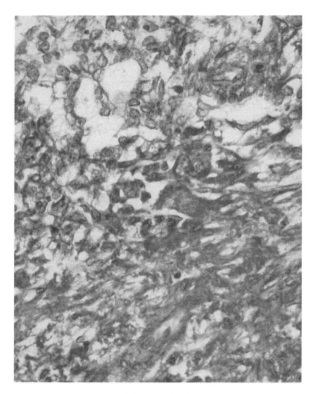

Figure 13-26
YOLK SAC TUMOR, PARIETAL PATTERN
Abundant basement membrane material is visible. (Periodic acid–Schiff stain)

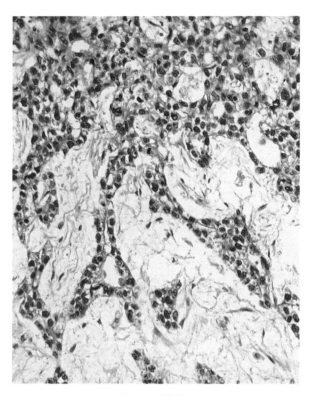

Figure 13-27
YOLK SAC TUMOR
The neoplastic cells are separated by a myxoid stroma.

carcinosarcoma (44). A third subtype of glandular yolk sac tumor is composed of small, rounded, nonspecific-appearing glands surrounded by a prominent fibromatous stroma, simulating a malignant adenofibroma.

Ulbright et al. (83) described "parietal" differentiation in the form of small, typically linear, extracellular accumulations of basement membrane material (fig. 13-26), usually within reticular and solid areas, in over 90 percent of yolk sac tumors. Parietal yolk sac differentiation is consistent with the observation that the parietal cells in the rat yolk sac synthesize a thick, eosinophilic basement membrane (Reichert's membrane). A parietal pattern may be the predominant feature of a recurrent yolk sac tumor even though it was not identified in the primary neoplasm (47). In such cases, the recurrence may not be associated with an elevated serum AFP level.

Teilum (82) described a loose stromal component of yolk sac tumors that he believed recapit-

ulated the appearance of extraembryonic mesenchyme (magma reticulare), and in occasional tumors, a myxoid or myxomatous pattern may be striking (fig. 13-27) (52). Michael and colleagues (61) described a "mesenchyme-like" component in yolk sac tumors consisting of a myxoid or collagenous stroma containing stellate or spindle-shaped cells and thin-walled blood vessels, and occasionally, skeletal muscle and cartilage. This pattern was more common and prominent after chemotherapy. The authors suggested that mesenchyme-like areas may be the site of origin of the sarcomas that occur in some patients after chemotherapy.

Nonspecific patterns that may occur in yolk sac tumors include solid (fig. 13-28) and papillary, which may simulate papillary adenocarcinoma of other types (figs. 13-29, 13-30). Cells with large intracellular vacuoles that displace the nucleus may be prominent in some cases, simulating liposarcoma or signet-ring cell carcinoma. Rare tumors contain small numbers of

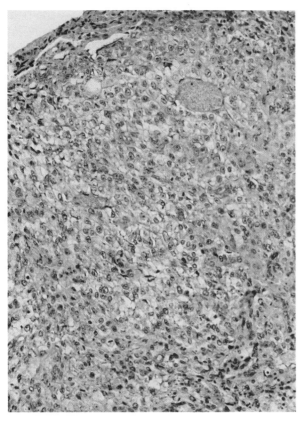

Figure 13-28
YOLK SAC TUMOR
The tumor cells have a solid pattern.

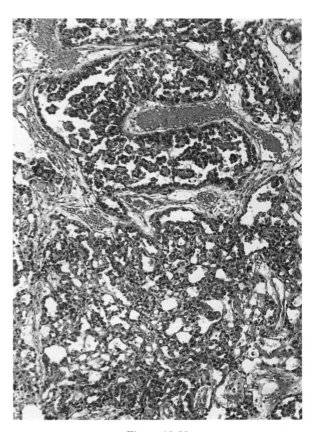

Figure 13-29
YOLK SAC TUMOR
A papillary pattern (above) merges with a reticular pattern (below).

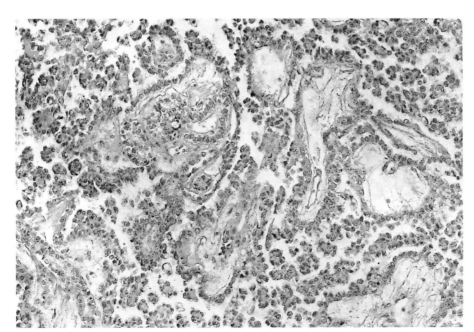

Figure 13-30
YOLK SAC TUMOR
Numerous small cellular papillae create an appearance resembling that of a serous carcinoma. (Fig. 17-23 from Young RH, Scully RE. Unusual patterns, subtypes, and differential diagnosis of gonadal yolk sac tumors. In: Nogales FF, ed. The human yolk sac and yolk sac tumors. Heidelberg: Springer-Verlag, 1993:309–42.)

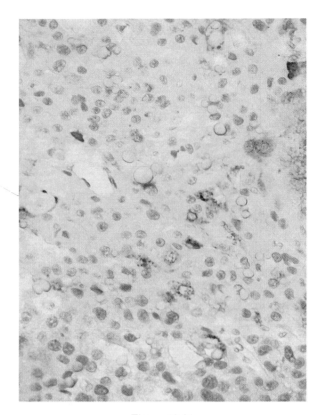

Figure 13-31
YOLK SAC TUMOR, HEPATOID VARIANT
The cytoplasm of the tumor cells is focally immunoreactive for alpha-fetoprotein.

brane antigen (58,62,65); the staining for the first two antigens may be focal (58). The contents of the cysts, acini, and glands within the poly-vesicular-vitelline, intestinal, and endometrioid-like patterns may also stain for AFP and alpha-1-antitrypsin. Most hyaline bodies are negative for AFP as well as for alpha-1-antitrypsin, albumin, and transferrin (78,83). The apical cytoplasm and the luminal contents of enteric glands typically stain for carcinoembryonic antigen (83). Basement membrane material in yolk sac tumors is immunoreactive for laminin and type IV collagen (83). Other antigens that have been demonstrated in yolk sac tumors include placental-like alkaline phosphatase, neuron-specific enolase, vimentin, and Leu-7 (65).

At least two types of distinctive material have been demonstrated ultrastructurally in yolk sac tumors (63,83). One of them, in the form of exclusively intracellular, uniformly electron-dense, spheroidal, nonmembrane-bound inclusions, corresponds to the hyaline bodies seen on light microscopic examination. Ultrastructurally, these inclusions are always surrounded by cytoplasm, which is sometimes scanty (83). The other deposit, which corresponds to basement membrane material and may be either intracellular or extracellular, is irregularly shaped, often linear, and of variable electron density (83). When intracellular, it is membrane-bound and in close association with cisternae of rough endoplasmic reticulin. Ultrastructural examination of hepatoid yolk sac tumors discloses features similar to those of hepatocellular carcinoma (72). The enteric nature of the sparsely distributed glands within typical yolk sac tumors, as well as those in the intestinal glandular variant, has been confirmed ultrastructurally by the presence of villi and subvillous rootlets (45,74,83).

Differential Diagnosis. The differential diagnosis of yolk sac tumors is extensive because of their numerous microscopic patterns (86). Their distinction from clear cell carcinomas, which cause the greatest confusion, is discussed on page 148, and the differences between endometrioid-like and hepatoid yolk sac tumors and endometrioid neoplasms and hepatoid carcinomas, respectively, are discussed on pages 124 and 324. Hepatoid yolk sac tumors must also be differentiated from many other ovarian tumors, both primary and metastatic, that are

syncytiotrophoblastic giant cells (59). Luteinized stromal cells, lymphocytes, granulomas, and erythropoietic foci are occasionally found within the stroma of yolk sac tumors (51,58,59).

Metastatic tumor usually has an appearance similar to that of the primary tumor, although in some cases, a predominantly solid pattern with the appearance of an undifferentiated malignant neoplasm is seen at autopsy (58). In some cases, this altered microscopic appearance may be related to chemotherapy (51).

Immunohistochemical staining may be useful in confirming a diagnosis of yolk sac tumor, particularly when unusual or nonspecific histologic patterns predominate. A variety of proteins synthesized by the normal yolk sac have been identified immunohistochemically within yolk sac tumors. The cytoplasm of the tumor cells is almost always immunoreactive for AFP (fig. 13-31), alpha-1-antitrypsin, and cytokeratin, but not epithelial mem-

characterized by large cells with abundant eosinophilic cytoplasm, including steroid cell tumors, oxyphilic endometrioid and clear cell carcinomas, metastatic melanoma, and metastatic hepatocellular carcinoma (see Table 6-1).

Yolk sac tumors should be distinguished from other germ cell tumors, including dysgerminoma (page 244) and the rare embryonal carcinoma. Embryonal carcinomas, although closely related to yolk sac tumors, lack the distinctive patterns of the latter and are composed of larger, more pleomorphic cells that line glands and papillae and grow as solid sheets. In addition, syncytiotrophoblastic cells are almost always present in embryonal carcinomas (resulting in an elevated serum hCG), in contrast to their rarity in yolk sac tumors. Because of their occurrence in young patients, yolk sac tumors may also be confused with a variety of other tumors (85,86), including the juvenile granulosa cell tumor (page 184), the small cell carcinoma of hypercalcemic type (page 316), and the Sertoli-Leydig cell tumor (page 218).

Treatment and Prognosis. The optimal therapy for a unilateral yolk sac tumor is unilateral salpingo-oophorectomy, cytoreduction of extraovarian tumor, and combination chemotherapy (51,54,58,77). In contrast to the dismal prognosis for patients in the prechemotherapy era (13 percent 3-year survival) (58), postoperative chemotherapy has achieved survival rates of 70 to 90 percent for patients with stage I tumors, and 30 to 50 percent for patients with higher stage tumors (50,51,54). Some successfully treated patients have had normal term pregnancies (51). Serial determination of AFP is useful in monitoring the effects of therapy and detecting recurrent tumor. Patients with microscopic residual tumor, however, may have normal AFP levels (46), and rarely, AFP-secreting yolk sac tumors convert to nonsecretory tumors during treatment (47). Adverse prognostic factors in one study included a tumor stage of II or greater, gross residual tumor after cytoreductive surgery, and more than 100 ml of ascitic fluid (54). Liver involvement, either at presentation or as recurrent disease, is also associated with a poor prognosis (84). One group found that patients with stage I tumors having three or four histologic patterns had a better prognosis than patients with tumors having only one or two patterns (75).

EMBRYONAL CARCINOMA

Definition. This rare germ cell tumor is characterized by large primitive cells resembling those of the embryonic germ disk and growing in solid, papillary, and glandular patterns.

General Features. Embryonal carcinomas are much rarer in the ovary than in the testis, accounting for only about 3 percent of primitive ovarian germ cell tumors; they are one fifth to one tenth as common as yolk sac tumors (89,90). The patients range in age from 4 to 28 years, with a median age of 12 years; approximately half the patients are prepubertal (88–90,93,95). The clinical presentation is usually as an adnexal mass, and in half the cases, as endocrine manifestations, including isosexual pseudoprecocity, irregular bleeding, amenorrhea, and hirsutism, alone or in combination. The serum hCG and AFP levels have been elevated in all the patients tested for these markers, although AFP has been measured in only a few cases (89,90,93,95). An elevation of both markers in a female with an adnexal mass should therefore suggest at least a component of embryonal carcinoma in the tumor. In several cases, the clinical presentation has mimicked that of an intrauterine or ectopic pregnancy (89). Laparotomy reveals spread to the peritoneum in 40 percent of the cases, sometimes accompanied by parenchymal involvement of pelvic or intra-abdominal viscera (89).

Pathologic Findings. The tumors are typically large (median diameter, 17 cm) with smooth external surfaces; in occasional cases, preoperative rupture occurs (89). In all the reported cases the tumor was unilateral. The cut surface is predominantly solid and variegated, with white, tan-grey, and yellow soft tissue alternating with cysts containing mucoid material. Foci of hemorrhage and necrosis are common.

Microscopic examination reveals solid sheets and nests of cells, often with central necrosis, gland-like spaces, and papillae composed of or lined by large primitive cells with amphophilic or sometimes clear cytoplasm and well-defined cell membranes (figs. 13-32–13-34) (89). The nuclei are round and vesicular with a coarse, irregular membrane and one or more prominent nucleoli (fig. 13-34). Mitotic figures, including atypical forms, are usually numerous. Eosinophilic hyaline droplets, identical to those occurring

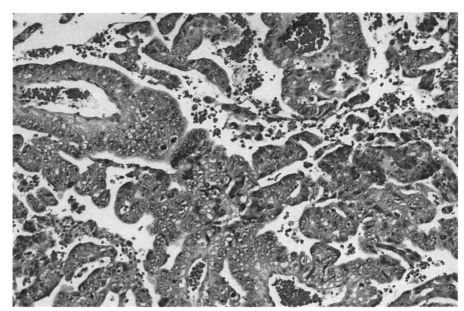

Figure 13-32
EMBRYONAL CARCINOMA
A papillary pattern is seen.

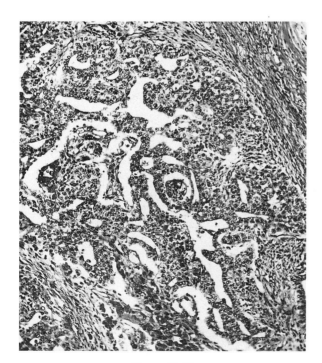

Figure 13-33
EMBRYONAL CARCINOMA

The tumor cells line irregular slit-like spaces and form papillae. (Fig. 1 from Kurman RJ, Norris HJ. Embryonal carcinoma of the ovary. A clinicopathologic entity distinct from endodermal sinus tumor resembling embryonal carcinoma of the adult testis. Cancer 1976;38:2420–33.)

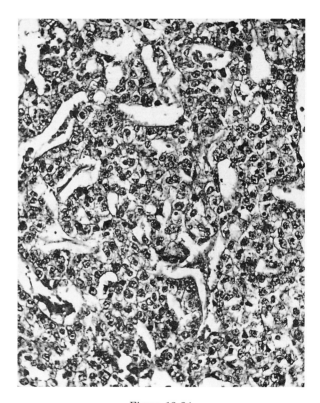

Figure 13-34
EMBRYONAL CARCINOMA
Cells with primitive-appearing nuclei form solid aggregates and line irregular gland-like spaces.

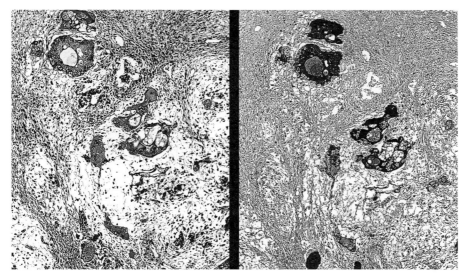

Figure 13-35
EMBRYONAL CARCINOMA
Left: Numerous syncytio-
trophoblastic giant cells are
present.
Right: The giant cells are immunoreactive for hCG.

in yolk sac tumors, are present in many of the cases. Syncytiotrophoblastic giant cells (fig. 13-35) were conspicuous in all the reported tumors, usually individually disposed within or at the periphery of the tumor nests, or within the stroma, which may vary from edematous to densely fibrous. Foci resembling intermediate trophoblast (91), embryoid bodies, enteric glands that may contain goblet cells, and minor foci of mature teratomatous elements (squamous epithelium, cartilage) are present in occasional cases (89).

The cytoplasm of the tumor cells is typically immunoreactive for cytokeratin, placental-like alkaline phosphatase, and neuron-specific enolase, and is almost always negative for epithelial membrane antigen (87,92,94). Immunoreactivity for AFP is seen in one third to half of the cases (89,94) although such immunoreactivity may reflect an admixture of unrecognized yolk sac neoplasia. The syncytiotrophoblastic cells are immunoreactive for hCG (fig. 13-35, right).

Differential Diagnosis. The distinction of embryonal carcinoma from other germ cell tumors (dysgerminoma, yolk sac tumor) and the juvenile granulosa cell tumor, has been discussed on pages 244, 255, and 184, respectively. Rarely, embryonal carcinoma may be confused microscopically with poorly differentiated adenocarcinomas or undifferentiated carcinomas in the surface epithelial–stromal category. Such tumors, however, in contrast to embryonal carcinomas, typically occur in the late reproductive and postmenopausal age groups, rarely elaborate AFP (with the exception of the rare hepatoid carcinoma), typically lack overt trophoblastic differentiation, and are immunoreactive for epithelial membrane antigen in most cases.

Treatment and Prognosis. The optimal therapy for embryonal carcinoma is unilateral salpingo-oophorectomy, cytoreduction of extraovarian tumor, and postoperative combination chemotherapy. Serial determinations of serum hCG and AFP are useful in monitoring the effects of chemotherapy and detecting recurrent tumor. The 5-year survival rate for patients with stage I disease in the series of Kurman and Norris (89) was only 50 percent, but most of those patients did not receive chemotherapy. Chemotherapy was curative, however, in other cases in that series as well as additional cases reported subsequently (88,93,95), including some with extraovarian spread.

POLYEMBRYOMA

Definition. This tumor is characterized by an exclusive or preponderant content of embryoid bodies, which resemble normal early embryos in various stages of development.

General Features. Ovarian polyembryomas are exceedingly rare, with less than 10 cases reported during the last four decades (96–100,102, 104–106). The patients are typically children or young women who present with manifestations related to the presence of a pelvic mass. At least

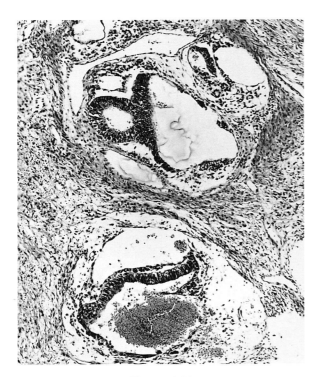

Figure 13-36
POLYEMBRYOMA
Several embryoid bodies are seen in different stages of development. The two large bodies contain an amniotic cavity, thick germ disc, and voluminous yolk sac cavity. (Fig. 94 from Serov SF, Scully RE, Sobin LH. Histological typing of ovarian tumours. International Histological Classification of Tumours No. 9. Geneva: World Health Organization, 1973.)

some patients have elevated serum levels of AFP, hCG, or both at presentation (96,97,105,106) although these tumor markers have not been measured in most of the reported cases. Occasional patients have evidence of extraovarian spread of tumor at presentation (104,106).

Pathologic Findings. On gross examination, polyembryomas are usually bulky tumors with sectioned surfaces that are typically spongy or microcystic, soft, reddish brown, and focally hemorrhagic. Microscopic examination reveals myriads of small structures resembling perfect or imperfect early embryos containing germ disks, amniotic cavities, yolk sacs, chorionic elements including syncytiotrophoblastic giant cells, and extraembryonic mesenchyme scattered in a fibrous or edematous stroma (fig. 13-36). Mature and immature teratomatous elements, predominantly of endodermal derivation, are usually also present. The embryoid bodies are often contiguous with

intestinal glands or embryonal or adult hepatic tissue, which may secrete bile (101–103). Foci of polyvesicular vitelline yolk sac tumor were present in one case (103), and in another, there was a prominent hemangioma-like vascular component (99). The yolk sac component of the embryoid bodies and the hepatic elements are immunoreactive for AFP and alpha-1-antitrypsin, and the syncytiotrophoblastic elements are immunoreactive for hCG (99,103,101,105).

Treatment and Prognosis. Polyembryomas behave like other primitive malignant germ cell tumors. Several patients who did not receive adjuvant chemotherapy died of tumor less than a year after presentation (98,104). Other patients, including some with extraovarian spread, have been treated successfully with combination chemotherapy (102,105). One patient with a stage IA tumor was treated only surgically; the serum AFP and hCG levels declined postoperatively and there was no evidence of disease 5 years later (97). Recurrent or metastatic tumor in two cases consisted of mature teratomatous elements; in one of these cases, the patient had not received any chemotherapy (99,106).

CHORIOCARCINOMA

Definition. This tumor is composed of an intimate admixture of either cytotrophoblast, intermediate trophoblast, or both, and syncytiotrophoblast.

General Features. Pure nongestational choriocarcinomas account for less than 1 percent of primitive germ cell tumors of the ovary (107,110, 111,115–118). More commonly, choriocarcinoma is a component of a mixed germ cell tumor, and was encountered in 20 percent of the latter in one series (112). The occurrence of choriocarcinoma in a prepubertal patient or the presence of other germ cell elements establishes a germ cell origin of the tumor. Gestational choriocarcinomas of the ovary are almost always metastatic from uterine, or rarely, tubal choriocarcinomas, but exceptionally complicate an ovarian pregnancy (page 331). In some cases, it may be impossible to prove a germ cell or gestational origin (107). The presence of paternal human leukocyte antigens (111) or a Y chromosome (109), which are characteristic of gestational choriocarcinomas but not of choriocarcinomas of germ cell lineage, may prove useful in establishing the origin of the tumor.

Ovarian choriocarcinomas typically occur in children and young adults. Patients present with an adnexal mass, pain, and in occasional cases, hemoperitoneum (107). The serum hCG levels are elevated, leading to isosexual pseudoprecocity in children, and menstrual abnormalities, breast enlargement (occasionally with colostrum secretion), androgenic changes, or combinations thereof, in adults. The clinical presentation may mimic that of a tubal pregnancy.

Pathologic Findings. On gross examination, the pure choriocarcinoma is typically solid, hemorrhagic, and friable. Bilateral involvement is rare. Microscopic examination reveals uninucleated trophoblastic cells with scanty or abundant clear cytoplasm (cytotrophoblast or intermediate trophoblast) admixed with syncytiotrophoblastic cells, which contain cytoplasmic vacuoles and many dark nuclei, and may form syncytial knots (fig. 13-37) (113). A plexiform pattern is often, but not invariably, present, and in areas the tumor may have a nonspecific poorly differentiated appearance. The neoplastic elements are frequently juxtaposed to dilated vascular sinusoids, which are the source of the massive hemorrhage that is typically present. Vascular invasion may be prominent.

The syncytiotrophoblastic cells are typically immunoreactive for cytokeratin, hCG, human placental lactogen (hPL), and pregnancy-specific beta-1 glycoprotein (SP1); the cytotrophoblast is typically immunoreactive for cytokeratin; and the intermediate trophoblast is usually immunoreactive for cytokeratin, hPL, and SP1 (113). Immunoreactivity for placental-like alkaline phosphatase, epithelial membrane antigen, neuron-specific enolase, alpha-1-antitrypsin, and carcinoembryonic antigen may be present as well (114).

Differential Diagnosis. Choriocarcinoma should be distinguished on histologic examination from malignant germ cell tumors in which isolated syncytiotrophoblastic cells may be encountered, such as embryonal carcinoma, dysgerminoma, and yolk sac tumor. The differential diagnosis also includes occasional poorly differentiated carcinomas of surface epithelial origin, usually occurring in older women, that exhibit trophoblastic differentiation (pages 167 and 379). These tumors range in appearance from carcinomas containing isolated giant cells resembling

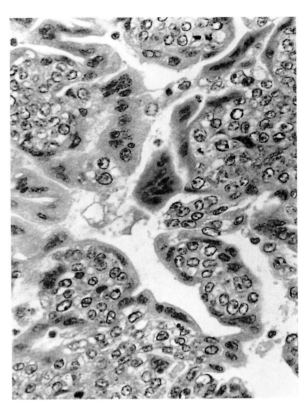

Figure 13-37
CHORIOCARCINOMA

Smaller cytotrophoblastic cells are growing with syncytiotrophoblastic cells in a plexiform pattern. (Fig. 95 from Serov SF, Scully RE, Sobin LH. Histological typing of ovarian tumours. International Histological Classification of Tumours No. 9. Geneva: World Health Organization, 1973.)

syncytiotrophoblastic giant cells to typical choriocarcinoma. Such tumors may secrete hCG and have endocrine manifestations (108,114a).

Treatment and Prognosis. Tumors reported in the prechemotherapy era were usually rapidly fatal, with spread throughout the abdomen and often to the lungs, although rare patients survived for many years after surgical removal alone (107). More recently, unilateral salpingo-oophorectomy combined with combination chemotherapy has markedly improved survival rates, with apparent cures or prolonged remissions in patients with extraovarian spread (107,110,111,118). Ovarian choriocarcinomas of germ cell origin, however, may be less responsive to chemotherapy than gestational choriocarcinomas (110,115,116). Moreover, it has been suggested that the former tumors should be treated with combination chemotherapy known to be effective against germ cell tumors rather than with the single agent therapy (methotrexate or actinomycin D) that is highly effective in the treatment of gestational choriocarcinomas (111).

MIXED MALIGNANT GERM CELL TUMORS

These tumors, which contain mixtures of two or more types of germ cell neoplasia (dysgerminoma, yolk sac tumor, embryonal carcinoma, polyembryoma, choriocarcinoma, immature teratoma) account for 8 to 10 percent of malignant primitive germ cell tumors of the ovary (122,123). Their occurrence emphasizes the importance of careful gross examination and judicious sampling of germ cell tumors. Each component should be named specifically in the diagnosis in the order of decreasing quantity, the components should be quantified as accurately as possible, and the tumor should be coded according to all the neoplastic types present. Kurman and Norris (122) found that the prognosis in cases of mixed germ cell neoplasia depended not only on the nature of the malignant elements identified, but also on the quantity of the most malignant components. A highly malignant component did not adversely affect the prognosis unless it accounted for more than one third of the tumor area. Most of the patients in their study, however, did not receive postoperative chemotherapy. In a second series of mixed germ cell tumors, in which most of the patients received chemotherapy, no correlation was found between the histologic composition of the tumor and its behavior (121). In the first study, size was also an important prognostic factor: all the patients whose neoplasm was less than 10 cm in diameter survived. If one combines the data from both series, dysgerminoma was present in approximately 73 percent of the cases, yolk sac tumor in 64 percent, immature teratoma in 58 percent, embryonal carcinoma in 15 percent, and choriocarcinoma in 14 percent (figs. 13-38–13-40). In both studies, most of the tumors contained only two components (most commonly dysgerminoma and yolk sac tumor), with the remaining tumors containing three to five.

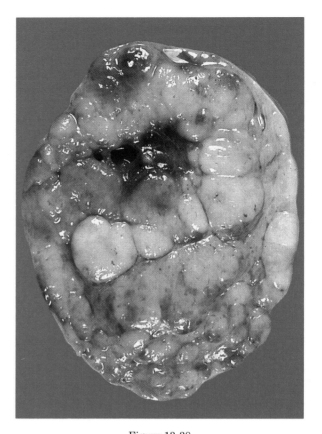

Figure 13-38
MIXED MALIGNANT GERM CELL TUMOR
The tumor has a lobulated, focally hemorrhagic sectioned surface. On microscopic examination, dysgerminoma, yolk sac tumor, embryonal carcinoma, and immature teratoma were found.

Rarer forms of mixed germ cell tumors have also been described. A distinctive pattern characterized by a diffuse intermingling of embryonal carcinoma and yolk sac tumor, designated diffuse embryoma, has been reported to occur in the testis (120) and has been encountered in the ovary as well. In this tumor, the yolk sac element consists of disseminated foci of pale cells growing in a reticular pattern and mingling in a repetitive manner with clusters of larger, darker embryonal carcinoma cells (figs. 13-41, 13-42). The yolk sac foci are often continuous with a thin layer of yolk sac cells that enclose nests of embryonal carcinoma in a necklace pattern (figs. 13-41, 13-42). Hepatoid cells and syncytiotrophoblastic cells may be present focally. Another unusual mixed germ cell tumor consisted predominantly

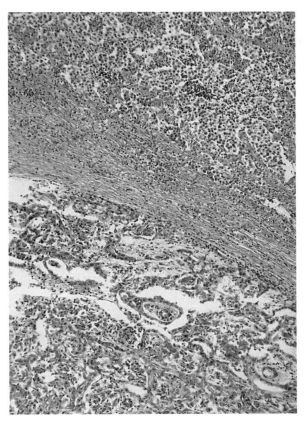

Figure 13-39
MIXED MALIGNANT GERM CELL TUMOR
Dysgerminoma (top) abuts yolk sac tumor (bottom).

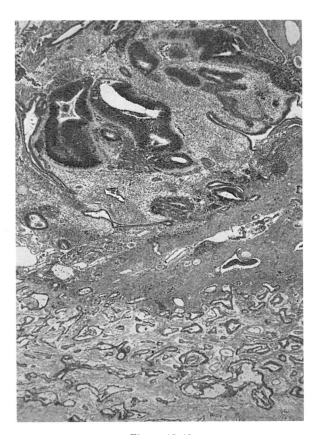

Figure 13-40
MIXED MALIGNANT GERM CELL TUMOR
Immature teratoma (top) abuts yolk sac tumor (bottom).

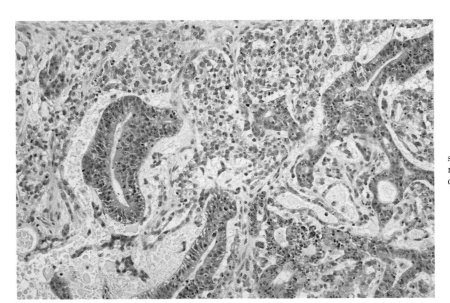

Figure 13-41
DIFFUSE EMBRYOMA
A network of spaces lined by yolk sac cells with small nuclei are admixed with acini lined by embryonal carcinoma cells with large nuclei.

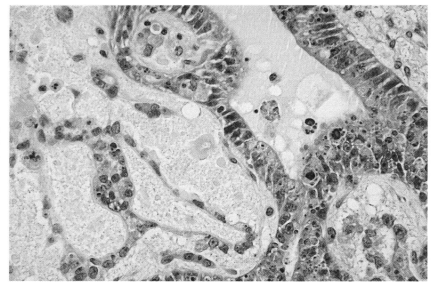

Figure 13-42
DIFFUSE EMBRYOMA
Embryonal carcinoma (columnar epithelium) is admixed with yolk sac epithelium (thin cords of cells) with small nuclei.

of immature pancreatic tissue, but also contained foci of benign and malignant mucinous epithelium, dysgerminoma, yolk sac tumor, and immature teratoma (124). Akhtar et al. (119) have reported a unique ovarian tumor composed of dysgerminoma and rhabdomyosarcoma.

REFERENCES

General Features

1. James PD, Taylor CW, Templeton AC. Tumours of the female genitalia. In: Templeton AC, ed. Tumours in a tropical country: a survey of Uganda 1964-1968. New York: Springer-Verlag, 1973:101–31.
2. Katsube Y, Berg JW, Silverberg SG. Epidemiologic pathology of ovarian tumors: a histopathologic review of primary ovarian neoplasms diagnosed in the Denver standard metropolitan statistical area, 1 July–31 December 1969 and 1 July–31 December 1979. Int J Gynecol Pathol 1982;1:3–16.
3. Koonings PP, Campbell K, Mishell DR Jr, Grimes DA. Relative frequency of primary ovarian neoplasms: a 10-year review. Obstet Gynecol 1989;74:921–6.
4. Kurman RJ, Norris HJ. Malignant mixed germ cell tumors of the ovary. A clinical and pathologic analysis of 30 cases. Obstet Gynecol 1976;48:579–89.
5. Lack EE, Goldstein DP. Primary ovarian tumors in childhood and adolescence. Current Prob Obstet Gynecol 1984;7:8.
6. Mandel M, Toren A, Kende G, Neuman Y, Kenet G, Rechavi G. Familial clustering of malignant germ cell tumors and Langerhans' histiocytosis. Cancer 1994;73:1980–3.
7. Nakashima N, Nagasaka T, Fukata S, et al. Study of ovarian tumors treated at Nagoya University Hospital, 1965-1988. Gynecol Oncol 1990;37:103–11.
8. Norris HJ, Jensen RD. Relative frequency of ovarian neoplasms in children and adolescents. Cancer 1972;30:713–9.
9. Sasano N, Tateno H, Takano A, Okuno Y. Ovarian cancers in Miyagi prefecture, Japan. An international survey of distributions of histologic types of tumours of the testis and ovary. UICC technical report series. 1983;75:193–8.
10. Shulman LP, Muram D, Marina N, et al. Lack of heritability in ovarian germ cell malignancies. Am J Obstet Gynecol 1994;170:1803–8.
11. Williams AO, Junaid TA. Ovarian tumours in Nigerian Africans. An international survey of distributions of histologic types of tumours of the testis and ovary. UICC technical report series. 1983;75:143–6.

Dysgerminoma

12. Altaras MM, Goldberg GL, Levin W, Darge L, Bloch B, Smith JA. The value of cancer antigen-125 as a tumor marker in malignant germ cell tumors of the ovary. Gynecol Oncol 1986;25:150–9.
13. Bailey D, Baumal R, Law J, et al. Production of a monoclonal antibody specific for seminomas and dysgerminomas. Proc Natl Acad Sci 1986;83:5291–5.

14. Beckstead JH. Alkaline phosphatase histochemistry in human germ cell neoplasms. Am J Surg Pathol 1983;7:341–9.
15. Bjorkholm E, Lundell M, Gyftodimos A, Silfversward C. Dysgerminoma. The Radiumhemmet series 1927-1984. Cancer 1990;65:38–44.
16. Buskirk SJ, Schray MF, Podratz KC, et al. Ovarian dysgerminoma: a retrospective analysis of results of treatment, sites of treatment failure, and radiosensitivity. Mayo Clin Proc 1987;62:1149–57.
17. De Palo G, Lattuada A, Kenda R, et al. Germ cell tumors of the ovary: the experience of the National Cancer Institute of Milan. I. Dysgerminoma. Int J Radiat Oncol Biol Phys 1987;13:853–60.
18. Dgani R, Shoham (Schwartz) Z, Czernobilsky B, Kaftori A, Borenstein R, Lancet M. Lactic dehydrogenase, alkaline phosphatase and human chorionic gonadotropin in a pure ovarian dysgerminoma. Gynecol Oncol 1988;30:44–50.
19. Dietl J, Horny HP, Kaiserling E. Frequent overexpression of p53 in dysgerminoma of the ovary. Gynecol Obstet Invest 1994;37:141–2.
20. Eglen DE, Ulbright TM. The differential diagnosis of yolk sac tumor and seminoma. Usefulness of cytokeratin, alpha-fetoprotein, and alpha-1-antitrypsin immunoperoxidase reactions. Am J Clin Pathol 1987;88:328–32.
21. Ferreiro JA. Ber-H2 expression in testicular germ cell tumors. Hum Pathol 1994;25:522–4.
22. Fujii S, Konishi I, Suzuki A, Okamura H, Okasaki T, Mori T. Analysis of serum lactic dehydrogenase levels and its isoenzymes in ovarian dysgerminoma. Gynecol Oncol 1985;22:65–72.
23. Gershenson DM. Update on malignant ovarian germ cell tumors. Cancer 1993;71:1581–90.
24. Gordon A, Lipton D, Woodruff JD. Dysgerminoma: a review of 158 cases from the Emil Novak Tumor Registry. Obstet Gynecol 1981;58:497–504.
25. Kawai M, Kano T, Kikkawa F, et al. Seven tumor markers in benign and malignant germ cell tumors of the ovary. Gynecol Oncol 1992;45:248–53.
26. Kawata M, Sekiya S, Hatakeyama R, Takamizawa H. Neuron-specific enolase as a serum marker for immature teratoma and dysgerminoma. Gynecol Oncol 1989;32:191–7.
27. Koide O, Iwai S, Kanno T, Kanda S. Isoenzymes of alkaline phosphatase in germinoma cells. Am J Clin Pathol 1988;89:611–6.
28. Krepart G, Smith JP, Rutledge F, Delclos L. The treatment for dysgerminoma of the ovary. Cancer 1978;41:986–90.
29. LaPolla JP, Benda J, Vigliotti AP, Anderson B. Dysgerminoma of the ovary. Obstet Gynecol 1987;69:859–67.
30. Lifschitz-Mercer B, Walt H, Kushnir I, et al. Differentiation potential in ovarian dysgerminoma: an immunohistochemical study of 15 cases. Hum Pathol 1995;26:62–6.
31. Miettinen M, Wahlstrom T, Virtanen I, Talerman A, Astengo-Osuna C. Cellular differentiation in ovarian sex-cord-stromal and germ-cell tumors studied with antibodies to intermediate-filament proteins. Am J Surg Pathol 1985;9:640–51.
32. Mullin TJ, Lankerani MR. Ovarian dysgerminoma: immunocytochemical localization of human chorionic gonadotropin in the germinoma cell cytoplasm. Obstet Gynecol 1986;68:80S–3S.
33. Niehans GA, Manivel JC, Copland GT, Scheithauer BW, Wick MR. Immunohistochemistry of germ cell and trophoblastic neoplasms. Cancer 1988;62:1113–23.
34. Oud PS, Soeters RP, Pahlplatz MM, et al. DNA cytometry of pure dysgerminoma of the ovary. Int J Gynecol Pathol 1988;7:258–67.
35. Palmquist MB, Webb MJ, Lieber MM, Gaffey TA, Nativ O. DNA ploidy of ovarian dysgerminomas: correlation with clinical outcome. Gynecol Oncol 1992;44:13–6.
36. Pressley RH, Muntz HG, Falkenberry S, Rice LW. Serum lactic dehydrogenase as a tumor marker in dysgerminoma. Gynecol Oncol 1992;44:281–3.
37. Rutgers JL, Scully RE. Functioning ovarian tumors with peripheral steroid cell proliferation: a report of twenty-four cases. Int J Gynecol Pathol 1986;5:319–37.
38. Schwartz PE, Chambers SK, Chambers JT, Kohorn E, McIntosh S. Ovarian germ cell malignancies: the Yale University experience. Gynecol Oncol 1992;45:26–31.
39. Schwartz PE, Morris JM. Serum lactic dehydrogenase: a tumor marker for dysgerminoma. Obstet Gynecol 1988;72:511–5.
40. Stewart CJ, Farquharson MA, Foulis AK. Characterization of the inflammatory infiltrate in ovarian dysgerminoma: an immunocytochemical study. Histopathology 1992;20:491–7.
41. Thomas GM, Dembo AJ, Hacker NF, DePetrillo AD. Current therapy for dysgerminoma of the ovary. Obstet Gynecol 1987;70:268–75.
42. Tsuura Y, Hiraki H, Watanabe K, et al. Preferential localization of c-kit product in tissue mast cells, basal cells of skin, epithelial cells of breast, small cell lung carcinoma and seminoma/dysgerminoma in human: immunohistochemical study on formalin-fixed, paraffin-embedded tissues. Virch Arch 1994;424:135–41.
43. Zaloudek CJ, Tavassoli FA, Norris HJ. Dysgerminoma with syncytiotrophoblastic giant cells. A histologically and clinically distinctive subtype of dysgerminoma. Am J Surg Pathol 1981;5:361–7.

Yolk Sac Tumor

44. Clement PB, Young RH, Scully RE. Endometrioid-like variant of ovarian yolk sac tumor. A clinicopathological analysis of eight cases. Am J Surg Pathol 1987;11:767–78.
45. Cohen MB, Friend DS, Molnar JJ, Talerman A. Gonadal endodermal sinus (yolk sac) tumor with pure intestinal differentiation: a new histologic type. Path Res Pract 1987;182:609–16.
46. Curtin JP, Rubin SC, Hoskins WJ, Hakes TB, Lewis JL Jr. Second-look laparotomy in endodermal sinus tumor: a report of two patients with normal levels of alpha-fetoprotein and residual tumor at reexploration. Obstet Gynecol 1989;73:893–5.
47. Damjanov I, Amenta PS, Zarghami F. Transformation of an AFP-positive yolk sac carcinoma into an AFP-negative neoplasm. Evidence for in vivo cloning of the human parietal yolk sac carcinoma. Cancer 1984;53:1902–7.
48. Dickersin GR, Oliva E, Young RH. Endometrioid-like variant of ovarian yolk sac tumor with foci of carcinoid: an ultrastructural study. Ultrastr Pathol 1995;19:421–9.
49. Farahmand SM, Marchetti DL, Asirwatham JE, Dewey MR. Ovarian endodermal sinus tumor associated with pregnancy: review of the literature. Gynecol Oncol 1991;41:156–60.

50. Fujita M, Inoue M, Tanizawa O, Minagawa J, Yamada T, Tani T. Retrospective review of 41 patients with endodermal sinus tumor of the ovary. Int J Gynecol Cancer 1993;3:329–35.

51. Gershenson DM, Del Junco G, Herson J, Rutledge FN. Endodermal sinus tumor of the ovary: the M.D. Anderson experience. Obstet Gynecol 1983;61:194–202.

52. Jacobsen GK, Talerman A, eds. Atlas of germ cell tumors. Copenhagen: Munksgaard, 1989.

53. Kawai M, Furuhashi Y, Kano T, et al. Alpha-fetoprotein in malignant germ cell tumors of the ovary. Gynecol Oncol 1990;39:160–6.

54. Kawai M, Kano T, Furuhashi Y, et al. Prognostic factors in yolk sac tumors of the ovary. A clinicopathologic analysis of 29 cases. Cancer 1991;67:184–92.

55. Kawai M, Kano T, Kikkawa F, et al. Seven tumor markers in benign and malignant germ cell tumors of the ovary. Gynecol Oncol 1992;45:248–53.

56. Kim CR, Hsiu JG, Given FT. Intestinal variant of ovarian endodermal sinus tumor. Gynecol Oncol 1989;33:379–81.

57. Kinoshita K. A 62-year-old woman with endodermal sinus tumor of the ovary. Am J Obstet Gynecol 1990;162:760-2.

58. Kurman RJ, Norris HJ. Endodermal sinus tumor of the ovary: a clinical and pathologic analysis of 71 cases. Cancer 1976;38:2404–19.

59. Langley FA, Govan AD, Anderson MC, Gowing NF, Woodcock AS, Harilal KR. Yolk sac and allied tumours of the ovary. Histopathology 1981;5:389–401.

60. Mazur MT, Talbot WH Jr, Talerman A. Endodermal sinus tumor and mucinous cystadenofibroma of the ovary. Occurrence in an 82-year-old woman. Cancer 1988;62:2011–5.

61. Michael H, Ulbright TM, Brodhecker CA. The pluripotential nature of the mesenchyme-like component of yolk sac tumor. Arch Pathol Lab Med 1989;113:1115–9.

62. Miettinen M, Wahlstrom T, Virtanen I, Talerman A, Astengo-Osuna C. Cellular differentiation in ovarian sex-cord-stromal and germ-cell tumors studied with antibodies to intermediate-filament proteins. Am J Surg Pathol 1985;9:640–51.

63. Nakanishi I, Kawahara E, Kajikawa K, Miwa A, Terahata S. Hyaline globules in yolk sac tumor. Histochemical, immunohistochemical and electron microscopic studies. Acta Pathol Jpn 1982;32:733–9.

64. Nakashima N, Fukatsu T, Nagasaka T, Sobue M, Takeuchi J. The frequency and histology of hepatic tissue in germ cell tumors. Am J Surg Pathol 1987;11:682–92.

65. Niehans GA, Manivel JC, Copland GT, Scheithauer BW, Wick MR. Immunohistochemistry of germ cell and trophoblastic neoplasms. Cancer 1988;62:1113–23.

66. Nogales FF. Embryologic clues to human yolk sac tumors: a review. Int J Gynecol Pathol 1993;12:101–7.

67. Nogales FF, ed. The human yolk sac and yolk sac tumors. Heidelberg: Springer-Verlag, 1993.

68. Nogales FF, Beltran E, Pavcovich M, Bustos M. Ectopic somatic endoderm in secondary human yolk sac. Hum Pathol 1992;23:921–4.

68a. Nogales FF, Bergeron C, Carvia RE, Alvaro T, Fulwood HR. Ovarian endometrioid tumors with yolk sac tumor component, an unusual form of ovarian neoplasm. Analysis of six cases. Am J Surg Pathol 1996;20:1056–66.

69. Nogales FF, Fernandez PL, Alvaro T. Alpha-fetoprotein-positive globules in involving human yolk sac [Letter]. Hum Pathol 1988;19:995.

70. Nogales FF, Matilla A, Nogales-Ortiz F, Galera-Davidson HL. Yolk sac tumors with pure and mixed polyvesicular vitelline patterns. Hum Pathol 1978;9:553–66.

71. Nogales FF, Silverberg SG, Bloustein PA, Martinez-Hernandez A, Pierce GB. Yolk sac carcinoma (endodermal sinus tumor). Ultrastructure and histogenesis of gonadal and extragonadal tumors in comparison with normal human yolk sac. Cancer 1977;39:1462–74.

72. Prat J, Bhan AK, Dickersin GR, Robboy SJ, Scully RE. Hepatoid yolk sac tumor of the ovary (endodermal sinus tumor with hepatoid differentiation): a light microscopic, ultrastructural and immunohistochemical study of seven cases. Cancer 1982;50:2355–68.

73. Rutgers JL, Young RH, Scully RE. Ovarian yolk sac tumor arising from an endometrioid carcinoma. Hum Pathol 1987;18:1296–9.

74. Salazar H, Kanbour A, Tobon H, Gonzalez-Angulo A. Endoderm cell derivatives in embryonal carcinoma of the ovary: an electron microscopic study of two cases. Am J Pathol 1973;74:108a.

75. Sasaki H, Furusato M, Teshima S, et al. Prognostic significance of histopathological subtypes in stage I pure yolk sac tumour of the ovary. Br J Cancer 1994;69:529–36.

76. Schiller W. Mesonephroma ovarii. Am J Cancer 1939;35:1–21.

77. Schwartz PE, Chambers SK, Chambers JT, Kohorn E, McIntosh S. Ovarian germ cell malignancies: the Yale University experience. Gynecol Oncol 1992;45:26–31.

78. Shirai T, Itoh T, Yoshiki T, Noro T, Tomino Y, Hayasaka T. Immunofluorescent demonstration of alpha-fetoprotein and other plasma proteins in yolk sac tumor. Cancer 1976;38:1661–7.

79. Takashina T, Kanda Y, Hayakawa O, Kudo R, Sagae S. Yolk sac tumors of the ovary and the human yolk sac. Am J Obstet Gynecol 1987;156:223–9.

80. Tavassoli FA, Yeh IT. Surgical pathology of the ovary: a review of selected tumors. Mod Pathol 1988;1:140–67.

82. Teilum G. Endodermal sinus tumors of the ovary and testis. Comparative morphogenesis of the so-called mesonephroma ovarii (Schiller) and extraembryonic (yolk sac-allantoic) structures of the rat's placenta. Cancer 1959;12:1092–105.

81. Teilum G. Gonocytoma. Homologous ovarian and testicular tumors. I. Acta Pathol Microbiol Scand 1946;23:242–51.

83. Ulbright TM, Roth LM, Brodhecker CA. Yolk sac differentiation in germ cell tumors. A morphologic study of 50 cases with emphasis on hepatic, enteric, and parietal yolk sac features. Am J Surg Pathol 1986;10:151–64.

84. Yazigi R, Sandstad J, Munoz A. Endodermal sinus tumor of the ovary: a paradoxical response to chemotherapy. Gynecol Oncol 1989;35:177–80.

85. Young RH. New and unusual aspects of ovarian germ cell tumors. Am J Surg Pathol 1993;17:1210–24.

86. Young RH, Scully RE. Unusual patterns, subtypes, and differential diagnosis of gonadal yolk sac tumors. In: Nogales FF, ed. The human yolk sac and yolk sac tumors. Heidelberg: Springer-Verlag, 1993:309–42.

Embryonal Carcinoma

87. Beckstead JH. Alkaline phosphatase histochemistry in human germ cell neoplasms. Am J Surg Pathol 1983;7:341–9.
88. Ibrahim EM, Al-Idrissi H, Al-Farag A, Al-Tamimi D, Perry W. Situs inversus totalis with embryonal cell carcinoma of ovaries. Gynecol Oncol 1984;18:270–3.
89. Kurman RJ, Norris HJ. Embryonal carcinoma of the ovary: a clinicopathologic entity distinct from endodermal sinus tumor resembling embryonal carcinoma of the adult testis. Cancer 1976;38:2420–33.
90. Langley FA, Govan AD, Anderson MC, Gowing NF, Woodcock AS, Harilal KR. Yolk sac and allied tumours of the ovary. Histopathology 1981;5:389–401.
91. Manivel JC, Niehans G, Wick MR, Dehner LP. Intermediate trophoblast in germ cell neoplasms. Am J Surg Pathol 1987;11:693–701.

92. Miettinen M, Wahlstrom T, Virtanen I, Talerman A, Astengo-Osuna C. Cellular differentiation in ovarian sex-cord-stromal and germ-cell tumors studied with antibodies to intermediate-filament proteins. Am J Surg Pathol 1985;9:640–51.
93. Nakakuma K, Tashiro S, Uemura K, Takayama K. Alpha-fetoprotein and human chorionic gonadotropin in embryonal carcinoma of the ovary. An 8-year survival case. Cancer 1983;52:1470–2.
94. Niehans GA, Manivel JC, Copland GT, Scheithauer BW, Wick MR. Immunohistochemistry of germ cell and trophoblastic neoplasms. Cancer 1988;62:1113–23.
95. Ueda G, Abe Y, Yoshida M, Fujiwara T. Embryonal carcinoma of the ovary: a six-year survival. Int J Gynecol Obstet 1990;31:287–92.

Polyembryoma

96. Beck JS, Fulmer HF, Lee ST. Solid malignant ovarian teratoma with "embryoid bodies" and trophoblastic differentiation. J Pathol 1969; 99:67–73.
97. Chapman DC, Grover R, Schwartz PE. Conservative management of an ovarian polyembryoma. Obstet Gynecol 1994;83:879–82.
98. Duhig JT. A unusual adenocarcinoma of the ovary. A case simulating Schiller's "mesonephroma." Am J Obstet Gynecol 1959;77:201–5.
99. King ME, Hubbell MJ, Talerman A. Mixed germ cell tumor of the ovary with a prominent polyembryoma component. Int J Gynecol Pathol 1991;10:88–95.
100. Marin-Padilla M. Origin, nature and significance of the embryoids of human teratomas. Virchows Arch Pathol Anat 1965;340:105–21.
101. Nakashima N, Fukatsu T, Nagasaka T, Sobue M, Takeuchi J. The frequency and histology of hepatic tissue in germ cell tumors. Am J Surg Pathol 1987;11:682–92.

102. Nakashima N, Murakami S, Fukatsu T, et al. Characteristics of embryoid body in human gonadal germ cell tumors. Hum Pathol 1988;19:1144–54.
103. Prat J, Matias-Guiu X, Scully RE. Hepatic yolk sac differentiation in an ovarian polyembryoma. Surg Pathol 1989;2:147–50.
104. Simard L. Polyembryonic embryoma of the ovary of pathogenetic origin. Cancer 1957;10:215–23.
105. Takeda A, Ishizuka T, Goto T, et al. Polyembryoma of ovary producing alpha-fetoprotein and HCG: immunoperoxidase and electron microscopic study. Cancer 1982;14:1878–89.
106. Tsukahara Y, Fukuta T, Yamada T, Nakai I. Retroperitoneal giant tumor formed by migrating polyembryoma with numerous embryoid bodies from an ovarian mixed germ cell tumor. Gynecol Obstet Invest 1991;31:58–60.

Choriocarcinoma

107. Axe SR, Klein VR, Woodruff JD. Choriocarcinoma of the ovary. Obstet Gynecol 1985;66:111–4.
108. Civantos F, Rywlin AM. Carcinomas with trophoblastic differentiation and secretion of chorionic gonadotrophins. Cancer 1972;29:789–98.
109. Davis JR, Surgit EA, Garay J, Fortier KJ. Sex assignment in gestational trophoblastic neoplasia. Am J Obstet Gynecol 1984;148:722–5.
110. Gerbie MV, Brewer JI, Tamimi H. Primary choriocarcinoma of the ovary. Obstet Gynecol 1975;46:720–3.
111. Jacobs AJ, Newland JR, Green RK. Pure choriocarcinoma of the ovary. Obstet Gynecol Surv 1982;37:603–9.
112. Kurman RJ, Norris HJ. Malignant mixed germ cell tumors of the ovary. A clinical and pathologic analysis of 30 cases. Obstet Gynecol 1976;48:579–89.
113. Manivel JC, Niehans G, Wick MR, Dehner LP. Intermediate trophoblast in germ cell neoplasms. Am J Surg Pathol 1987;11:693–701.

114. Niehans GA, Manivel JC, Copland GT, Scheithauer BW, Wick MR. Immunohistochemistry of germ cell and trophoblastic neoplasms. Cancer 1988;62:1113–23.
114a. Oliva E, Andrada E, Pezzica E, Prat J. Ovarian carcinomas with choriocarcinomatous differentiation. Cancer 1993;72:2441–6.
115. Vance RP, Geisinger KR. Pure nongestational choriocarcinoma of the ovary. Report of a case. Cancer 1985;56:2321–5.
116. Vogler C, Schmidt WA, Edwards CL. Primary ovarian nongestational choriocarcinoma. Report of a case in a young woman of childbearing age. Diagn Gynecol Obstet 1981;3:331–6.
117. Wheeler CA, Davis S, Degefu S, Thorneycroft IH, O'Quinn AG. Ovarian choriocarcinoma: a difficult diagnosis of an unusual tumor and a review of the hook effect. Obstet Gynecol 1990;75:547–9.
118. Wider JA, Marshall JR, Bardin CW, Lipsett MB, Ross GT. Sustained remissions after chemotherapy for primary ovarian cancers containing choriocarcinoma. N Engl J Med 1969;280:1439–42.

Mixed Malignant Germ Cell Tumors

119. Akhtar M, Bakri Y, Rank F. Dysgerminoma of the ovary with rhabdomyosarcoma. Report of a case. Cancer 1989;64:2309–12.

120. Cardoso de Almeida PC, Scully RE. Diffuse embryoma of the testis. A distinctive form of mixed germ cell tumor. Am J Surg Pathol 1983;7:633–42.

121. Gershenson DM, Del Junco G, Copeland LJ, et al. Mixed germ cell tumors of the ovary. Obstet Gynecol 1984;64:200–6.

122. Kurman RJ, Norris HJ. Malignant mixed germ cell tumors of the ovary. A clinical and pathologic analysis of 30 cases. Obstet Gynecol 1976;48:579–89.

123. Schwartz PE, Chambers SK, Chambers JT, Kohorn E, McIntosh S. Ovarian germ cell malignancies: the Yale University experience. Gynecol Oncol 1992;45:26–31.

124. Ueda G, Yamasaki M, Inoue M, et al. A rare malignant ovarian mixed germ cell tumor containing pancreatic tissue with islet cells. Int J Gynecol Pathol 1984;3:220–31.

14
TERATOMAS (EXCLUDING MONODERMAL)

Teratomas are germ cell tumors composed of a variety of tissues usually representing two or three embryonic layers (ectoderm, mesoderm, endoderm), but occasionally made up of elements derived from one layer other than mesoderm. If the neoplastic tissue is uniformly mature, the tumor is designated mature teratoma, which is almost always a dermoid cyst. The presence of any immature tissue warrants a diagnosis of immature teratoma. An exception to the foregoing statement is the rare, otherwise typical dermoid cyst that contains tiny foci of immature tissue (page 275); the benign behavior in the relatively few reported cases of this type does not support the diagnosis of immature teratoma (44). Teratomas with a predominant or exclusive component of endodermal or ectodermal tissue are referred to as *monodermal teratomas.*

The presence of nuclear sex chromatin (Barr bodies) and a 46,XX karyotype in most mature ovarian teratomas is consistent with an origin through parthenogenetic development of ova (5). Chromosomal abnormalities such as trisomy, tetraploidy, and mosaicism, however, have been found in 7 percent of cases (7). Almost all dermoid cysts are probably of postmeiotic origin. Surti et al. (7) found that 65 percent of teratomas are derived from a single germ cell after the first meiotic division (meiosis I) as the result of either failure of meiosis II (type II) or endoreduplication of a mature ovum (type III); 35 percent arise by failure of meiosis I (type I) or mitotic division of premeiotic germ cells (type IV). Other studies have found that multiple dermoid cysts from the same individual as well as immature teratomas frequently exhibit both premeiotic (heterozygous) and postmeiotic (homozygous) patterns (1,3,4,6). Gibas et al. (2) found that the chromosomal abnormalities present in an immature teratoma were also present in its metastases, despite the presence of more mature elements in the latter after chemotherapy.

IMMATURE TERATOMA

Definition. Immature teratomas contain variable quantities of immature tissues that resembles those of the embryo; mature elements are also present in most of the cases. Although immature teratomas have been referred to as solid teratomas in the past, such tumors are occasionally predominantly cystic, and their separation from mature teratomas rests exclusively on their microscopic appearance.

General Features. Although only 3 percent of ovarian teratomas are immature, immature teratomas are the third most common primitive germ cell tumor, accounting for almost 20 percent of them, 1 percent of ovarian cancers in general (18), and 10 to 20 percent of ovarian cancers occurring in the first two decades. The tumors are most common in young adults and children; the median age in three large studies was 17, 19, and 21 years (17,24,31). The clinical presentation is typically that of an abdominal or pelvic mass, frequently accompanied by pain. Rarely, an immature teratoma is preceded by an ipsilateral dermoid cyst that was resected months to years previously (9,44). The risk of development of an immature teratoma in patients with dermoid cysts may be increased, particularly if the cysts are bilateral or multiple, or have ruptured (9,44).

Sixty-five percent of the patients with immature teratoma have an elevated serum level of alpha-fetoprotein at presentation (20,22), although the levels are only rarely as high as those encountered in patients with yolk sac tumors (20,33,34). Other serum markers that may be elevated include: human chorionic gonadotropin (hCG), sometimes associated with isosexual pseudoprecocity (22); neuron-specific enolase (23); CA125 (8,20,22); CA19-9 (22); and carcinoembryonic antigen (CEA) (22).

Approximately one third of immature teratomas have spread outside the ovary at the time of surgery, usually in the form of peritoneal implants, less commonly as lymph node metastases, and rarely as hematogenous metastases (11,17, 21,24,30,31,34). The risk of peritoneal implants appears to be increased with tumors that have ruptured preoperatively or are adherent (30,35).

Gross Findings. Immature teratomas are usually large (median diameter, 18 cm [31]), encapsulated masses with a smooth glistening

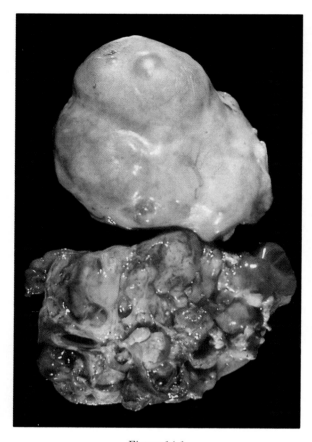

Figure 14-1
IMMATURE TERATOMA
The sectioned surface is composed of a mixture of solid and cystic tissues.

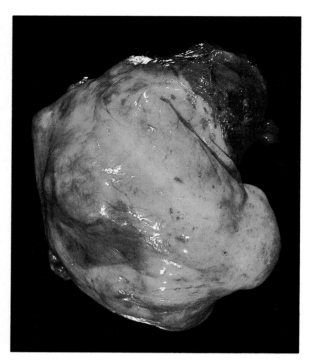

Figure 14-2
IMMATURE TERATOMA
Tumor has extended through a capsular defect (upper right).

outer surface (fig. 14-1). Capsular rupture, sometimes with herniation of tumor through the defect, is seen in almost half the cases (fig. 14-2) (28,35). The sectioned surfaces are predominantly solid but small cysts containing mucinous, serous, or bloody fluid or hair are frequently present, and occasionally, one or more large cysts occupy most of the specimen (fig. 14-3). Grossly evident dermoid cysts can be identified in approximately 25 percent of the cases (44). The solid areas within immature teratomas, which are usually composed predominantly of neural tissue, are typically soft, fleshy, and gray to pink (fig. 14-1), and may be focally hemorrhagic or necrotic. Foci of melanotic pigmentation may be present, and areas of bone and cartilage may be visible or palpable. Bilateral involvement is rare in the absence of extraovarian spread, but there

is a dermoid cyst or less often, another benign tumor in the contralateral ovary in approximately 10 percent of the cases (44).

Microscopic Findings. *Primary Tumor.* The amount of immature tissue varies from rare foci to a predominant component. Most or all of the immature tissue is composed of immature neuroectodermal tissue, which typically takes the form of primitive neuroepithelial rosettes and tubules, cellular foci of mitotically active glia (figs. 14-4–14-6), and in occasional cases, small areas resembling glioblastoma or neuroblastoma. The neuroepithelium may be pigmented. Immature or embryonal epithelium of various types, both ectodermal and endodermal, including hepatic tissue (27,34), as well as immature mesenchymal elements, such as cartilage (fig. 14-7) and skeletal muscle, are also common. Mature tissues identical to those encountered in mature teratomas (page 273) are typically present. Uncommon findings include immature renal tissue (30), isolated syncytiotrophoblastic giant cells, and yolk sac–like tissue (34). Nogales et al. (29) described

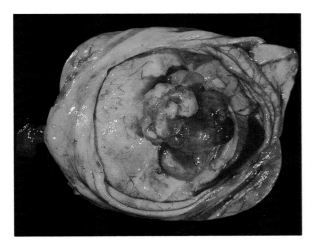

Figure 14-3
IMMATURE TERATOMA
The tumor is predominantly cystic. (Fig. 16 from Scully RE. Recent progress in ovarian cancer. Hum Pathol 1970;1:73–98.)

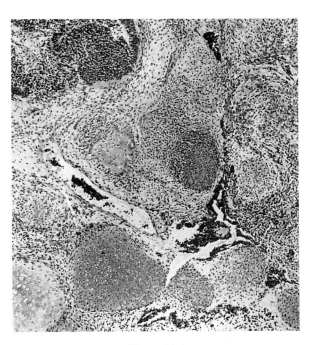

Figure 14-4
IMMATURE TERATOMA
Cellular foci of immature neuroectodermal tissue (upper left) and nodules of immature cartilage (lower half) are separated by immature mesenchyme.

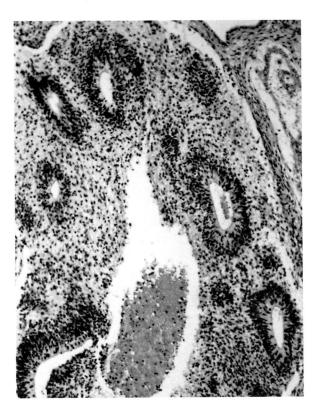

Figure 14-5
IMMATURE TERATOMA
Centrally necrotic cellular glial tissue envelops six neuroepithelial rosettes. (Fig. 17 from Scully RE. Recent progress in ovarian cancer. Hum Pathol 1970;1:73-98.)

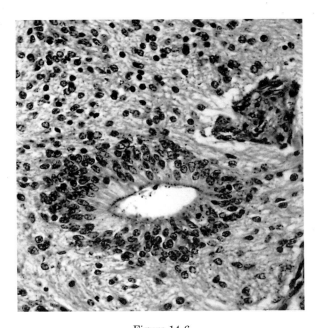

Figure 14-6
IMMATURE TERATOMA
A neuroepithelial rosette lies in cellular glial tissue; the lining cells contain mitotic figures. (Fig. 2 from Thurlbeck WM, Scully RE. Solid teratomas of the ovary. A clinicopathological analysis of 9 cases. Cancer 1960;13:804-11.)

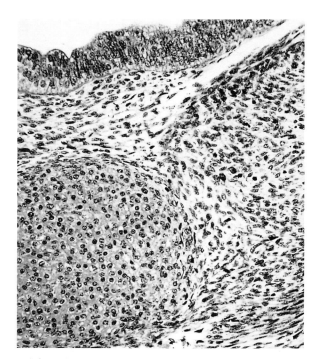

Figure 14-7
IMMATURE TERATOMA
Embryonal epithelium lines a cyst. An island of immature cartilage is seen below. (Fig. 5 from Thurlbeck WM, Scully RE. Solid teratomas of the ovary. A clinicopathological analysis of 9 cases. Cancer 1960;13:804-11.)

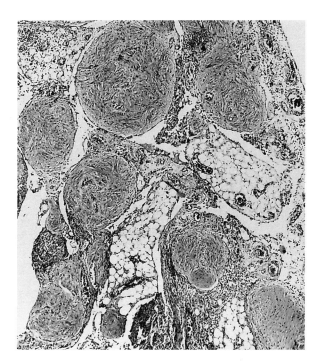

Figure 14-8
PERITONEAL GLIOMATOSIS
Multiple nodules of mature (grade 0) glial tissue involve the omentum. Some nodules are surrounded by a cuff of lymphocytes. The primary tumor was a grade 1 immature teratoma. (Fig. 1 from Robboy SJ, Scully RE. Ovarian teratoma with glial implants on the peritoneum. Hum Pathol 1970;16:

two unusual immature teratomas composed predominantly of endodermal structures without neuroectodermal elements.

Primary and metastatic immature teratomas are graded histologically on the basis of the amount of immature tissue present. The grading almost always depends on examination of the immature neuroectodermal tissue described above. Rare immature teratomas may have sparse or absent neuroectodermal tissue, and in such cases the grading may be based on the amount of immature non-neural tissue, such as cellular mesenchyme, that is present. Accurate grading depends on thorough sampling of the tumor, optimally one block per centimeter of tumor diameter. Grade 1 has been applied to tumors with rare foci of immature neural tissue, occupying less than one low-power field (40x) in any slide; grade 2 to tumors with moderate quantities of immature neural tissue, occupying more than 1 and less than 4 LPFs in any slide; and grade 3 to tumors with immature neural tissue occupying 4 or more

LPFs in any slide (31). O'Connor and Norris (32) have proposed that the three-grade system be replaced by a two-grade system, in which grade 1 is left unchanged but grades 2 and 3, which have a much poorer prognosis, are combined. We prefer the three-grade system.

Implants. Rarely, immature teratomas, as well as mature solid teratomas, are associated with peritoneal implants composed exclusively or mainly of mature (grade 0) glial tissue (peritoneal gliomatosis) (figs. 14-8, 14-9) (10,14,28,30,35). Mature epithelial elements or mature cartilage are also occasionally present. In some cases, the glial implants have been intimately admixed with foci of endometriosis (10,14,15). Similar glial tissue is sometimes encountered in pelvic and para-aortic lymph nodes, either in association with peritoneal implants or in their absence (34,35). It is important to sample the implants of immature teratomas generously as immature implants (fig. 14-10) may coexist with mature implants.

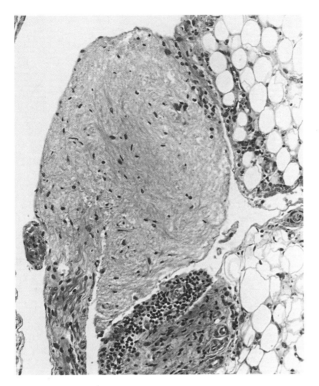

Figure 14-9
PERITONEAL GLIOMATOSIS
The omental implant consists of mature glial tissue (grade 0). (Fig. 103 from Serov SF, Scully RE, Sobin LH. Histological typing of ovarian tumours. International Histological Classification of Tumours No. 9. Geneva: World Health Organization, 1973.)

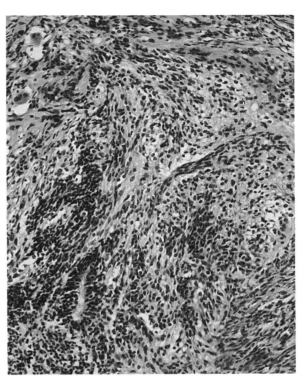

Figure 14-10
IMPLANT OF IMMATURE TERATOMA
ON PERITONEUM
The implant is composed exclusively of immature neuroectodermal tissue. The primary tumor was a grade 3 immature teratoma.

Immunohistochemical Findings. The neuroectodermal tissues are variably immunoreactive for one or more of a variety of neural markers, including glial fibrillary acidic protein, neuron-specific enolase, S-100 protein, neurofilament protein, synaptophysin, nerve growth factor receptor, glial filament protein, myelin basic protein, and polysialic acid (12,13,23,25,26,36,39,41,42). Alpha-fetoprotein immunoreactivity in immature teratoma is typically confined to hepatic tissue, yolk sac–like vesicles, and intestinal-type epithelium (27,33). Syncytiotrophoblastic elements, if present, are immunoreactive for hCG (12,13). Additional histochemical and immunohistochemical findings that may be encountered in mature tissues within immature teratomas are discussed on page 277.

Differential Diagnosis. Distinction from mature solid teratoma is based on the identification of even minor foci of immature tissue. The presence of fetal-type tissue such as cartilage, and developing cerebral cortex and cerebellum is not diagnostic of immature teratoma (40); brain tissue normally continues to develop with mitotic activity into the early postnatal months. As noted above (page 267), the rare otherwise typical dermoid cysts that contain microscopic foci of immature neural tissue should not be considered immature teratomas (44). Distinction of immature teratomas from heterologous malignant mesodermal mixed tumors and primitive neuroectodermal tumors is discussed on pages 130 and 303, respectively.

Treatment and Prognosis. Before the use of combination chemotherapy, the survival of patients with high-grade immature teratomas, particularly those with high-grade implants, was poor. In contrast, 90 to 100 percent of the patients in subsequent studies who had received combination chemotherapy achieved a sustained remission (11,

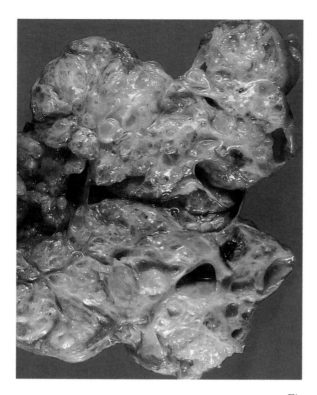 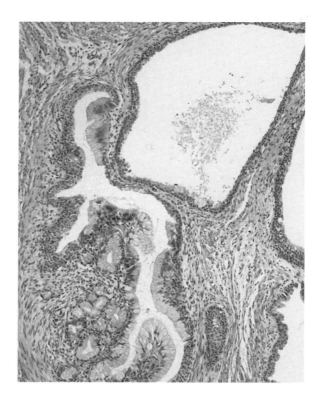

Figure 14-11
RECURRENT TERATOMA, POSTCHEMOTHERAPY (GROWING TERATOMA SYNDROME)
Left: The sectioned surface of the pelvic mass is solid and cystic.
Right: The mass is composed entirely of mature tissues (grade 0), consisting predominantly of cysts lined by mucinous epithelium and separated by mature fibrous tissue.

17,21,24). Chemotherapy typically is followed by disappearance of high-grade implants; the remaining implants are composed exclusively of mature tissue, necrotic tumor, fibrous tissue, or combinations thereof. Mature implants may continue to grow and occasionally invade local structures, requiring reoperation (growing teratoma syndrome) (fig. 14-11) (11,16,19,43). Patients who present with exclusively mature implants, which, as noted above, are typically glial, almost always have a benign clinical course even without postoperative treatment (28,35). Three cases of apparent transformation of mature peritoneal gliomatosis to tumor resembling glioblastoma multiforme have been reported (14a,28,38). In one of these cases (28), however, the interval between the two lesions was only 1 month, suggesting the possibility of incomplete sampling of the peritoneal implants at the time of the first procedure.

The initial treatment of patients with a unilateral immature teratoma should include unilat-eral salpingo-oophorectomy and removal of as much extraovarian tumor as considered feasible. Patients with grade 2 or 3 stage I tumors or those with immature metastases should receive combination chemotherapy. Patients with stage IA, grade 1 tumors or those with exclusively mature glial implants need no adjuvant chemotherapy (11, 30,35,37). Treatment recommendations for patients with stage IC, grade 1 tumors, or those with grade 1 metastases are unavailable because of the small numbers of such cases in the literature.

MATURE TERATOMA, SOLID

Definition. This tumor is solid or predominantly solid and is composed exclusively of mature elements.

General Features. The frequency of this tumor among all solid teratomas is difficult to determine as most investigators have included it indiscriminately in series of "solid" or "malignant"

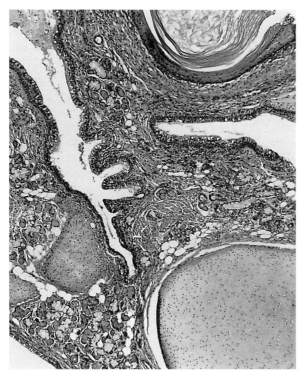

Figure 14-12
MATURE TERATOMA, SOLID
Tubular structures lined by respiratory epithelium, a keratinizing squamous cyst, islands of cartilage, and small groups of fat cells are visible. (Fig. 100 from Serov SF, Scully RE, Sobin LH. Histological typing of ovarian tumours. International Histological Classification of Tumours No. 9. Geneva: World Health Organization, 1973.)

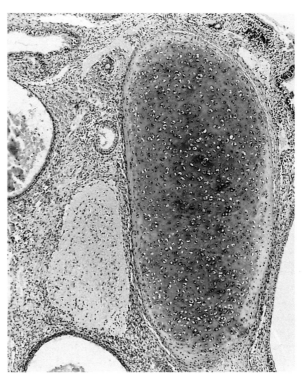

Figure 14-13
MATURE TERATOMA, SOLID
Islands of cartilage and glia as well as several cysts are visible. (Fig. 101 from Serov SF, Scully RE, Sobin LH. Histological typing of ovarian tumours. International Histological Classification of Tumours No. 9. Geneva: World Health Organization, 1973.)

teratomas. In four small unselected series, it accounted for 15 to 20 percent of solid teratomas (45–47,50). Patients have the same age distribution as those with immature teratomas, and in contrast to patients with dermoid cysts, are never postmenopausal. The occasional patients who have mature peritoneal glial implants at presentation are younger (mean age, 12 years) than those without implants (mean age, 19 years) (49).

Gross Findings. The macroscopic appearance is similar to that of immature teratoma except that soft areas and foci of necrosis and hemorrhage are much less common (51).

Microscopic Findings. Mature tissues representing all three germ layers and resembling fetal as well as adult tissues are present (figs. 14-12, 14-13). Well-differentiated glia may be the predominant element; small foci of hepatic, renal, or retinal tissue may also be seen. Squa-

mous, respiratory, and intestinal types of epithelium are common, and rudimentary organ formation is occasionally observed. Mitotic figures are absent or exceedingly rare.

Differential Diagnosis. Mature solid teratomas should be distinguished from immature teratomas. As noted above, even a small focus of immature tissue justifies a diagnosis of grade 1 immature teratoma, as such tumors may have a low malignant potential.

Treatment and Prognosis. The treatment is that for any benign ovarian neoplasm. Any associated implants should be excised if technically feasible and examined microscopically to confirm their maturity, and to avoid reoperation if they continue to grow (49). All patients, including those with mature implants, have had a benign clinical course (49), except for one whose tumor was probably inadequately sampled (48).

DERMOID CYST
(MATURE CYSTIC TERATOMA)

Definition. A dermoid cyst is a mature teratoma composed predominantly of a cyst lined entirely or partly by epithelium resembling the epidermis with its appendages. Mesodermal, endodermal, and other ectodermal derivatives are also present in most cases. Rarely, a mature cystic teratoma is lined by mature tissues other than those resembling epidermis, and in such cases the designation "dermoid cyst" is not appropriate.

General Features. The dermoid cyst is the most common type of ovarian tumor, accounting for 27 to 44 percent of all primary ovarian tumors and for 35 to 58 percent of the benign forms (64,68). Over 80 percent of dermoid cysts occur during the reproductive years. They account for half the ovarian neoplasms that appear in the first two decades (69) and over two thirds of those in children under the age of 15 years (61). In some cases the tumor is not detected until years after the menopause. In rare cases the tumor is familial (66).

In addition to their usual occurrence in pure form, dermoid cysts may be components of complex ovarian tumors in which struma, various forms of carcinoid tumor, solid teratoma, or rarely, a primitive germ cell tumor are also present. Also, dermoid cysts are found in the ovary contralateral to a yolk sac tumor or immature teratoma in 5 to 10 percent of the cases.

Dermoid cysts are usually associated with the typical symptoms and signs of benign ovarian tumors, although approximately 25 percent of them are asymptomatic (74). Because the sebaceous content of the cyst typically forms a rounded or ovoid mass of abnormally low density surrounded by a ring of increased capsular density, and because calcified structures, including bone and teeth, are often present, a radiologic diagnosis of dermoid cyst can be made in a high proportion of the cases (80). Rarely, teeth have been demonstrated to develop on serial X-ray films. As many as 50 percent and 30 percent of dermoid cysts have been associated with elevated serum levels of CA19-9 and CEA, respectively (65,67).

Dermoid cysts are prone to a variety of complications (55,59,73,74) and may be associated with a number of unusual clinical manifestations. Four to 15 percent of the tumors undergo torsion, which may be complicated by infarction,

perforation, hemoperitoneum, or autoamputation, alone or in combination (59,74). Infection occurs in approximately 2 percent of dermoid cysts; the organisms may reach the ovary by lymphatic, hematogenous, or direct routes. Perforation into the peritoneal cavity or a hollow viscus is encountered in 1 to 2 percent of the cases and is more likely to occur during pregnancy. Slow leakage into the abdominal cavity results in a localized or generalized granulomatous peritonitis, which may mimic metastatic carcinoma or tuberculosis at operation. Rarely, sudden rupture leads to an acute abdominal crisis with shock, related to the expulsion of the irritating cyst contents into the peritoneal cavity. Exceptionally, the cyst ruptures into the urinary bladder, vagina, or bowel, or through the anterior abdominal wall, leading to unusual manifestations that include the passage of hair, teeth, bony fragments, or gas in the urine; the formation of urinary calculi containing hair or teeth; and the passage of hair, teeth, or even an intact cyst through the vagina or rectum. In four cases pigmentation of the peritoneum (melanosis) was associated with dermoid cysts (52,63,70,76); in two of these cases, the cysts had ruptured preoperatively. At laparotomy, focal or diffuse, tan to black peritoneal staining or similarly pigmented tumor-like nodules were seen within the pelvis, and in some cases, the omentum. Hemolytic anemia associated with dermoid cysts is discussed on page 385.

Gross Findings. Dermoid cysts are globular or ovoid, with a white to gray external surface; most of them are less than 15 cm in diameter (figs. 14-14, 14-15). They are bilateral in approximately 15 percent of the cases (fig. 14-15), and are occasionally multiple in one ovary (79). Yellow to brown sebaceous material and hair fill one, or occasionally several lumens. The cysts are typically lined by tissue resembling skin (figs. 14-14, 14-15). One or more rounded, polypoid masses, designated mamillae or Rokitansky's protuberances and usually composed predominantly of fat, typically protrude into the lumen. Teeth are present in one third of the cases, either in the cyst wall or cavity; occasionally they are embedded in a rudimentary mandible or maxilla. Bone, cartilage, mucinous cysts, adipose tissue, thyroid, and soft brain tissue may be seen grossly. Rarely, partially developed organs and tissues such as bowel, appendix, skull, vertebrae, limb

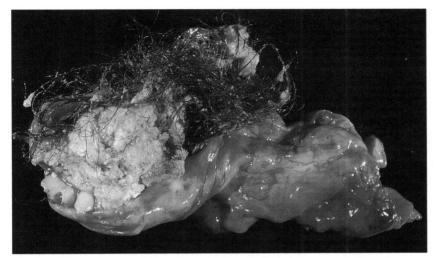

Figure 14-14
DERMOID CYST, OPENED
The cyst is filled with hair and sebaceous material. Several teeth are visible.

Figure 14-15
DERMOID CYST,
BILATERAL
A tooth is visible in the cyst on the left.

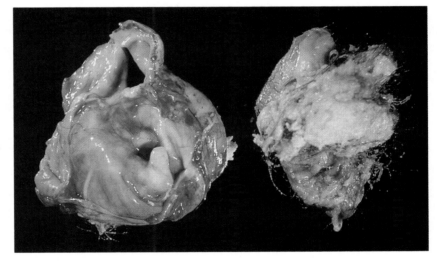

buds, external genitalia, and eyes are present. Some of the locules within the dermoid cysts associated with peritoneal melanosis have pigmented contents and lining.

Microscopic Findings. The tumors are typically composed of adult-type tissues, usually representing all three germ layers (figs. 14-16–14-20). Microscopic foci of immature or fetal-type tissues, however, are occasionally seen (79). Ectodermal derivatives predominate in almost all cases, with the cyst lining composed of epidermis and underlying skin appendages (figs. 14-16, 14-17); salivary gland tissue may be detected. Neuroectodermal elements, usually glia and peripheral nervous tissue, are typically present, but cerebrum, cerebellum (fig. 14-18), and choroid

plexus are also common. Mesodermal derivatives in the form of smooth muscle, bone, teeth, cartilage (figs. 14-17, 14-19), and fat (fig. 14-17) are usually present. Common endodermal derivatives include respiratory and gastrointestinal epithelium (fig. 14-20), as well as thyroid tissue (fig. 14-19). Rare constituents resemble retina, pancreas, thymus, adrenal gland, pituitary gland, kidney, lung, breast, and prostate gland (72). Respiratory epithelium or glial tissue occasionally lines portions of the cyst. Mitotic figures are absent or rare. The tissues are often arranged in an organoid fashion, exemplified by cartilage and mucinous glands beneath respiratory epithelium, and layers of bowel wall, including Auerbach's plexus, underlying intestinal epithelium (78).

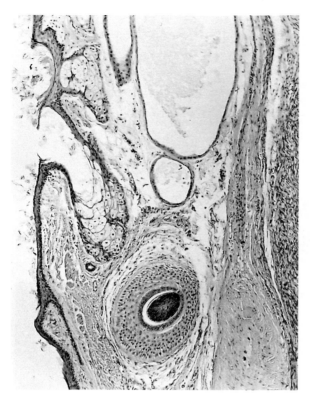

Figure 14-16
DERMOID CYST

Skin with its appendages lines the cyst. (Fig. 104 from Serov SF, Scully RE, Sobin LH. Histological typing of ovarian tumors. International Histological Classification of Tumours No. 9. Geneva: World Health Organization, 1973.)

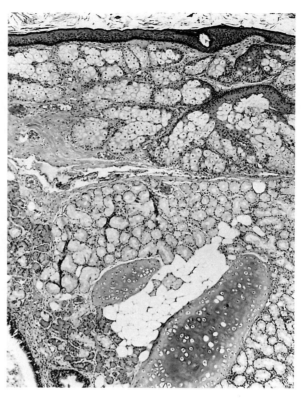

Figure 14-17
DERMOID CYST

Beneath the skin and its appendages are mucinous glands, fat, two islands of cartilage, and two cysts lined by respiratory epithelium. (Fig. 105 from Serov SF, Scully RE, Sobin LH. Histological typing of ovarian tumors. International Histological Classification of Tumours No. 9. Geneva: World Health Organization, 1973.)

Figure 14-18
DERMOID CYST

Cerebellar tissue is well developed. (Fig. 106 from Serov SF, Scully RE, Sobin LH. International histological classification of tumours no. 9. Histological typing of ovarian tumors. International Histological Classification of Tumours No. 9. Geneva: World Health Organization, 1973.)

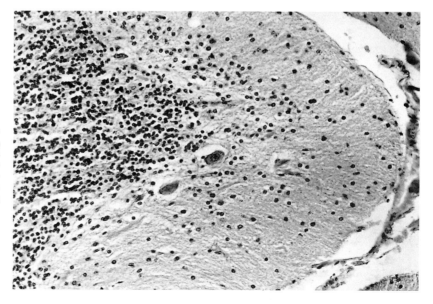

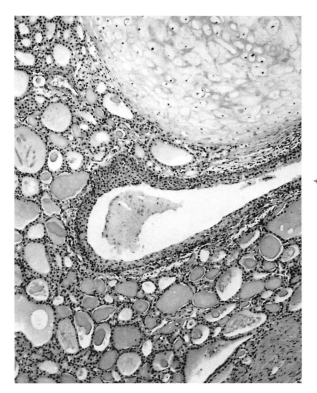

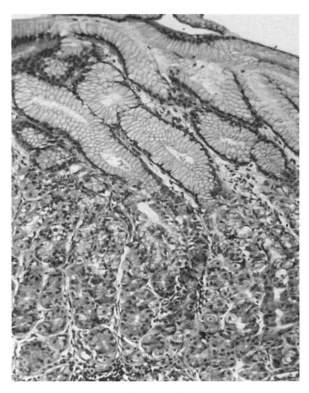

Figure 14-19
DERMOID CYST
Thyroid tissue and cartilage envelop a collapsed cyst lined by respiratory epithelium with focal squamous metaplasia.

Figure 14-20
DERMOID CYST
Gastric mucosa is present.

Rare lesions encountered in the tissues within dermoid cysts include compound nevi (53), thyroiditis (62), lactational changes in breast tissue (77), dental caries, and peptic ulceration of gastric mucosa (76).

Focal cyst rupture often results in a foreign body reaction to keratin, hair (fig. 14-21), or the oily cyst contents. The latter incites a lipogranulomatous response in the wall of the cyst or the surrounding ovarian tissue, in which variably sized, clear spaces are surrounded by inflammatory cells, including histiocytes and foreign body–type giant cells, often accompanied by dense fibrosis (fig. 14-22) (75).

In the cases of peritoneal "melanosis," the ovarian and peritoneal pigmentation is characterized by pigment-laden histiocytes in a fibrous stroma (fig. 14-23). In at least three of the reported cases (52,63,76) and in a fourth case we have encountered, gastric mucosa was prominent within an otherwise typical dermoid cyst; no obvious source

for the pigment could be identified in any of the cases. The nature of the pigment, although considered melanin in some reports, is not clear (76).

Argyrophil and argentaffin cells are frequently found in respiratory and intestinal epithelium in teratomas (56–58). These cells may be immunoreactive for a wide variety of neurohormonal polypeptides, including glucagon, secretin, gastrin, insulin, somatostatin, and pancreatic polypeptide (56–58). Growth hormone, prolactin, and thyroid-stimulating hormone have been identified immunohistochemically in the anterior pituitary gland tissue found rarely within teratomas (71). The wide variety of antigens that have been demonstrated within neuroectodermal tissue in teratomas are discussed on page 271.

Treatment and Prognosis. Unless the patient is perimenopausal or postmenopausal, dermoid cysts are usually resected, with conservation of the adjacent ovarian tissue (59). Although they are often bilateral, bisection of the contralateral ovary in search of an occult tumor, once a common

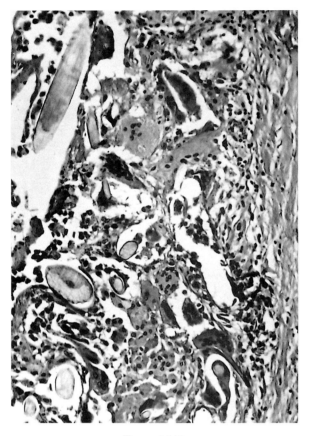

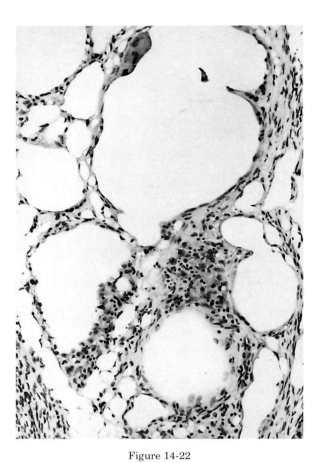

Figure 14-21
DERMOID CYST
A foreign-body giant cell reaction has developed around extruded hair shafts in the wall of a ruptured dermoid cyst.

Figure 14-22
DERMOID CYST
A lipogranulomatous reaction has developed in the wall of a ruptured dermoid cyst.

Figure 14-23
DERMOID CYST
WITH MELANOSIS
One cyst is lined by mucinous epithelium; the other is lined by melanin-laden histiocytes.

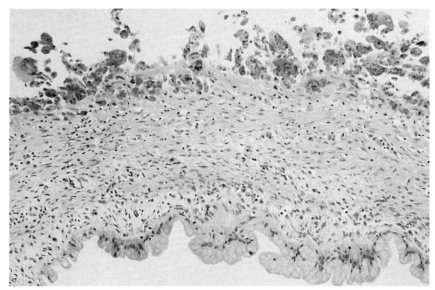

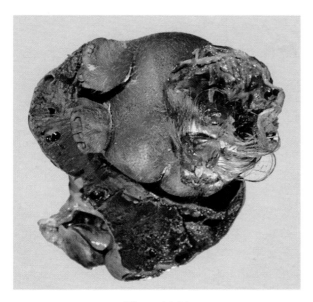

Figure 14-24
HOMUNCULUS
A fetus-like structure lies within an ovarian cyst, which has undergone torsion and hemorrhagic infarction.

practice, is now considered of little value (59). Doss et al. (60), for example, reported that incisional biopsy or excision of a visually normal contralateral ovary in 90 patients revealed no tumor, and a dermoid cyst later developed in only one of 58 patients in whom biopsy or removal of the contralateral ovary was not performed. Similar findings were reported in another study (55).

With the exception of cases of malignant transformation (below) dermoid cysts are clinically benign even if they contain microscopic foci of immature tissue (79). Rare dermoid cysts, however, are followed by the development of immature teratoma in the ipsilateral residual ovarian tissue; in such cases the cysts were multiple or had ruptured more often than in cases unassociated with that sequela (54,79).

FETIFORM TERATOMA (HOMUNCULUS)

This rare form of teratoma resembles a malformed human fetus (fig. 14-24) (81,83). Twenty-two cases have been reported in patients ranging in age from 9 to 65 years; most were diagnosed in the third or fourth decade (81). The caudal region of the homunculus, including the lower extremities, is typically more highly developed than the cephalic portion. This tumor should be distinguished from the more highly developed fetus-in-fetu, a parasitic monozygotic twin that develops within the upper retroperitoneal space of its partner (82). Most cases of fetus-in-fetu have occurred in infants less that 1 year of age, and no examples have been reported within the ovary (81). In additional contrast to a homunculus, the fetus-in-fetu typically contains a highly developed, segmented vertebral column.

DERMOID CYSTS WITH SECONDARY MALIGNANT TUMORS

Definition. These are dermoid cysts in which a malignant neoplasm of adult type arises from a constituent of the cyst. Several of these tumors are discussed in chapter 15, which covers carcinoid tumors, struma ovarii, and other monodermal teratomas (84,91,97). Also excluded from this section are two hemangiomas that arose in a dermoid cyst (89,93) and the primitive germ cell tumors that are occasionally associated with a dermoid cyst (see chapter 13).

General Features. As many as 1 to 2 percent of mature teratomas harbor a cancer of adult type, accounting for approximately 1 percent of all ovarian cancers in some studies (98,103). In one large study, however, malignant transformation was found in only 0.17 percent of dermoid cysts (88). Although dermoid cysts with malignant transformation are found in patients in every decade of life, over 75 percent of the cases, and an even higher proportion of the squamous cell carcinomas, are detected between the ages of 30 and 70 years, with most patients between 40 and 60 years (98,98a). The mean age of patients with squamous cell carcinomas in one large study was 59 years (90). If a woman 70 years of age or older has a dermoid cyst, there is an approximately 15 percent chance that it will contain a secondary malignant tumor (103). Cancer rarely develops in a dermoid cyst during the first two decades.

The clinical presentation varies from that of a typical dermoid cyst to that of an advanced ovarian cancer, depending on the tumor stage. Malignant change in a dermoid cyst should be suspected at the time of laparotomy if the patient is over the age of 40 years, especially when the cyst is adherent or has areas of nodularity, thickening

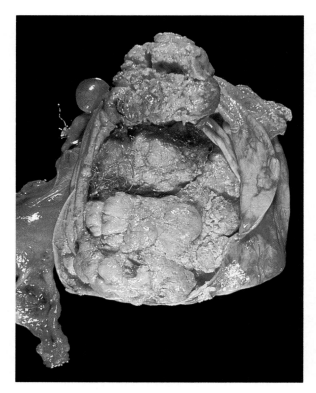

Figure 14-25
SQUAMOUS CELL CARCINOMA
ARISING IN DERMOID CYST
A fungating yellow tumor fills the cyst lumen.

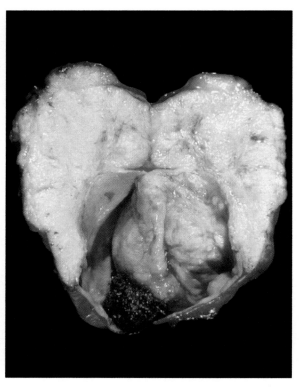

Figure 14-26
SQUAMOUS CELL CARCINOMA
ARISING IN DERMOID CYST
A solid white tumor occupies one pole and thickens the wall of a dermoid cyst. (Fig. 1 from Pins MR, Young RH, Daly WJ, Scully RE. Primary squamous cell carcinoma of the ovary. Report of 37 cases. Am J Surg Pathol 1996;20:823–33.)

of its wall, hemorrhage, or necrosis. In many cases, the tumor has already spread to adjacent organs or throughout the abdomen. Hematogenous metastases are associated with sarcomas more often than with carcinomas.

Miyazaki et al. (95) found that the serum level of squamous cell carcinoma antigen (SCCA) is elevated in patients with squamous cell carcinomas arising in dermoid cysts, including three stage I cases in which the level became normal postoperatively. In another study (92), serum levels of CA19-9 and CA125 were elevated in over 50 percent of cases of dermoid cyst with malignant transformation.

Gross Findings. Dermoid cysts harboring a malignant tumor tend to be larger than benign dermoid cysts; over 90 percent of the former have a maximal dimension of 10 to 20 cm (103). Squamous cell carcinomas and other forms of cancer may appear as cauliflower-like masses protruding into the cavity of the cyst (fig. 14-25), as a

mural nodule or plaque (fig. 14-26), or if extensive, a solid tumor mass that almost obliterates the cyst. Foci of hemorrhage and necrosis within the malignant component are common. Smaller cancers may not be apparent on gross examination. In all of the reported cases the cancer was unilateral, although a dermoid cyst without malignant change was present in the opposite ovary in 10 to 15 percent of the cases (98).

Microscopic Findings. Approximately 80 percent of malignant tumors arising in dermoid cysts are squamous cell carcinomas, almost always invasive, but occasionally in situ (figs. 14-27, 14-28) (90,98,98a). The invasive squamous cell carcinoma rarely has the appearance of a spindle cell carcinoma. Hirakawa et al. (90) found that the squamous cell carcinoma usually arises from columnar epithelium (fig. 14-27) or metaplastic squamous epithelium rather than

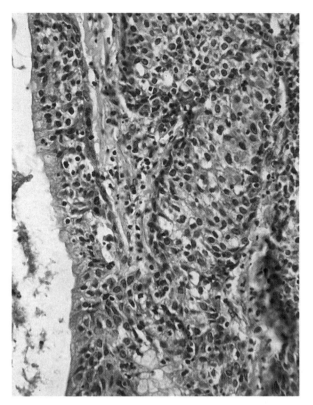

Figure 14-27
SQUAMOUS CELL CARCINOMA
ARISING IN DERMOID CYST
Atypical squamous cells, which are intimately associated with columnar epithelium, merge with invasive squamous cell carcinoma (right).

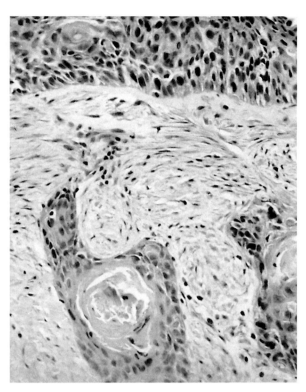

Figure 14-28
SQUAMOUS CELL CARCINOMA
ARISING IN DERMOID CYST
In situ squamous cell carcinoma (top) overlies nests of invasive squamous cell carcinoma.

from epidermis. The remainder of the adult cancers arising in dermoid cysts include: adenocarcinomas, including Paget's disease; adenosquamous carcinoma; undifferentiated carcinomas, including small cell carcinoma; sarcomas (fibrosarcoma, leiomyosarcoma, chondrosarcoma, osteosarcoma, malignant fibrous histiocytoma, rhabdomyosarcoma); and malignant melanoma (85–87,88a,94,96,98,99,101–103). Evidence for origin of a malignant melanoma within a dermoid cyst includes an absence of an extraovarian primary melanoma and the presence of junctional activity within the epidermal lining of the cyst. There have also been rare examples of lymphoma or basal cell carcinoma arising within dermoid cysts (98,100).

Treatment and Prognosis. The treatment is the same as for ovarian cancer in general. In one study, the 5-year survival rate for patients with a stage I squamous cell carcinoma was 77 percent, but it was only 11 percent for patients with higher stage tumors (90). Prognostic factors for stage I tumors in the same study included grade and vascular invasion. Well-differentiated tumors were associated with a 78 percent survival rate, whereas none of the patients with moderately or poorly differentiated tumors survived. The tumors without vascular invasion were associated with a 100 percent survival rate in contrast to no survival in the presence of vascular invasion. Adenocarcinomas behave like squamous cell carcinomas (102). In contrast, almost all patients with sarcomas die of tumor (87,96,98). Carlson and Wheeler (85) found that approximately half of the patients with malignant melanomas with follow-up data died from tumor progression.

REFERENCES

Teratomas

1. Carritt B, Parrington JM, Welch HM, Povey S. Diverse origins of multiple ovarian teratomas in a single individual. Proc Natl Acad Sci USA 1992;79:7400–4.
2. Gibas Z, Talerman A, Faruqi S, Carlson J, Noumoff J. Cytogenetic analysis of an immature ovarian teratoma of the ovary and its metastases after chemotherapy-induced maturation. Int J Gynecol Pathol 1993;12:276–80.
3. Ihara T, Ohama K, Satoh H, Fujii T, Nomura K, Fujiwara A. Histologic grade and karyotype of immature teratoma of the ovary. Cancer 1984;54:2988–94.
4. King ME, DiGiovanni LM, Yung JF, Clarke-Pearson DL. Immature teratoma of the ovary grade 3, with karyotype analysis. Int J Gynecol Pathol 1990;9:178–84.
5. Linder D, McCaw BK, Hecht F. Parthenogenic origin of benign ovarian teratomas. N Engl J Med 1975;292:63–6.
6. Ohama K, Nomura K, Okamoto E, Fukuda Y, Ihara T, Fujiwara A. Origin of immature teratoma of the ovary. Am J Obstet Gynecol 1985;152:896–900.
7. Surti U, Hoffner L, Chakravarti A, Ferrell RE. Genetics and biology of human ovarian teratomas. I. Cytogenetic analysis and mechanism of origin. Am J Hum Genet 1990;47:635–43.

Immature Teratoma

8. Altaras MM, Goldberg GL, Levin W, Darge L, Bloch B, Smith JA. The value of cancer antigen-125 as a tumor marker in malignant germ cell tumors of the ovary. Gynecol Oncol 1986;25:150–9.
9. Anteby EY, Ron M, Revel A, Shimonovitz S, Ariel I, Hurwitz A. Germ cell tumors of the ovary arising after dermoid cyst resection: a long term follow-up study. Obstet Gynecol 1994;83:605–8.
10. Bassler R, Theele C, Labach H. Nodular and tumorlike gliomatosis peritonei with endometriosis caused by a mature ovarian teratoma. Path Res Pract 1982;175:392–403.
11. Bonazzi C, Peccatori F, Colombo N, Lucchini V, Cantu MG, Mangioni C. Pure ovarian immature teratoma, a unique and curable disease: 10 years' experience of 32 prospectively treated patients. Obstet Gynecol 1994;84:598–604.
12. Calame J, Bosman FT, Schaberg A, Louwerens JW. Immunocytochemical localization of neuroendocrine hormones and oncofetal antigens in ovarian teratomas. Int J Gynecol Pathol 1984;3:92–100.
13. Calame J, Schaberg A. Solid teratomas and mixed mullerian tumors of the ovary: a clinical, histological, and immunocytochemical comparative study. Gynecol Oncol 1989;33:212–21.
14. Calder CJ, Light AM, Rollason TP. Immature ovarian teratoma with mature peritoneal metastatic deposits showing glial, epithelial, and endometrioid differentiation: a case report and review of the literature. Int J Gynecol Pathol 1994;13:279–82.
14a. Dadmanesh F, Miller DM, Swenerton KD, Clement PB. Gliomatosis peritonei with malignant transformation. Mod Pathol 1997;10:597–601.
15. Dworak O, Knopfle G, Varchmin-Schultheiss K, Meyer G. Gliomatosis peritonei with endometriosis externa. Gynecol Oncol 1988;29:263–6.
16. Geisler JP, Goulet R, Foster RS, Sutton GP. Growing teratoma syndrome after chemotherapy for germ cell tumors of the ovary. Obstet Gynecol 1994;84:719–21.
17. Gershenson DM, Del Junco G, Silva EG, Copeland LJ, Wharton JT, Rutledge FN. Immature teratoma of the ovary. Obstet Gynecol 1986;68:624–9.
18. Katsube Y, Berg JW, Silverberg SG. Epidemiologic pathology of ovarian tumors: a histopathologic review of primary ovarian neoplasms diagnosed in the Denver standard metropolitan statistical area, 1 July–31 December 1969 and 1 July–31 December 1979. Int J Gynecol Pathol 1982;1:3–16.
19. Kattan J, Droz JP, Culine S, Duvillard P, Thiellet A, Peillon C. The growing teratoma syndrome: a woman with nonseminomatous germ cell tumor of the ovary. Gynecol Oncol 1993;49:395–9.
20. Kawai M, Furuhashi Y, Kano T, et al. Alpha-fetoprotein in malignant germ cell tumors of the ovary. Gynecol Oncol 1990;39:160–6.
21. Kawai M, Kano T, Furuhashi Y, et al. Immature teratoma of the ovary. Gynecol Oncol 1991;40:133–7.
22. Kawai M, Kano T, Kikkawa F, et al. Seven tumor markers in benign and malignant germ cell tumors of the ovary. Gynecol Oncol 1992;45:248–53.
23. Kawata M, Sekiya S, Hatakeyama R, Takamizawa H. Neuron-specific enolase as a serum marker for immature teratoma and dysgerminoma. Gynecol Oncol 1989;32:191–7.
24. Koulos JP, Hoffman JS, Steinhoff MM. Immature teratoma of the ovary. Gynecol Oncol 1989;34:46–9.
25. Metzman RA, Warhol MJ, Gee B, Roth J. Polysialic acid as a marker of both immature and mature neural tissue in human teratomas. Mod Pathol 1991;4:491–7.
26. Miettinen M, Wahlstrom T, Virtanen I, Talerman A, Astengo-Osuna C. Cellular differentiation in ovarian sex-cord-stromal and germ-cell tumors studied with antibodies to intermediate-filament proteins. Am J Surg Pathol 1985;9:640–51.
27. Nakashima N, Fukatsu T, Nagasaka T, Sobue M, Takeuchi J. The frequency and histology of hepatic tissue in germ cell tumors. Am J Surg Pathol 1987;11:682–92.
28. Nielsen SN, Scheithauer BW, Gaffey TA. Gliomatosis peritonei. Cancer 1985;56:2499–503.
29. Nogales FF Jr, Avila IR, Concha A, del Moral E. Immature endodermal teratoma of the ovary: embryologic correlations and immunohistochemistry. Hum Pathol 1993;24:364–70.
30. Nogales FF Jr, Favara BE, Major FJ, Silverberg SG. Immature teratoma of the ovary with a neural component ("solid" teratoma). A clinicopathologic study of 20 cases. Hum Pathol 1976;7:625–42.
31. Norris HJ, Zirkin HJ, Benson WL. Immature (malignant) teratoma of the ovary: a clinical and pathologic study of 58 cases. Cancer 1976;37:2359–72.
32. O'Connor DM, Norris HJ. The influence of grade on the outcome of stage I ovarian immature (malignant) teratomas and the reproducibility of grading. Int J Gynecol Pathol 1994;13:283–9.

33. Perrone T, Steeper TA, Dehner LP. Alpha-fetoprotein localization in pure ovarian teratoma. An immunohistochemical study of 12 cases. Am J Clin Pathol 1987;88:713–7.

34. Perrone T, Steiner M, Dehner LP. Nodal gliomatosis and alpha-fetoprotein production. Two unusual facets of grade I ovarian teratoma. Arch Pathol Lab Med 1986;110:975–7.

35. Robboy SJ, Scully RE. Ovarian teratoma with glial implants on the peritoneum. An analysis of 12 cases. Hum Pathol 1970;1:643–53.

36. Sangruchi T, Sobel RA. Microglial and neural differentiation in human teratomas. Acta Neuropathol 1989;78:258–63.

37. Schwartz PE, Chambers SK, Chambers JT, Kohorn E, McIntosh S. Ovarian germ cell malignancies: the Yale University experience. Gynecol Oncol 1992;45:26–31.

38. Shefren G, Collin J, Soreiro O. Gliomatosis peritonei with malignant transformation: a case report and review of the literature. Am J Obstet Gynecol 1991;164:1617–21.

39. Steeper TA, Mukai K. Solid ovarian teratomas: an immunocytochemical study of thirteen cases with clinicopathologic correlation. Pathol Annu 1984;19:81–92.

40. Thurlbeck WM, Scully RE. Solid teratoma of the ovary. A clinicopathological analysis of 9 cases. Cancer 1960;13:804–11.

41. Trojanowski JQ, Hickey WF. Human teratomas express differentiated neural antigens. An immunohistochemical study with anti-neurofilament, anti-glial filament, and anti-myelin basic protein monoclonal antibodies. Am J Pathol 1984;115:383–9.

42. Vance RP, Geisinger KR, Randall MB, Marshall RB. Immature neural elements in immature teratomas. Am J Clin Pathol 1988;90:397–411.

43. Williams SD, Blessing JA, DiSaia PJ, Major FJ, Ball HG III, Liao S. Second-look laparotomy in ovarian germ cell tumors: the Gynecologic Oncology Group experience. Gynecol Oncol 1994;52:287–91.

44. Yanai-Inbar I, Scully RE. Relation of ovarian dermoid cysts and immature teratomas: an analysis of 350 cases of immature teratoma and 10 cases of dermoid cyst with microscopic foci of immature tissue. Int J Gynecol Pathol 1987;6:203–12.

Mature Solid Teratoma

45. Beilby JO, Parkinson C. Features of prognostic significance in solid ovarian teratoma. Cancer 1975;36:2147–59.

46. Calame JJ, Schaberg A. Solid teratomas and mixed mullerian tumors of the ovary: a clinical, histological, and immunocytochemical comparative study. Gynecol Oncol 1989;33:212–21.

47. diZerega G, Acosta AA, Kaufman RH, Kaplan AL. Solid teratoma of the ovary. Gynecol Oncol 1975;3:93–102.

48. Peterson WF. Solid, histologically benign teratomas of the ovary. A report of four cases and review of the literature. Am J Obstet Gynecol 1956;72:1094–102.

49. Robboy SJ, Scully RE. Ovarian teratoma with glial implants on the peritoneum. An analysis of 12 cases. Hum Pathol 1970;1:643–53.

50. Steeper TA, Mukai K. Solid ovarian teratomas: an immunocytochemical study of thirteen cases with clinicopathologic correlation. Pathol Ann 1984;19:81–92.

51. Thurlbeck WM, Scully RE. Solid teratoma of the ovary. A clinicopathological analysis of 9 cases. Cancer 1960;13:804–11.

Mature Cystic Teratoma

52. Afonso JF, Martin GM, Nisco FS, De Alvarez RR. Melanogenic ovarian tumors. Am J Obstet Gynecol 1962;84:667–76.

53. Amortegui AJ, Kanbour AI. Compound nevus in a cystic teratoma of the ovary [Letter]. Arch Pathol Lab Med 1981;105:115–6.

54. Anteby EY, Ron M, Revel A, Shimonovitz S, Ariel I, Hurwitz A. Germ cell tumors of the ovary arising after dermoid cyst resection: a long term follow-up study. Obstet Gynecol 1994;83:605–8.

55. Ayhan A, Aksu T, Develioglu O, Tuncer S, Ayhan A. Complications and bilaterality of mature ovarian teratomas (clinicopathological evaluation of 286 cases). Aust NZ J Obstet Gynaecol 1991;31:83–5.

56. Bosman FT, Louwerens JK. APUD cells in teratomas. Am J Pathol 1981;104:174–80.

57. Calame J, Bosman FT, Schaberg A, Louwerens JW. Immunocytochemical localization of neuroendocrine hormones and oncofetal antigens in ovarian teratomas. Int J Gynecol Pathol 1984;3:92–100.

58. Calame J, Schaberg A. Solid teratomas and mixed mullerian tumors of the ovary: a clinical, histological, and immunocytochemical comparative study. Gynecol Oncol 1989;33:212–21.

59. Comerci JT Jr, Licciardi F, Bergh PA, Gregori C, Breen JL. Mature cystic teratoma: a clinicopathologic evaluation of 517 cases and review of the literature. Obstet Gynecol 1994;84:22–8.

60. Doss N Jr, Forney JP, Vellios F, Nalick RH. Covert bilaterality of mature ovarian teratomas. Obstet Gynecol 1977;50:651–3.

61. Ein SH. Malignant ovarian tumors in children. J Pediatr Surg 1973;8:539–42.

62. Farrell DJ, Bloxham CA, Scott DJ. Hashimoto's disease in a benign cystic treatoma of the ovary. Histopathology 1991;19:283–4.

63. Fukushima M, Sharpe L, Okagaki T. Peritoneal melanosis secondary to a benign dermoid cyst of the ovary: a case report with ultrastructural study. Int J Gynecol Pathol 1984;2:403–9.

64. Katsube Y, Berg JW, Silverberg SG. Epidemiologic pathology of ovarian tumors: a histopathologic review of primary ovarian neoplasms diagnosed in the Denver standard metropolitan statistical area, 1 July–31 December 1969 and 1 July–31 December 1979. Int J Gynecol Pathol 1982;1:3–16.

65. Kawai M, Kano T, Kikkawa F, et al. Seven tumor markers in benign and malignant germ cell tumors of the ovary. Gynecol Oncol 1992;45:248–53.

66. Kim R, Bohm-Velez M. Familial ovarian dermoids. J Ultrasound Med 1994;13:225–8.

67. Konishi I, Fujii S, Okumura H, et al. Analysis of serum CA125, CEA, AFP, LDH levels and LDH isoenzymes in patients with ovarian tumors—correlation between tumor markers and histological types of ovarian tumors. Acta Obstet Gynaecol Jpn 1986;38:827–36.

68. Koonings PP, Campbell K, Mishell DR Jr, Grimes DA. Relative frequency of primary ovarian neoplasms: a 10-year review. Obstet Gynecol 1989;74:921–6.

69. Lack EE, Goldstein DP. Primary ovarian tumors in childhood and adolescence. Current Prob Obstet Gynecol 1984;7:8–90.

70. Lee D, Pontifex AH. Melanosis peritonei. Am J Obstet Gynecol 1975;122:526–7.

71. McKeel DW Jr, Askin FB. Ectopic hypophyseal hormonal cells in benign cystic teratoma of the ovary. Light microscopic histochemical dye staining and immunoperoxidiase cytochemistry. Arch Pathol Lab Med 1978;102:122–8.

72. Nogales FF, Vergara E, Medina MT. Prostate in ovarian mature cystic teratoma. Histopathology 1995;26:373–5.

73. Pantoja E, Noy MA, Axtmayer RW, Colon FE, Pelegrina I. Ovarian dermoids and their complications. Comprehensive historical review. Obstet Gynecol Surv 1975;30:1–20.

74. Peterson WF, Prevost EC, Edmunds FT, Hundley JM Jr, Morris FK. Benign cystic teratomas of the ovary. Am J Obstet Gynecol 1955;70:368–82.

75. Rubin A, Papadaki L. Multicystic structures appearing in mature cystic teratomas of the ovary: an immunohistochemical and ultrastructural study. Histopathology 1990;17:359-63.

76. Sahin AA, Ro JY, Chen J, Ayala AG. Spindle cell nodule and peptic ulcer arising in a fully developed gastric wall in a mature cystic teratoma. Arch Pathol Lab Med 1990;114:529-31.

77. Ulirsch RC, Goldman RL. An unusual teratoma of the ovary: neurogenic cyst with lactating breast tissue. Obstet Gynecol 1982;60:400-2.

78. Woodfield B, Katz DA, Cantrell CJ, Bogard PJ. A benign cystic teratoma with gastrointestinal tract development. Am J Clin Pathol 1985;83:236–40.

79. Yanai-Inbar I, Scully RE. Relation of ovarian dermoid cysts and immature teratomas: an analysis of 350 cases of immature teratoma and 10 cases of dermoid cyst with microscopic foci of immature tissue. Int J Gynecol Pathol 1987;6:203–12.

80. Zakin D. Radiologic diagnosis of dermoid cysts in the ovary. Obstet Gynecol Surv 1976;31:165–84.

Fetiform Teratoma (Homunculus)

81. Abbott TM, Hermann WJ Jr, Scully RE. Ovarian fetiform teratoma (homunculus) in a 9-year-old girl. Int J Gynecol Pathol 1984;2:392–402.

82. Lord JM. Intra-abdominal foetus-in-fetu. J Pathol Bacteriol 1956;72:627–41.

83. Miyake J, Ireland K. Ovarian mature teratoma with homunculus coexisting with an intrauterine pregnancy. Arch Pathol Lab Med 1986;110:1192–4.

Dermoid Cysts with Secondary Tumors

84. Axiotis CA, Lippes HA, Merino MJ, deLanerollo NC, Stewart AF, Kinder B. Corticotroph cell pituitary adenoma within an ovarian teratoma. A new cause of Cushing's syndrome. Am J Surg Pathol 1987;11:218–24.

85. Carlson JA Jr, Wheeler JE. Primary ovarian melanoma arising in a dermoid stage IIIC: long-term disease-free survival with aggressive surgery and platinum therapy. Gynecol Oncol 1993;48:397-401.

86. Chang DH, Hsueh S, Soong Y. Small cell carcinoma with neurosecretory granules arising in an ovarian dermoid cyst. Gynecol Oncol 1992;46:246–50.

87. Climie AR, Heath LP. Malignant degeneration of benign cystic teratomas of the ovary. Review of the literature and report of a chondrosarcoma and carcinoid tumor. Cancer 1968;22:824–32.

88. Comerci JT Jr, Licciardi F, Bergh PA, Gregori C, Breen JL. Mature cystic teratoma: a clinicopathologic evaluation of 517 cases and review of the literature. Obstet Gynecol 1994;84:22–8.

88a. Davis GL. Malignant melanoma arising in mature ovarian cystic teratoma (dermoid cyst). Report of two cases and literature analysis. Int J Gynecol Pathol 1996;15:356–62.

89. Feuerstein IM, Aronson BL, McCarthy EF. Bilateral ovarian cystic teratomata mimicking bilateral pure ovarian hemangiomata: case report. Int J Gynecol Pathol 1984;3:393–7.

90. Hirakawa T, Tsuneyoshi M, Enjoji M. Squamous cell carcinoma arising in mature cystic teratoma of the ovary. Clinicopathologic and topographic analysis. Am J Surg Pathol 1989;13:397-405.

91. Kallenberg GA, Pesce CM, Norman B, Ratner RE, Silverberg SG. Ectopic hyperprolactinemia resulting from an ovarian teratoma. JAMA 1990;263:2472–82.

92. Kawai M, Kano T, Kikkawa F, et al. Seven tumor markers in benign and malignant germ cell tumors of the ovary. Gynecol Oncol 1992;45:248–53.

93. Madison JF, Cooper PH. A histiocytoid (epithelioid) vascular tumor of the ovary: occurrence within a benign cystic teratoma. Mod Pathol 1989;2:55–8.

94. Manson CM, Cross PA, Herd ME, Wake CR. Mixed adeno- and squamous carcinoma in a mature cystic teratoma in a young woman. Histopathology 1993;23:481–2.

95. Miyazaki K, Tokunaga T, Katabuchi H, Ohba T, Tashiro H, Okamura H. Clinical usefulness of serum squamous cell carcinoma antigen for early detection of squamous cell carcinoma arising in mature cystic teratoma of the ovary. Obstet Gynecol 1991;78:562–6.

96. Ngwalle KE, Hirakawa T, Tsuneyoshi M, Enjoji M. Osteosarcoma arising in a benign dermoid cyst of the ovary. Gynecol Oncol 1990;37:143–7.

97. Palmer PE, Bogojavlensky S, Bhan AK, Scully RE. Prolactinoma in wall of ovarian dermoid cyst with hyperprolactinemia. Obstet Gynecol 1990;75:540–3.

98. Peterson WF. Malignant degeneration of benign cystic teratomas of the ovary. A collective review of the literature. Obstet Gynecol Surv 1957;12:793–830.

98a. Pins MR, Young RH, Daly WJ, Scully RE. Primary squamous cell carcinoma of the ovary. Report of 37 cases. Am J Surg Pathol 1996;20:823–33.

99. Randall BJ, Ritchie C, Hutchison RS. Paget's disease and invasive undifferentiated carcinoma occurring in a mature cystic teratoma of the ovary. Histopathology 1991;18:469–70.

100. Seifer DB, Weiss LM, Kempson KL. Malignant lymphoma arising within thyroid tissue in a mature cystic teratoma. Cancer 1986;58:2459–61.

101. Shimizu S, Kobayashi H, Suchi T, Torii Y, Narita K, Aoki S. Extramammary Paget's disease arising in mature cystic teratoma of the ovary. Am J Surg Pathol 1991;15:1002–6.

102. Ueda G, Fujita M, Ogawa H, Sawada M, Inoue M, Tanizawa O. Adenocarcinoma in a benign cystic teratoma of the ovary: report of a case with a long survival period. Gynecol Oncol 1993;48:259–63.

103. Waxman M, Deppisch LM. Malignant alteration in benign teratomas. In: Damjanov I, Knowles B, Solter D, eds. The human teratomas. Experimental and clinical biology. Clifton NJ: Humana Press, 1983:105–36.

15

MONODERMAL TERATOMAS

STRUMA OVARII

Definition. This is a teratoma in which thyroid tissue is the predominant or sole component, or forms a grossly recognizable component of a more complex teratoma. Neoplasms composed of struma and carcinoid tumor are classified separately as strumal carcinoids (page 295).

General Features. Although meticulous examination of dermoid cysts has revealed thyroid tissue in 20 percent of the cases, this component is recognized grossly in considerably less than 5 percent of the cases. The peak frequency of struma ovarii is in the fifth decade, although occasional cases have been reported in prepubertal and postmenopausal females.

In addition to symptoms and signs caused by the presence of a mass, struma may be associated with a number of unusual clinical manifestations. Ascites occurs in approximately one third of the cases, and occasionally, Meigs' syndrome (ascites and hydrothorax associated with a benign ovarian tumor) is present (page 389) (5). Although many, if not most strumas probably produce thyroid hormones at subclinical levels, clinical evidence of hormone production occurs in only about 5 percent of cases (8,10). Factors complicating accurate determination of the frequency of struma-related hyperthyroidism include the presence of an enlarged thyroid gland in approximately one sixth of patients with struma ovarii (8) and an absence of confirmation of hyperthyroidism by modern laboratory tests in most of the reported cases. In some patients with clinical or laboratory evidence of hyperthyroidism, the preoperative diagnosis of hyperfunctioning struma ovarii has been based on a high ^{131}I uptake in the pelvis (fig. 15-1) with low uptake in the neck. This technique is not entirely reliable in establishing the presence of function, however, since in one case a false-positive result was caused by a hemorrhagic cyst (10a). In other cases function of a tumor was not recognized until symptoms of hyperthyroidism regressed after removal of an ovarian tumor; in some of these cases, a prior thyroidectomy had had no effect on the symptoms. Occasionally, oophorectomy for struma is followed by compensatory enlargement of the thyroid gland with increased uptake of radioactive iodine or an episode of thyrotoxicosis (8,10). Torsion of an ovary containing a struma precipitated striking hyperthyroxinemia in a pregnant patient (7).

Gross Findings. The thyroid tissue is usually recognizable as brown or greenish brown, predominantly solid, gelatinous tissue, usually in pure form (fig. 15-2), and less often associated with a dermoid cyst (fig. 15-3) or mixed with a solid carcinoid tumor as a strumal carcinoid. Some strumas appear as unilocular or multilocular cysts containing brown to green, mucoid or gelatinous fluid (fig. 15-4) (14). Although rare strumas occur in the wall of a mucinous cystadenoma or are admixed with a Brenner tumor (9), the association of approximately one third of strumas with a serous cystadenoma

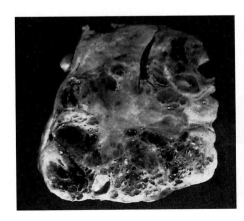 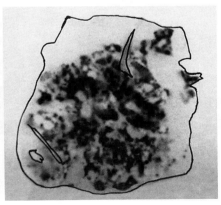

Figure 15-1
STRUMA OVARII,
HYPERFUNCTIONING

Sectioned surface of the gross specimen (left) and the corresponding specimen autoradiograph (right) are shown. (Fig. 2 from Clement PB, Young RH, Scully RE. Clinical syndromes associated with tumors of the female genital tract. Semin Diagn Pathol 1991;8:204-33.)

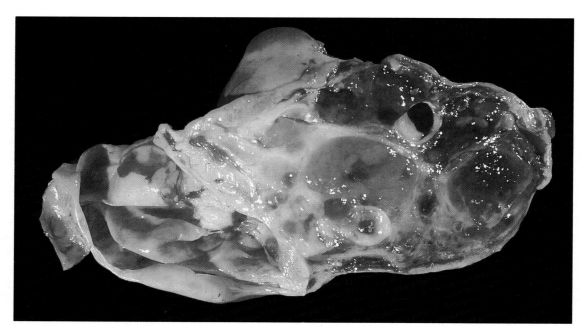

Figure 15-2
STRUMA OVARII
The sectioned surface is solid and cystic. The solid tissue is red to brown with foci of white fibrotic tissue.

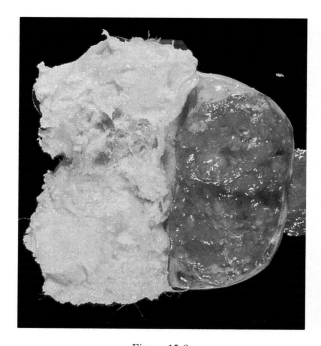

Figure 15-3
STRUMA OVARII
The struma forms a reddish brown solid mass adjacent to a dermoid cyst.

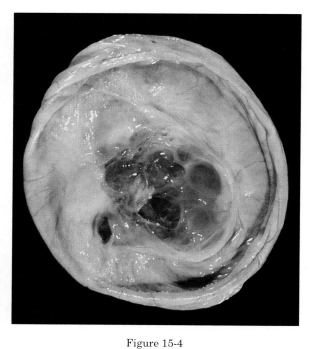

Figure 15-4
STRUMA OVARII, CYSTIC
The largest locule has been opened to reveal a number of smaller locules that contained greenish gelatinous material.

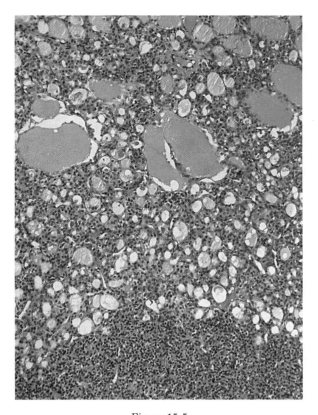

Figure 15-5
STRUMA OVARII
Macrofollicular, microfollicular, and solid areas are seen.

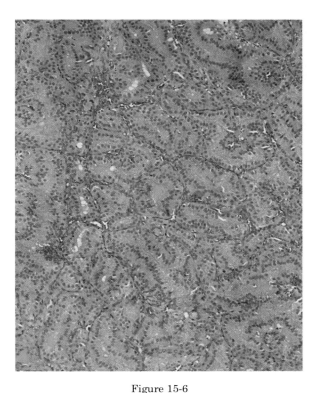

Figure 15-6
STRUMA OVARII
The solid tubular pattern resembles that of a Sertoli cell tumor. (Fig. 105 from Young RH, Clement PB, Scully RE. Pathology of the ovary. In: Sternberg SS, ed. Diagnostic surgical pathology, Vol 2, 2nd ed. New York: Raven Press, 1994:2253.)

reported in the older literature may be due to misinterpretation of the cysts lined by thyroid-type epithelium as serous cysts (14). Occasionally, the contralateral ovary contains a dermoid cyst, and rarely, another struma.

Microscopic Findings. The struma may resemble normal thyroid tissue; a thyroid adenoma, with patterns including macrofollicular, microfollicular, pseudotubular, trabecular, and solid (nests or sheets), alone or in combination (figs. 15-5–15-8); or a thyroid carcinoma. The neoplastic cells typically have bland or minimally atypical nuclei; mitotic figures are sporadic in most cases, although as many as 5 mitotic figures per 10 high-power fields have been encountered in rare cases (14). Colloid within the follicles often contains birefringent calcium oxalate crystals. Oxyphil cells may be present, and occasionally the tumor has the appearance of an oxyphilic thyroid tumor (fig. 15-7). Rare strumas are composed of a prominent or predominant component of clear cells (fig. 15-8) (15). In strumas that are predominantly cystic, the cysts are often lined by nonspecific-appearing, flat to cuboidal epithelial cells, and typical follicles of thyroid type may be only sparsely and focally distributed in the cyst wall or interlocular fibrous septa (fig. 15-9) (14). Occasionally, a struma is admixed with mucinous neoplasia or contains luminal mucin, as might be expected in a mixed endodermal teratoma. Focal "thyroiditis" is an occasional finding. Immunoreactivity of the tumor cell cytoplasm and colloid for thyroglobulin is useful in establishing the diagnosis of struma, especially in cases with unusual patterns or cell types (fig. 15-10) (15).

Uniformly accepted criteria for malignant change in struma have not been established. As in the thyroid gland, a papillary pattern with typical nuclear characteristics of carcinoma (fig. 15-11) or a follicular pattern with few papillae and similar nuclear features provides microscopic evidence of carcinoma.

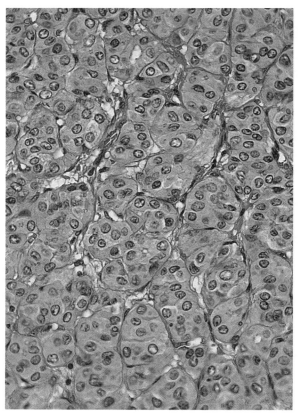

Figure 15-7
STRUMA OVARII
Oxyphilic cells are arranged in nests. (Figures 15-7 and 15-10 are from the same case.)

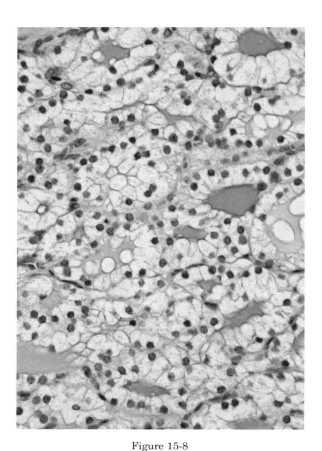

Figure 15-8
STRUMA OVARII
The tumor cells, some of which surround spaces filled with colloid, contain moderate amounts of clear cytoplasm, simulating a clear cell carcinoma (see figure 6-9).

Figure 15-9
STRUMA OVARII, CYSTIC
A cyst is lined by nonspecific-appearing epithelium (arrow). A few small thyroid-type follicles are present within the cyst wall.

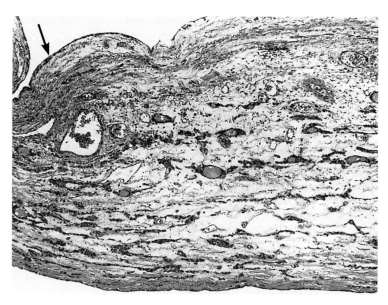

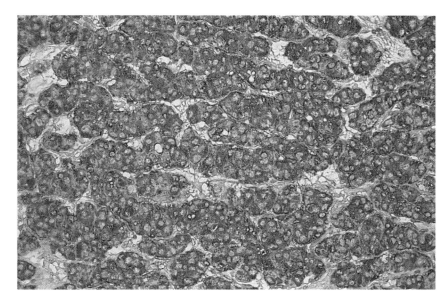

Figure 15-10
STRUMA OVARII
The cells are strongly immunore-
active for thyroglobulin.

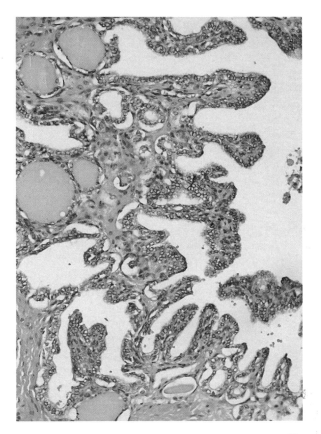 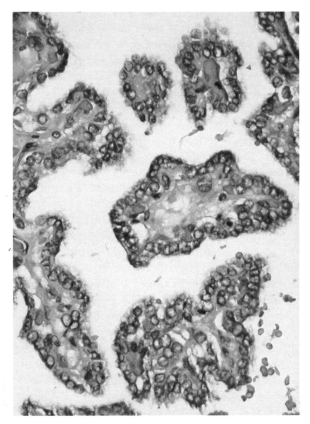

Figure 15-11
STRUMA OVARII WITH PAPILLARY CARCINOMA
Left: The carcinoma (right) merges with thyroid follicles (left).
Right: The characteristic nuclear features of papillary carcinoma are present.

Differential Diagnosis. On gross examination, cystic strumas can be mistaken for mucinous or serous cystic tumors, depending on their content of mucoid or watery fluid, respectively. The green to brown color of the fluid, and on microscopic examination, the focal presence of thyroid follicles in the wall or septa of the cyst, the additional presence of typical struma in some cases, and the occasional association with a dermoid cyst facilitate the diagnosis (14). Rare oxyphilic and clear cell strumas containing few typical thyroid follicles may be mistaken for a variety of oxyphilic cell tumors (see Table 6-1), clear cell carcinomas, and metastatic renal cell carcinomas (15). The tumor may have a solid tubular pattern indistinguishable from that of a well differentiated Sertoli cell tumor, and a prominent microfollicular pattern has occasionally resulted in confusion with the Call-Exner bodies of a granulosa cell tumor (15). In these and other problematic cases, an association with a dermoid cyst or teratomatous elements of another type, the demonstration of foci of typical thyroid follicles, the presence in the eosinophilic secretion of birefringent calcium oxalate crystals, and immunoreactivity for thyroglobulin may be helpful in confirming the thyroid nature of the tumor. Additionally, many of the above tumors in the differential diagnosis have distinctive features inconsistent with a diagnosis of struma.

Just as struma ovarii can mimic a variety of other ovarian tumors, the converse is also true. Clear cell carcinomas, endometrioid carcinomas, Sertoli-Leydig cell tumors, and pregnancy luteomas may contain cystic glands or follicle-like spaces filled with secretion resembling thyroid colloid, but other features of such tumors almost always permit their identification.

A final consideration in the differential diagnosis is the rare follicular carcinoma of the thyroid gland metastatic to the ovary (17). This differential diagnosis is facilitated by knowledge of a primary tumor, the typical patterns of metastatic tumor in the ovary (pages 325 and 357), and the absence of an adjacent dermoid cyst.

Treatment and Prognosis. The treatment of benign struma is oophorectomy. Cases of malignant struma should be treated by oophorectomy and the removal of any extraovarian tumor to the extent that is technically feasible. Some cases of malignant struma with extraovarian spread have been treated successfully with [131]I (16).

Although 5 to 10 percent of strumas have been considered malignant, less than half of such tumors have spread beyond the ovary. Sites of spread include the peritoneum, the contralateral ovary, regional lymph nodes, bone, liver, brain, lungs, and mediastinum (3,6,11,13,16). "Malignant" strumas confined to the ovary have been diagnosed by microscopic criteria alone, and some such cases are now known to be strumal carcinoids. Devaney et al. (2) found that most cases of struma with atypical or malignant features on microscopic examination are not associated with a malignant course. These investigators studied 54 cases of struma, which were subdivided into proliferative (41 cases) and malignant forms (13 cases). A feature of the former group was the presence of densely packed follicles or papillary formations without the distinctive nuclear features of papillary carcinoma, vascular invasion, or mitotic activity. After a mean follow-up interval of 8.7 years, all the patients were clinically free of disease. Eleven of the 13 "malignant" strumas were papillary carcinomas; the others resembled follicular carcinoma with "capsular" and vascular invasion. One of the patients with papillary carcinoma had peritoneal involvement at the time of oophorectomy; the peritoneal lesions were incompletely resected. None of the patients received adjuvant therapy. On follow-up examination (mean follow-up interval, 7.3 years), none of the patients had clinical evidence of disease, including the patient with stage III tumor.

Preliminary data from another study (12) suggest that tumor size, the presence of adhesions or ascites, and a solid microscopic architecture may be associated with an increased frequency of recurrence. Some of the tumors recurred late, one 27 years postoperatively. Another observation from this and other studies (4,6) is that occasional cases of struma associated with extraovarian spread have a histologically benign appearance. In some of these cases, the term "strumosis" has been applied to benign-appearing peritoneal implants detected during oophorectomy or at a later operation (1,4,6). Peritoneal strumosis may be associated with an indolent clinical course, with the implants appearing many years after oophorectomy, and with prolonged survival. No study of an unselected series of cases of struma has been reported to date to determine the frequency of malignant behavior.

CARCINOID TUMORS

Primary carcinoid tumors of the ovary, most forms of which are similar microscopically to those of the gastrointestinal tract, are associated with other teratomatous components in 85 to 90 percent of the cases. In the remainder, the carcinoid component is the exclusive element of the tumor. The impure forms are most often combined with a dermoid cyst, and less commonly, with a struma (strumal carcinoid), a mature solid teratoma, or a cystic mucinous tumor. Tumors containing isolated argentaffin cells that are not aggregated to form a mass, such as some mucinous cystic tumors and heterologous Sertoli-Leydig cell tumors, are not classified as carcinoid tumors. Four types of carcinoid tumor of germ cell origin have sufficiently distinctive clinicopathologic features to warrant specific designations: insular, trabecular, strumal, and goblet cell (mucinous).

Insular Carcinoid Tumor

Definition. This tumor is characterized by a predominant pattern of discrete islands of neoplastic cells, and resembles the intestinal carcinoid tumor that arises in midgut derivatives. The tumor may be pure but is much more often mixed with other components of a teratoma.

General Features. The insular carcinoid is the most common type of primary ovarian carcinoid tumor; approximately 75 cases have been reported. The patients range in age from approximately 30 to 80 years and may present with any of the signs or symptoms of a slow-growing ovarian tumor. In approximately one third of the reported cases the patients had preoperative clinical evidence of the carcinoid syndrome, which disappeared after removal of the tumor. In some patients the syndrome is the presenting manifestation (34). It typically occurs in the absence of extraovarian spread because the ovarian venous drainage, unlike that of the intestine, bypasses the liver, which inactivates the hormones responsible for the syndrome. Patients with the syndrome are almost always over 50 years of age and have larger tumors (over 7 cm in diameter) than those without the syndrome. The manifes-

tations in decreasing order of frequency are: flushing, which may be mistaken for menopausal hot flashes; diarrhea; a murmur of pulmonary stenosis or tricuspid insufficiency, or both; and peripheral edema. Urinary 5-hydroxyindole acetic acid (5-HIAA) levels are typically elevated. The tumor is almost always confined to the ovary at the time of laparotomy, although tumor cells were found in ascitic fluid in one patient (26). Ascites has been noted in occasional other patients, both with and without the syndrome (34). One patient who presented with the carcinoid syndrome also had elevated serum levels of calcitonin (39), and another patient with a mixed insular and trabecular carcinoid tumor had recurrent hyperinsulinemic hypoglycemia (page 381) (31).

Gross Findings. The tumor may appear as a small nodule that protrudes into the lumen or thickens the wall of a dermoid cyst, or rarely, a mucinous cystic tumor (33); may lie within a mature solid teratoma; or may form a large homogenous mass that replaces the ovary (fig. 15-12). The sectioned surfaces are predominantly solid, firm, tan to yellow, and variably fibrous. Cysts filled with clear fluid are occasionally present, and rarely, the tumor is predominantly cystic (fig. 15-12). All the tumors have been unilateral, although the contralateral ovary has contained a dermoid cyst, mucinous tumor, or Brenner tumor in about 15 percent of the cases.

Microscopic Findings. The tumor is characterized by discrete cellular masses and nests separated by a scanty to abundant fibromatous stroma, resembling a midgut carcinoid (fig. 15-13) (34). The tumor cells have round, uniform nuclei containing coarse chromatin and no or rare mitotic figures (figs. 15-14, 15-15). The peripheral cells of the islands typically have abundant cytoplasm that frequently contains prominent red, orange, or brown argentaffin granules (fig. 15-15). Small round acini lined by columnar cells with copious cytoplasm commonly puncture the cellular islands, particularly at their periphery (fig. 15-14). An eosinophilic secretion, which may undergo psammomatous calcification, is typically present in the glandular lumens. The lining cells have a brush border, and may contain argentaffin granules. An intimate relation of the tumor to respiratory (fig. 15-16) or gastrointestinal epithelium is evident in some cases; in other cases, the

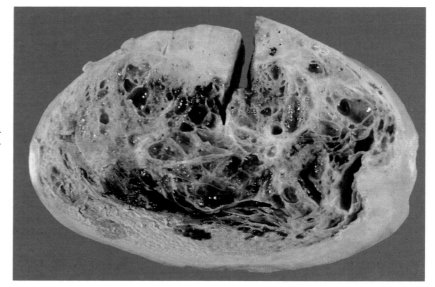

Figure 15-12
INSULAR CARCINOID
The sectioned surface is predominantly cystic, although solid tan-yellow areas are present.

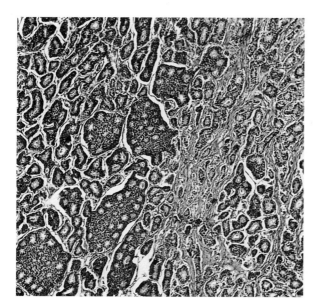

Figure 15-13
INSULAR CARCINOID
Islands perforated by multiple lumens and small, simple glands are characteristic features. The tumor was associated with the carcinoid syndrome. (Fig. 4B from Robboy SJ, Norris HJ, Scully RE. Insular carcinoid primary in the ovary. A clinicopathologic analysis of 48 cases. Cancer 1975;36:404-18.)

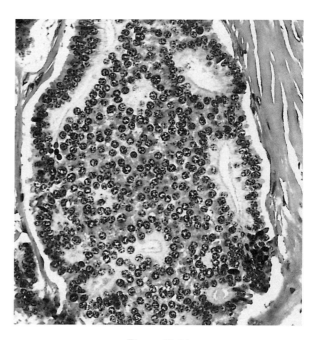

Figure 15-14
INSULAR CARCINOID
Multiple glands lined by columnar cells are present within the periphery of an otherwise solid island. The round nuclei with stippled chromatin are characteristic.

neoplastic tissue is admixed with or abuts a mucinous cystic tumor (33).

Neuron-specific enolase (27), serotonin (45), and chromogranin have been demonstrated immunohistochemically within the tumor cells. In less than 10 percent of the cases, the neoplastic cells are immunoreactive for one or more peptide hormones (43). Pleomorphic, reniform, or dumbbell-shaped dense core granules are present on ultrastructural examination (34).

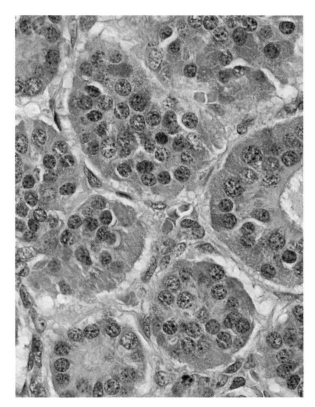

Figure 15-15
INSULAR CARCINOID
Reddish brown cytoplasmic (argentaffin) granules are visible.

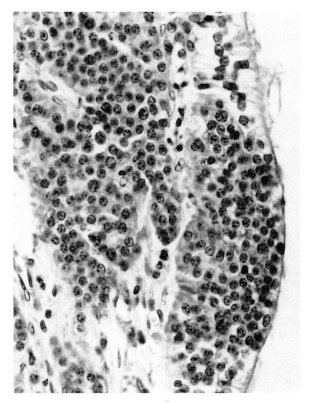

Figure 15-16
INSULAR CARCINOID IN TERATOMA
Carcinoid is present in and to the left of respiratory epithelium that was present in a dermoid cyst. (Fig. 111 from Serov SF, Scully RE, Sobin LH. Histological typing of ovarian tumours. International Histological Classification of Tumours No. 9. Geneva: World Health Organization, 1973.)

Differential Diagnosis. In the absence of teratomatous elements, the tumor can be difficult to distinguish from a metastatic insular carcinoid, which is usually of ileal origin. Evidence favoring or establishing the diagnosis of metastasis in such cases includes the probable or certain presence of an intestinal carcinoid tumor, bilateral involvement, intraovarian growth as multiple nodules, extraovarian metastases particularly to mesenteric lymph nodes and liver, and postoperative clinical or laboratory evidence of the carcinoid syndrome.

The primary tumor most often confused with the insular carcinoid tumor is the microfollicular granulosa cell tumor. This differential is discussed on page 178. Sertoli-Leydig cell tumors may have tubules that simulate the acini of insular carcinoids and their heterologous forms may contain small carcinoid tumors. Other features of the Sertoli-Leydig cell tumor, however, almost always permit a correct diagnosis. Occa-

sionally, a carcinoid tumor is mistaken for adenocarcinoma, a benign or malignant adenofibroma, a Brenner tumor, or a low-grade transitional cell carcinoma, particularly when the fibromatous component of the tumor is abundant, but careful examination of the epithelial elements of each of these tumors enables its identification. In difficult cases, the demonstration of argentaffin or argyrophil granules in a characteristic distribution, immunostaining for chromogranin or a wide variety of peptide hormones, and the electron microscopic demonstration of dense core granules strongly favor or establish the diagnosis of a carcinoid tumor.

Treatment and Prognosis. A primary ovarian carcinoid tumor can be treated as an ovarian cancer with a limited potential for spread. Unilateral salpingo-oophorectomy, however, is only rarely indicated because the tumor almost always occurs in women in the late reproductive and postmenopausal age groups. The postoperative course can be monitored by urinary 5-HIAA determinations.

In cases associated with the carcinoid syndrome, most clinical manifestations disappear after removal of the tumor, with the associated cardiac murmurs decreasing in intensity in a few cases, and elevated 5-HIAA levels returning to normal. Tricuspid insufficiency, however, has persisted or progressed postoperatively in several patients despite the absence of persistent or recurrent tumor (26,33,52). Rare patients have died of intra-abdominal recurrent tumor (33,34, 39) and in one exceptional case, in which systemic metastasis was the presenting manifestation, the tumor was rapidly fatal (39). Two patients with the carcinoid syndrome in whom the tumor was diagnosed at autopsy had ascites and a thick, pearly white, fibrous coating of the visceral and parietal peritoneal surfaces (21,49).

Trabecular Carcinoid Tumor

Definition. This carcinoid tumor resembles those arising in hindgut derivatives, and is characterized by a predominant pattern of elongated, thin trabeculae or ribbons. The tumor almost always contains other teratomatous elements, but when associated with a struma is classified separately as a strumal carcinoid.

General Features. Approximately 25 cases have been reported, almost all in women in the third to sixth decades (24,25,32,36,46). The presenting manifestations are typically related to the presence of a slowly growing neoplasm in the absence of the carcinoid syndrome. Some patients have severe chronic constipation, which is relieved postoperatively (32,54). One patient with a tumor interpreted as a primary trabecular carcinoid had Cushing's syndrome due to adrenocorticotropic hormone (ACTH) production by the tumor (38), but the systemic distribution of that tumor at autopsy, including involvement of the mediastinum and bronchial lymph nodes, suggests that the ovarian tumor was metastatic from an undetected primary pulmonary or thymic carcinoid tumor. Another patient with a mixed insular-trabecular ovarian carcinoid detected at autopsy had a 12-year history of episodic hyperinsulinemic hypoglycemia (31).

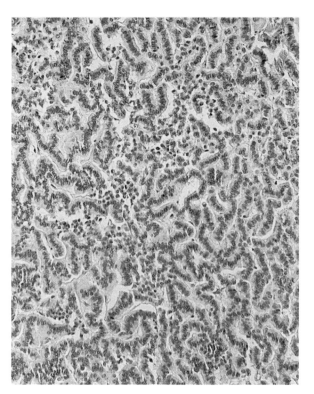

Figure 15-17
TRABECULAR CARCINOID
The winding-ribbon pattern is characteristic.

Gross Findings. The gross findings are similar to those of insular carcinoid. In two cases, a squamous cell carcinoma occurred in the same ovary. None of the tumors have been bilateral, but in a few cases, the contralateral ovary was the site of another type of tumor, usually a dermoid cyst.

Microscopic Findings. This tumor is characterized by long, wavy, parallel ribbons of cells separated by a scanty to abundant fibromatous stroma, creating an appearance similar to that of hindgut carcinoids (figs. 15-17, 15-18). The ribbons are composed of columnar cells, usually one or two cells thick, with oblong nuclei oriented perpendicular to the axis of the ribbons (fig. 15-18). The moderately abundant eosinophilic cytoplasm typically contains argyrophilic granules, and much less commonly, argentaffin granules. The nuclei contain finely dispersed chromatin and occasional mitotic figures. An insular pattern is observed as a minor feature in about 20 percent of the cases. Other teratomatous elements are present in almost all the cases.

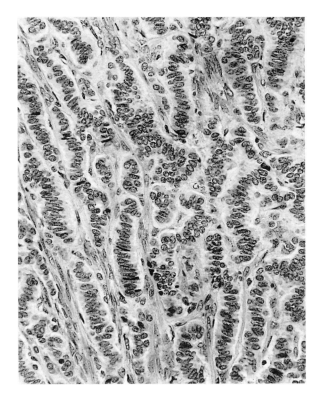

Figure 15-18
TRABECULAR CARCINOID
(Fig. 114 from Serov SF, Scully RE, Sobin LH. Histological typing of ovarian tumours. International Histological Classification of Tumours No. 9. Geneva: World Health Organization, 1973.)

The tumor cells are immunoreactive for chromogranin and synaptophysin in most cases. One or a combination of peptide hormones have been demonstrated in approximately half the cases, including somatostatin, glucagon, pancreatic polypeptide, vasoactive intestinal polypeptide, neurotensin, enkephalin, calcitonin, and ACTH (43). Peptide YY, which has an inhibitory effect on intestinal motility, has been found in four cases, including three cases in which chronic constipation was relieved by oophorectomy (24,32,54). Insulin was found in the cells of the mixed insular-trabecular carcinoid tumor in the patient with hypoglycemia noted above (31). The dense core granules are small, round, and uniform in contrast to those in insular carcinoids (26,47).

Differential Diagnosis. Primary trabecular carcinoids are distinguished from metastatic tumors of the same type by criteria similar to those used for distinguishing primary from metastatic insular carcinoids. A strumal carcinoid can be excluded only by extensive sampling to exclude the presence of thyroid tissue. In an occasional case, the ribbons of a trabecular carcinoid can be confused with unusually long sex cord formations of a Sertoli-Leydig cell tumor, but other features of the latter almost always allow distinction (page 216). Argyrophilia or argentaffinity of the cytoplasm is also helpful in confirming the diagnosis of carcinoid in these cases.

Treatment and Prognosis. The treatment is the same as that for an ovarian cancer with a low malignant potential. No patient with a trabecular carcinoid has died from spread of tumor, although a peritoneal implant was discovered in one patient 2 years after oophorectomy (36).

Strumal Carcinoid Tumor

Definition. This tumor is composed of thyroid tissue and carcinoid, almost always intimately admixed in at least a portion of the specimen. Other teratomatous elements are also present in most of the cases.

General Features. Approximately 80 cases have been reported (19,23,28,30,35,37,40,42,44, 48,50,51). Almost all the patients have been between 30 and 60, with a range of 20 to 78, years of age. The clinical presentation is usually related to the presence of a mass. Only one patient had the carcinoid syndrome, although in 8 percent of the cases various manifestations suggested function of the thyroid component (35). Three patients had chronic constipation relieved by removal of the tumor (32). In one patient, a strumal carcinoid was associated with hyperinsulinemic hypoglycemia and cutaneous melanosis (20) and another patient had multiple endocrine neoplasia, type IIA (Sipple's syndrome) (48). Extraovarian spread at presentation has been documented in only one case, in which multiple nodules of benign-appearing thyroid tissue were found on the pelvic peritoneum at the time of oophorectomy (19).

Gross Findings. In over one third of cases, the tumor appears as a yellow or tan, solid nodule or mass protruding into the cavity of a dermoid cyst or thickening its wall. Somewhat more often, the combination of thyroid and carcinoid components is pure, or almost pure, with varying proportions of each; in some cases, each component

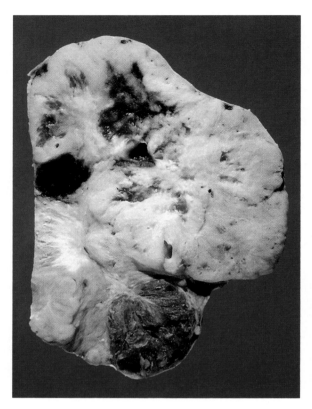

Figure 15-19
STRUMAL CARCINOID
A 4 cm, rounded, brown nodule of struma (bottom) is sharply demarcated from white carcinoid tissue; foci of hemorrhage are present. (Courtesy of Dr. Norval Mortensen, Portsmouth, Va; also fig. 19-1 from Proceedings Thirty-seventh Seminar of the American Society of Clinical Pathologists. Hartman WH, ed. Chicago: American Society of Clinical Pathologists, 1971.)

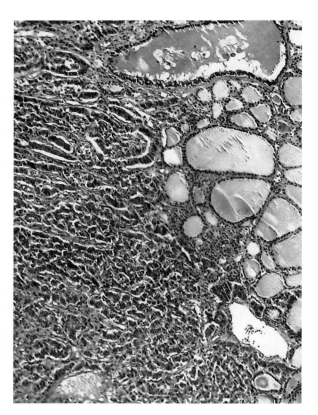

Figure 15-20
STRUMAL CARCINOID
Struma on right merges with trabecular carcinoid on left. (Fig. 70 from Morris JM, Scully RE. Endocrine pathology of the ovary. St. Louis: CV Mosby Co, 1958.)

is recognizable grossly (fig. 15-19). In the remaining cases, the tumor is the predominant constituent of a mature solid teratoma or is a microscopic focus within a mature teratoma. Rarely, the tumor is almost entirely cystic. In one case, the tumor was associated with a mucinous tumor of borderline malignancy (50).

Microscopic Findings. The two components may be only contiguous, but in most cases are intimately admixed; either component may predominate (figs. 15-20, 15-21). The carcinoid exhibits a trabecular pattern in half the cases, a mixed trabecular-insular pattern with the former predominating in most of the remainder, and a pure insular pattern in an occasional specimen. Rarely, the carcinoid component has a solid tubular appearance. The thyroid element usually re-

sembles normal thyroid tissue or a follicular adenoma, and may contain calcium oxalate crystals. In areas where the two components are admixed, carcinoid cells may replace the original epithelial lining of colloid-filled spaces. As a result, argyrophil, and in half the cases, argentaffin granules, are present not only within cells forming trabeculae, but also within those lining adjacent thyroid follicles. Small foci of glands or cysts lined by mucinous epithelium were seen in almost half the tumors in one study (35), and occasional strumal carcinoids contain a component of goblet cell carcinoid (29,35). Rare strumal carcinoids have amyloid in their stroma (30).

The neoplastic cells, particularly within the carcinoid component, are variably immunoreactive for neuron-specific enolase, chromogranin (fig. 15-22, top), synaptophysin, serotonin, and enigmatically, as in some intestinal carcinoid tumors, prostatic acid phosphatase (27,28,41,42,44).

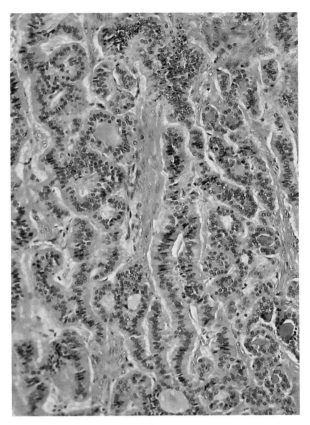

Figure 15-21
STRUMAL CARCINOID
There is an intimate admixture of trabecular carcinoid with a few microfollicles containing colloid.

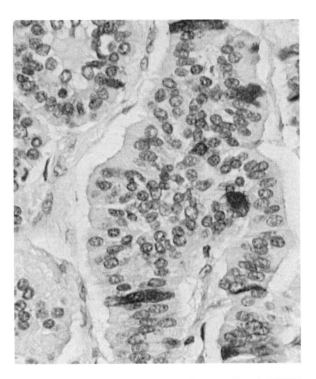

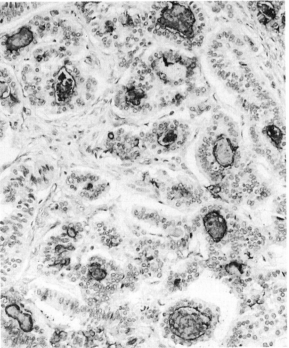

Figure 15-22
STRUMAL CARCINOID
Top: The carcinoid component is immunoreactive for chromogranin.
Bottom: The strumal component is immunoreactive for thyroglobulin.

In 42 percent of the cases in one series, the neoplastic cells were immunoreactive for one or a combination of peptide hormones (43). In another series, all five tumors were positive for one or more peptide hormones, including somatostatin, glucagon, insulin, gastrin, and calcitonin (44). In contrast to medullary carcinoma of the thyroid, the last hormone has been found in only rare cases of strumal carcinoid. Peptide YY was found in the carcinoid component in the three aforementioned patients with chronic constipation (32). The tumor that was associated with hypoglycemia and cutaneous melanosis (page 295) was immunoreactive for insulin and alpha–melanocyte–stimulating hormone (20). Both the strumal component and, occasionally, foci within the carcinoid component of strumal carcinoids are immunoreactive for thyroglobulin (fig. 15-22, bottom). Ultrastructural examination reveals uniform, round, dense core granules within the trabecular cells; the follicles are lined by similar cells of neuroendocrine type, cells of thyroid epithelial type, or a mixture of the two (42,44). In addition, hybrid cells with ultrastructural evidence of both thyroid and carcinoid differentiation have been identified (28,42).

Differential Diagnosis. The pattern of the strumal carcinoid is so distinctive that it is usually easy to distinguish from other neoplasms. Occasional strumal carcinoids with a minor component of thyroid tissue may be misdiagnosed as pure trabecular carcinoids. Because the latter are about one third as common as strumal carcinoids, they should be thoroughly sampled to exclude a strumal component before a diagnosis of pure trabecular carcinoid is rendered. In the older literature, strumal carcinoid was most frequently mislabelled as malignant struma even though it does not resemble closely any of the forms of carcinoma encountered in the thyroid gland, including medullary carcinoma. The ovarian tumor, however, shares some features with the latter; the major differences between the two tumors are summarized elsewhere (35,44).

Treatment and Prognosis. The treatment is that for an ovarian tumor with a very low malignant potential. The tumor extended beyond the ovary in only two reported cases (19,35): one woman, in whom the metastatic tumor consisted only of benign-appearing thyroid tissue, was alive with tumor 1 year after presentation (19); the other patient died from tumor 2.5 years postoperatively (35).

Goblet Cell Carcinoid Tumor

Definition. This tumor is characterized by small acini or solid nests containing a prominent population of goblet and neuroendocrine cells. The tumor resembles the goblet cell or mucinous carcinoid of the appendix.

General Features. Primary goblet cell carcinoids of the ovary are rare and knowledge of them is still incomplete (18,45,53): only two cases have been reported in detail (18,53). The age distribution and clinical presentation are similar to those of other types of ovarian carcinoid tumor. At the time of laparotomy there may be evidence of extraovarian spread. None of these tumors have been associated with the carcinoid syndrome.

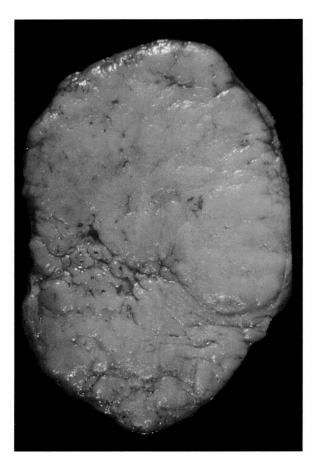

Figure 15-23
GOBLET CELL CARCINOID
The sectioned surface is solid and cream colored.

Pathologic Findings. The tumors resemble other ovarian carcinoid tumors on gross examination (fig. 15-23). They may occur in pure form or be associated with a mature teratoma or an epidermoid cyst. The typical microscopic appearance is that of glands with small or inconspicuous lumens or nests sometimes floating in pools of mucin; the stroma may be scanty or abundant and fibromatous (fig. 15-24). The acini and nests are composed of varying numbers of goblet cells and argyrophil cells, some of which may also be argentaffin (fig. 15-25). Hybrid cells containing both mucin and granules may be present. The nuclei are uniform, small, and round to oval. Small pools of mucin may lie within cystically dilated glands or within the stroma. More poorly differentiated cells, often of signet-ring type, may invade the stroma, singly or in small nests,

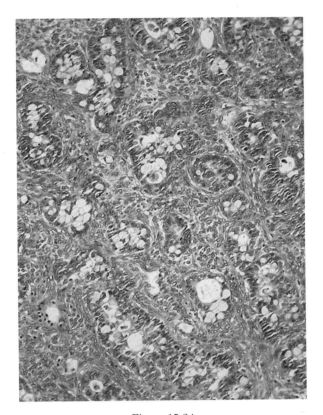

Figure 15-24
GOBLET CELL CARCINOID
Uniform small nests and glands containing goblet cells
lie within a cellular stroma.

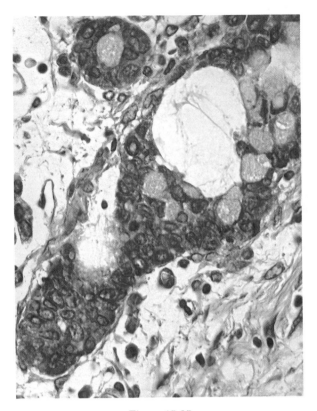

Figure 15-25
GOBLET CELL CARCINOID
Goblet cells and cells filled with reddish brown
(argentaffin) granules are visible.

mimicking the pattern of a Krukenberg tumor. As noted above, occasional mixed goblet cell-strumal carcinoids have been reported (29). Dense core granules have been identified on ultrastructural examination in one of the reported cases (18). Two tumors have been positive immunohistochemically for at least three of the following antigens: carcinoembryonic antigen, pancreatic polypeptide, serotonin, and gastrin (18,53). We have also observed immunoreactivity for chromogranin (fig. 15-26).

Differential Diagnosis. Goblet cell carcinoid metastatic from the appendix or elsewhere is differentiated from the primary form on the basis of operative and pathologic criteria similar to those used for distinguishing metastatic from primary insular carcinoids. Most of the same criteria facilitate the distinction of a primary mucinous carcinoid with a signet-ring carcinomatous component from a Krukenberg tumor. Mucinous tumors of

the ovary, unlike mucinous carcinoid tumors, are typically predominantly cystic on gross examination and are composed of large glands or cysts lined by mucinous epithelium, which frequently contains argyrophil and argentaffin cells. These cells tend to be less numerous than in mucinous carcinoid tumors.

Treatment and Prognosis. The treatment is that of an ovarian tumor with a malignant potential. Although only a small number of cases have been studied, the risk of extraovarian spread is probably greater than in cases of other types of primary ovarian carcinoid tumor. Staging therefore should be performed if the diagnosis is suspected or confirmed by intraoperative frozen section examination. In one of the reported cases, which contained a signet-ring carcinomatous component within the primary tumor, metastatic signet-ring carcinoma was found in the contralateral ovary and the pelvic lymph nodes at the time of

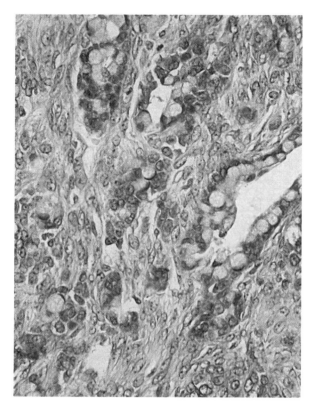

Figure 15-26
GOBLET CELL CARCINOID
Some of the cells are immunoreactive for chromogranin.

exploration (18). The appendix should also be removed for thorough pathologic examination.

Rare Carcinoid Tumors

Rare ovarian carcinoids include those of spindle cell type that resemble their pulmonary counterparts and those with nonspecific, sometimes poorly differentiated patterns (22). These tumors may merge morphologically with ovarian small cell carcinomas of pulmonary type (page 320). Rare carcinoid tumors have a solid tubular pattern, resembling that of a Sertoli cell tumor, or have cells with abundant oxyphilic cytoplasm (see Table 6-1).

NEUROECTODERMAL TUMORS

Definition. These tumors closely resemble neoplasms of the central nervous system, with a similar spectrum of differentiation, ranging from "primitive" and "anaplastic" tumors to differentiated gliomas.

General Features. Less than 50 cases have been reported (55,61). In the only large reported series (61), the patients ranged in age from 6 to 69 years, with differences in the mean age according to the subcategory of tumor: anaplastic (16 years), primitive (23 years), and differentiated (30 years). The presenting symptoms were usually those of a pelvic mass. At laparotomy, 14 of the 25 tumors were stage II or III, usually in the form of peritoneal implants.

Gross Findings. The tumors vary from cystic to solid, ranging from 4 to 20 (mean, 14) cm in diameter (61). Intracystic or surface papillary excrescences are present in some cases. The neoplastic tissue is typically soft and gray-tan, gray-pink, or yellow, often with areas of hemorrhage and necrosis. One tumor (an ependymoma) was bilateral (58), and in several other cases, the contralateral ovary contained a dermoid cyst (57,61).

Microscopic Findings. The 25 cases in the large series mentioned above (61) were subdivided into three categories: differentiated (6 cases), primitive (12 cases), and anaplastic (7 cases). The differentiated tumors were ependymomas; four other ovarian ependymomas have also been described (57,58,60,62). These tumors closely resemble ependymomas of the central nervous system, containing cells with fibrillary cytoplasmic processes (fig. 15-27), which may form perivascular pseudorosettes in addition to occasional true rosettes. Other findings include cysts with a sieve-like appearance, intracystic polypoid structures, papillae (fig. 15-28), tubules and glands, ribbons or columns of cells, and psammoma bodies. In occasional cases, some of the tumor cells have vacuoles that displace the nucleus. Mitotic activity ranges from 1 to 3 per 10 high-power fields. One tumor had a prominent additional component of grade 2 gemistocytic astrocytoma. No teratomatous elements have been identified in any of the reported cases. Metastases generally resemble the primary tumors, but in one of our cases there was a more complex papillary pattern with numerous psammoma bodies, resembling that of a low-grade serous carcinoma.

The primitive tumors resemble primitive neuroectodermal tumors of the central nervous system (figs. 15-29, 15-30). They are typically highly cellular; are composed of small cells with hyperchromatic, round to oval nuclei and scanty

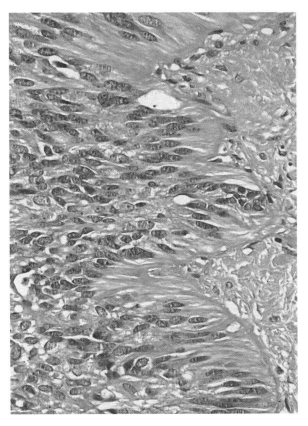

Figure 15-27
EPENDYMOMA
Fibrillary cytoplasmic processes abut a fibrovascular septum.

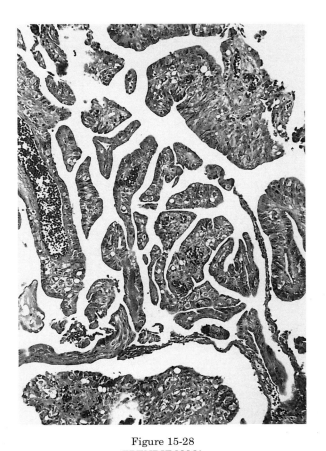

Figure 15-28
EPENDYMOMA
The tumor has a papillary pattern. (Fig. 9 from Kleinman GM, Young RH, Scully RE. Primary neuroectodermal tumors of the ovary. A report of 25 cases. Am J Surg Pathol 1993;17:764-78.)

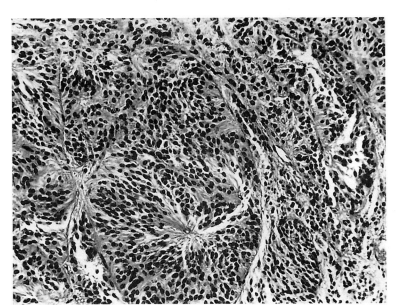

Figure 15-29
PRIMITIVE
NEUROECTODERMAL TUMOR
The tumor is composed of primitive small cells; perivascular rosettes are present.

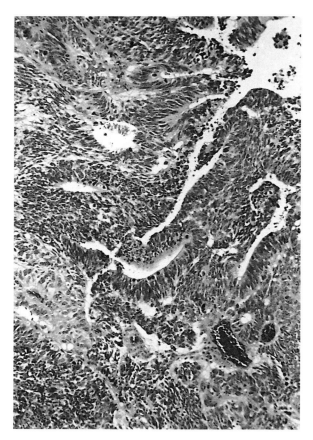

Figure 15-30
PRIMITIVE NEUROECTODERMAL TUMOR
The tumor has a medulloepitheliomatous pattern. (Fig. 12A from Kleinman GM, Young RH, Scully RE. Primary neuroectodermal tumors of the ovary. A report of 25 cases. Am J Surg Pathol 1993;17:764-78.)

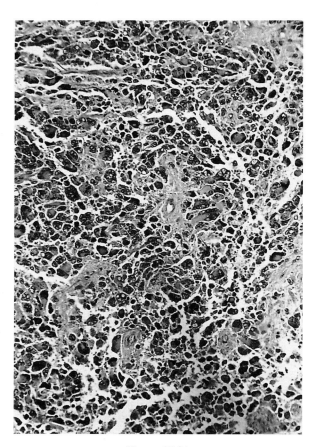

Figure 15-31
ANAPLASTIC NEUROECTODERMAL TUMOR
The tumor resembles a glioblastoma multiforme.

cytoplasm containing varying numbers of finely fibrillar cell processes; and have numerous mitotic figures. The tumor cells are arranged in patternless sheets or lobules separated by fibrovascular septa. Central luminal or central fibrillary rosettes (fig. 15-29) or ribbons reminiscent of embryonal neural tube may be seen. Necrosis, which may be extensive, is common. In the large study cited above, the 12 primitive tumors were subclassified as medulloepithelioma (4 cases) (fig. 15-30), neuroblastoma (3 cases), ependymoblastoma (3 cases), and medulloblastoma (2 cases). Almost half the tumors contained teratomatous elements, usually minor in amount; one tumor was associated with a dermoid cyst. Extraovarian tumor typically resembled the primary tumor, although in one case a medullo-

epithelioma recurred as a mixed astrocytoma and ependymoma.

The anaplastic tumors are moderately to highly cellular and resemble glioblastoma multiforme (fig. 15-31), with areas of necrosis, sometimes surrounded by palisading tumor cells. The tumors cells are arranged in sheets or lobules and contain varying amounts of cytoplasm with eosinophilic fibrillary processes. The nuclei are more pleomorphic than in other neuroectodermal tumors, and multinucleated giant cells are characteristically present. Mitotic figures are numerous, and abnormal forms are usually seen. Minor teratomatous elements are typically encountered.

The fibrillary processes and the tumor cell cytoplasm of ependymomas were immunoreactive for glial fibrillary acidic protein (GFAP) in all the reported cases in which this stain was performed (57,58,60,61). Two anaplastic tumors were also GFAP positive (61). Progesterone receptors were demonstrated immunohistochemically in the primary and recurrent tumor in one case of ependymoma (58).

Differential Diagnosis. Ovarian neuroectodermal tumors should be distinguished from teratomas in which neuroectodermal tissue not resembling tumors of the central nervous system is abundant within the tumor. Rare mature teratomas of the ovary contain large masses composed of several neuroectodermal cell types such as astrocytes, oligodendroglial cells, and ganglion cells. These masses resemble malformations or hamartomas of the central nervous system rather than true neoplasms, and have been interpreted as focal overgrowths within teratomas rather than neuroectodermal tumors (61).

Ovarian neuroectodermal tumors may mimic a variety of primary and metastatic ovarian tumors, most of which are more common. Ependymomas can be mistaken for surface epithelial–stromal tumors, specifically serous and endometrioid borderline tumors and carcinomas; sex cord–stromal tumors, including Sertoli-Leydig cell tumors and granulosa cell tumors; and ovarian tumors of probable wolffian origin. The presence of the characteristic long fibrillary cytoplasmic processes, the perivascular rosettes, and immunoreactivity for GFAP establish the diagnosis of ependymoma in problem cases. The features differentiating ependymomas from other tumors with which they may be confused are discussed in more detail elsewhere (61).

The differential diagnosis of the primitive and anaplastic tumors is generally with grade 2 or 3 immature teratomas. The latter, however, characteristically show a greater spectrum and diversity of neuroepithelial differentiation and a more extensive and varied admixture of endodermal, mesodermal, and other ectodermal tissues. Primitive tumors may also be mistaken for small cell malignant tumors of other types that occur in the ovary of young women (see Table 4-4). Clinical information, thorough sampling of the tumor, and immunohistochemical staining, especially for GFAP, facilitate the diagnosis. Finally, ovarian tumors that are not of germ cell origin, such as malignant mesodermal mixed tumors (59) and heterologous Sertoli-Leydig cell tumors, may contain neuroectodermal tissue (61) (pages 130 and 215).

Treatment and Prognosis. Unilateral salpingo-oophorectomy is probably sufficient for a stage Ia neuroectodermal tumor in a young woman in whom preservation of fertility is desired. The presence of progesterone receptors in the ependymoma noted above, as well as the demonstration of estrogen and progesterone receptors in the cytosol of another ependymoma (56), suggests the possibility that hormone replacement therapy may stimulate growth of the tumor. Stage I as well as higher stage primitive neuroectodermal tumors have been treated with postoperative chemotherapy regimens of the types successfully used for other primitive germ cell tumors, but the results have been disappointing. It seems logical to treat patients with such tumors like patients with similar tumors arising elsewhere, with the inclusion of radiation therapy (61).

The subclassification of ovarian neuroectodermal tumor has important prognostic implications. Ovarian ependymomas tend to have an indolent behavior even when extraovarian spread has occurred. Only one tumor, which was stage III, was fatal (61). In eight other cases with follow-up data, including five stage II or III tumors, the patients were alive, some after successful treatment of one or more recurrences (57,58, 60,62). In contrast, patients with primitive and anaplastic tumors have a poor prognosis if extraovarian spread has occurred. Of those with follow-up data, only one of six patients with stage I disease died of tumor, whereas the 10 patients with stage II or III tumors died of their disease or were alive with tumor at the time of reporting (61).

SEBACEOUS TUMORS

Nine ovarian sebaceous neoplasms, eight of which arose within a dermoid cyst, have been reported (63–65). The women were 31 to 79 years of age (mean, 60 years); all of them had symptoms referable to a pelvic mass. In one case, there was local extension of the tumor into the rectosigmoid (65). On gross examination, the tumors were usually predominantly cystic, containing solid, yellow to tan, nodular or papillary masses projecting into the lumen. All the tumors were unilateral, although the contralateral ovary contained a typical dermoid cyst in some cases. On microscopic examination, the tumors were similar to cutaneous sebaceous neoplasms and included

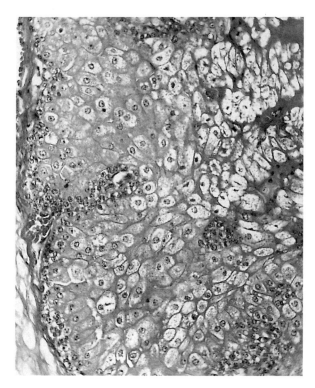

Figure 15-32
SEBACEOUS ADENOMA
Note the orderly maturation from germinative cells (left) to mature, spongy sebaceous cells (center) to holocrine necrobiosis (right).

sebaceous adenoma (5 cases) (fig. 15-32), basal cell carcinoma with sebaceous differentiation (2 cases), and sebaceous carcinoma (2 cases) (63–65). Abundant eosinophilic necrobiotic material with ghost outlines of mature sebaceous cells were present in at least five tumors. One patient with basal cell carcinoma with sebaceous differentiation had a pelvic recurrence 2.5 years after the diagnosis, but in the other cases there were no recurrences or metastases during follow-up periods of 1 to 6 years.

The histologic diagnosis of sebaceous tumor of the ovary is generally not difficult. The presence of large numbers of mature spongy sebaceous cells in a tumor arising within a dermoid cyst is diagnostic. One sebaceous carcinoma, however, was originally misinterpreted as a clear cell adenocarcinoma. The diagnosis of a sebaceous neoplasm should be considered for an ovarian tumor con-

taining spongy or basaloid cells, and in such cases evidence of an origin in a dermoid cyst should be sought.

OTHER MONODERMAL TERATOMAS

Two malignant ovarian tumors interpreted as retinal anlage tumor have been described (69,71). One of them, from a 17-year-old, was a 4-cm pigmented nodule in a stage Ic immature teratoma. Eight months later there was widespread abdominal tumor, and biopsy revealed recurrent retinal anlage tumor. The patient died of disease 30 months after presentation (71). In the other case, a 64-year-old woman had an ovarian tumor with extensive intra-abdominal spread. Only a biopsy of the primary tumor was performed, and the patient died of tumor 5 weeks later. Microscopic examination of the pigmented nodule in the first case and of the biopsy specimen in the second case revealed malignant elements resembling retinal anlage, with mitotically active, melanin-laden cells that formed solid nests and lined tubules, clefts, and cysts. Some of the tubules and cysts contained solid or papillary projections of similar cells. Fibrillary areas with glial cells immunoreactive for GFAP were also present in the first case (71). In another reported case, a benign lesion in the retinal anlage category designated as "pigmented progonoma," was an incidental microscopic finding within a dermoid cyst in an 8-year-old girl (72). A short follow-up interval was uneventful. On microscopic examination, nests and gland-like arrangements of pigmented cuboidal cells were found adjacent to dental elements; nests of small, hyperchromatic, nonpigmented cells occupied some of the gland-like spaces.

Other rare monodermal teratomas include tumors arising from pituitary tissue in dermoid cysts and associated with hyperprolactinemia (page 383) or Cushing's syndrome (page 381), and cysts lined predominantly or exclusively by mature glial tissue (68,70), ependymal epithelium (73), respiratory epithelium (67), or melanotic epithelium (66). Epidermoid cysts, which are lined exclusively by mature squamous epithelium, are placed in the epithelial-stromal category, although there is evidence that at least some of them may be monodermal teratomas (page 162).

REFERENCES

Struma Ovarii

1. Balasch J, Pahisa J, Marquez M, et al. Metastatic ovarian strumosis in an in-vitro fertilization patient. Hum Reprod 1993;8:2075–7.
2. Devaney K, Snyder R, Norris HJ, Tavassoli FA. Proliferative and histologically malignant struma ovarii—a clinicopathologic study of 54 cases. Int J Gynecol Pathol 1993;12:333–43.
3. Hasleton PS, Kelehan P, Whittaker JS, Burslem RW, Turner L. Benign and malignant struma ovarii. Arch Pathol Lab Med 1978;102:180–4.
4. Karseladze AI, Kulinitch SI. Peritoneal strumosis. Pathol Res Pract 1994;190:1086–8.
5. Kempers RD, Dockerty MB, Hoffman DL, Bartholomew LG. Struma ovarii —ascitic, hyperthyroid, and asymptomatic syndromes. Ann Intern Med 1970;72:883–93.
6. Kragel PJ, Devaney K, Merino MJ. Struma ovarii with peritoneal implants: a case report with lectin histochemistry. Surg Pathol 1991;4:274–81.
7. Kung AW, Ma JT, Wang C, Young RT. Hyperthyroidism during pregnancy due to coexistence of struma ovarii and Graves' disease. Postgrad Med J 1990;66:132–3.
8. Marcus CC, Marcus SL. Struma ovarii. A report of 7 cases and a review of the subject. Am J Obstet Gynecol 1961;81:752–62.
9. Moon S, Waxman M. Mixed ovarian tumor composed of Brenner and thyroid elements. Cancer 1976;38:1997–2001.
10. Nieminen U, Von Numers C, Widholm O. Struma ovarii. Acta Obstet Gynecol Scand 1963;42:399–424.
10a. Nodine JH, Maldia G. Pseudostruma ovarii. Obstet Gynecol 1961;17:460–3.
11. Pardo-Mindan FJ, Vazquez JJ. Malignant struma ovarii. Light and electron microscopic study. Cancer 1983;51:337–43.
12. Robboy SJ, Krigman HR, Donohue J, Scully RE. Prognostic indices in malignant struma ovarii: clinicopathologic analysis of 36 patients with 20+ year followup. Mod Pathol 1995;8:95A.
13. Rosenblum NG, LiVolsi VA, Edmonds PR, Mikuta JJ. Malignant struma ovarii. Gynecol Oncol 1989;32:224–7.
14. Szyfelbein WM, Young RH, Scully RE. Cystic struma ovarii: a frequently unrecognized tumor. A report of 20 cases. Am J Surg Pathol 1994;18:785–8.
15. Szyfelbein WM, Young RH, Scully RE. Struma ovarii simulating ovarian tumors of other types. A report of 30 cases. Am J Surg Pathol 1995;19:21–9.
16. Willemse PH, Oosterhuis JW, Aalders JG, et al. Malignant struma ovarii treated by ovariectomy, thyroidectomy, and 131I administration. Cancer 1987;60:178–82.
17. Young RH, Jackson A, Wells M. Ovarian metastasis from thyroid carcinoma 12 years after partial thyroidectomy mimicking struma ovarii: report of a case. Int J Gynecol Pathol 1994;13:181–5.

Carcinoid Tumors

18. Alenghat E, Okagaki T, Talerman A. Primary mucinous carcinoid tumor of the ovary. Cancer 1986;58:777–83.
19. Armes JE, Ostor AG. A case of malignant strumal carcinoid. Gynecol Oncol 1993;51:419–23.
20. Ashton MA. Strumal carcinoid of the ovary associated with hyperinsulinemic hypoglycemia and cutaneous melanosis. Histopathology 1995;27:463–7.
21. Bancroft JH, O'Brien DJ, Tickner A. Carcinoid syndrome due to carcinoid tumor of the ovary. Br Med J 1964;2:1440–1.
22. Czernobilsky B, Segal M, Dgani R. Primary ovarian carcinoid with marked heterogeneity of microscopic features. Cancer 1984;54:585–9.
23. De Wilde R, Raas P, Zubke W, Trapp M, Weidenhammer HG, Luis W. A strumal carcinoid primary in the ovary. Eur J Gynecol Reprod Biol 1986;21:237–40.
24. Fukuda T, Ohnishi Y, Terashima T, Iwafuchi M, Itoh S. Peptide tyrosine-positive ovarian carcinoid tumor arising from a dermoid cyst. Acta Pathol Jpn 1991;41:394–8.
25. Hayashi M, Yabuki Y, Asamoto A, Kohno N, Ohta G. Primary trabecular carcinoid of the ovary. Acta Pathol Jpn 1987;37:837–42.
26. Hilton P, Tweddell A, Wright A. Primary insular argentaffin carcinoma of ovary. Case report and literature review. Br J Obstet Gynaecol 1988;95:1324–31.
27. Inoue M, Ueda G, Nakajima T. Immunohistochemical demonstration of neuron-specific enolase in gynecologic malignant tumors. Cancer 1985;55:1686–90.
28. Kimura N, Sasano N, Namiki T. Evidence of hybrid cell of thyroid follicular cell and carcinoid cell in strumal carcinoid. Int J Gynecol Pathol 1986;5:269–77.
29. Matias-Guiu X, Forteza J, Prat J. Mixed strumal and mucinous carcinoid tumor of the ovary. Int J Gynecol Pathol 1995;14:179–83.
30. Morgan K, Wells M, Scott JS. Ovarian strumal carcinoid tumor with amyloid stroma—report of a case with 20-year follow-up. Gynecol Oncol 1985;22:121–8.
31. Morgello S, Schwartz E, Horwith M, King ME, Gorden P, Alonso DR. Ectopic insulin production by a primary ovarian carcinoid. Cancer 1988;62:800–5.
32. Motoyama T, Katayama Y, Watanabe H, Okazaki E, Shibuya H. Functioning ovarian carcinoids induce severe constipation. Cancer 1992;70:513–8.
33. Robboy SJ. Insular carcinoid of ovary associated with malignant mucinous tumors. Cancer 1984;54:2273–6.
34. Robboy SJ, Norris HJ, Scully RE. Insular carcinoid primary in the ovary. A clinicopathologic analysis of 48 cases. Cancer 1975;36:404–18.
35. Robboy SJ, Scully RE. Strumal carcinoid of the ovary: an analysis of 50 cases of a distinctive tumor composed of thyroid tissue and carcinoid. Cancer 1980;46:2019–34.
36. Robboy SJ, Scully RE, Norris HJ. Primary trabecular carcinoid of the ovary. Obstet Gynecol 1977;49:202–7.
37. Sakura H, Hamada Y, Tsuruta S, Okamoto K, Nakamura S. Large glucagon-like immunoreactivity in a primary ovarian carcinoid. Cancer 1985;55:1001–6.
38. Schlaghecke R, Kreuzpainter G, Burrig KF, Juli E, Kley HK. Cushing's syndrome due to ACTH-production by an ovarian carcinoid. Klin Wochenschr 1989;67:640–4.
39. Sens MA, Levenson TB, Metcalf JS. A case of metastatic carcinoid arising in an ovarian teratoma. Case report with autopsy findings and review of the literature. Cancer 1982;49:2541–6.

40. Senterman MK, Cassidy PN, Fenoglio CM, Ferenczy A. Histology, ultrastructure, and immunohistochemistry of strumal carcinoid: a case report. Int J Gynecol Pathol 1984;3:232–40.

41. Sidhu J, Sanchez RL. Prostatic acid phosphatase in strumal carcinoids of the ovary. An immunohistochemical study. Cancer 1993;72:1673–8.

42. Snyder RR, Tavassoli FA. Ovarian strumal carcinoid: immunohistochemical, ultrastructural, and clinicopathologic observations. Int J Gynecol Pathol 1986;5:187–201.

43. Sporrong B, Falkmer S, Robboy SJ, et al. Neurohormonal peptides in ovarian carcinoids: an immunohistochemical study of 81 primary carcinoids and of intraovarian metastases from six mid-gut carcinoids. Cancer 1982;49:68–74.

44. Stagno PA, Petras RE, Hart WR. Strumal carcinoids of the ovary. An immunohistologic and ultrastructural study. Arch Pathol Lab Med 1987;111:440–6.

45. Talerman A. Carcinoid tumors of the ovary. J Cancer Res Clin Oncol 1984;107:125–35.

46. Talerman A, Evans MI. Primary trabecular carcinoid tumor of the ovary. Cancer 1982;50:1403–7.

47. Talerman A, Okagaki T. Ultrastructural features of primary trabecular carcinoid tumor of the ovary. Int J Gynecol Pathol 1985;4:153–60.

48. Tamsen A, Mazur MT. Ovarian strumal carcinoid in association with multiple endocrine neoplasia, type IIA. Arch Pathol Lab Med 1992;116:200–3.

49. Torvik A. Carcinoid syndrome in a primary tumour of the ovary. Report of a case with extensive peritoneal fibrosis resembling Pick's syndrome. Acta Pathol Microbiol Scand 1960;48:81–8.

50. Tsubura A, Sasaki M. Strumal carcinoid of the ovary. Ultrastructural and immunohistochemical study. Acta Pathol Jpn 1986;36:1383–90.

51. Ulbright TM, Roth LM, Ehrlich CE. Ovarian strumal carcinoid. An immunocytochemical and ultrastructural study of two cases. Am J Clin Pathol 1982;77:622–31.

52. Wilkowske MA, Hartmann LC, Mullany CJ, Behrenbeck T, Kvols LK. Progressive carcinoid heart disease after resection of primary ovarian carcinoid. Cancer 1994;73:1889–91.

53. Wolpert HR, Fuller AF, Bell DA. Primary mucinous carcinoid tumor of the ovary. A case report. Int J Gynecol Pathol 1989;8:156–62.

54. Yaegashi N, Tsuiki A, Shimizu T et al. Ovarian carcinoid with severe constipation due to peptide YY production. Gynecol Oncol 1995;56:302–6.

Neuroectodermal Tumors

55. Aguirre P, Scully RE. Malignant neuroectodermal tumor of the ovary, a distinctive form of monodermal teratoma: report of five cases. Am J Surg Pathol 1982;6:282–92.

56. Auerbach R, Mittal K, Schwartz PE. Estrogen and progestin receptors in an ovarian ependymoma. Obstet Gynecol 1988;71:1043–5.

57. Carlsson B, Havel G, Kindblom LG, Knutson F, Mark J. Ependymoma of the ovary. APMIS 1989;97:1007–12.

58. Carr KA, Roberts JA, Frank TS. Progesterone receptors in bilateral ovarian ependymoma presenting in pregnancy. Hum Pathol 1992;23:962–5.

59. Ehrmann RL, Weidner N, Welch WR, Gleiberman I. Malignant mixed mullerian tumor of the ovary with prominent neuroectodermal differentiation (teratoid carcinosarcoma). Int J Gynecol Pathol 1990;9:272–82.

60. Guerrieri C, Jarlsfelt I. Ependymoma of the ovary. A case report with immunohistochemical, ultrastructural, and DNA cytometric findings, as well as histogenetic considerations. Am J Surg Pathol 1993;17:623–32.

61. Kleinman GM, Young RH, Scully RE. Primary ovarian neuroectodermal tumors. A report of 25 cases. Am J Surg Pathol 1993;17:764–78.

62. Selvaggi SM. Cytologic features of malignant ovarian monodermal teratoma with an ependymal component in peritoneal washings. Int J Gynecol Pathol 1992;11:299–303.

Sebaceous Tumors

63. Chumas JC, Scully RE. Sebaceous tumors arising in ovarian dermoid cysts. Int J Gynecol Pathol 1991;10:356–63.

64. Kaku T, Toyoshima S, Hachisuga T, Enjoji M, Tanaka M. Sebaceous gland tumor of the ovary. Gynecol Oncol 1987;26:398–402.

65. Papadopoulos AJ, Ahmed H, Pakarian FB, Caldwell CJ, McNicholas J, Raju KS. Sebaceous carcinoma arising within an ovarian cystic mature teratoma. Int J Gynecol Cancer 1995;5:76–9.

Other Monodermal Teratomas

66. Anderson MC, McDicken IW. Melanotic cyst of the ovary. J Obstet Gynecol Brit Commonwth 1971;78:1047–9.

67. Clement PB, Dimmick JE. Endodermal variant of mature cystic teratoma of the ovary: report of a case. Cancer 1979;43:383–5.

68. Fogt F, Vortmeyer AO, Ahn G, et al. Neural cyst of the ovary with central nervous system microvasculature. Histopathology 1994;24:477–80.

69. Hameed K, Burslem MR. A melanotic ovarian neoplasm resembling the "retinal anlage" tumor. Cancer 1970;25:564–7.

70. Karten G, Sher JH, Marsh MR, Caruso P, Minkowitz S. Neurogenic cyst of the ovary. A rare form of benign cystic teratoma. Arch Path 1968;86:563–7.

71. King ME, Micha JP, Mouradian JA, Allen SL, Chaganti RS. Immature teratoma of the ovary with predominant malignant retinal anlage component. A parthenogenically derived tumor. Am J Surg Pathol 1985;9:221–31.

72. Sinniah R, O'Brien FV. Pigmented progonoma in a dermoid cyst of the ovary. J Pathol 1973;109:357–9.

73. Tiltman AJ. Ependymal cyst of the ovary. A case report. S Afr Med J 1985;68:424–5.

16
MIXED GERM CELL–SEX CORD–STROMAL TUMORS

These rare tumors are composed of two or three gonadal cell types. The two elements essential for the diagnosis are germ cells and cells of sex cord derivation, which resemble immature Sertoli or granulosa cells. Cells having the appearance of lutein or Leydig cells are also present in most of the cases. These neoplasms can be divided into two categories: gonadoblastoma and an unclassified heterogeneous group.

GONADOBLASTOMA

Definition. This mixed germ cell-sex cord-stromal tumor is composed of germ cells and smaller cells resembling immature sex cord cells; the two cell types are admixed in several distinctive patterns within discrete nests; cells resembling lutein and Leydig cells are usually present between the nests. The germ cells may invade beyond the nests, most commonly as germinoma, and occasionally, as another type of malignant germ cell tumor. The gonadoblastoma almost always occurs in individuals with abnormal gonadal development and a karyotype containing Y-chromosome material.

General Features. The gonadoblastoma occurs almost exclusively in patients with an underlying gonadal disorder, accounting for two thirds of gonadal tumors in such individuals (9). The affected patients are typically children or young adults: about one third of the tumors are detected before the age of 15 years. The clinical picture depends not only on the presence of a tumor mass and its occasional secretion of steroid hormones, but also on the abnormal nature of the underlying gonads and the secondary sex organs. The type of gonadal abnormality may be impossible to determine in cases in which one or both gonads are replaced by tumor. When the underlying sexual disorder is identifiable, it is almost always pure or mixed gonadal dysgenesis (page 399); a Y chromosome is detected in over 90 percent of the cases. Patients with gonadoblastoma are usually phenotypic females, who are typically virilized; a minority are phenotypic males with varying degrees of feminization. Enigmatically, one gonadoblastoma was found to produce prolactin (5).

Gross Findings. The gross appearance of the tumor varies with its size and the presence or absence of an associated malignant germ cell tumor, calcification, or both (figs. 16-1, 16-2). The tumor may be soft and fleshy, firm and cartilaginoid, flecked with calcium or totally calcified, and brown to yellow to grey. Pure gonadoblastomas are typically less than 8 cm in diameter, and 25 percent of them are microscopic; those with germinomatous overgrowth may be

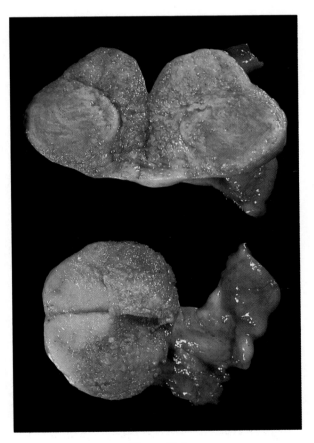

Figure 16-1
GONADOBLASTOMA, BILATERAL,
WITH GERMINOMA
The tumors occurred in a patient with 46,XY pure gonadal dysgenesis. The coarsely granular, pale yellow surfaces of both tumors are due to extensive calcification. In the left pole of the lower tumor, a cream-colored nodule, which was soft, is a germinoma.

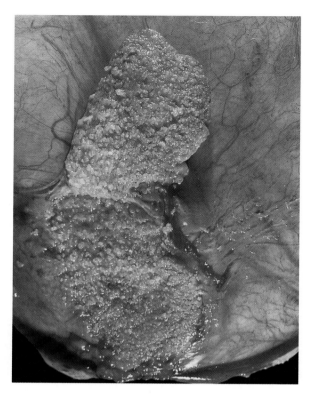

Figure 16-2
GONADOBLASTOMA WITH GERMINOMA
The bisected, calcified, yellow nodule is in the wall of a germinoma, the capsule of which is visible.

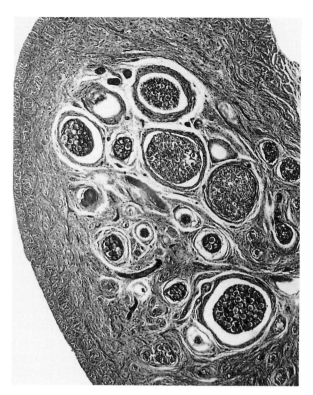

Figure 16-3
GONADOBLASTOMA
Nests of tumor are present within a streak gonad.

much larger. The contralateral gonad contains gonadoblastoma in approximately one third of the cases (fig. 16-1); less often it harbors a malignant germ cell tumor, usually a germinoma, with no trace of underlying gonadoblastoma. The gonad in which a gonadoblastoma develops is of unknown nature in 60 percent of cases, an abdominal or inguinal testis in 20 percent, and a gonadal streak in 20 percent. Extremely rare tumors arise in an apparently normal ovary (7).

Microscopic Findings. The cardinal feature is the presence of discrete or, rarely, diffuse cellular aggregates composed of an intimate admixture of germ cells and smaller epithelial cells of sex cord type (figs. 16-3–16-6) (9). The most common type of germ cell is similar to that of a germinoma (dysgerminoma, seminoma) and usually exhibits mitotic activity; other types of germ cell, some resembling normal immature testicular germ cells and others resembling spermatogonia, have also been described (5a). The smaller, round to oval epithelial cells have pale nuclei, are mitotically inactive, and resemble immature Sertoli or granulosa cells. These cells are immunoreactive for cytokeratin and vimentin, and on ultrastructural examination may contain bundles of Charcot-Bottcher filaments (8), consistent with a Sertoli cell nature. The sex cord–type cells surround circular spaces filled with eosinophilic basement membrane material, line the periphery of nests that contain germ cells centrally, or envelop individual germ cells (figs. 16-5, 16-6). The epithelial nests are separated by a scanty to abundant fibrous stroma. Stromal Leydig or lutein cells are present in two thirds of the cases (fig. 16-5). Rare, otherwise typical gonadoblastomas have focal patterns of the types encountered in the unclassified mixed germ cell-sex cord-stromal tumors discussed in the next section (1).

The typical histologic appearance of a gonadoblastoma can be altered or obliterated by: an

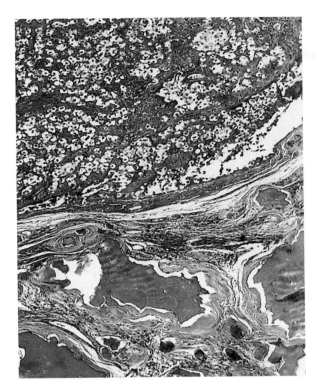

Figure 16-4
GONADOBLASTOMA WITH GERMINOMA
Calcified plaques are present in the gonadoblastoma
component in the lower half.

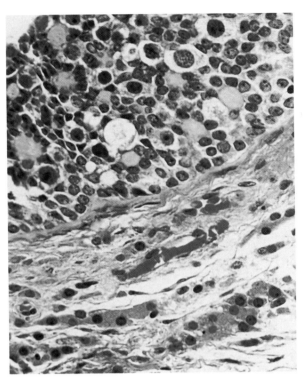

Figure 16-5
GONADOBLASTOMA
Small sex cord–type cells surround germ cells as well as
rounded spaces filled with eosinophilic basement membrane
material. Nests of steroid-type cells are present within the
adjacent stroma. (Fig. 116 from Serov SF, Scully RE, Sobin
LH. Histological typing of ovarian tumours. International
Histological Classification of Tumours No. 9. Geneva: World
Health Organization, 1973.)

extensive deposition of hyalinized basement
membrane material; calcification, which is present in over 80 percent of the cases, typically as
laminated plaques and mulberry-like masses
(fig. 16-4); or overgrowth by a malignant germ
cell tumor, which occurs in approximately 60
percent of the cases. In over 80 percent of the
cases, the associated malignant tumor is a
germinoma (figs. 16-4, 16-6), which may vary in
extent from microscopic penetration into the
stroma to massive replacement of the gonad. Less
commonly, one or more other types of primitive
germ cell tumor such as yolk sac tumor, embryonal carcinoma, choriocarcinoma, or immature
teratoma overgrow the gonadoblastoma (2,4,10).

Differential Diagnosis. Gonadoblastoma
can be confused with a pure dysgerminoma and
a sex cord tumor with annular tubules (SCTAT)
(page 220). The presence of a dysgerminoma or
seminoma in a patient with abnormal gonads
should raise the suspicion of its origin in a gonadoblastoma; the only clue to the presence of the

latter may be a tiny focus of calcification or a rare
nest of typical gonadoblastoma. The SCTAT resembles the gonadoblastoma because of its similar growth pattern and the presence of basement membrane material and calcification, but
it contains no germ cells. Gonadoblastoma
should also be distinguished from the unclassified germ cell-sex cord-stromal tumors discussed
below. Finally, microscopic gonadoblastoma-like
foci have been found in 15 percent of normal
fetuses and newborn infants in one study (6).

Treatment and Prognosis. Gonadoblastoma
without an invasive germ cell component is clinically benign, but due to the high frequency with
which it gives rise to a malignant germ cell tumor,
it should be regarded as an in situ malignant germ
cell tumor. The treatment is bilateral gonadec-
tomy except in the very rare cases in which the

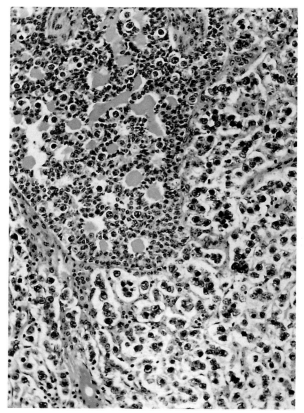

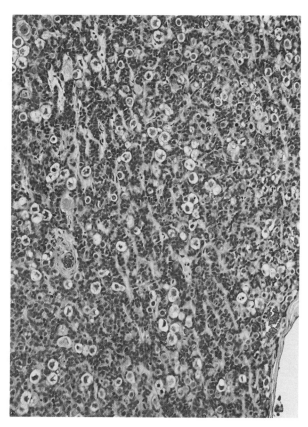

Figure 16-6
GONADOBLASTOMA AND GERMINOMA
The gonadoblastoma is in the upper left. (Fig. 117 from Serov SF, Scully RE, Sobin LH. Histological typing of ovarian tumours. International Histological Classification of Tumours No. 9. Geneva: World Health Organization, 1973.)

Figure 16-7
GERM CELL–SEX CORD TUMOR, UNCLASSIFIED
Cells with abundant clear cytoplasm are scattered within long, anastomosing cords and trabeculae composed predominantly of smaller cells.

tumor has arisen within an otherwise normal ovary in a woman with a normal karyotype and no underlying gonadal disorder (3,7).

GERM CELL–SEX CORD–STROMAL TUMORS, UNCLASSIFIED

This category includes all tumors that contain germ cells, sex cord elements, and occasionally, lutein or Leydig-type cells, but lack the distinctive patterns of the gonadoblastoma (11–18). These neoplasms usually occur in infants or girls under the age of 10 years with normal gonadal development and a normal karyotype. Occasional examples have caused isosexual precocity (12,15), and one bilateral tumor has been reported (11).

The few such tumors that have been observed in the ovary have varied in appearance. Exami-

nation reveals an infiltrative growth of sex cord and germ cell elements, with each component varying widely in amount from one case to another (figs. 16-7–16-9). The combination of cells may grow in diffuse masses, broad cords likened to the Pfluger tubules (sex cords) of the developing ovary, or small solid tubules similar to those of the Sertoli cell adenoma of the androgen insensitivity syndrome. Rarely, the sex cord cells grow in retiform patterns (17). The sex cord elements may be less mature than in the gonadoblastoma. The germ cells have large round nuclei without prominent nucleoli in most cases (fig. 16-8), but in some cases they resemble closely the cells of a dysgerminoma (fig. 16-9, right). Hyaline bodies and calcified foci, characteristic of gonadoblastoma, are few or absent. An associated dysgerminoma, or

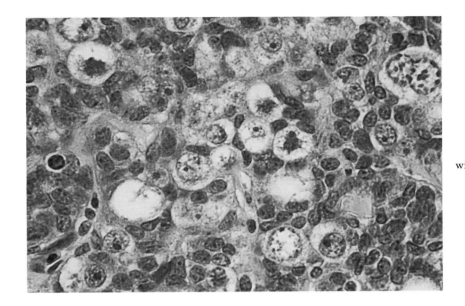

Figure 16-8
GERM CELL–SEX CORD
TUMOR, UNCLASSIFIED
The large germ cells are admixed
with the smaller sex cord–type cells.

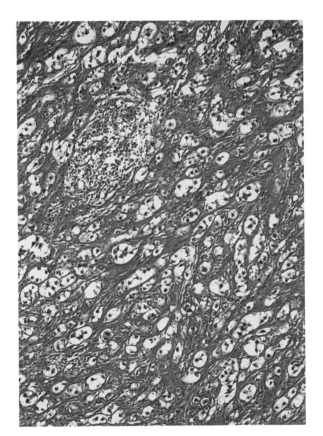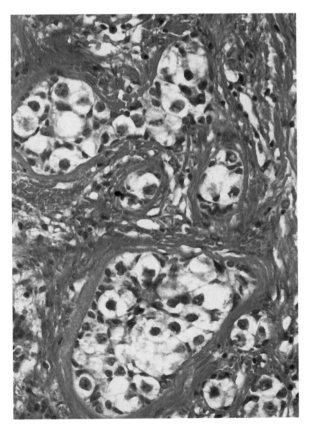

Figure 16-9
GERM CELL–SEX CORD TUMOR, UNCLASSIFIED
Left: Clusters of clear germ cells and small sex cord–type cells lie in a dense fibrous stroma.
Right: The germ cells have the appearance of dysgerminoma cells.

rarely a more malignant germ cell tumor, has been encountered in some cases.

Two otherwise typical tumors of this type also had a component that the authors interpreted as surface epithelial (16,18). In one of these cases (16), however, it was considered to be a retiform sex cord component by another observer (14). In the second case, mucinous epithelium lined glands and cysts of intestinal type (18).

The tumors are usually clinically benign, but two of them, one of which was fatal, metastasized (12). The metastases had a microscopic appearance similar to that of the primary tumor.

REFERENCES

Gonadoblastoma

1. Bhathena D, Haning RV Jr, Shapiro S. Coexistence of a gonadoblastoma and mixed germ cell-sex cord stroma tumor. Path Res Pract 1985;180:203–8.
2. Bremer GL, Land JA, Tiebosch A, Van Der Putten HW. Five different histological subtypes of germ cell malignancies in an XY female. Gynecol Oncol 1993;50:247–8.
3. Erhan Y, Toprak AS, Ozdemir N, Tiras B. Gonadoblastoma and fertility. J Clin Pathol 1992;45:828–9.
4. Hart WR, Burkons DM. Germ cell neoplasms arising in gonadoblastomas. Cancer 1979;43:669–78.
5. Hoffman WH, Gala RR, Kovacs K, Subramanian MG. Ectopic prolactin secretion from a gonadoblastoma. Cancer 1987;60:2690–5.
5a. Jorgensen N, Müller J, Jaubert F, Clausen OP Skakkebaek NE. Heterogeneity of gonadoblastoma germ cells: similarities with immature germ cells, spermatogonia and testicular carcinoma in situ cells. Histopathology 1997;30:177–86.
6. Kedzia H. Gonadoblastoma: structures and background of development. Am J Obstet Gynecol 1983;147:81–5.
7. Nakashima K, Nagasaka T, Fukata S, et al. Ovarian gonadoblastoma with dysgerminoma in a woman with two normal children. Hum Pathol 1989;20:814–6.
8. Roth LM, Eglen DE. Gonadoblastoma. Immunohistochemical and ultrastructural observations. Int J Gynecol Pathol 1989;8:72–81.
9. Scully RE. Gonadoblastoma. A review of 74 cases. Cancer 1970;25:1340–56.
10. Talerman A. Gonadoblastoma associated with embryonal carcinoma. Obstet Gynecol 1974;43:138–42.

Mixed Germ Cell-Sex Cord-Stromal Tumors, Unclassified

11. Jacobsen GK, Braendstrup O, Talerman A. Bilateral mixed germ cell sex-cord stroma tumour in a young adult woman. Case report. APMIS Suppl 1991;23:132–7.
12. Lacson AG, Gillis DA, Shawwa A. Malignant mixed germ cell-sex cord-stromal tumors of the ovary associated with isosexual precocious puberty. Cancer 1988;61:2122–33.
13. Talerman A. A distinctive gonadal neoplasm related to gonadoblastoma. Cancer 1972;30:1219–24.
14. Talerman A. A combined germ cell-gonadal stromal-epithelial tumor of the ovary or a hamartoma [Letter]. Am J Surg Pathol 1984;8:638–9.
15. Talerman A, van der Harten JJ. A mixed cell-sex cord stroma tumor of the ovary associated with isosexual precocious puberty in a normal girl. Cancer 1977;40:889–94.
16. Tavassoli FA. A combined germ cell-gonadal stromal-epithelial tumor of the ovary. Am J Surg Pathol 1983;7:73–84.
17. Tokuoka S, Aoki Y, Hayaski Y, et al. A mixed germ cell-sex cord-stromal tumor of the ovary with retiform tubular structure: a case report. Int J Gynecol Pathol 1985;4:161–70.
18. Zuntova A, Motlik K, Horejsi J, Eckschlager T. Mixed germ cell-sex cord stromal tumor with heterologous structures. Int J Gynecol Pathol 1992;11:227–33.

17
MISCELLANEOUS PRIMARY TUMORS

Although most primary ovarian tumors belong in the surface epithelial, sex cord–stromal, or germ cell category, a great variety of rarer neoplasms are of other or uncertain lineage. These tumors are the subject of this chapter.

SOFT TISSUE–TYPE TUMORS

Leiomyoma

Approximately 40 ovarian leiomyomas have been reported, (4,6,8,9,12,13,17,18) and we have seen 14 additional cases. The tumors have occurred in patients from the second through eighth decades; approximately 80 percent arise in premenopausal women. The tumors are incidental findings in most of the cases. Two tumors were associated with ascites and hydrothorax (Meigs' syndrome) (18) and one woman, whose tumor was accompanied by adjacent hilus cell hyperplasia, experienced virilization due to an elevated plasma testosterone level (12). On gross examination the tumors usually do not exceed 5 cm in diameter but occasional massive tumors have been described (6). The tumors resemble their uterine counterparts (fig. 17-1) and like them, may undergo cystic degeneration. Histologically, they are also similar to leiomyomas encountered elsewhere (fig. 17-2) and can show many of the

variations observed in uterine smooth muscle tumors (8). Mitotic activity may be seen but because of the rarity of mitotically active smooth muscle tumors of the ovary and the absence of long-term follow-up data on a significant number of cases (13), a mitotic count that justifies a diagnosis of sarcoma is currently unknown. On the basis of our experience with mitotically active cellular fibromas (page 197) we advise long-term follow-up to detect possible late recurrence of mitotically active leiomyomas. Leiomyomas may arise from smooth muscle in the hilus or blood vessel walls or from foci of smooth muscle metaplasia of the ovarian stroma, which are occasionally evident in regions of the ovary uninvolved by a leiomyoma.

The diagnosis of leiomyoma is usually straightforward. Typically the cells have fibers emanating from either end of a cigar-shaped nucleus. The abundant intercellular collagen seen in fibromas as well as their frequent storiform pattern are typically absent in leiomyomas. Epithelioid leiomyomas can simulate a variety of other neoplasms composed of oxyphilic or clear cells; in some cases immunostaining for desmin and other smooth muscle markers may be crucial in establishing the diagnosis. We have seen a symplastic (bizarre) leiomyoma of the ovary, large ovarian leiomyomas in a case of leiomyomatosis

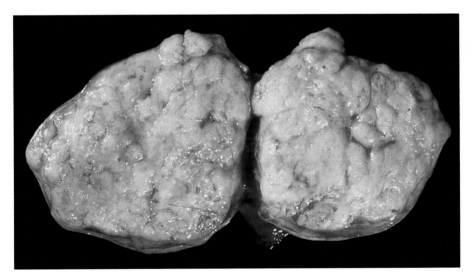

Figure 17-1
LEIOMYOMA
The tumor has a lobulated sectioned surface.

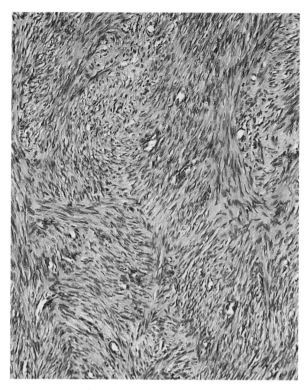

Figure 17-2
LEIOMYOMA
Spindle cells are arranged in intersecting fascicles.

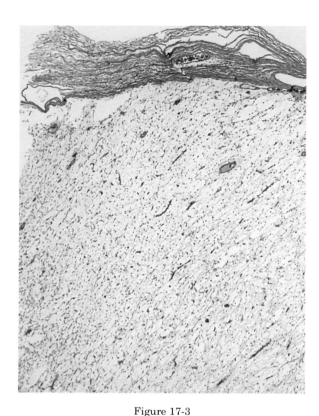

Figure 17-3
MYXOMA
The weakly basophilic tumor is well circumscribed and contains numerous fine blood vessels.

peritonealis disseminata, and a case of intravenous leiomyomatosis in which the ovarian mass was considered the probable source of the intravenous extension.

Myxoma

Sixteen ovarian neoplasms have been reported under the designation "myxoma" (1–3,11a,16). Almost all of them occurred in patients in the reproductive age group who had an asymptomatic unilateral adnexal mass. The tumors were 11 cm in average diameter and usually had soft sectioned surfaces, often with foci of cystic degeneration. Microscopic examination shows the characteristic features of a myxoma (figs. 17-3, 17-4): small tumor cells widely scattered on a background of pale basophilic to eosinophilic fluid. The tumors contain a prominent plexus of vessels (fig. 17-4) resembling those of a myxoid liposarcoma, but lipoblasts are absent. The neoplastic cells are bland and spindle shaped (fig.

17-4) or stellate with long tapering cytoplasmic processes. Tumors in the thecoma-fibroma group may contain minor foci consistent with myxoma, and we have seen one myxoma mixed with a sclerosing stromal tumor, suggesting that at least some myxomas are of ovarian stromal cell origin (1). One myxoma contained several nodules of typical leiomyoma. Ultrastructural and immunohistochemical studies show the cells to have features of myofibroblasts (2).

The differential diagnosis of ovarian myxoma includes other ovarian lesions characterized by abundant intercellular fluid such as massive edema and various low-grade sarcomas with myxoid features. Recognition of bland cytologic features, including a virtual absence of mitotic figures, should permit the distinction of a myxoma from a myxoid sarcoma. The diagnosis of myxoma should be made with caution in the presence of even slight cytologic atypia and occasional mitoses in view of recurrence in one case with such

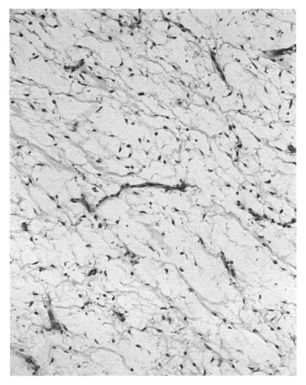

Figure 17-4
MYXOMA
The small cells have bland nuclear features. Numerous delicate blood vessels are present.

features after 19 years (16). Distinction of a myxoma from massive edema (page 416) depends on the recognition of the typical features of a myxoma, including staining of the intercellular material with colloidal iron and alcian blue and abolition of staining by pretreatment with hyaluronidase, as well as the absence of follicles and their derivatives within the tumor.

Hemangioma

A small number of ovarian hemangiomas have been reported. A few have been associated with isolated hemangiomas elsewhere or generalized hemangiomatosis (10); some have been incidental findings at autopsy. One patient with bilateral hemangiomas also had thrombocytopenia, which was cured by removal of the tumors (7). A few tumors have been reported to contain lutein cells in their stroma with associated evidence of hormonal function (14). One hemangioma lay adja-

cent to a mixed germ cell tumor in a patient with Turner's syndrome (15). An infantile hemangioendothelioma from a newborn has been reported (13a). Hemangiomas are most commonly situated in the medulla and hilus and are usually of the cavernous type. They must be distinguished from the large collections of closely packed vessels in the ovarian medulla that are present normally in older women and from the spaces containing red blood cells that may be seen in degenerating steroid cell tumors (pages 227, 230, and 236).

Other Benign Soft Tissue–Type Tumors

One or a few benign neural tumors, lipomas, lymphangiomas, chondromas, osteomas, and ganglioneuromas have been described in the ovary (5,11,14a). Their features are as seen elsewhere in the body.

Sarcomas

Rare pure or apparently pure sarcomas such as fibrosarcomas (20,27,28,31,34,36,38), leiomyosarcomas including the myxoid variant (21,23,29, 32,35), malignant schwannomas (39), lymphangiosarcomas, angiosarcomas (30a,33), and osteosarcomas (25,26,37) may arise from the ovarian stroma or the nonspecific supporting tissue of the ovary. Other tumors of these types as well as rhabdomyosarcomas, which are mostly embryonal but may be alveolar (22,24); chondrosarcomas (40); and at least one osteogenic sarcoma (30) result from overgrowth of one component of a complex malignant tumor such as a malignant mesodermal mixed tumor, adenosarcoma, immature teratoma, or heterologous Sertoli-Leydig cell tumor; or arise in a dermoid cyst. Some apparently pure sarcomas may reflect incomplete sampling of more complex tumors. Rare sarcomas of various types have been associated with surface epithelial–stromal tumors, particularly serous, mucinous, and clear cell carcinomas (pages 72, 94, and 144) (19, 41,42). The clinical picture is usually that of a rapidly growing adnexal mass. An unusual manifestation of alveolar rhabdomyosarcoma of the ovary is clinical simulation of leukemia caused by diffuse bone marrow involvement (30b).

The appearances of ovarian sarcomas are similar to those seen in other organs and tissues and similar diagnostic criteria apply in their differential diagnosis. The distinction of a fibrosarcoma

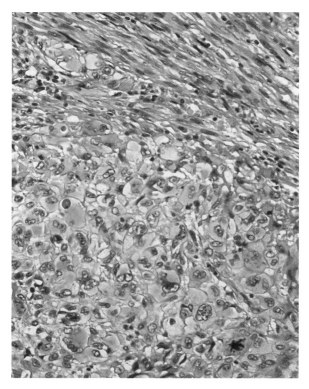

Figure 17-5
EPITHELIOID LEIOMYOSARCOMA
Typical leiomyosarcoma is seen above and epithelioid cells with abundant eosinophilic cytoplasm below. An atypical mitotic figure is evident.

from a cellular fibroma is discussed on page 197. Exceptionally, soft tissue-type fibromatosis presents as an ovarian mass, but it extensively involves adjacent tissues as well (30c).

The criteria for separating cellular leiomyomas from leiomyosarcomas in the ovary are not well established due to the paucity of cases of each that have been investigated. Some leiomyosarcomas with high mitotic activity contain only minimally atypical nuclei and lack coagulative tumor cell necrosis, and infarct-type necrosis is not particularly helpful in the differential diagnosis of large cellular ovarian tumors. Most leiomyosarcomas, however, have obviously malignant microscopic features. Epithelioid leiomyosarcomas (fig. 17-5) may cause an additional problem by resembling other clear cell or oxyphilic tumors (see Table 6-1). A yolk sac tumor with prominent myxoid areas (32) is occasionally confused with a myxoid leiomyosarcoma but the variety of pat-

terns and primitive appearance of the former, and if necessary, immunostaining for alpha-fetoprotein, should resolve the problem.

SMALL CELL CARCINOMA, HYPERCALCEMIC TYPE

Definition. This undifferentiated carcinoma is composed predominantly of small cells with scanty cytoplasm in most cases although large cells with abundant cytoplasm coexist in some cases and occasionally predominate. The tumor is usually associated with paraendocrine hypercalcemia.

General Features. The tumor occurs in females from 2 to 46 (average, 24) years of age (43, 45,50,51,53,54). Rarely, it is familial, as was exemplified in one family by its occurrence in three sisters (54). Those tumors were all bilateral in contrast to the 1 percent frequency of bilaterality in general. Approximately two thirds of the tumors are accompanied by paraendocrine hypercalcemia, accounting for half the ovarian tumors associated with this disorder in the literature. Approximately 50 percent of small cell carcinomas of hypercalcemic type have spread beyond the ovary at the time of laparotomy.

Gross Findings. The tumors are usually large and predominantly solid, cream-colored (fig. 17-6) to gray masses, closely resembling ovarian lymphomas and dysgerminomas. Areas of necrosis and hemorrhage are often present. Cystic degeneration is common but only rare neoplasms are predominantly cystic; one tumor was a unilocular cyst (50).

Microscopic Findings. The most common pattern is a diffuse arrangement of small, closely packed epithelial cells (fig. 17-7) with scanty cytoplasm and small round, ovoid, or rarely, spindle-shaped nuclei containing single small nucleoli (fig. 17-8). Mitotic figures are frequent. The tumor cells also grow in small islands (fig. 17-9), clusters, cords, and trabeculae. Follicle-like structures lined by tumor cells are present in 80 percent of the cases (fig. 17-10) (54). These spaces almost always contain eosinophilic fluid (fig. 17-10) but rarely their content is basophilic. In approximately half the tumors a small, or occasionally, large proportion of the neoplastic cells have abundant eosinophilic cytoplasm (fig. 17-11), which sometimes takes the form of a pale eosinophilic globule (fig. 17-12) (54). The large cells have larger, paler nuclei with

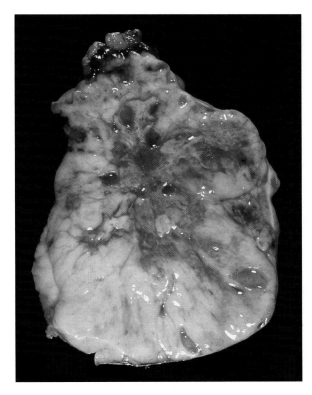

Figure 17-6
SMALL CELL CARCINOMA,
HYPERCALCEMIC TYPE
The sectioned surface is lobulated and composed of fleshy cream-colored tissue resembling that of a dysgerminoma or lymphoma, with focal hemorrhage and necrosis. (Fig.1 from Young RH, Oliva E, Scully RE. Small cell carcinoma of the ovary, hypercalcemic type. A clinicopathological analysis of 150 cases. Am J Surg Pathol 1994;18:1102–16.)

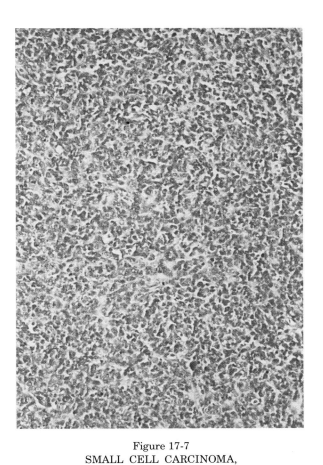

Figure 17-7
SMALL CELL CARCINOMA,
HYPERCALCEMIC TYPE
There is a diffuse growth of small cells with scanty cytoplasm.

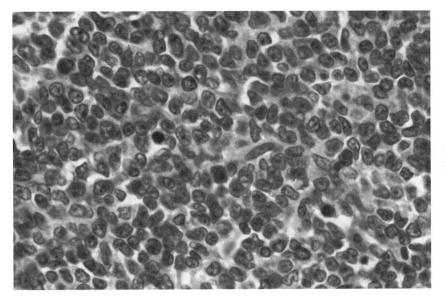

Figure 17-8
SMALL CELL CARCINOMA,
HYPERCALCEMIC TYPE
The tumor cells have hyperchromatic nuclei and scanty cytoplasm; nucleoli are evident in some of the nuclei.

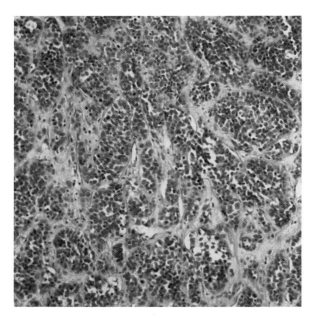

Figure 17-9
SMALL CELL CARCINOMA,
HYPERCALCEMIC TYPE
The tumor cells are growing in nests.

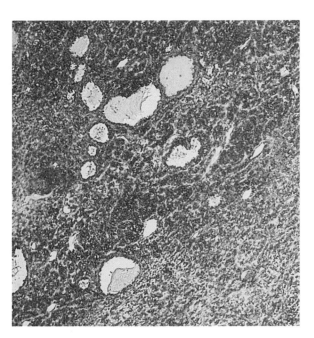

Figure 17-10
SMALL CELL CARCINOMA,
HYPERCALCEMIC TYPE
Follicle-like structures of varying sizes containing eosinophilic material are present within a densely cellular tumor.

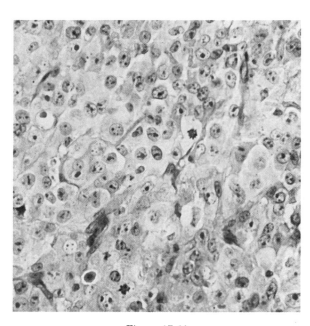

Figure 17-11
SMALL CELL CARCINOMA, HYPERCALCEMIC
TYPE, LARGE CELL VARIANT
The tumor cells have abundant eosinophilic cytoplasm and central nuclei, many of which have prominent nucleoli. (Fig. 12 from Young RH, Oliva E, Scully RE. Small cell carcinoma of the ovary, hypercalcemic type. A clinicopathological analysis of 150 cases. Am J Surg Pathol 1994;18:1102–16.)

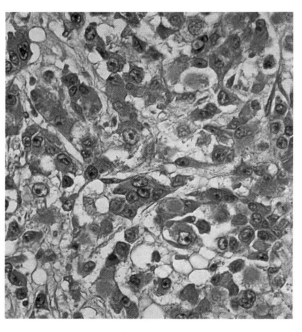

Figure 17-12
SMALL CELL CARCINOMA, HYPERCALCEMIC
TYPE, LARGE CELL VARIANT
The cells have eosinophilic cytoplasm, which forms globules in some cells. A few cells have eccentric nuclei.

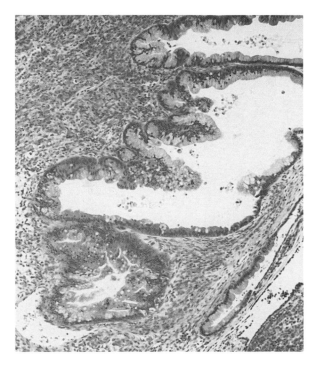

Figure 17-13
SMALL CELL CARCINOMA,
HYPERCALCEMIC TYPE
Several mucinous glands, some of which are lined by atypical epithelium, are present.

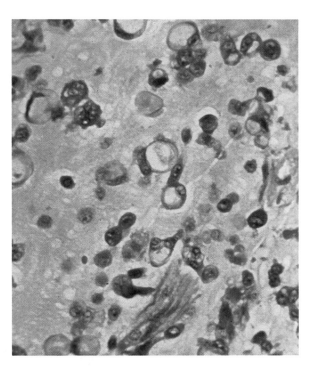

Figure 17-14
SMALL CELL CARCINOMA,
HYPERCALCEMIC TYPE
Signet-ring cells lie in a sea of basophilic mucin. (Fig. 9 from Young RH, Oliva E, Scully RE. Small cell carcinoma of the ovary, hypercalcemic type. A clinicopathological analysis of 150 cases. Am J Surg Pathol 1994;18:1102–16.)

prominent nucleoli. In approximately 10 percent of the tumors small foci of benign-appearing mucinous epithelium lining glands or cysts, malignant-appearing mucin-containing cells admixed with mucin-free neoplastic cells, or isolated signet-ring cells are seen (figs. 17-13–17-15) (54). The tumor stroma is typically inconspicuous but is occasionally prominent and may be edematous or myxoid. In most cases electron microscopic examination has shown an epithelial appearance of the tumor cells, which characteristically contain abundant dilated rough endoplastic reticulin (46,52). Large tumor cells may contain whorls of microfilaments; dense core granules are absent or rare. The cells stain variably for vimentin, cytokeratin, and epithelial membrane antigen (44). Flow cytometry on paraffin-embedded material has shown that the tumor cells are diploid (47).

Differential Diagnosis. Small cell carcinoma is most commonly misinterpreted as a granulosa cell tumor of either the adult or juvenile type. Differentiation of the latter tumors

from small cell carcinoma has been discussed on pages 177 and 185. Small cell carcinomas can also be confused with malignant lymphomas, particularly when the former have a diffuse pattern or when the latter have an insular pattern or rarely, form spaces simulating follicles. The much more common presence of epithelial growth patterns, including follicle-like structures in the small cell carcinoma, and the differing clinical, cytologic, immunohistochemical, and ultrastructural features of the two tumors permit their distinction. Small cell carcinomas are occasionally misinterpreted as other small cell malignant tumors that involve the ovary (see Table 5-4) such as primitive neuroectodermal tumors (page 300), primary or metastatic malignant melanoma (page 354), metastatic alveolar rhabdomyosarcoma (page 356), and desmoplastic small round cell tumor (page 357), but a variety of clinical and pathologic features generally facilitate these diagnoses.

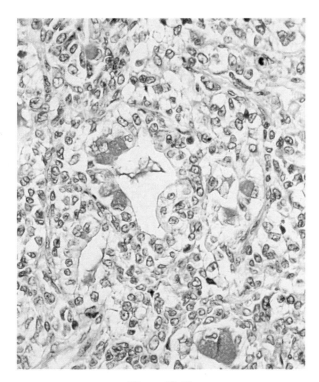

Figure 17-15
SMALL CELL CARCINOMA,
HYPERCALCEMIC TYPE
Several glands are lined by tumor cells, some of which
contain mucin. (Mucicarmine stain)

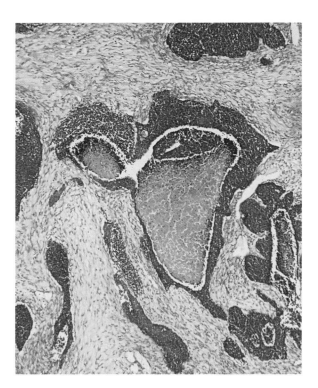

Figure 17-16
SMALL CELL CARCINOMA, PULMONARY TYPE
Large nests of small cells are centrally necrotic.

The designation "small cell carcinoma" must not lead to its confusion with the better known small cell carcinoma of pulmonary type, which may be seen in the ovary as a primary (see below) (49) or metastatic tumor (page 353) (48).

Treatment and Prognosis. Small cell carcinomas of hypercalcemic type have a very poor prognosis. In a recent large study only one third of patients with stage IA tumors had a disease-free follow-up, which ranged from 1 to 13 (average, 5.7) years (54). Most of the patients with higher stage tumors died of their disease, usually within 2 years, and the remainder had progressive disease at relatively short postoperative intervals. Rare patients with high-stage tumors who received intensive chemotherapy, radiation therapy, or both were alive up to 6.5 years postoperatively. Features in stage IA cases that appear to be associated with a more favorable outcome include a patient age greater than 30 years, a normal preoperative calcium level, a tumor

diameter under 10 cm, an absence of large cells, an operation that includes bilateral oophorectomy, and postoperative radiation therapy (54).

SMALL CELL CARCINOMA, PULMONARY TYPE

Definition. This tumor is composed of cells similar to those of the typical small cell undifferentiated carcinoma of the lung.

General Features. The 11 reported tumors of this type occurred in women 28 to 85 (mean, 59) years of age; the clinical presentation was similar to that of other ovarian cancers (49). At laparotomy five tumors were bilateral and most had spread beyond the ovary.

Gross Findings. The tumors are typically large, with a mean diameter of 13.5 cm, and solid, occasionally with a minor cystic component.

Microscopic Findings. Microscopic examination shows sheets, closely packed islands (fig. 17-16), and trabeculae composed of small to medium-sized round to spindle cells, which have

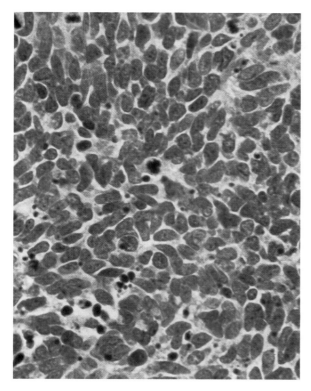

Figure 17-17
SMALL CELL CARCINOMA, PULMONARY TYPE
The tumor cells have scanty cytoplasm and hyperchromatic nuclei, which are molded and mostly lack recognizable nucleoli.

scanty cytoplasm and hyperchromatic nuclei with stippled chromatin and inconspicuous nucleoli (fig. 17-17). A component of endometrioid carcinoma was present in four tumors, another neoplasm had foci of squamous differentiation, another contained a cyst lined by atypical mucinous cells, and two others were associated with a Brenner tumor. Argyrophil granules were present focally in two of six tumors and immunohistochemical staining showed that six of nine tumors were immunoreactive for keratin, five for epithelial membrane antigen, seven for neuron-specific enolase, two for chromogranin, and one for Leu-7; vimentin staining was absent (49). Flow cytometry disclosed that five tumors were aneuploid and three diploid. Electron microscopic examination was not performed in the reported series of cases.

Differential Diagnosis. The many differing clinical and pathologic features of small cell carcinomas of pulmonary and hypercalcemic types (page 316) should permit their differentiation.

Primary ovarian small cell carcinomas of pulmonary type must also be distinguished from metastatic tumors from the lung and, occasionally, other sites. The distinction is made mainly on the basis of the usual association of the primary form with neoplastic elements of surface epithelial type (49) and clinical identification of an extraovarian primary tumor. As with the hypercalcemic form of small cell carcinoma, the differential diagnosis of the pulmonary form includes many other primary and metastatic ovarian tumors that are characterized by small cells with scanty cytoplasm (see Table 5-4).

Prognosis. Five of 10 patients with follow-up information died of, or with, disease at 1 to 13 (mean, 8) months; one died after an unknown interval. Three other patients had recurrent or residual disease after a follow-up period of less than 1 year; only one was alive after a long interval (7 1/2 years) (49).

UNDIFFERENTIATED CARCINOMA, NON-SMALL CELL NEUROENDOCRINE TYPE

Eight of these tumors, each of which was admixed with a surface epithelial tumor (seven mucinous and one endometrioid), have been reported in women 22 to 77 years of age (55–58). The neuroendocrine component of the mixed tumors, which are typically unilateral, usually has gross features indistinguishable from those of other ovarian cancers. Six of the tumors were stage I; one, stage II, and one, stage III.

On microscopic examination the neuroendocrine component is composed predominantly of sheets, closely packed islands, and cords and trabeculae of epithelial cells with little intervening stroma. The tumor cells are of medium to large size and contain scanty to moderate amounts of cytoplasm (fig. 17-18) and large nuclei, which may have central macronuclei. In most of the cells staining was positive for argyrophil granules and immunostaining was positive for chromogranin (fig. 17-19), neuron-specific enolase, and serotonin; neuropeptide hormones were detected in scattered cells in a number of the tumors. The prognosis was poor in all the cases with follow-up information; some of the patients had hematogenous metastases composed of the undifferentiated neuroendocrine component of the tumor.

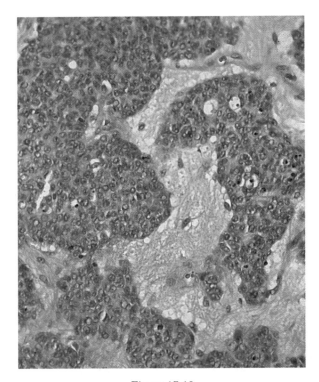

Figure 17-18
UNDIFFERENTIATED CARCINOMA,
NON-SMALL CELL NEUROENDOCRINE TYPE
Tumor cells of moderate size are growing in nests and trabeculae.

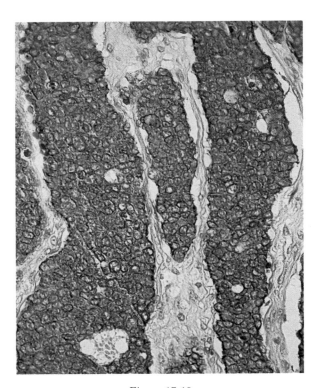

Figure 17-19
UNDIFFERENTIATED CARCINOMA,
NON-SMALL CELL NEUROENDOCRINE TYPE
The tumor cells are strongly immunoreactive for chromogranin.

The diagnosis of this type of tumor is usually suggested by orderly trabecular and insular growth patterns, and the uniform malignant nuclei. It is important that the tumor be distinguished from the less malignant carcinoid tumor by the greater atypia of the former, but distinction from small cell carcinoma of the pulmonary type, which is based on nuclear size, does not appear to have prognostic significance. The association with surface epithelial neoplasia is a strong clue to the primary nature of the neoplasm but if such a component were absent, use of other criteria to exclude a metastatic non-small cell carcinoma of neuroendocrine type would be necessary (see chapter 18).

"ADENOID CYSTIC"
AND BASALOID CARCINOMAS

Eight ovarian tumors with an exclusive or conspicuous component resembling adenoid cystic carcinoma (see page 71; figs. 3-42, 17-20) and six other tumors with an exclusive or predominant component resembling basal cell carcinoma (fig. 17-21) have been reported (59,59a,59b). Six of the seven tumors in the adenoid cystic category, five of which were stage III, contained a component of surface epithelial neoplasia (serous, endometrioid, mixed clear cell and endometrioid carcinomas, and a serous borderline tumor) (59). These tumors were designated "adenoid cystic" because unlike salivary gland adenoid cystic carcinomas they were negative immunohistochemically for S-100 protein and actin, indicating absence of a myoepithelial component. One tumor was designated adenoid cystic because it contained myoepithelial cells (59a), and another tumor, which also contained myoepithelial-like cells, was interpreted as either an adenoid cystic carcinoma or a basal cell adenoma of salivary gland type (59b). Almost all the patients were in the seventh to eighth decade. The prognosis was

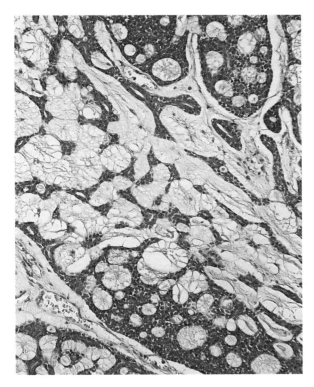

Figure 17-20
OVARIAN CARCINOMA
RESEMBLING ADENOID CYSTIC CARCINOMA

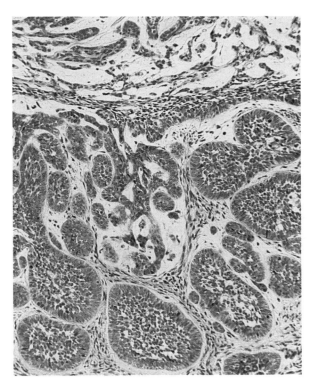

Figure 17-21
OVARIAN CARCINOMA WITH BASALOID
AND AMELOBLASTOMA-LIKE FEATURES

poor except in one case in which the surface epithelial component was a serous borderline tumor, and another tumor that was pure and occurred in a 45-year-old woman (59a).

The patients whose carcinomas were predominantly or entirely basaloid presented at an age range of 19 to 65 years. Several of the tumors contained foci of squamous differentiation and gland formation and one had a minor component of endometrioid adenocarcinoma. In three cases the carcinomas had an ameloblastoma-like pattern. Most of the tumors were stage IA; the prognosis was excellent with relatively limited follow-up periods (16 to 71 months).

The evidence suggests that most tumors in this category are variants of surface epithelial carcinomas. Rarely, however, prominent stromal hyalinization in a sex cord-stromal tumor results in a resemblance to an adenoid cystic carcinoma. In such cases other more characteristic patterns of sex cord neoplasia facilitate the diagnosis.

HEPATOID CARCINOMA

Definition. This tumor resembles hepatocellular carcinoma and hepatoid carcinoma of the stomach, and stains immunohistochemically for alpha-fetoprotein (AFP).

General Features. Six of the seven known patients with this tumor were postmenopausal and one was in the reproductive age group (60–61a). The symptoms were nonspecific. Five of the seven tumors had spread beyond the ovary at the time of presentation.

Pathologic Findings. The tumor has no distinctive gross features. Microscopic examination reveals sheets, trabeculae, and cords of cells with moderate to large amounts of eosinophilic cytoplasm and round to oval central nuclei resembling, to varying extents, hepatocytes (fig. 17-22); hyaline bodies may be conspicuous. Some of the tumor cells can be stained immunohistochemically for AFP (fig. 17-23). An admixture with serous (fig. 17-24) or another surface epithelial carcinoma in some cases supports a surface epithelial lineage of the tumor.

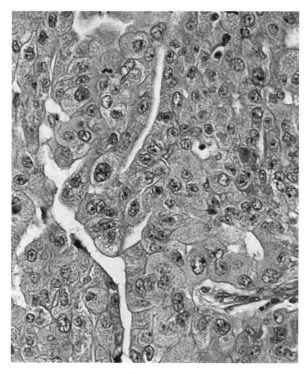

Figure 17-22
HEPATOID CARCINOMA
The tumor cells have abundant eosinophilic cytoplasm and nuclei with prominent nucleoli.

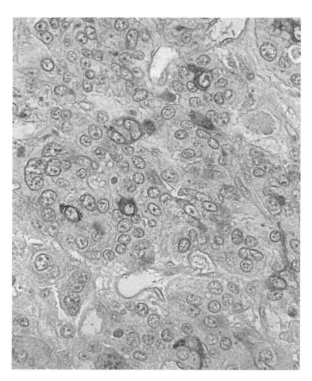

Figure 17-23
HEPATOID CARCINOMA
Several of the tumor cells are immunoreactive for alpha-fetoprotein.

Differential Diagnosis. This tumor must be distinguished from hepatocellular carcinoma metastatic to the ovary (62) (page 348) and other ovarian tumors characterized by cells with abundant eosinophilic cytoplasm (see Table 6-1), particularly the hepatoid yolk sac tumor (page 247). Most women with hepatocellular carcinoma and clinical manifestations of metastatic disease in the ovary are under 40 years of age, younger than the typical age of women with hepatoid carcinoma (page 323). The presence of a liver mass compatible with a primary tumor is strong evidence in favor of a hepatocellular carcinoma; however, in one case the liver mass was discovered only after bilateral ovarian metastases had been resected. The finding of bile in the tumor favors metastatic hepatocellular carcinoma. Hepatoid yolk sac tumor occurs typically in young women and microscopic examination usually reveals foci of the more common forms of yolk sac neoplasia, which are absent in hepatoid carcinoma. There is also greater nuclear pleomorphism in hepatoid carcinoma than in hepatoid yolk

sac tumor. Finally, hepatoid carcinoma must be distinguished from the oxyphilic variants of endometrioid and clear cell carcinomas (pages 142 and 116) and oxyphilic (lipid-poor or lipid-free) steroid cell tumors (see chapter 12).

TUMOR OF PROBABLE WOLFFIAN ORIGIN

Definition. This is an epithelial tumor with a characteristic admixture of patterns, some of which mimic those of surface epithelial tumors and others, those of sex cord tumors. The tumor is thought to be of wolffian origin because of its relatively frequent occurrence in the broad ligament, where wolffian remnants are present, and its distinctive microscopic features that differ from mullerian-type tumors of surface epithelial origin.

General Features. The tumors are rare; the 17 reported examples have occurred in women 28 to 79 years of age (63,63b,64). They are associated with the usual symptoms of an ovarian

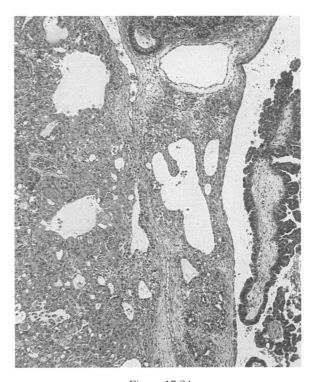

Figure 17-24
HEPATOID CARCINOMA
The hepatoid component is seen at the left and a small
component of serous adenocarcinoma at the right.

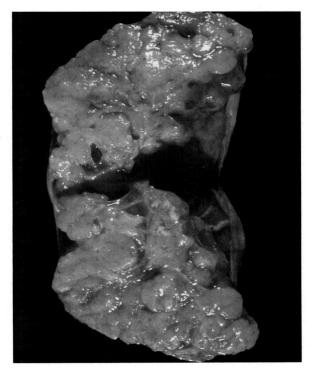

Figure 17-25
OVARIAN TUMOR OF
PROBABLE WOLFFIAN ORIGIN
The sectioned surfaces are lobulated.

tumor. In one unreported case luteinization of the adjacent ovarian stroma was associated with endometrial hyperplasia manifested clinically by irregular uterine bleeding.

Gross Findings. The tumors are almost invariably unilateral, average 12 cm in diameter, and are solid and often lobulated, or solid and cystic (fig. 17-25). The solid tissue varies from gray-white to tan or yellow and may be rubbery or firm.

Microscopic Findings. The low-power pattern may be solid, cystic, or solid and cystic (fig. 17-26). The solid areas may be diffuse or composed of closely packed tubules (fig. 17-27). A prominent fibrous stroma may result in a lobulated pattern. The cysts, which may result in a sieve-like appearance (fig. 17-26), typically contain eosinophilic secretion. The tubules are solid or hollow and are usually closely packed, but may be separated by considerable fibrous stroma (fig. 17-27). In some cases in which the pattern is apparently diffuse a tubular pattern may be unmasked by a periodic acid–Schiff (PAS) or reticulin stain. The tumor cells typically have the appearance of epithelial cells, and usually contain small amounts of eosinophilic cytoplasm, but may be spindle shaped (fig. 17-28). The nuclei are typically uniform and pale with no or few mitotic figures. Rare tumors contain high-grade areas and have a metastatic potential. The neoplastic cells often stain weakly immunohistochemically for α-inhibin (63a)

Differential Diagnosis. This tumor is often misinterpreted as a tumor in the Sertoli-stromal cell category since the tubules of the two tumors may be indistinguishable. The differential diagnosis is discussed on page 218. Tumors with a diffuse pattern can be misinterpreted as undifferentiated carcinomas on low-power microscopic examination but high-power evaluation reveals cells that almost always have bland or only slightly atypical nuclear features and few mitotic figures. Occasional ependymomas of the ovary have cysts and may focally superficially resemble a wolffian tumor (page 303). Differentiation of a wolffian

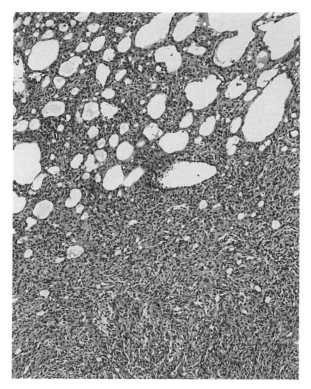

Figure 17-26
OVARIAN TUMOR OF
PROBABLE WOLFFIAN ORIGIN
A sieve-like pattern is present at the top and a solid
pattern at the bottom.

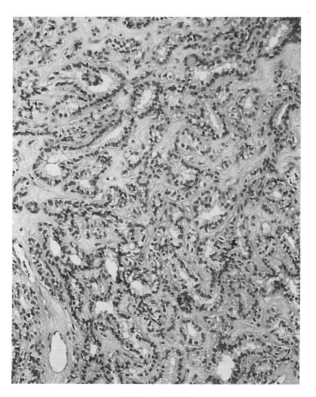

Figure 17-27
OVARIAN TUMOR OF
PROBABLE WOLFFIAN ORIGIN
This hollow tubular pattern simulates that of a Sertoli
cell tumor.

tumor from endometrioid adenocarcinoma is discussed on page 124.

Treatment and Prognosis. These tumors are typically associated with a benign course. One that had obvious malignant features microscopically was associated with pulmonary metastases.

RETE CYSTS AND TUMORS

Definition. These lesions are located in the ovarian hilus, lined by nonciliated epithelium, and characterized by crevices along their inner surfaces and smooth muscle in their walls. Adenomas and rare carcinomas originate in the rete.

General Features. Rete cysts and cystadenomas (cysts greater than 1 cm in diameter) occur in patients 23 to 80 (average, 59) years of age (65). The patients with cystadenomas usually have a palpable mass on pelvic examination. Androgenic manifestations related to adjacent hilus cell hyperplasia may develop; in two cases

it was associated with elevated testosterone levels (see chapter 19).

Although the largest series of rete cystadenomas in the literature comprised only 16 cases, 7 of them were identified in a review of 126 cysts that had been misinterpreted as simple cysts or serous cystadenomas, leading the authors to conclude that the occurrence of rete cystadenomas is more frequent than the paucity of reported cases suggests (65).

Less than 10 rete adenomas, usually occurring in middle-aged or elderly patients, have been reported; almost all of them have been incidental microscopic findings. The one well-documented rete adenocarcinoma occurred in a 52-year-old woman with abdominal swelling due to ascites (65).

Gross Findings. Rete cystadenomas have ranged up to 24 (mean, 8.7) cm in diameter. They are usually unilocular but may be multilocular. The cyst fluid is typically clear and yellow, or

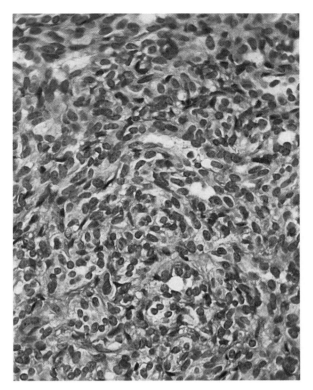

Figure 17-28
OVARIAN TUMOR OF
PROBABLE WOLFFIAN ORIGIN
The tumor cells, some of which are spindle shaped, have
bland nuclear features.

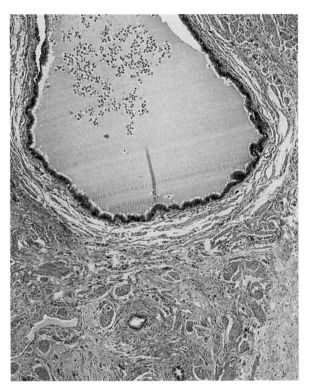

Figure 17-29
RETE CYST
A small cyst in the hilus is lined by cuboidal epithelial
cells. Wolffian remnants are visible below.

rarely, mucoid. The cysts walls are typically thin and have a smooth lining. The single patient with rete adenocarcinoma had bilateral solid and cystic tumors without specific gross features (65).

Microscopic Findings. Rete cysts are located in the hilus and are lined by epithelium similar to that of the larger cystadenomas (fig. 17-29). Rete cystadenomas are also situated in the hilus but may expand into the adjacent medulla. Their walls are composed of fibrovascular tissue containing fascicles of smooth muscle and little or no stroma of ovarian type. Over 80 percent of them have irregularly spaced, shallow crevices along their inner surfaces (fig. 17-30). They are typically lined by bland cuboidal cells (fig. 17-30) but the cells may be columnar or flattened. They have scanty eosinophilic cytoplasm in most cases but occasionally the cytoplasm is clear. In 3 of 16 cases in one series (65) rare ciliated cells were present. Hilus cells have been identified in the cyst walls in slightly more than half the cases, and are

typically hyperplastic and arranged in prominent bands subjacent to the epithelial lining.

Rete adenomas are well-circumscribed hilar lesions composed of closely packed, elongated small tubules, some of which are dilated and contain simple papillae. The tubules and papillae are lined by a single layer of cuboidal or columnar cells resembling that of the normal rete. The rete adenocarcinoma had a predominant pattern of branching tubules and cysts containing simple papillae with fibrovascular or hyalinized cores. Some cysts contained eosinophilic material. A solid tubular pattern was present focally. The tubules and papillae were lined by atypical, cuboidal, nonciliated cells, and areas of transitional-like cells were identified. Mitotic figures were numerous and nucleoli were prominent in some cells.

Differential Diagnosis. Rete cysts and cystadenomas are distinguished from other benign ovarian and paraovarian cysts on the basis of

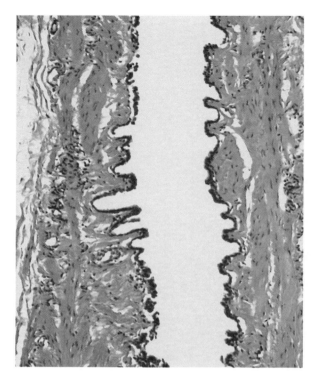

Figure 17-30
RETE CYSTADENOMA
Numerous small crevices are seen along the epithelial lining. A layer of smooth muscle is present in the wall. (Fig. 88 from Young RH, Clement PB, Scully RE. Pathology of the ovary. In: Sternberg SS, ed. Diagnostic surgical pathology, Vol 2, 2nd ed. New York: Raven Press, 1994:2243.)

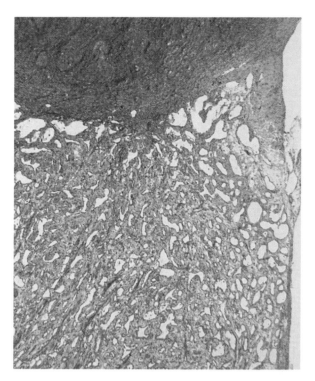

Figure 17-31
ADENOMATOID TUMOR
The tumor is well circumscribed in the hilus and contains scattered cysts. Ovarian stroma is visible in the upper portion.

their location in the hilus, the muscular tissue or hilus cells in their walls, the typical presence of crevices along their inner surfaces, and an absence or rarity of cilia in their lining cells. Serous cystadenomas, with which they are most likely to be confused, do not have a hilar location, rarely, if ever, have prominent smooth muscle or hilus cells in their walls, characteristically are ciliated, and generally lack crevices in their walls.

Rete adenomas may be confused with female adnexal tumors of probable wolffian origin but the adenomas, in contrast to the latter, typically have a uniform tubular pattern, lacking the sieve-like and solid components of wolffian tumors.

The diagnosis of rete adenocarcinoma is suggested when the tumor has a hilar location and a predominant pattern of slit-like retiform tubules with cysts containing papillae lined by cells similar to those of the normal rete. The tumor is distinguished from a retiform Sertoli-Leydig cell

tumor primarily on the basis of greater nuclear atypia and an absence of other patterns more typical of retiform Sertoli-Leydig cell tumors.

ADENOMATOID TUMOR

This benign tumor is characterized by tubules, cysts, and solid proliferations of mesothelial cell origin. Only 10 well-documented cases have been reported, all in adults; only 2 were symptomatic (66–68). Eight of them were located predominantly in the hilus and were 3 cm or less in diameter, but 2 were 6 and 8 cm. Nine were solid and one was multicystic.

Microscopic examination reveals a characteristic pattern of round, oval, elongated and occasionally slit-like tubules (fig. 17-31), which are mostly small but may undergo focal cystic dilatation. Small clusters of cells and individual cells may be present as well, and one neoplasm had a diffuse pattern. The tumor cells range from flat to columnar, and contain scanty to moderate amounts of

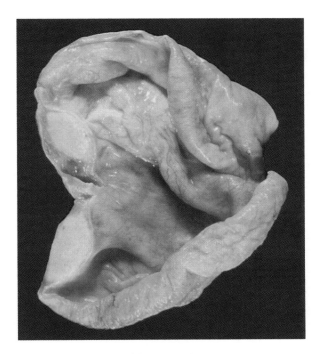

Figure 17-32
MALIGNANT MESOTHELIOMA
The unilocular cystic neoplasm has a solid mural nodule and tumor visible on the cyst lining. (Courtesy of Dr. A. Asher, Flint, MI.)

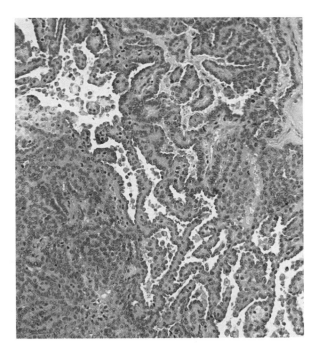

Figure 17-33
MALIGNANT MESOTHELIOMA
The tumor has solid and tubulopapillary patterns, and the cells are typical of mesothelioma.

eosinophilic to pale, vacuolated cytoplasm and nuclei that lack significant atypia or mitotic activity. The cytoplasm of single cells is often distended by a large oval vacuole. PAS-positive hyaline bodies were present in one case (68). The stroma is typically scanty.

Although the distinctive microscopic features should facilitate the diagnosis, the rarity of adenomatoid tumors in the ovary may cause them to be misinterpreted. One such tumor was misdiagnosed as a multilocular peritoneal inclusion cyst (page 440). Confusion with a yolk sac tumor is possible because the adenomatoid tumor may have a similar reticular pattern, and the rare presence of hyaline bodies in the latter may compound the problem (68). However, the nuclei in the adenomatoid tumor lack the primitive appearance of those in a yolk sac tumor, and other patterns of the latter neoplasm are lacking. A cystic adenomatoid tumor may be misinterpreted as a lymphangioma. In difficult cases immunohistochemical staining should exclude yolk sac tumors and lymphangiomas from the differential diagnosis.

MALIGNANT MESOTHELIOMA

The ovary may be involved focally in cases of peritoneal well-differentiated papillary and diffuse malignant mesothelioma (see chapter 18). Occasionally, the ovary is extensively involved, and the clinical presentation is that of an ovarian cancer (71,72). In one series, ovarian involvement was present in 10 of 13 patients with peritoneal mesothelioma (72) and another series of abdominal malignant mesotheliomas comprised nine that presented as ovarian masses (71). Two of the nine tumors, occurring in patients 16 and 52 years of age, were interpreted as primary ovarian mesotheliomas because of confinement of the tumor to the ovaries (fig. 17-32). An additional case of primary mesothelioma of the ovary in a 67-year-old woman has been reported (69). In these three cases, the microscopic features of the ovarian tumors were similar to those of peritoneal malignant mesothelioma. The distinctive patterns of malignant mesothelioma (fig. 17-33) and the characteristic uniform cells that typically contain considerable

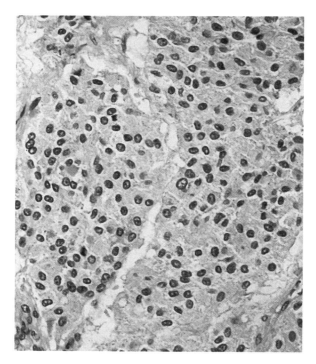

Figure 17-34
PARAGANGLIOMA
Nests are composed of tumor cells that contain abundant eosinophilic cytoplasm.

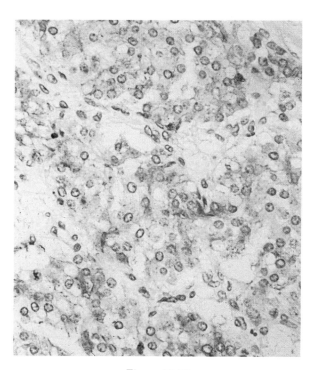

Figure 17-35
PARAGANGLIOMA
Most of the tumor cells are immunoreactive for chromogranin.

eosinophilic cytoplasm, facilitate differentiation from serous carcinoma in routinely stained sections, although occasionally, histochemical and immunohistochemical staining are necessary to confirm the diagnosis (page 73) (72).

ONCOCYTOMA

One tumor interpreted as an oncocytoma and another as an oncocytic adenocarcinoma have been described in women 22 and 39 years of age, respectively (74,75). The first neoplasm was composed of solid sheets of cells with oxyphilic cytoplasm, and electron microscopy demonstrated numerous mitochondria. The second tumor was similar except for the additional presence of focal glandular and papillary differentiation. The differential diagnosis of these neoplasms involves numerous other ovarian tumors containing oxyphilic cells, which in some cases are oncocytic. The "oncocytic adenocarcinoma" may be the same type of tumor as one reported as an oxyphilic (oncocytic) endometrioid adenocarcinoma (73). Before a diagnosis of

oncocytoma of the ovary is rendered extensive sampling and immunohistochemical evaluation, if necessary, should be undertaken to exclude a specific tumor type (see Table 6-1).

PARAGANGLIOMA

One tumor of this type was reported in a 15-year-old girl with hypertension (76). The tumor was large and unilateral and had the typical microscopic appearance of a pheochromocytoma. Epinephrine and norepinephrine were extracted from the tumor tissue. After removal of the tumor the symptoms disappeared, and follow-up evaluation after 1 year was uneventful. We have seen two additional unpublished cases of ovarian paraganglioma (fig. 17-34). The tumor must be distinguished from other tumors containing oxyphilic cells (see Table 6-1). Immunohistochemical staining for chromogranin should be helpful in the diagnosis (fig. 17-35) and the characteristic sustentacular cells can be highlighted by a S-100 stain.

WILMS' TUMOR

A single ovarian Wilms' tumor was reported in a 56-year-old woman whose tumor was confined to the ovary. She received adjuvant radiation therapy and chemotherapy, and was well 9 years postoperatively (77). The neoplasm had the typical features of Wilms' tumor on microscopic examination, including small tubules, glomeruloid formations, and prominent blastema. An important tumor to be distinguished from Wilms' tumor is the retiform Sertoli-Leydig cell tumor (page 213), which, although rare, is much more common than the Wilms' tumor, typically occurs in young females, may be virilizing, has a variety of distinctive patterns, and usually contains at least minor foci of more typical Sertoli-Leydig cell tumor. Although the retiform tumor may contain glomeruloid structures, it does not have areas of typical renal blastema.

GESTATIONAL TROPHOBLASTIC DISEASE

The diagnosis of primary gestational trophoblastic disease of the ovary can be made only after spread from an extraovarian lesion has been excluded. Most of the reported cases of primary ovarian gestational trophoblastic disease have been choriocarcinomas (78) but sporadic cases of hydatidiform mole have been reported as well (79). On gross examination the choriocarcinoma appears as a solid hemorrhagic mass, and the hydatidiform mole as a hemorrhagic mass containing vesicles.

Gestational choriocarcinoma must also be distinguished from a choriocarcinoma of germ cell (page 258), and rarely, somatic cell origin (page 167). In one review of the reported cases of ovarian choriocarcinoma (80), 18 were considered gestational; 6, nongestational; and 11 of uncertain origin. Patients with gestational choriocarcinoma typically have symptoms caused by large hemorrhagic ovarian masses, which sometimes rupture, with resultant hemoperitoneum. The microscopic findings are identical to those of uterine choriocarcinoma. The specimens must be sectioned extensively to exclude a germ cell or, in an older patient, a surface epithelial origin. Six of the 15 patients with follow-up data in one review (80) were free of disease 1 to 5 1/2 years postoperatively. Three of the survivors had stage IA or IIB tumors and were treated before the advent of modern chemotherapy.

REFERENCES

Benign Mesenchymal Tumors

1. Costa MJ, Morris R, DeRose PB, Cohen C. Histologic and immunohistochemical evidence for considering ovarian myxoma as a variant of the thecoma-fibroma group of ovarian stromal tumors. Arch Pathol Lab Med 1993;117:802–8.
2. Costa MJ, Thomas W, Majmudar B, Hewan-Lowe K. Ovarian myxoma: ultrastructural and immunohistochemical findings. Ultrastruct Pathol 1992;16:429–38.
3. Eichhorn JH, Scully RE. Ovarian myxoma: clinicopathologic and immunocytologic analysis of five cases and a review of the literature. Int J Gynecol Pathol 1991;10:156–69.
4. Fallahzadeh H, Dockerty MB, Lee RA. Leiomyoma of the ovary: report of five cases and review of the literature. Am J Obstet Gynecol 1972;113:394–8.
5. Hegg CA, Flint A. Neurofibroma of the ovary. Gynecol Oncol 1990;37:437–68.
6. Kandalaft PL, Esteban JM. Bilateral massive ovarian leiomyomata in a young woman: a case report with review of the literature. Mod Pathol 1992;5:586–9.
7. Lawhead RA, Copeland LJ, Edwards CL. Bilateral ovarian hemangiomas associated with diffuse abdominopelvic hemangiomatosis. Obstet Gynecol 1985;65:597–9.
8. Matamala MF, Nogales FF, Aneiros J, Herraiz MA, Caracuel MD. Leiomyomas of the ovary. Int J Gynecol Pathol 1988;7:190–6.
9. Mira JL. Lipoleiomyoma of the ovary: report of a case and review of the English literature. Int J Gynecol Pathol 1991;10:198–202.

10. Miyauchi J, Mukai M, Yamazaki K, Kiso I, Higashi S, Hori S. Bilateral ovarian hemangiomas associated with diffuse hemangioendotheliomatosis: a case report. Acta Pathol Jpn 1987;37:1347–55.
11. Nogales FF. Letter to the editor. Histopathology 1982;6:376.
11a. Pai S, Naresh KN, Desai PB, Borges AM. Ovarian myxoma in a premenarchal girl. Gynecol Oncol 1994;55:453–5.
12. Parish JM, Lufkin EG, Lee RA, Gaffey TA. Ovarian leiomyoma with hilus cell hyperplasia that caused virilization. Mayo Clin Proc 1984;59:275–7.
13. Prayson RA, Hart WR. Primary smooth-muscle tumors of the ovary. A clinicopathologic study of four leiomyomas and two mitotically active leiomyomas. Arch Pathol Lab Med 1992;116:1068–71.
13a. Prus D, Rosenberg AE, Blumenfeld A, et al. Infantile hemangioendothelioma of the ovary: a monodermal teratoma or a neoplasm of ovarian somatic cells? Am J Surg Pathol 1997;21:1231–5.

14. Savargaonkar PR, Wells S, Graham I, Buckley CH. Ovarian hemangiomas and stromal luteinization. Histopathology 1994;25:185–8.
14a. Talerman A. Nonspecific tumors of the ovary, including mesenchymal tumors and malignant lymphoma. In Kurman RJ, ed. Blaustein's pathology of the female genital tract. New York: Springer-Verlag, 1994:915–37.
15. Tanaka Y, Sasaki Y, Tachibana K, et al. Gonadal mixed germ cell tumor combined with a large hemangiomatous lesion in a patient with Turner's syndrome and 45,X/46,X, +mar karyotype. Arch Pathol Lab Med 1994;118:1135–8.
16. Tetu B, Bonenfant JL. Ovarian myxoma. A study of two cases with long-term follow-up. Am J Clin Pathol 1991;95:340–6.
17. Tsalacopoulos G, Tiltman AJ. Leiomyoma of the ovary. A report of 3 cases. S Afr Med J 1981;59:574–5.
18. Van Winter JT, Stanhope CR. Giant ovarian leiomyoma associated with ascites and polymyositis. Obstet Gynecol 1992;80:560–3.

Sarcomas

19. Allen C, Stephens M, Williams J. Combined high grade sarcoma and serous ovarian neoplasm. J Clin Pathol 1992;45:263–4.
20. Anderson B, Turner DA, Benda J. Ovarian sarcoma. Gynecol Oncol 1987;26:183–92.
21. Balaton A, Vaury P, Imbert MC, Mussy MA. Primary leiomyosarcoma of the ovary: a histological and immunocytochemical study. Gynecol Oncol 1987;28:116–20.
22. Chen YF, Leung CS, Ma L. Primary embryonal rhabdomyosarcoma of the ovary in a 4-year-old girl. Histopathology 1989;15:309–11.
23. Friedman HD, Mazur MT. Primary ovarian leiomyosarcoma. An immunohistochemical and ultrastructural study. Arch Pathol Lab Med 1991;115:941–5.
24. Guerard MJ, Arguelles MA, Ferenczy A. Rhabdomyosarcoma of the ovary: ultrastructural study of a case and review of the literature. Gynecol Oncol 1983;15:325–39.
25. Hines JF, Compton DM, Stacy CC, Potter ME. Pure primary osteosarcoma of the ovary presenting as an extensively calcified adnexal mass: a case report and review of the literature. Gynecol Oncol 1990;39:259–63.
26. Hirakawa T, Tsuneyoshi M, Enjoji M, Shigyo R. Ovarian sarcoma with histologic features of telangiectatic osteosarcoma of bone. Am J Surg Pathol 1988;12:567–72.
27. Kraemer BB, Silva EG, Sniege N. Fibrosarcoma of ovary. A new component in the nevoid basal-cell carcinoma syndrome. Am J Surg Pathol 1984;8:231–6.
28. Miles PA, Kiley KC, Mena H. Giant fibrosarcoma of the ovary. Int J Gynecol Pathol 1985;4:83–7.
29. Monk BJ, Nieberg R, Berek JS. Primary leiomyosarcoma of the ovary in a perimenarchal female. Gynecol Oncol 1993;48:389–93.
30. Ngwalle KE, Hirakawa T, Tseuneyoshi M, Enjoji M. Osteosarcoma arising in a benign dermoid cyst of the ovary. Gynecol Oncol 1990;37:143–7.
30a. Nielsen GP, Young RH, Prat J, Scully RE. Primary angiosarcoma of the ovary. A report of seven cases and review of the literature. Int J Gynecol Pathol 1997;16:378–82.

30b. Nielsen GP, Young RH, Rosenberg AE, Oliva E, Prat J, Scully RE. Primary ovarian rhabdomyosarcoma. A report of 13 cases. Int J Gynecol Pathol 1998;17:113–9.
30c. Nielsen GP, Young RH. Fibromatosis (soft tissue type) of the female genital tract. A report of two cases primarily involving the vulva and ovary. Int J Gynecol Pathol 1997;16:383–6.
31. Nieminen V, von Numers C, Purola E. Primary sarcoma of the ovary. Acta Obstet Gynecol Scand 1969;48:423–32.
32. Nogales FF, Ayala A, Ruiz-Avila I, Sirvent JJ. Myxoid leiomyosarcoma of the ovary: analysis of three cases. Hum Pathol 1991;22:1268–73.
33. Ongkasuwan C, Taylor JE, Tang CK, Prempree T. Angiosarcomas of the uterus and ovary: clinicopathologic report. Cancer 1982;49:1469–75.
34. Prat J, Scully RE. Cellular fibromas and fibrosarcomas of the ovary: a comparative clinicopathologic analysis of seventeen cases. Cancer 1981;47:2663–70.
35. Reddy SA, Poon TP, Ramaswamy G, Tchertkoff V. Leiomyosarcoma of the ovary. N Y State J Med 1985;85:218–20.
36. Sahin A, Benda JA. An immunohistochemical study of primary ovarian sarcoma. An evaluation of nine tumors. Int J Gynecol Pathol 1988;7:268–79.
37. Sakata H, Hirahara T, Ryu A, Sawada T, Yamamoto M, Sakurai I. Primary osteosarcoma of the ovary. A case report. Acta Pathol Jpn 1991;41:311–7.
38. Shakfeh SM, Woodruff JD. Primary ovarian sarcomas: report of 46 cases and review of the literature. Obstet Gynecol Surv 1987;42:331–49.
39. Stone GC, Bell DA, Fuller A, Dickersin GR, Scully RE. Malignant schwannoma of the ovary. Report of a case. Cancer 1986;58:1575–82.
40. Talerman A, Auerbach WM, Van Meurs AJ. Primary chondrosarcoma of the ovary. Histopathology 1981;5:319–24.
41. Tsujimura T, Kawano K. Rhabdomyosarcoma coexistent with ovarian mucinous cystadenocarcinoma: a case report. Int J Gynecol Pathol 1992;11:58–62.
42. Walts AE, Lichtenstein I. Primary leiomyosarcoma associated with serous cystadenocarcinoma of the ovary. Gynecol Oncol 1977;5:81–6.

Small Cell Carcinoma, Hypercalcemic and Pulmonary Types

43. Abeler V, Kjorstad KE, Nesland JM. Small cell carcinoma of the ovary: a report of six cases. Int J Gynecol Pathol 1988;7:315–29.

44. Aguirre P, Thor AD, Scully RE. Ovarian small cell carcinoma. Histogenetic considerations based on immunohistochemical and other findings. Am J Clin Pathol 1989;92:140–9.

45. Dickersin GR, Kline IW, Scully RE. Small cell carcinoma of the ovary with hypercalcemia: a report of eleven cases. Cancer 1982;49:188–97.

46. Dickersin GR, Scully RE. An update on the electron microscopy of small cell carcinoma of the ovary with hypercalcemia. Ultrastruct Pathol 1993;17:411–22.

47. Eichhorn JH, Bell DA, Young RH, et al. DNA content and proliferative activity in ovarian small cell carcinomas of the hypercalcemic type. Implications for diagnosis, prognosis, and histogenesis. Am J Clin Pathol 1992;98:579–86.

48. Eichhorn JH, Young RH, Scully RE. Non-pulmonary small cell carcinomas of extragenital origin metastatic to the ovary. Cancer 1993;71:177–86.

49. Eichhorn JH, Young RH, Scully RE. Primary ovarian small cell carcinoma of pulmonary type. A clinicopathologic, immunohistologic and flow cytometric analysis of 11 cases. Am J Surg Pathol 1992;16:926–38.

50. Jensen ML, Rasmussen KL, Jacobsen M. Ovarian small cell carcinoma. A case report with histologic, immunohistochemical and ultrastructural findings. APMIS Suppl 1991;23:126–31.

51. Matias-Guiu X, Prat J, Young RH, Capen CC, Rosol TJ, DeLellis RA, Scully RE. Human parathyroid hormone-related protein in ovarian small cell carcinoma. An immunohistochemical study. Cancer 1994;73:1878–81.

52. McMahon JT, Hart WR. Ultrastructural analysis of small cell carcinomas of the ovary. Am J Clin Pathol 1988;90:523–9.

53. Ulbright TM, Roth LM, Stehman FB, Talerman A, Senekjian EK. Poorly differentiated (small cell) carcinoma of the ovary in young women: evidence supporting a germ cell origin. Hum Pathol 1987;18:175–84.

54. Young RH, Oliva E, Scully RE. Small cell carcinoma of the ovary, hypercalcemic type. A clinicopathologic analysis of 150 cases. Am J Surg Pathol 1994;18:1102–16.

Ovarian Carcinoma (Non-small Cell Type) with Neuroendocrine Differentiation

55. Collins R, Cheung A, Ngan H, Wong L, Chan S, Mah H. Primary mixed neuroendocrine carcinoma of the ovary. Arch Gynecol Obstet 1991;248:139–43.

56. Eichhorn JH, Lawrence WD, Young RH, Scully RE. Ovarian neuroendocrine carcinomas of non-small cell type associated with surface epithelial adenocarcinomas. A study of five cases and review of the literature. Int J Gynecol Pathol 1996;15:303–14.

57. Jones K, Diaz JA, Donner LR. Neuroendocrine carcinoma arising in an ovarian mucinous cystadenoma. Int J Gynecol Pathol 1996;15:167–70.

58. Khurana KK, Tornos C, Silva EG. Ovarian neuroendocrine carcinoma associated with a mucinous neoplasm. Arch Pathol Lab Med 1994;118:1032–4.

"Adenoid Cystic" and Basaloid Carcinomas

59. Eichhorn JH, Scully RE. "Adenoid cystic" and basaloid carcinomas of the ovary: evidence for a surface epithelial lineage. A report of 12 cases. Mod Pathol 1995;8:731–40.

59a. Feczko JD, Jentz DL, Roth LM. Adenoid cystic ovarian carcinoma compared with other adenoid cystic carcinomas of the female genital tract. Mod Pathol 1996;9:413–7.

59b. Russell P, Wills EJ, Watson G, Lee J, Geraghty T. Monomorphic (basal cell) salivary adenoma of ovary: report of a case. Ultrastruct Pathol 1995;19:431–8.

Hepatoid Carcinoma

60. Ishikura H, Scully RE. Hepatoid carcinoma of the ovary: a report of five cases of a newly described tumor. Cancer 1987;60:2775–84.

61. Matsuta M, Ishikura H, Murakami K, Kagabu T, Nishiya I. Hepatoid carcinoma of the ovary: a case report. Int J Gynecol Pathol 1991;10:302–10.

61a. Scurry JP, Brown RW, Jobling T. Combined ovarian serous papillary and hepatoid carcinoma. Gynecol Oncol 1996;63:138–42.

62. Young RH, Gersell DJ, Clement PB, Scully RE. Hepatocellular carcinoma metastatic to the ovary: a report of three cases discovered during life with discussion of the differential diagnosis of hepatoid tumors of the ovary. Hum Pathol 1992;23:574–80.

Wolffian Tumors

63. Hughesdon PE. Ovarian tumours of wolffian or allied nature: their place in ovarian oncology. J Clin Pathol 1982;35:526–35.

63a. Kommoss F, Oliva E, Bhan AK, Young RH, Scully RE. Inhibin expression in ovarian tumors and tumor-like lesions. An immunohistochemical study. Mod Pathol 1998;11:656–64.

63b. Tavassoli FA, Andrade R, Merino M. Retiform wolffian adenoma. In: Fenoglio-Preiser CM, Wolff M, Rilke F, eds. Progress in surgical pathology. New York: Field & Wood Medical Publishers, 1990;11:121–36.

64. Young RH, Scully RE. Ovarian tumors of probable wolffian origin. A report of 11 cases. Am J Surg Pathol 1983;7:125–35.

Rete Cysts and Tumors

65. Rutgers JL, Scully RE. Cysts (cystadenomas) and tumors of the rete ovarii. Int J Gynecol Pathol 1988;7:330–42.

Adenomatoid Tumor

66. Hirakawa T, Tsuneyoshi M, Enjoji M. Adenomatoid tumor of the ovary: an immunohistochemical and ultrastructural study. Jpn J Clin Oncol 1988;18:159–66.
67. Kupryjanczyk J. Adenomatoid tumour of the ovary and uterus in the same patient. Zentralbl Allg Pathol 1989;135:437–44.

68. Young RH, Silva EG, Scully RE. Ovarian and juxtaovarian adenomatoid tumors: a report of six cases. Int J Gynecol Pathol 1991; 10:364–71.

Malignant Mesothelioma

69. Addis BJ, Fox H. Papillary mesothelioma of the ovary. Histopathology 1983;7:287–98.
70. Bollinger DJ, Wick MR, Dehner LP, Mills SE, Swanson PE, Clark RE. Peritoneal malignant mesothelioma versus serous papillary adenocarcinoma. A histochemical and immunohistochemical comparison. Am J Surg Pathol 1989;13:659–70.
71. Clement PB, Young RH, Scully RE. Malignant mesotheliomas presenting as ovarian masses: a report of nine cases, including two primary ovarian mesotheliomas. Am J Surg Pathol 1996;20:1067–80.
72. Goldblum J, Hart WR. Localized and diffuse mesotheliomas of the genital tract and peritoneum in women. A clinicopathologic study of nineteen true mesothelial neoplasms, other than adenomatoid tumors, multicystic mesotheliomas and localized fibrous tumors. Am J Surg Pathol 1995;19:1124–37.

Oncocytoma

73. Pitman MB, Young RH, Clement PB, Dickersin GR, Scully RE. Endometrioid carcinoma of the ovary and endometrium, oxyphilic cell type: a report of nine cases. Int J Gynecol Pathol 1994;13:290–301.
74. Takeda A, Matsuyama M, Sugimoto Y, et al. Oncocytic adenocarcinoma of the ovary. Virchows Arch [A] 1983; 399:345–53.
75. Yoshida Y, Tenzaki T, Ishiguro T, Kawanami D, Oshima M. Oncocytoma of the ovary: light and electron microscopic study. Gynecol Oncol 1984;18:109–14.

Paraganglioma

76. Fawcett FJ, Kimbell NK. Phaeochromocytoma of the ovary. J Obstet Gynecol Brit Cmwlth 1971;78:458–9.

Wilms' Tumor

77. Sahin A, Benda JA. Primary ovarian Wilms' tumor. Cancer 1988;61:1460–3.

Gestational Trophoblastic Disease

78. Axe SR, Klein VR, Woodruff JD. Choriocarcinoma of the ovary. Obstet Gynecol 1985;66:111–4.
79. D'Aguillo AF, Goldberg MI, Kamalamma M, Yuliano SE, Scully JT. Primary ovarian hydatidiform mole. Hum Pathol 1982;13:279–81.
80. Jacobs AJ, Newland JR, Green RK. Pure choriocarcinoma of the ovary. Obstet Gynecol Surv 1982;37:603–9.

18
SECONDARY (INCLUDING HEMATOPOIETIC) TUMORS

It is difficult to establish the frequency of metastatic tumors in the ovary as some studies have been based on autopsy findings, others on surgical specimens, and still others on both (1–12). In addition, some series have included clinically silent metastases such as those of breast carcinoma found in prophylactic or therapeutic oophorectomy specimens and small metastases detected incidentally during surgery for gastrointestinal carcinomas. Some studies have included as metastases ovarian carcinomas associated with uterine cancers of similar histologic type, but present evidence indicates that many of these ovarian tumors are independent primary neoplasms (page 125). The frequency that is most meaningful in clinical practice is the 6 to 7 percent possibility that a cancer found in the ovary on exploration of a pelvic or abdominal mass is metastatic (9).

Geographically, individual types of ovarian metastatic tumors vary in frequency because of differences in their prevalence at their primary sites. For example, metastatic gastric carcinoma accounts for a high percentage of ovarian cancers in Japan, where gastric carcinoma is common, but this type of metastasis is uncommon in black Africa. The average age of patients with ovarian involvement for each of the most common forms of cancer that spread to the ovary (intestinal, gastric, and mammary) is significantly lower than that of patients without ovarian spread, presumably because of the greater vascularity of the ovary of younger women.

Tumors spread to the ovary by various routes. The frequent association of ovarian metastases with other blood-borne metastases and the common finding of vascular invasion on microscopic examination of metastatic tumors are consistent with the important role of hematogenous spread. Transcelomic dissemination is another frequent route by which intra-abdominal cancers spread to the ovary. Foci of metastatic carcinoma on the surface of the ovary or within the superficial cortex are characteristic of this mode of spread. Direct extension is an important pathway for cancers of the fallopian tube and uterus, mesotheliomas, occasional colonic and appendiceal carcinomas, and retroperitoneal sarcomas. Genital tract carcinomas also spread through the lumen of the fallopian tube and onto the ovarian surface. An extensive anastomosis between uterine and ovarian blood vessels in the upper portion of the broad ligament facilitates spread of tumors from one organ to the other. Lymphatic connections between the two ovaries may also have a role in dissemination from one to the other.

Because of the approximately 70 percent frequency with which metastases are bilateral, the possibility of metastasis should be seriously considered when evaluating bilateral cancers. Almost 10 percent of bilateral ovarian cancers presenting as adnexal masses prove to be metastatic. Two gross findings that are suggestive, but not pathognomonic, of metastasis are the presence of multiple discrete nodules within the ovary and the location of tumor deposits on its surface. Although usually predominantly solid, some ovarian metastases are predominantly cystic, and rare cysts are uniformly thin-walled, with an appearance grossly indistinguishable from that of a cystadenoma. On microscopic examination the presence of implants on the surface of the ovary, growth in the form of multiple nodules, and lymphatic or blood vessel invasion strongly suggest metastasis. The surface implants are typically focal and commonly contain tumor cells embedded in a desmoplastic stroma. An additional finding suggestive of metastasis is the presence within an ovarian tumor specimen of a variation in growth pattern from one nodule to another. For example, within some metastatic mucinous adenocarcinomas benign-appearing glands and cysts may be present in one nodule and small, irregular, infiltrating glands haphazardly arranged in a reactive stroma in an adjacent nodule. Many types of metastatic tumor are found on microscopic examination to contain follicle-like spaces (13), simulating patterns of a variety of primary ovarian cancers. Recognition of the metastatic nature of an ovarian tumor depends to varying extents in individual cases on an adequate clinical history, a thorough clinical and intraoperative search for a primary tumor elsewhere, and a careful evaluation of the gross and microscopic features of the ovarian tumor. Sometimes, special stains, either conventional or immunohistochemical, and rarely, electron microscopy, have a role. Occasionally, a primary tumor may not be discovered until several years after removal of the metastatic ovarian tumor. In one series of 82 cases of metastasis to the ovary, 11 of the primary tumors were not discovered until autopsy (8).

GASTRIC CARCINOMA, INCLUDING KRUKENBERG TUMOR

General Features. Most ovarian metastases of gastric origin are Krukenberg tumors (14–27), i.e., carcinomas containing a significant component of mucin-filled signet-ring cells typically lying within a cellular stroma derived from the ovarian stroma. Some metastatic signet-ring cell tumors do not have a cellular stroma or contain it only focally, however, and in current practice the term is applied to any metastatic signet-ring cell adenocarcinoma whether or not the typical cellular stroma is present. The source of a Krukenberg tumor in over 70 percent of the cases is a gastric carcinoma, usually arising in the pylorus (15,17, 19,21,23,26,27). Carcinomas of the intestine, appendix, breast, gallbladder, biliary tract, pancreas, urinary bladder, and cervix are the primary tumors in the remaining cases, in an estimated descending order of frequency. Gastric signet-ring cell carcinomas metastasize to the ovary more than twice as often as intestinal-type carcinomas of the stomach (16). Saphir (23) similarly found a higher frequency of ovarian metastasis in association with signet-ring cell carcinomas of the breast and intestine than with carcinomas of these organs without signet-ring cells. The average age of patients with a Krukenberg tumor is about 45 years; it is the most common form of ovarian metastatic carcinoma in young women, often found in the fourth decade and occasionally in the third decade.

Almost 80 percent of patients with Krukenberg tumors have symptoms related to ovarian involvement, the most common of which are abdominal pain and swelling; occasionally, there is abnormal uterine bleeding and rarely, there are androgenic manifestations, particularly during pregnancy (see chapter 19). In some cases symptoms related to the primary tumor, which are usually upper abdominal because of the gastric origin of most tumors, are present. In most cases the diagnosis of the gastric carcinoma is made preoperatively, during surgery for the ovarian tumor, or within a few months thereafter, but sometimes the primary tumor is too small to be detected during surgery (19) or by radiographic examination of the upper gastrointestinal tract. Rarely, a gastric carcinoma is not detected until 5 or more years, and even up to 12 years, after discovery of the ovarian metastatic tumor (17). The primary carcinoma in a few cases of Krukenberg tumor, particularly those arising in the stomach and breast, has been tiny, requiring exhaustive sectioning for detection, even at autopsy. Almost all the patients die within a year of the diagnosis of the ovarian metastasis, with an average survival of 7 months (17), but a rare patient has survived free of clinical evidence of tumor for more than 5 years after gastrectomy and bilateral oophorectomy (19), and in one case a 16-year survival was reported (24).

Gross Findings. Approximately 80 percent of metastatic gastric carcinomas are bilateral. Gross examination reveals typically rounded or reniform, firm, white to pale yellow, solid masses that may be bosselated (fig. 18-1). The sectioned surfaces are basically white or pale yellow but usually contain focal or diffuse areas of purple, red, or brown discoloration (fig. 18-2); the consistency may be firm, fleshy, gelatinous, or spongy. Occasionally, the tumor contains large, thin-walled cysts filled with mucinous or watery fluid, separated by relatively small amounts of solid tissue. Metastatic gastric adenocarcinomas that are not Krukenberg tumors may be predominantly solid or predominantly cystic (fig. 18-3).

Microscopic Findings. Microscopic examination typically reveals mucin-laden, signet-ring cells (figs. 18-4–18-6) strewn individually, in small clusters, or in large aggregates within a cellular ovarian stroma (fig. 18-4); occasionally the stroma has a storiform pattern. Frequent variations from the typical appearance include small glands, a prominent tubular architecture (figs. 18-7, 18-8) (14), mucin-poor tumor cells singly or in clusters, trabeculae or large masses, abundant collagen formation, marked stromal edema (fig. 18-6), and cell-free pools of mucin in the stroma. Occasionally, small or large cysts

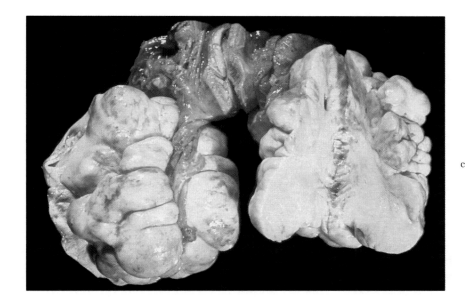

Figure 18-1
KRUKENBERG TUMOR
The bilateral bosselated masses are composed of solid yellow-white tissue.

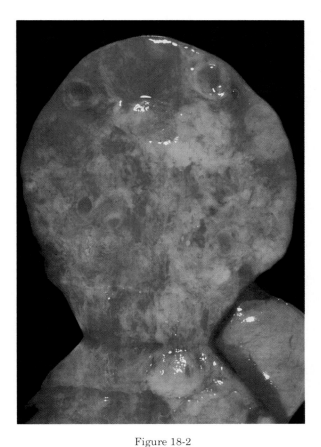

Figure 18-2
KRUKENBERG TUMOR
The sectioned surface exhibits focal hemorrhage. The tumor tissue was soft.

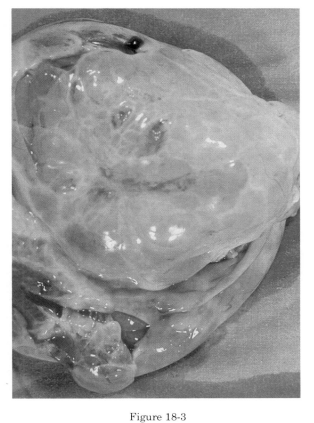

Figure 18-3
METASTATIC ADENOCARCINOMA
FROM THE STOMACH
A multiloculated cystic neoplasm simulates a primary mucinous cystic tumor.

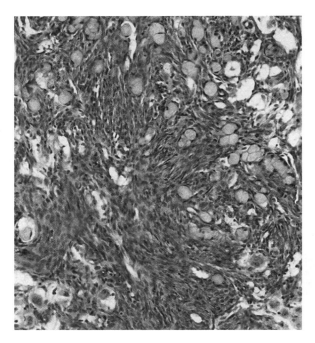

Figure 18-4
KRUKENBERG TUMOR
Signet-ring cells are distributed irregularly within a cellular stroma.

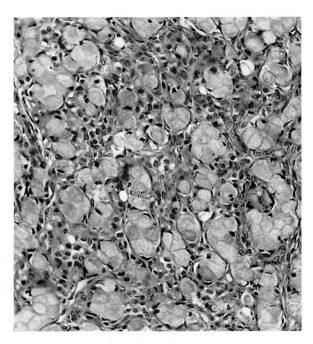

Figure 18-5
KRUKENBERG TUMOR
Numerous signet-ring cells with eccentric nuclei and abundant pale cytoplasm are present.

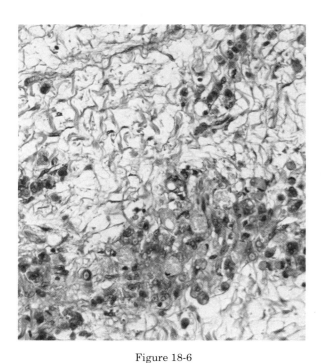

Figure 18-6
KRUKENBERG TUMOR
Nests of cells and single cells, some of signet-ring cell type, lie within an edematous stroma.

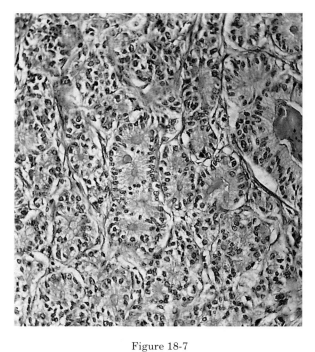

Figure 18-7
KRUKENBERG TUMOR, TUBULAR
Numerous small tubules lined by cells with abundant pale cytoplasm impart a striking resemblance to a Sertoli cell tumor (see figure 11-3).

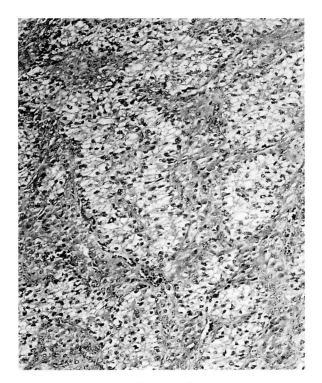

Figure 18-8
KRUKENBERG TUMOR, TUBULAR
The abundant cytoplasm and antipodal arrangement of the nuclei of the tumor cells suggest a lipid-rich Sertoli cell tumor (see figure 11-2). (Fig. 21 from Young RH, Scully RE. Metastatic tumors in the ovary. A problem oriented approach with review of the recent literature. Semin Diagn Pathol 1991;8:250–76.)

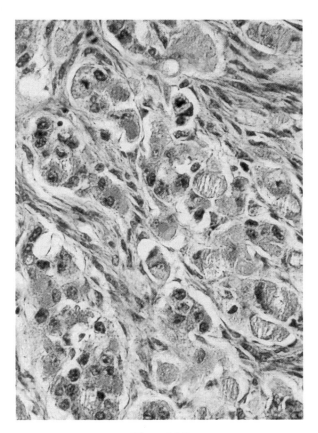

Figure 18-9
KRUKENBERG TUMOR
A mucicarmine stain demonstrates the mucin in the signet-ring cells.

lined by minimally atypical-appearing mucinous epithelium form a conspicuous component of the tumor, with more characteristic areas separating the cysts. The cytoplasm of the signet-ring cells is occasionally granular and eosinophilic rather than pale and vacuolated (25); it often has a bull's-eye appearance, with a clear vacuole containing a central eosinophilic body. The mucin in the signet-ring cells is usually easily demonstrable by mucin stains such as periodic acid–Schiff (PAS) or mucicarmine (fig. 18-9). Blood vessel and lymphatic invasion are common, particularly at the periphery of the tumor. Lutein cells are occasionally present in the stroma, particularly if the patient is pregnant. Some metastatic gastric carcinomas are composed of glands and cysts of intestinal type showing varying degrees of differentiation (fig. 18-10) as well as sheets and irregular aggregates of poorly differentiated epithelial cells.

Differential Diagnosis. An occasional Krukenberg tumor has a paucity of signet-ring cells and may superficially resemble a fibroma (19). Careful search for signet-ring cells is crucial in such cases. A frequent misinterpretation of the tubular form of Krukenberg tumor is as a Sertoli-Leydig cell tumor, particularly when luteinization of the stroma is present (14). Mucin-filled cells, however, are not a feature of Sertoli-Leydig cell tumors except for the heterologous subtype that contains mucinous glands and cysts (page 213); in such cases typical patterns of Sertoli-Leydig cell tumor are also present. Clear cell carcinomas occasionally contain mucin-filled signet-ring cells typically in rounded nests or masses but other characteristic patterns and cell types are almost always present (page 142). Very rare primary Krukenberg tumors and goblet cell

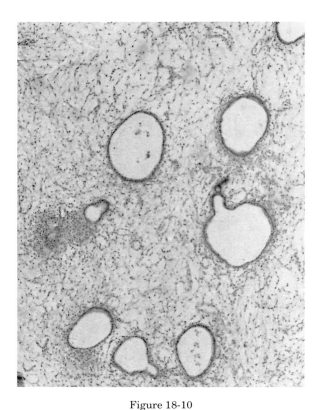

Figure 18-10
METASTATIC ADENOCARCINOMA
FROM STOMACH
Cystic glands are present within an edematous stroma.

carcinoid tumors that contain large numbers of signet-ring cells must be distinguished from Krukenberg tumors (pages 92 and 298). The sclerosing stromal tumor may contain cells resembling signet-ring cells but they contain lipid rather than mucin (page 198). The rare signet-ring stromal tumor also may enter the differential diagnosis but the vacuolated cells in this tumor also fail to react with mucin stains (page 200).

The rare non-neoplastic lesion, mucicarminophilic histiocytosis (page 442), is characterized by signet-ring–like cells and may involve numerous tissues and organs, including the ovaries. However, the cells are PAS negative in contrast to the Krukenberg tumor in which PAS staining is typically extensive. Surface epithelial cystic or solid inclusions in the ovarian cortex rarely show a vacuolar, presumably hydropic, cytoplasmic change that mimics that of signet-ring cells. The vacuolar material, however, is negative with mucin stains (page 442).

INTESTINAL CARCINOMA

General Features. Approximately 4 percent of women with intestinal cancer have ovarian metastases at some time in the course of their disease (28–30,32–39,42–45,47–51). These tumors occur more often in women under 40 years of age than in older women. In one series (43) the mean age of the patients with colorectal carcinoma in whom ovarian metastases developed was 51 years in contrast to 62 years for all patients with that type of cancer. Abu-Rustum et al. (27a) reported that of 35 women with a history of colorectal cancer who had undergone adnexectomy for a new pelvic mass, 26 percent had a benign ovarian tumor, 17 percent a primary ovarian cancer, and 57 percent a metastatic colorectal cancer. Despite the frequency of metastasis in this setting, however, Lash and Hart (39) estimated that up to 45 percent of colorectal cancer metastases to the ovary are misinterpreted clinically as primary ovarian tumors, and many are misdiagnosed as such on microscopic examination, even when the existence of an intestinal cancer is known. In one study 77 percent of the intestinal primary tumors were in the rectum or sigmoid colon, 5 percent in the descending colon, 9 percent in the ascending colon, and 9 percent in the cecum (39). The tumors may also originate in the transverse colon (50) or the small intestine (44, 52a). The primary tumors may be very small and yet account for large, bilateral ovarian tumors (49).

Patients with metastatic intestinal carcinoma fall into three categories: 1) those who present with an intestinal carcinoma (50 to 75 percent of the cases), which antedates the diagnosis of the ovarian tumor by up to 3 years in 90 percent of the cases; 2) those in whom ovarian involvement is found unexpectedly during an operation for resection of an intestinal carcinoma (15 to 20 percent of the cases); and 3) those with initial manifestations of an ovarian tumor (3 to 20 percent of the cases). Except for those in the sex cord–stromal category, metastatic intestinal carcinomas are among the most common ovarian tumors associated with estrogenic or androgenic manifestations, which result from stimulation of the ovarian stroma by the neoplastic cells (see chapter 19). Almost all patients with intestinal carcinoma metastatic to the ovary die within 3 years of detection of ovarian involvement; the mean survival period in one series was 16 months (43).

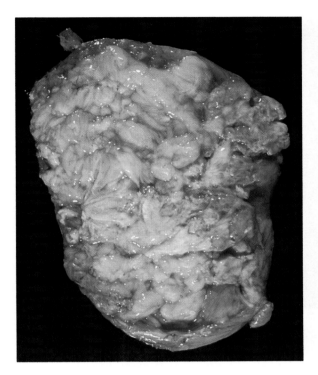

Figure 18-11
METASTATIC ADENOCARCINOMA FROM COLON
The sectioned surface is composed mostly of yellow necrotic tissue.

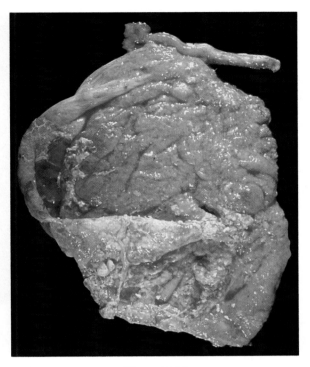

Figure 18-12
METASTATIC ADENOCARCINOMA FROM COLON
The cystic tumor is lined by shaggy necrotic tissue.

Gross Findings. Metastatic intestinal carcinomas are bilateral in approximately 60 percent of the cases. They may form solid masses, but are more often predominantly cystic. They are frequently large, with a median largest dimension of 11 cm in one series (39), and commonly rupture preoperatively or during their removal. Sectioning typically reveals friable or mushy yellow (fig. 18-11), red, or gray tissue, with cysts that contain necrotic tumor, mucinous or clear fluid, or fresh or old blood (fig. 18-12). An occasional tumor contains multiple, thin-walled cysts filled with mucinous or clear fluid, simulating closely a mucinous cystadenoma or cystadenocarcinoma (fig. 18-13).

Microscopic Findings. The tumor cells typically form small or large glands, which are often arranged in a cribriform pattern (fig. 18-14); mucin-containing goblet cells are occasionally scattered among mucin-free cells, but are often absent. Cysts lined by well differentiated mucin-rich epithelium form a prominent component of the tumor in up to 20 percent of the cases (fig. 18-15) (33,39). Rarely, the tumor has the pattern

of colloid carcinoma. Necrosis is common and often extensive, forming eosinophilic masses containing nuclear debris within cyst and gland lumens (dirty necrosis) (figs. 18-14, 18-16); this finding was present in all the cases in one series (39). Two other features of the tumor are the frequent disposition of glands in a ring at the edge of the necrotic material (likened to a garland) and focal segmental necrosis of the glandular epithelium (39). The glands are typically lined by stratified cells with moderate to severe cytologic atypia and frequent mitotic figures (fig. 18-16). The stroma may be desmoplastic, edematous, or mucoid, but often simulates ovarian stroma, containing cells resembling theca externa cells or theca lutein cells in approximately 30 percent of the cases (39).

We have seen several cases in which the rare clear cell adenocarcinoma of the intestine (37a) metastasized to the ovary (52a).

Differential Diagnosis. The most difficult tumors to exclude on microscopic examination are primary endometrioid and mucinous adenocarcinomas. In two series totaling 50 cases of metastatic

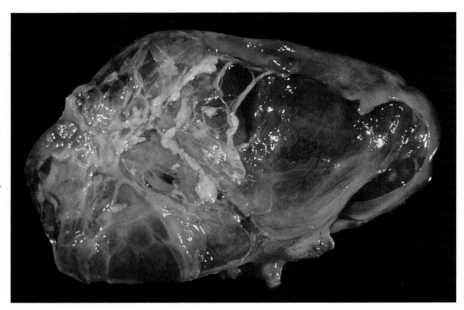

Figure 18-13
METASTATIC
ADENOCARCINOMA
FROM COLON
A multilocular cystic tumor with necrotic tissue focally adherent to the lining simulates a primary mucinous cystic tumor. (Fig. 123 from Young RH, Clement PB, Scully RE. Pathology of the ovary. In: Sternberg SS, ed. Diagnostic surgical pathology, Vol 2, 2nd ed. New York: Raven Press, 1994;2266.)

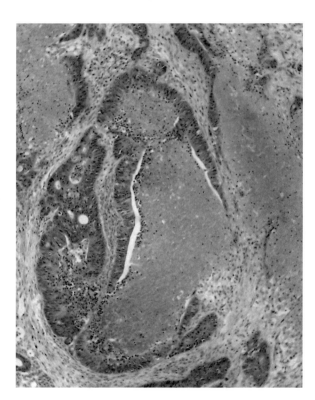

Figure 18-14
METASTATIC ADENOCARCINOMA FROM COLON
There is extensive "dirty" necrosis of tumor, with nuclear debris within amorphous necrotic tissue, which was eosinophilic.

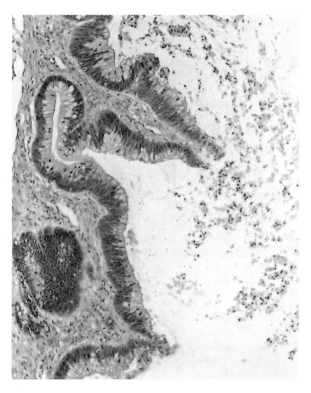

Figure 18-15
METASTATIC ADENOCARCINOMA FROM COLON
The mucinous epithelium is indistinguishable from that of a mucinous borderline tumor of intestinal type. Fig. 9 from Young RH, Scully RE. Metastatic tumors in the ovary. A problem oriented approach with review of the recent literature. Semin Diagn Pathol 1991;8:250–76.)

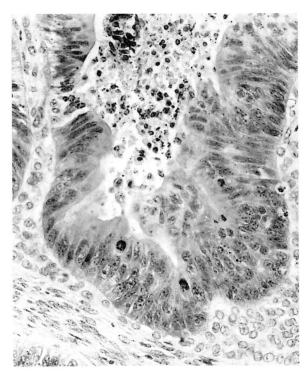

Figure 18-16
METASTATIC ADENOCARCINOMA FROM COLON
A gland lined by stratified cells with prominent nuclear atypia and mitotic activity contains "dirty" necrotic debris. (Fig. 8 from Young RH, Scully RE. Metastatic tumors in the ovary. A problem oriented approach with review of the recent literature. Semin Diagn Pathol 1991;8:250–76.)

intestinal cancers, 35 mimicked endometrioid carcinoma, 6 mucinous carcinoma, and 9 mixed endometrioid and mucinous carcinoma (33,39). The frequent bilaterality of metastatic intestinal carcinomas contrasts with the less than 15 percent frequency of bilateral involvement in cases of primary endometrioid and mucinous carcinomas. Endometrioid adenocarcinomas are often cystic, like metastatic intestinal adenocarcinomas, but the cysts in the former are sometimes filled with chocolate fluid, usually related to a background of endometriosis, and the solid component of the tumor is usually more homogeneous and less often necrotic.

On microscopic examination the glands of metastatic intestinal adenocarcinoma are typically lined by more poorly differentiated cells with greater nuclear hyperchromatism, loss of polarity, and mitotic activity than those of endometrioid adenocarcinomas with similar de-

grees of glandular differentiation. In addition, "dirty" necrosis is usually more extensive in metastatic intestinal carcinomas, but it may also be seen in endometrioid adenocarcinomas. Focal segmental necrosis of glandular lining epithelium is considerably more frequent in the former tumors as well. Foci of squamous differentiation occur in approximately one third of endometrioid carcinomas, but are rare in intestinal carcinomas; adjacent adenofibromatous neoplasia or endometriosis strongly favors endometrioid carcinoma. Immunostaining may be additionally helpful, although not definitive, in the differential diagnosis. Carcinoembryonic antigen (CEA) and especially some of its epitopes, are demonstrable much more often and more diffusely in colorectal adenocarcinomas than in endometrioid adenocarcinomas (33,33b,46) and the reverse is true for CA125 (31) and HAM-56 (33b, 40,41,52). Also, vimentin antibodies have been shown to decorate diffusely approximately one third of endometrioid adenocarcinomas but vimentin is rare and then only focal in colonic adenocarcinomas that resemble endometrioid adenocarcinomas (32a). Finally, a cytokeratin 7-positive/cytokeratin 20-negative immunophenotype has been demonstrated in 86 percent of endometrioid carcinomas in contrast to none of 16 metastatic colorectal carcinomas; and conversely, a cytokeratin 7-negative/cytokeratin 20-positive immunophenotype was demonstrated in 94 percent of the metastatic colorectal carcinomas in contrast to none of 64 endometrioid carcinomas (40a).

Primary mucinous carcinomas of the ovary have a range of microscopic appearances that do not suggest an intestinal carcinoma in most cases. In the minority of cases that resemble bowel cancers microscopically several criteria distinguish the primary tumors: 1) the much lower frequency of bilaterality, multinodularity, vascular-space invasion, and surface involvement; and 2) less variation in pattern within the tumor in most of the cases. Such variation is often striking in metastatic intestinal carcinomas (fig. 18-17). An admixture of carcinoma with benign-appearing and borderline-appearing mucinous epithelium lining glands and cysts would seem theoretically to favor a mucinous carcinoma arising on the background of a more benign neoplastic process, but use of such a criterion to exclude metastatic intestinal adenocarcinoma is

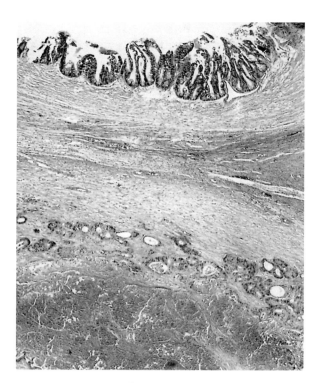

Figure 18-17
METASTATIC ADENOCARCINOMA FROM COLON
The upper part of the tumor is a cyst lined by papillae, and the lower part is a centrally necrotic array of small glands lying in a desmoplastic stroma.

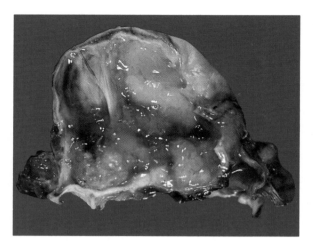

Figure 18-18
MUCINOUS TUMOR OF OVARY IN PATIENT WITH MUCINOUS CYSTIC TUMOR OF APPENDIX
The large and small cystic locules were filled with jelly-like material.

APPENDICEAL TUMORS

Ovarian metastases from appendiceal tumors may be seen in cases of adenocarcinoma, including tumors of typical intestinal (59a,61), colloid, and signet-ring cell types (57,59a); carcinoid tumors, which are almost always of the goblet cell type (53–56); and mucinous epithelial tumors of low-grade or borderline malignancy. The largest group of tumors that spread from the appendix to the ovary are in the last category in the opinion of some investigators (58,59b,62) but others interpret the ovarian tumors in such cases as independent primary tumors (60) (page 100). If these low-grade appendiceal tumors are excluded, only about 40 appendiceal carcinomas with ovarian metastases have been reported. In about one third of the cases the ovarian involvement accounted for the presenting manifestation.

Patients with low-grade mucinous tumors of the appendix, which typically appear as mucoceles on gross examination but can appear grossly normal, may have microscopically similar tumors in one or both ovaries accompanied by "pseudomyxoma peritonei" (58,60,62). Laparotomy in such cases typically discloses large cystic ovarian tumors, which are frequently bilateral and multilocular (fig. 18-18). The relations among the ovarian tumors, appendiceal tumors, and peritoneal disease in such cases are discussed on page 99.

unreliable. The latter occasionally contains a similar admixture of epithelia as a result of remarkable degrees of morphologic maturation of the tumor cells. The criterion may be helpful, however, near one end of the spectrum of admixed epithelia in which a small area of carcinoma is encountered on the background of a large, otherwise benign-appearing mucinous tumor. Such an admixture would strongly favor a primary carcinoma, as it would be unusual for a metastatic intestinal carcinoma to appear benign to such an extent. It occasionally, however, has very large areas simulating a primary borderline tumor of intestinal type. The rare metastatic intestinal clear cell carcinoma is distinguished from secretory endometrioid carcinoma and primary clear cell carcinoma of the ovary by the usual criteria for differentiating primary and metastatic tumors (page 335), as well as by immunohistochemical differences (page 343) (52a).

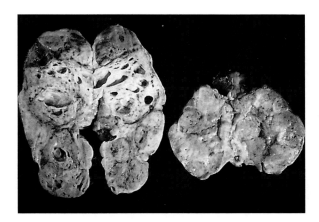

Figure 18-19
METASTATIC CARCINOID TUMOR
The smaller tumor is solid; the larger one contains numerous cysts, which were lined by the tumor cells. (Fig. 25 from Scully RE. Recent progress in ovarian cancer. Human Pathol 1970;1:73–98.)

CARCINOID TUMORS

General Features. In the largest series of pure carcinoid tumors metastatic to the ovary the age of the 35 patients ranged from 21 to 82 years, with a median of 57 years; 10 of the tumors were found at autopsy (59). Forty percent of the women whose metastases were discovered at operation had the carcinoid syndrome, and some of them also had signs and symptoms referable to intestinal or ovarian involvement. Extraovarian metastases were found in at least 90 percent of the cases. One third of the patients died within 1 year, and three fourths within 5 years; 6 patients, however, were asymptomatic for a median period of 5 years postoperatively. All 4 patients with the carcinoid syndrome had postoperative relief, 2 for periods of over 3 years after removal of the ovarian tumors. Although the primary tumors were mostly of small-intestinal origin in that series, on occasion they have been located in the colon, stomach, pancreas, or bronchus (59).

Goblet cell carcinoid tumors of the appendix spread to the ovary in approximately one third of the cases, and in over half these cases the patient presents with an ovarian mass (53–56). Typical carcinoid tumors of the appendix almost never spread to the ovary.

Gross Findings. Most metastatic carcinoid tumors are bilateral. They may be large and are typically predominantly solid, with smooth or

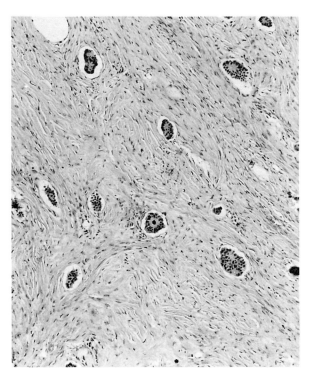

Figure 18-20
METASTATIC CARCINOID TUMOR
Small glands are scattered in a dense fibrous stroma. (Fig. 123 from Serov SF, Scully RE, Sobin LH. Histological typing of ovarian tumours. International Histological Classification of Tumours No. 9. Geneva: World Health Organization, 1973.)

bosselated surfaces. Sectioning reveals single or confluent, firm, white or yellow nodules, which may resemble ovarian fibromas or thecomas. Cysts of varying size are occasionally present and are typically filled with clear, watery fluid, resulting in a gross appearance similar to that of a cystadenofibroma (fig. 18-19). Necrosis and hemorrhage may occur but are usually only focal. Rare carcinoid tumors form predominantly cystic ovarian metastases. Cyst formation is more common in metastatic goblet cell carcinoid tumors than in other types.

Microscopic Findings. An insular pattern, similar to that of midgut carcinoid tumors, is most common, but glandular, trabecular (ribbonlike), mixed, and rarely, solid tubular patterns (figs. 18-20, 18-21) are also encountered. Acini, which are characteristically uniformly small and round, are common, distributed particularly at the periphery of islands of tumor cells (fig. 18-22); the lumens typically contain a homogeneous

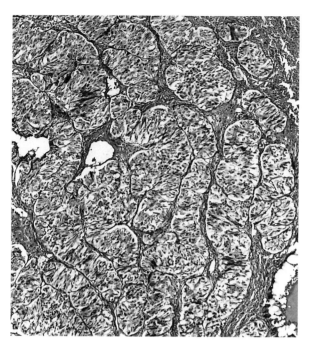

Figure 18-21
METASTATIC CARCINOID TUMOR
The tumor cells form solid tubular structures, simulating a Sertoli cell tumor (see figure 11-4). (Fig. 22.35 from Young RH, Scully RE. Metastatic tumors of the ovary. In: Kurman RJ, ed. Blaustein's pathology of the female genital tract, 4th ed. New York: Springer-Verlag, 1994:960.)

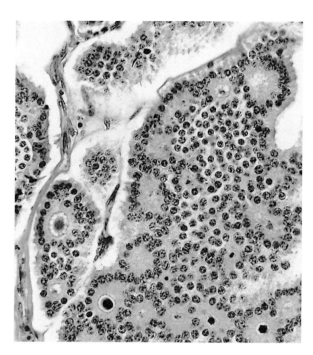

Figure 18-22
METASTATIC CARCINOID TUMOR
The gland lumens are round; the nuclei are round with coarse, stippled chromatin. (Fig. 122 from Serov SF, Scully RE, Sobin LH. Histological typing of ovarian tumours. International Histological Classification of Tumours No. 9. Geneva: World Health Organization, 1973.)

eosinophilic secretion which may undergo calcification, sometimes in the form of psammoma bodies. Cysts and follicle-like spaces lined by one or a few layers of neoplastic cells are sometimes seen (fig. 18-23). Occasionally, nests of tumor cells disintegrate, with the cells separating from one another; this phenomenon may be the forerunner of cyst formation. With rare exceptions, the carcinoid tumor is the only ovarian metastatic tumor that elicits an extensive stromal proliferation that closely resembles an ovarian fibroma (fig. 18-20); occasionally, the stroma becomes extensively hyalinized. The cytologic features of the tumors are as seen elsewhere; in occasional tumors the cells have abundant eosinophilic cytoplasm (fig. 18-24), resembling oxyphilic tumors of other types (see Table 6-1).

Metastatic goblet cell carcinoid tumors have rounded nests and glands containing both goblet cells and argentaffin or argyrophil cells (fig. 18-25). These tumors may also contain aggregates of signet-ring cells closely resembling a Kruken-

berg tumor, tubules, cysts filled with mucin, and nests of tumor cells lying in pools of mucin.

Differential Diagnosis. Metastatic carcinoid tumors are similar microscopically to primary ovarian tumors of the same type. The differential diagnosis has been discussed on page 293. Metastatic carcinoid tumors may be confused also with adult granulosa cell tumors (page 178); Sertoli or Sertoli-Leydig cell tumors; Brenner tumors; benign, borderline, and malignant adenofibromas and cystadenofibromas; and adenocarcinomas of various types. The sex cord–like formations of Sertoli-Leydig cell tumors may resemble the ribbons of the trabecular carcinoid but the latter are usually longer and thicker and have a more orderly architecture. Confusion may be caused by the occasional presence of a carcinoid component, which is usually minor in extent, in Sertoli-Leydig cell tumors with mucinous heterologous elements. We have seen only two heterologous Sertoli-Leydig cell tumors with a carcinoid component that was large enough to be visible on gross examination.

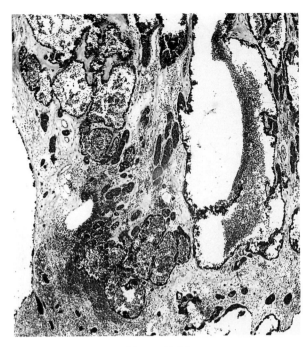

Figure 18-23
METASTATIC CARCINOID TUMOR
Follicle-like spaces are present. (Fig. 25 from Young RH, Scully RE. Metastatic tumors in the ovary. A problem oriented approach with a review of the recent literature. Semin Diagn Pathol 1991;8:250–76.)

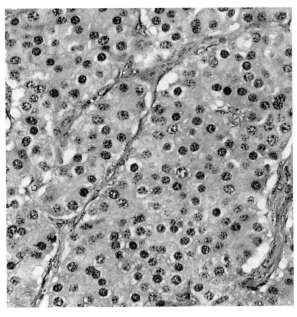

Figure 18-24
METASTATIC CARCINOID TUMOR
The tumor cells have abundant cytoplasm, which was eosinophilic. The nuclei are round with stippled chromatin. (Fig. 31 from Young RH, Scully RE. Metastatic tumors in the ovary. A problem oriented approach with a review of the recent literature. Semin Diagn Pathol 1991;8:250–76.)

Even in such tumors the finding of distinctive patterns of Sertoli-Leydig cell tumor enable one to make the correct diagnosis.

The fibromatous stroma of a Brenner tumor may be indistinguishable from that of an occasional metastatic carcinoid tumor but the epithelial nests of the former contain cells of urothelial type, with oval, pale, grooved nuclei, rather than the cells of carcinoid tumors with their characteristic round nuclei containing stippled chromatin. Benign and malignant adenofibromas and endometrioid adenocarcinomas containing small acini are generally readily distinguished from carcinoid tumors by the differing patterns and cytologic features of these tumors. A metastatic breast carcinoma with a prominent insular pattern may simulate a carcinoid tumor.

If a carcinoid tumor is difficult to diagnose, more thorough sampling; histochemical staining for argentaffin and argyrophil granules; immunohistochemical staining for chromogranin, neuron-specific enolase, peptide hormones, and

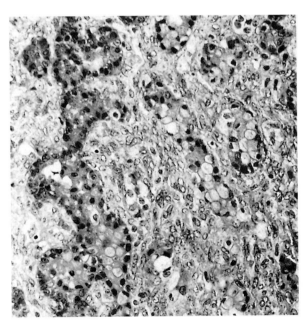

Figure 18-25
METASTATIC GOBLET CELL CARCINOID TUMOR
Solid tubules contain goblet cells and cells with dense cytoplasm, which were argentaffin.

serotonin; and an electron microscopic search for dense core granules should resolve the problem. Some of the above-mentioned tumors in the differential diagnosis, however, may stain similarly, contain occasional dense core granules, or both. Adenocarcinomas of the stomach, intestine, and ovary may contain scattered argentaffin or argyrophil cells but the diagnosis of goblet cell carcinoid tumor should be reserved for cases in which the distinctive pattern of small nests characteristic of that tumor is present. Distinction of a metastatic goblet cell carcinoid tumor from the rare primary form may be difficult and depends on knowledge of the distribution of disease and the presence or absence of a dermoid or epidermoid cyst, which may be associated with the latter tumor; bilaterality and extraovarian spread strongly favor metastasis. Metastatic goblet cell carcinoid tumors of the ovary have been reported much more often than primary tumors of the same type.

TUMORS OF THE PANCREAS, BILIARY TRACT, AND LIVER

Pancreatic adenocarcinomas account for up to 10 percent of ovarian metastases that present clinically as ovarian masses (66a,66c). These tumors are typically bilateral, large, cystic, and multiloculated, and may mimic closely primary mucinous tumors of the ovary (fig. 18-26) (68). Microscopic examination of metastatic pancreatic tumors, which are usually ductal adenocarcinomas, shows varying degrees of differentiation, with cysts resembling those of ovarian mucinous cystadenomas (fig. 18-27), borderline tumors, and well differentiated cystadenocarcinomas as well as areas of infiltrating small glands and single cells. The features that are helpful in identifying a mucinous tumor as metastatic from the pancreas are similar to those used for recognizing metastatic intestinal carcinomas, with surface implantation being an important criterion (fig. 18-28). Adenocarcinomas of the pancreas with a microglandular pattern (65a) may spread to the ovary and mimic a primary or metastatic ovarian carcinoid tumor (fig. 18-29), but do not contain argyrophil cells. Six percent of Krukenberg tumors in one series were primary in the pancreas (66b).

Metastatic tumors from the gallbladder and bile ducts are rarely encountered by the surgeon.

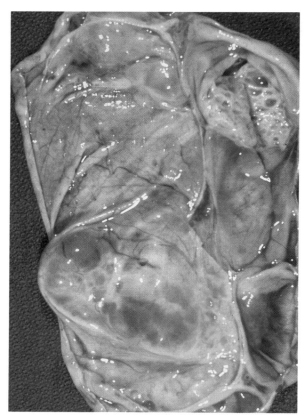

Figure 18-26
METASTATIC ADENOCARCINOMA FROM PANCREAS
The appearance is indistinguishable from that of a primary mucinous cystic tumor.

They are typically solid. Microscopic examination may disclose the characteristic small irregular glands that are present in the primary tumor or an appearance that simulates a primary endometrioid or mucinous carcinoma, or even a cystadenofibroma of the ovary (fig. 18-30) (69). Rarely, the ovarian metastatic tumor is of the Krukenberg type (64,65).

Spread of hepatocellular carcinoma to the ovary is unusual and is most often an incidental autopsy finding, but a few clinically important cases have been reported (66,67). One patient had bilateral ovarian tumors discovered at the same time as the hepatic tumor. In another woman the hepatic tumor was detected by radiologic investigation after bilateral ovarian tumors had been removed (fig. 18-31). In two other cases unilateral ovarian tumors were discovered within 1 year after the hepatic tumor was diagnosed.

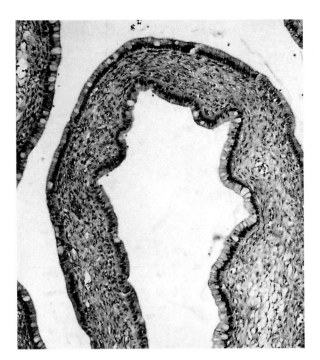

Figure 18-27
METASTATIC ADENOCARCINOMA FROM PANCREAS
The lining epithelium is indistinguishable from that of a slightly atypical mucinous cystadenoma. (Fig. 11 from Young RH, Scully RE. Metastatic tumors in the ovary. A problem oriented approach with review of recent literature. Semin Diagn Pathol 1991;8:250–76.)

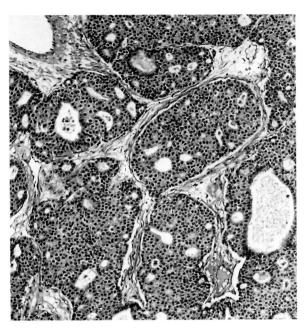

Figure 18-29
METASTATIC PANCREATIC ADENOCARCINOMA WITH MICROGLANDULAR PATTERN
Islands of tumor cells contain numerous small acini. The tumor mimics a carcinoid tumor (see figure 18-22). (Fig. 20 from Young RH, Scully RE. Metastatic tumors in the ovary. A problem oriented approach with review of recent literature. Semin Diagn Pathol 1991;8:250–76.)

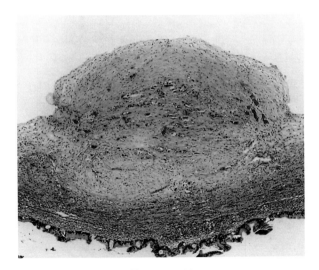

Figure 18-28
METASTATIC ADENOCARCINOMA
FROM PANCREAS
A surface implant with a desmoplastic stroma is present. The intraovarian tumor was a large cyst lined by moderately differentiated cells (bottom).

Microscopic examination has shown features characteristic of hepatocellular carcinoma except for one case in which cysts were prominent. Rare cholangiocarcinomas (67) and at least one hepatoblastoma (63) have metastasized to the ovary.

The major differential diagnosis of metastatic hepatocellular carcinoma involves hepatoid yolk sac tumor (page 247), primary hepatoid carcinoma (page 323), and metastatic hepatoid carcinomas from the stomach and lung. The finding of bile in the ovarian tumor favors the diagnosis of metastatic hepatocellular carcinoma.

BREAST CARCINOMA

General Features. Ovarian metastases are found at autopsy in 10 to 20 percent of patients with breast cancer (74,84,85) and in approximately 30 percent of patients who have had therapeutic oophorectomy for metastatic breast cancer (75, 77,78,80,81). In one series of cases, 17 percent of the ovarian metastases clinically simulated a

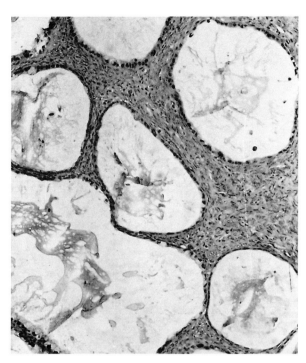

Figure 18-30
METASTATIC ADENOCARCINOMA
FROM GALLBLADDER
Cystically dilated glands lined by minimally atypical epithelium lie in a fibromatous stroma, mimicking a cystadenofibroma (see figure 6-5).

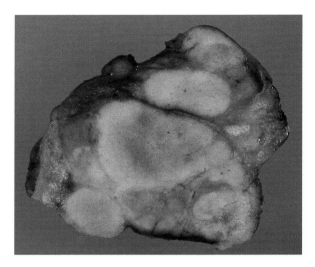

Figure 18-31
METASTATIC HEPATOCELLULAR CARCINOMA
Pale yellow and green nodules are seen on the sectioned surface.

primary ovarian tumor, a frequency surpassed only by that of colon cancer as a mimic of a primary ovarian tumor (87a). Sometimes, the ovarian metastatic tumor is evident before the detection of the primary tumor (87); 9 of 76 cases in one study, which included numerous consultation cases, were in this category (72). Although ovarian metastases of breast cancer are usually accompanied by other intra-abdominal metastases, involvement was limited to the ovary in 13 percent of the cases in one series (73). Lobular carcinomas, including those of signet-ring cell type, spread to the ovary more frequently than ductal carcinomas; in one study 36 percent of the former metastasized to the ovaries in contrast to only 2.6 percent of the latter (74). Because of the greater frequency of ductal carcinoma, however, approximately 75 percent of ovarian metastases of breast cancer are of the ductal type (72).

Gross Findings. Both ovaries are involved in approximately two thirds of the cases (fig. 18-32)

(70,72,73,76,83). The surfaces are often irregular due to the presence of discrete or confluent nodules (fig. 18-32), and sectioning reveals typically firm or gritty, white nodules of various sizes. When the organ is replaced by tumor, it is transformed into a smooth-surfaced or bosselated mass; cysts are present in about 20 percent of the cases (fig. 18-33) (72), and rarely, the tumor is entirely cystic. Exceptionally, papillae are evident on gross examination. Tumors larger than 5 cm accounted for only 15 percent of the cases in one study, which included both autopsy and therapeutic-oophorectomy cases (73).

Microscopic Findings. In cases of metastatic ductal carcinoma, tubular glands, islands, and small clusters of cells are common (fig. 18-34); in cases of lobular carcinoma parallel cords of cells are frequent (fig. 18-35). Lobular carcinomas may also have an insular pattern (fig. 18-36). A pure cribriform pattern is infrequent but focal cribriform areas are common in ductal-type metastases, and rarely, such tumors contain papillae. In approximately half the cases, at least a portion of the tumor has a diffuse pattern, which is more common in cases of metastatic lobular carcinoma.

Occasionally, the tumor cells of either subtype grow as single cells. Admixtures of several patterns may be seen. In premenopausal women, small deposits are often seen in the highly vascular theca interna of a graafian follicle or in the

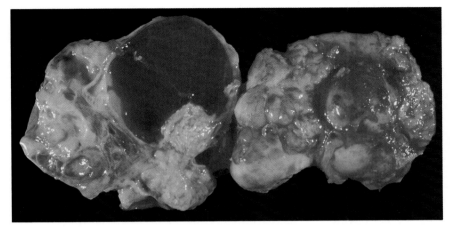

Figure 18-32
METASTATIC CARCINOMA
FROM BREAST
Multiple confluent nodules of
tumor are present on the external
(right) and sectioned (left) surfaces.

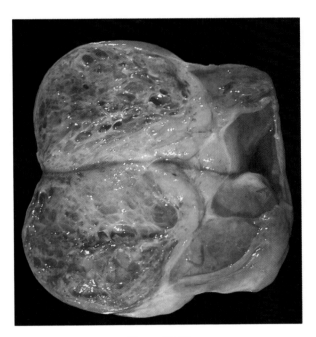

Figure 18-33
METASTATIC CARCINOMA FROM BREAST
The sectioned surface shows predominantly solid tissue
containing numerous small cysts.

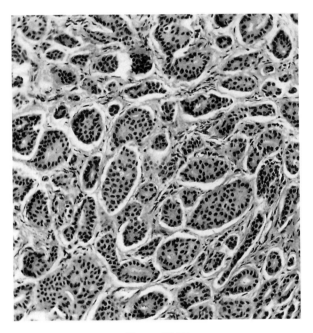

Figure 18-34
METASTATIC CARCINOMA
FROM BREAST, DUCTAL TYPE
The tumor cells are growing as small nests and glands.
(Fig. 19 from Young RH, Scully RE. Metastatic tumors in the
ovary. A problem oriented approach with review of the recent
literature. Semin Diagn Pathol 1991;8:250–76.)

granulosa or theca layer of a corpus luteum.
Signet-ring cells are usually not conspicuous unless the primary tumor contains them, but occasionally, a metastatic breast cancer is a Krukenberg tumor (78,82). The stroma of the tumor
varies from sparse to abundant; it is rarely luteinized in contrast to metastatic colorectal carcinoma.
Lymphatic invasion in the ovary was seen in 15
percent of the cases in one series (73).

Differential Diagnosis. Rare predominantly
glandular metastatic breast cancers resemble surface epithelial adenocarcinomas, particularly
those of endometrioid type; other metastatic breast
cancers simulate undifferentiated carcinomas.
With regard to these differential diagnoses, the
authors of one study (71) reported that a patient

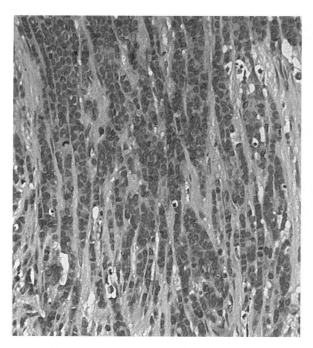

Figure 18-35
METASTATIC CARCINOMA
FROM BREAST, LOBULAR TYPE
The tumor cells are growing in cords. (Fig. 22.11 from Young RH, Scully RE. Metastatic tumors of the ovary. In: Kurman RJ, ed. Blaustein's pathology of the female genital tract. New York: Springer-Verlag, 1994;948.)

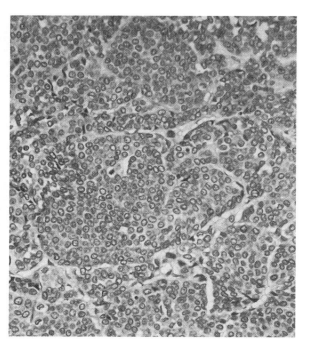

Figure 18-36
METASTATIC CARCINOMA
FROM BREAST, LOBULAR TYPE
The tumor cells are growing in closely packed islands, which resemble those of an insular granulosa cell tumor. (Fig. 22.12 from Young RH, Scully RE. Metastatic tumors of the ovary. In: Kurman RJ, ed. Blaustein's pathology of the female genital tract. New York: Springer-Verlag, 1994;948.)

with breast carcinoma and a subsequent carcinoma in the ovary was three times as likely to have a primary ovarian carcinoma as a metastatic tumor from the breast. Occasionally, other neoplasms enter the differential diagnosis. An insular pattern may mimic that of a carcinoid tumor (page 291) or a metastatic desmoplastic small round cell tumor with divergent differentiation (page 357). A metastatic breast carcinoma with a diffuse or insular pattern, particularly one of the lobular type, may also simulate a granulosa cell tumor (page 170). Staining of an ovarian neoplasm immunohistochemically for gross cystic disease fluid protein-15 (GCDFP-15) (fig. 18-37) may help to distinguish metastatic breast carcinoma from a primary ovarian carcinoma and other neoplasms with which it may be confused (79). In one study, 11 of 14 ovarian metastatic breast carcinomas exhibited strong cytoplasmic staining, usually in a paranuclear pattern; in contrast, 7 ovarian metastases of other tumors and 32 primary ovarian carcinomas failed to stain (79). In a similar

study only 4 percent of primary ovarian carcinomas were positive in contrast to 53 percent of primary lobular carcinomas and 77 percent of primary ductal carcinomas of the breast (86). Staining for GCDFP-15 and an absence of staining for desmin establishes the diagnosis of metastatic breast carcinoma when the differential diagnosis involves desmoplastic small round cell tumor with divergent differentiation. Rarely, the diffuse patterns and occasional cord-like patterns of malignant lymphoma and leukemic infiltration of the ovary cause a problem in diagnosis (pages 363 and 366).

RENAL TUMORS

Ten cases of clinically detected ovarian metastases of renal cell carcinoma have been reported (90,91). In six patients, the ovarian tumor was discovered first, leading to an initial misdiagnosis of primary ovarian clear cell carcinoma in

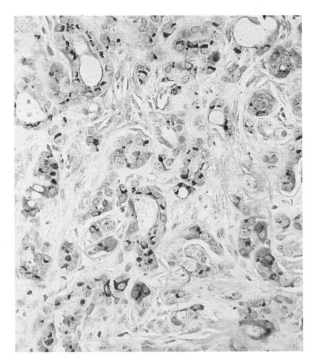

Figure 18-37
METASTATIC CARCINOMA
FROM BREAST, DUCTAL TYPE

The tumor cells are immunoreactive for gross cystic disease fluid protein (GCDFP)-15.

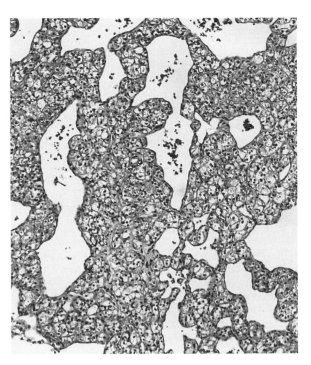

Figure 18-38
METASTATIC RENAL CELL CARCINOMA

The tumor cells have abundant clear cytoplasm; the pattern of dilated sinusoids is characteristic. (Fig. 16 from Young RH, Scully RE. Metastatic tumors in the ovary. A problem oriented approach with review of the recent literature. Semin Diagn Pathol 1991;8:250–76.)

three cases. The renal tumors were discovered within a short interval in most of these cases but one remained undetected for 8 years. The renal tumors were usually well differentiated clear cell carcinomas. Microscopic examination of the ovarian metastases showed diffuse sheets or nests of clear cells or tubules lined by clear cells and filled with eosinophilic fluid or blood; a prominent sinusoidal vascular pattern was almost always present (fig. 18-38). One patient with a renal-pelvic transitional cell carcinoma had an ovarian metastatic tumor at presentation (88) and another had ovarian spread after 4 years (89). One child with a renal rhabdoid tumor presented with an ovarian metastasis initially misinterpreted as a granulosa cell tumor (92).

In contrast to metastatic renal cell carcinomas, primary clear cell carcinomas of the ovary have an additional tubulocystic or papillary component, or both; hobnail cells; and intraluminal mucin in most of the cases. The latter two features, in contrast, are exceptional in renal cell carcinomas. In addition, the typical sinusoidal vascular framework of renal cell carcinoma is not a feature of ovarian clear cell carcinoma. In cases of clear cell carcinoma of the ovary without hobnail cells or mucin secretion, radiologic evaluation of the kidney may be necessary to exclude a renal cell carcinoma. Differentiation of ovarian transitional cell carcinomas from metastatic renal tumors of the same cell type is based on the same criteria used in distinguishing the former from metastatic transitional cell carcinomas of the urinary bladder (page 356).

PULMONARY AND MEDIASTINAL TUMORS

Approximately 5 percent of women with lung cancer have ovarian metastases at autopsy, and rarely, the metastatic tumor precedes the discovery of the pulmonary tumor or is found simultaneously (97). Small cell carcinoma accounts for most metastatic tumors from the lung (fig. 18-39),

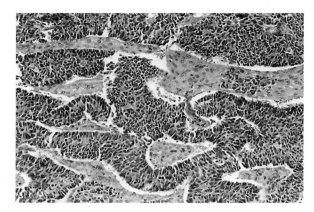

Figure 18-39
METASTATIC SMALL CELL CARCINOMA FROM LUNG
The tumor has a trabecular pattern. (Fig. 24 from Young RH, Scully RE. Metastatic tumors in the ovary. A problem oriented approach with review of the recent literature. Semin Diagn Pathol 1991;8:250–76.)

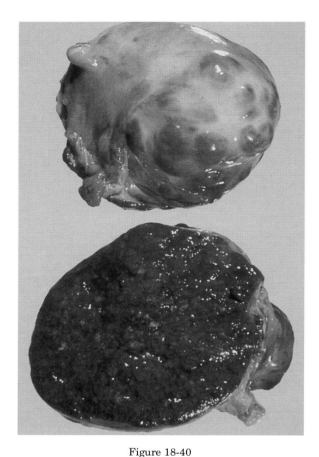

Figure 18-40
METASTATIC MELANOMA
The tumor has a bosselated external surface; the sectioned surface is black.

followed by adenocarcinoma and large cell carcinoma. When a patient has a pulmonary and ovarian neoplasm it can be difficult to decide which tumor is primary (97). When the histologic features are typical of a lung carcinoma, a pulmonary origin is probable. Small cell carcinomas of pulmonary type may be primary in the ovary (94) but are generally unassociated with pulmonary metastasis (page 320). The usual presence of a surface epithelial component in the ovarian tumor provides strong evidence for an ovarian origin.

Three patients have had mediastinal small cell carcinoma, apparently of thymic origin, and ovarian metastasis at the time of presentation (93). Rare thymomas (95) and one neuroblastoma of the posterior mediastinum (96) have metastasized to the ovary.

MALIGNANT MELANOMA

Patients with malignant melanoma have ovarian involvement at autopsy in almost 20 percent of the cases (98); ovarian metastasis from malignant melanoma that is detectable during life is much less common. Although some patients have a known primary tumor and evidence of metastasis elsewhere, isolated ovarian spread is seen occasionally, sometimes with a negative or remote history of a primary melanoma (100). Ovarian metastatic melanomas are bilateral in 45 percent of the cases (99,100). On gross examination there are no dis-

tinctive features except for black or brown coloration in some cases (figs. 18-40, 18-41). The most common of the many microscopic appearances is a diffuse proliferation of large cells with abundant eosinophilic cytoplasm (fig. 18-42) and nuclei with prominent nucleoli. Occasional tumors, in contrast, have a predominant or even exclusive population of small cells with scanty cytoplasm (fig. 18-43). Although spindle cells may be seen, they are generally inconspicuous. In one series of metastatic melanomas prominent nucleoli were seen in 65 percent of the cases and numerous intranuclear pseudoinclusions of cytoplasm in 25 percent (100). Melanin pigment was inconspicuous or absent in approximately half the cases in two large series (99,100). A helpful diagnostic feature of many metastatic melanomas is the presence of discrete rounded aggregates with a nevoid

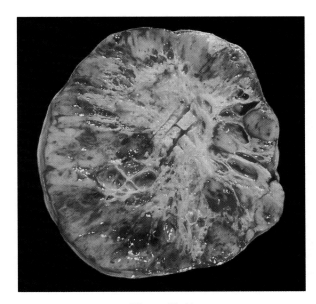

Figure 18-41
METASTATIC MELANOMA
The sectioned surface is pale yellow with focal hemorrhage.

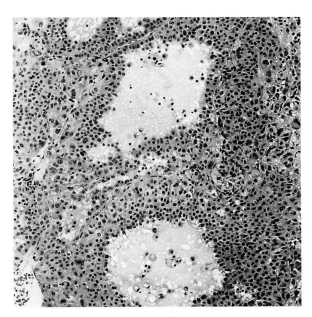

Figure 18-42
METASTATIC MELANOMA
The tumor contains several follicle-like spaces and the tumor cells have abundant cytoplasm, which was eosinophilic, imparting a resemblance to a juvenile granulosa cell tumor (see figure 9-23). (Fig. 26 from Young RH, Scully RE. Metastatic tumors in the ovary. A problem oriented approach with review of the recent literature. Semin Diagn Pathol 1991;8:250–76.)

appearance. One confusing feature of metastatic melanoma in the ovary, seen in approximately 40 percent of the cases, is the presence of follicle-like spaces (figs. 18-42, 18-43) (100).

Metastatic melanoma must be distinguished from the rare primary malignant melanoma, which usually arises in the wall of a dermoid cyst. The cyst may show junctional activity beneath its squamous lining cells; rarely, another teratomatous component, such as struma ovarii, accompanies the primary melanoma. In cases of apparently pure ovarian melanoma without an obvious primary tumor elsewhere an occult primary tumor should be searched for. If there is no evidence of the latter it remains possible that a primary cutaneous melanoma that had regressed was the source of the ovarian tumor. In such cases bilaterality, growth of the ovarian tumor in the form of multiple nodules, or both strongly suggest metastasis even in the absence of a known primary tumor.

The presence of follicle-like spaces in some metastatic melanomas has suggested the diagnosis of granulosa cell tumor (fig. 18-42) (100); this differential diagnosis is discussed on pages 178 and 186. When follicle-like spaces are found in a metastatic melanoma with small cells, the

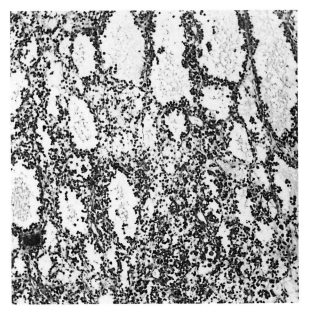

Figure 18-43
METASTATIC MELANOMA
The tumor contains many follicle-like spaces and the cells are small with scanty cytoplasm, imparting a resemblance to a small cell carcinoma of hypercalcemic type (see figure 17-10).

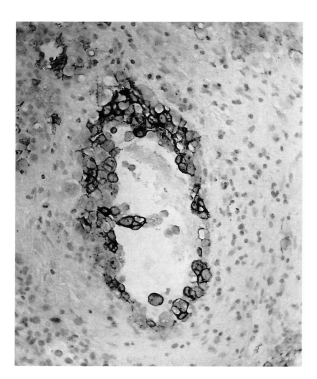

Figure 18-44
METASTATIC MELANOMA
The cells surrounding a follicle-like space are immunoreactive for HMB-45. (Fig. 27 from Young RH, Scully RE. Metastatic tumors in the ovary. A problem oriented approach with review of the recent literature. Semin Diagn Pathol 1991;8:250–76.)

diagnosis of small cell carcinoma of hypercalcemic type may be suggested (fig. 18-43) (page 316). Metastatic melanoma, particularly if it is amelanotic, may resemble a lipid-poor steroid cell tumor if the cells have abundant cytoplasm, or an adult granulosa cell tumor if they do not (99); in a pregnant patient pregnancy luteoma, which may also be in the form of multiple nodules, may be suggested. Also, melanin can be misinterpreted as lipochrome pigment, which may be present in steroid cell tumors and impart a dark green-brown or almost black color to the neoplasm. Some metastatic melanomas mimic surface epithelial carcinomas, especially transitional cell and undifferentiated carcinomas. The diagnosis of metastatic melanoma may be confirmed in these problem cases by the immunohistochemical demonstration of S-100 protein and HMB-45 (fig. 18-44) and a failure to stain for various antigens characteristic of other neoplasms in the differential diagnosis.

MISCELLANEOUS TUMORS

Urinary Tract Tumors

It may be difficult to distinguish between a rare metastatic urothelial tumor and a primary transitional cell neoplasm (113). In borderline and malignant Brenner tumors, however, foci of benign Brenner tumor are also present, often accompanied by benign mucinous epithelium. In primary transitional cell carcinomas components of other surface epithelial carcinomas are also detectable in most cases. If a urinary tract carcinoma is present, the extent of its invasion, as well as various features that favor a primary or metastatic ovarian tumor, have to be considered in the differential diagnosis. Finally, primary urinary tract transitional cell tumors are almost always stained by cytokeratin-20, whereas ovarian tumors of this type are very rarely stained (107). Three signet-ring cell carcinomas of the bladder have been the source of Krukenberg tumors (111), and we have also seen two metastatic urachal adenocarcinomas that simulated primary mucinous cystic tumors (107a).

Neuroblastoma

Twenty-five to 50 percent of females with adrenal neuroblastoma have ovarian involvement at autopsy, and clinically significant metastases are occasionally seen (110). In one case there was bilateral ovarian involvement at presentation, and in two other cases ovarian metastatic tumor caused the initial clinical manifestations. Bilaterality, absence of an association with a teratoma, and the presence of a known primary tumor elsewhere are helpful in the recognition of an ovarian neuroblastoma as metastatic. The prominent fibrillary background of neuroblastoma and the presence of Wright pseudorosettes should aid in the distinction of neuroblastoma from other small cell tumors (see Table 5-4), and immunohistochemical staining and electron microscopic examination may be helpful in difficult cases.

Rhabdomyosarcoma

Eleven rhabdomyosarcomas metastatic to the ovary, over half of which were of the alveolar type (fig. 18-45), have been reported (112). The ovarian tumors have rarely caused symptoms. Primary alveolar rhabdomyosarcoma of the ovary is very rare (page 315). Embryonal rhabdomyosarcoma

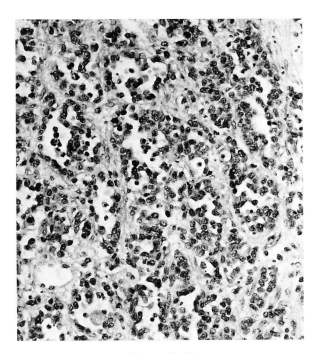

Figure 18-45
METASTATIC ALVEOLAR RHABDOMYOSARCOMA
Diagnostic rhabdomyoblasts are not visible. (Fig. 29 from Young RH, Scully RE. Metastatic tumors in the ovary. A problem oriented approach with review of the recent literature. Semin Diagn Pathol 1991;8:250–76.)

metastatic to the ovary must be distinguished from the primary form, the most common subtype of primary rhabdomyosarcoma of the ovary (page 315). All these tumors must be differentiated from other highly malignant primary and metastatic small cell tumors of the ovary, most of which occur in young patients (see Table 5-4). The ovary may be involved also by rhabdomyosarcoma in patients with bone marrow involvement and a clinical picture simulating that of acute leukemia (112).

Other Sarcomas

Rarely, hemangiosarcomas, several of which were primary in the breast (105,106), have metastasized to the ovaries, as have a few Ewing sarcomas. Also reported are four metastatic leiomyosarcomas (one primary in the stomach, two in the small intestine, and the fourth in the retrovesical area), and single examples of fibrosarcoma of the anterior abdominal wall, mesenteric sarcoma of smooth muscle or neural type,

osteosarcoma of the maxilla, chondrosarcoma of the rib, and chordoma (112,114). The only tumor in this group that caused diagnostic difficulty was an epithelioid leiomyosarcoma of the stomach with a unilateral ovarian metastatic tumor that presented as an ovarian mass and was confused with a Sertoli cell tumor (110). Clinical findings as well as the results of immunohistochemical staining help in the diagnosis of the above tumors.

Miscellaneous Carcinomas

Rare thyroid carcinomas have spread to the ovary, including one case in which ovarian involvement was detected 12 years after resection of the primary tumor (109). Isolated examples of head and neck carcinoma metastatic to the ovary have been documented. One 30-year-old woman had symptomatic ovarian metastases 10 years after resection of an adenoid cystic carcinoma of the submandibular gland (104) and we have seen an unpublished case of a young woman who had bilateral symptomatic ovarian metastases 11 years after treatment of a similar tumor of the parotid gland. Two Merkel cell tumors primary in the skin of the groin metastasized to the ovary (102).

Peritoneal Tumors

Secondary ovarian involvement by malignant mesothelioma is common (101,103). In most cases the tumor is confined to the surface of the ovary (fig. 18-46), but parenchymal invasion may be prominent (fig. 18-47). When ovarian involvement dominates the clinical presentation, differentiation from a primary ovarian cancer may be a problem. In one series of cases (101), most of the ovarian tumors were initially misinterpreted as primary neoplasms of various types, ranging from surface epithelial carcinomas to germ cell tumors to steroid cell tumors. Immunohistochemical staining may be necessary to distinguish among these various tumors (page 73). Rarely, malignant mesothelioma is primary in the ovary (101) (page 329). The differentiation of primary peritoneal and ovarian serous carcinomas is discussed on page 451.

A peritoneal tumor that may cause a major problem in differential diagnosis is the intra-abdominal desmoplastic small round cell tumor with divergent differentiation, which has been associated with ovarian involvement at presentation

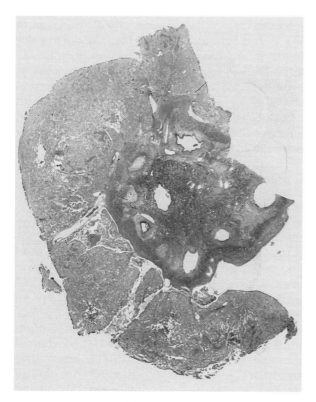

Figure 18-46
MESOTHELIOMA INVOLVING OVARY
The tumor coats the surface of the ovary.

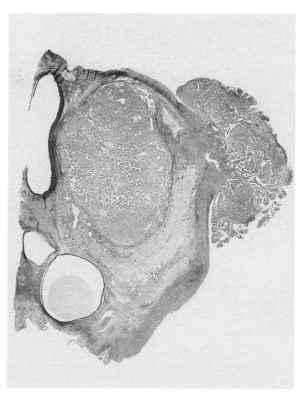

Figure 18-47
MESOTHELIOMA INVOLVING OVARY
Tumor is present on the surface; a large nodule occupies the parenchyma. (Fig. 1 from Young RH, Gersell DJ, Roth LM, Scully RE. Ovarian metastases from cervical carcinomas other than pure adenocarcinomas. A report of 12 cases. Cancer 1993;71:407–18.)

in several cases (108). In two cases the ovarian tumor was initially thought to be the primary neoplasm; in all the cases there was also extensive extraovarian tumor at the time of presentation. Microscopic examination of the ovarian metastases (figs. 18-48–18-53) shows nodules composed predominantly of nests of mitotically active small cells with hyperchromatic nuclei and scanty cytoplasm surrounded by a prominent desmoplastic stroma (figs. 18-48, 18-49). In some areas, however, the stroma may be scanty or the cells may have moderate to large amounts of cytoplasm. Small clusters or cords of tumor cells may be present (fig. 18-51). Gland-like structures are occasionally identified (fig. 18-52) as well as other epithelial-like formations that are diagnostically confusing. In some cases there is a biphasic appearance of the tumor due to the presence of nests of small rounded cells on a background of malignant-appearing spindle cells (fig. 18-50). These neoplasms exhibit a characteristic immu-

nohistochemical staining profile, with many of the tumor cells staining for cytokeratin, epithelial membrane antigen, vimentin, and particularly, desmin (fig. 18-53). The differential diagnosis is extensive and includes the many other primary and secondary small cell tumors that may involve the ovary, the features of which are described elsewhere (see Table 5-4).

UTERINE TUMORS

Endometrial Carcinoma

Although endometrial carcinomas of endometrioid type have often spread to the ovary by the time of autopsy (115,116) and metastatic ovarian involvement is occasionally encountered during life, endometrioid carcinoma of the ovary associated with a similar tumor of the endometrium is

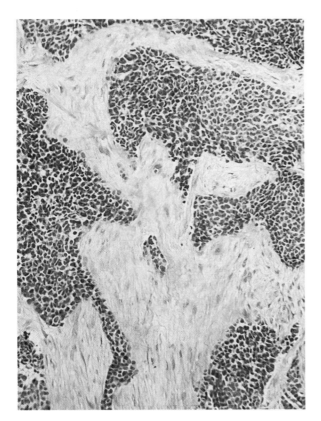

Figure 18-48
DESMOPLASTIC SMALL ROUND
CELL TUMOR INVOLVING OVARY
Discrete aggregates of small cells are embedded in a desmoplastic stroma.

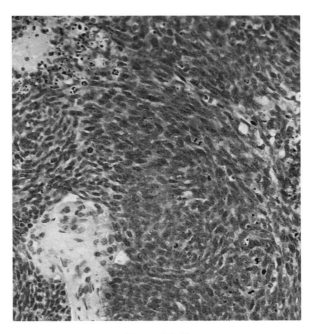

Figure 18-49
DESMOPLASTIC SMALL ROUND
CELL TUMOR INVOLVING OVARY
The cells are small and spindle shaped, with scanty cytoplasm. Mitotic figures are visible.

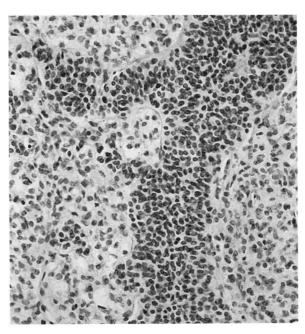

Figure 18-50
DESMOPLASTIC SMALL ROUND
CELL TUMOR INVOLVING OVARY
The trabeculae are surrounded by a diffuse cellular proliferation. This pattern resembles that of a carcinosarcoma.

often independently primary (117,121,124). Criteria helpful in distinguishing between independently primary neoplasia of both organs and metastasis from one organ to the other are discussed on page 125 and outlined in Tables 5-1, 5-2, and 5-3. Associations of endometrial and ovarian serous and clear cell carcinomas are less common (117); in some cases the presence of fragments of tumor within the tubal lumen or striking surface involvement (fig. 18-54) suggests spread of tumor from one organ to the other. Many of the criteria used for determining the site of origin of endometrioid carcinoma involving both organs can be used for serous and clear cell carcinomas. Rarely, ovarian surface lesions secondary to endometrioid adenocarcinoma with squamous differentiation takes the form of deposits of keratin or ghosts of mature squamous cells eliciting a foreign-body giant cell response (119) (page 127).

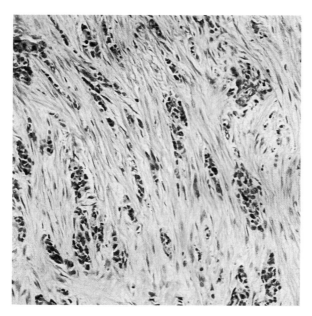

Figure 18-51
DESMOPLASTIC SMALL ROUND
CELL TUMOR INVOLVING OVARY
Small clusters of cells in a desmoplastic stroma simulate metastatic breast carcinoma. (Fig. 35 from Young RH, Scully RE. Metastatic tumors in the ovary. A problem oriented approach with review of the recent literature. Semin Diagn Pathol 1991;8:250–76.)

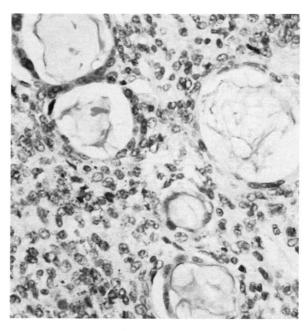

Figure 18-52
DESMOPLASTIC SMALL ROUND
CELL TUMOR INVOLVING OVARY
Gland-like structures contain mucin.

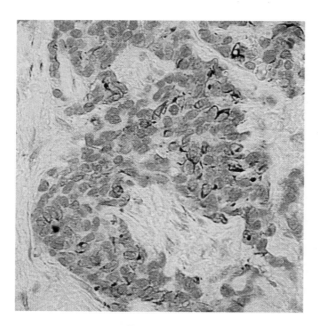

Figure 18-53
DESMOPLASTIC SMALL ROUND
CELL TUMOR INVOLVING OVARY
Many tumor cells are immunoreactive for desmin.

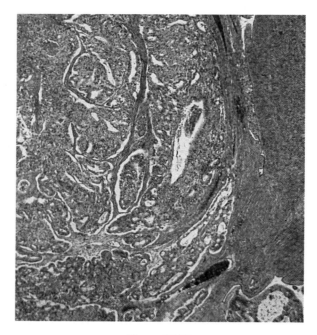

Figure 18-54
METASTATIC ENDOMETRIAL
ADENOCARCINOMA, ENDOMETRIOID TYPE
The tumor is adherent to the surface of the ovary.

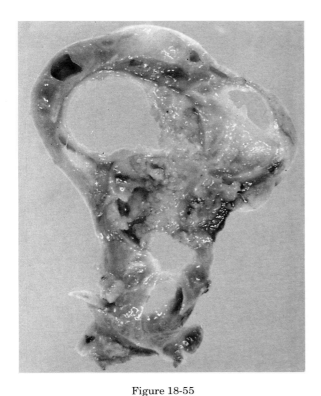

Figure 18-55
METASTATIC SQUAMOUS CELL
CARCINOMA FROM CERVIX
Several cysts and solid white tissue are visible. (Courtesy
of Dr. Deborah Gersell, St. Louis, MO.)

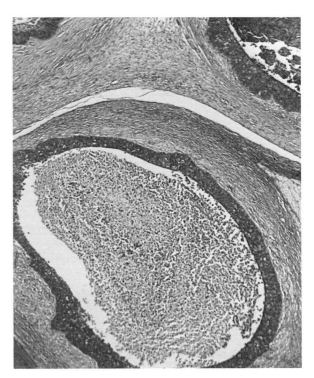

Figure 18-56
METASTATIC SQUAMOUS CELL
CARCINOMA FROM CERVIX
Large pseudocysts contain necrotic material.

Cervical Carcinoma

At autopsy, the frequency of ovarian metastasis of squamous cell carcinoma of the cervix is approximately 3 percent; the figure for adenocarcinoma is somewhat higher (122,123). Ovarian spread is discovered less often during life (fig. 18-55), with most of the reported examples having been adenocarcinomas. When cervical and ovarian mucinous adenocarcinomas coexist, it may be difficult to determine whether they are independent primary tumors (118,120) or metastatic from one organ to the other (126). Consideration of the different features of primary and metastatic ovarian tumors in general is usually helpful in this situation.

Most ovarian squamous cell carcinomas diagnosed during life arise in dermoid or endometriotic cysts (pages 279 and 162), and in most cases of squamous cell carcinoma metastatic to the ovary the primary site is evident clinically. If an ovarian squamous cell carcinoma cannot be shown to originate in a pre-existent benign ovarian lesion after adequate sampling, and a primary site elsewhere is not obvious, the cervix and other potential sources of the tumor should be investigated before a diagnosis of primary squamous cell carcinoma of the ovary is made (125). In rare cases, an in situ or microinvasive cervical squamous cell carcinoma spreads upward to involve the endometrial and tubal mucosae, and can spread onto the ovarian surface or to the parenchyma (figs. 18-56, 18-57) (120a,125).

Uterine Sarcomas and Choriocarcinoma

In one series of 11 uterine sarcomas metastatic to the ovary, 8 were endometrial stromal sarcomas and 3, leiomyosarcomas (127). The ovarian metastases accounted for the clinical presentation in 3 of the former group; in 2 of these cases, the primary uterine tumors were not discovered until 7 and 10 months after the ovarian tumors had

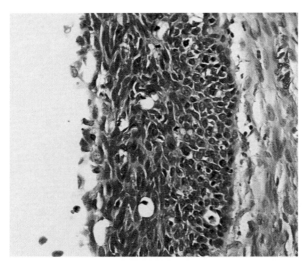

Figure 18-57
METASTATIC SQUAMOUS CELL
CARCINOMA FROM CERVIX
A cyst is lined by neoplastic squamous epithelium (high-power view of figure 18-56).

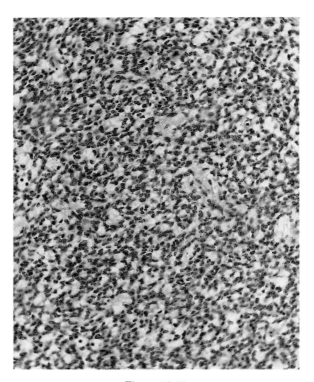

Figure 18-58
METASTATIC ENDOMETRIAL STROMAL SARCOMA
Small cells have uniform nuclei and scanty cytoplasm. In this area the characteristic arterioles are inconspicuous.

been removed. The differentiation of metastatic endometrial stromal sarcoma (figs. 18-58, 18-59) from primary endometrioid stromal sarcoma and sex cord–stromal tumors of the ovary is discussed on pages 136 and 135. Ovarian metastasis of uterine choriocarcinoma is rare and must be distinguished from a primary ovarian choriocarcinoma of gestational or germ cell origin (pages 331 and 258).

FALLOPIAN TUBE TUMORS

Tubal carcinomas may involve the ovary by direct extension or surface implantation; the distinction between a tubal carcinoma with spread to the ovary and vice versa is sometimes difficult (pages 464 and 471).

MALIGNANT LYMPHOMA

General Features. Although up to 25 percent of women with lymphoma have ovarian involvement at autopsy (134,149,151,162,163), lymphoma rarely presents clinically as an ovarian mass (158), and in most cases of that type it is only one component of intra-abdominal or generalized lymphoma. Despite its rarity, involvement of the ovary is more frequent than that of other female

genital organs (151). The rare long-term survival of a patient with ovarian lymphoma after oophorectomy indicates that it can be primary in the ovary in occasional cases (161,164).

One exception to the rarity of ovarian lymphoma is seen in countries where Burkitt's lymphoma is endemic and may account for approximately half the cases of malignant ovarian tumors in childhood (fig. 18-60). In such cases enlargement of one or both ovaries is second only to involvement of the jaw as the presenting manifestation of the disease. When Burkitt's lymphoma occurs in non-endemic areas, it often involves the ovaries as well (141,145).

Ovarian involvement by lymphoma in general may occur at any age, but the peak age incidence is in the fourth and fifth decades (136,138,143, 161). The most common presenting manifestations are similar to those of most ovarian masses (143, 151,163); a minority of the patients have generalized symptoms or abnormal vaginal bleeding.

At laparotomy both ovaries are involved in about half the cases (138,143,160,163). In two series the disease was confined to the ovaries in 10 and 21 percent of the cases (143,155). Extraovarian disease most often involves the pelvic or para-aortic lymph nodes, or both; occasionally, the peritoneum and the fallopian tubes; and less often, the uterus and miscellaneous other sites. Ascites, which is often bloody, is common (161).

Gross Findings. Ovarian lymphomas have an average diameter of 10 to 15 cm. They typically have an intact external surface, which may be smooth (fig. 18-60), nodular, or bosselated. The consistency ranges from soft and fleshy to firm and rubbery. The sectioned surfaces are usually white (fig. 18-61), tan, or gray-pink, occasionally with areas of cystic degeneration, hemorrhage, or necrosis.

Microscopic Findings. The microscopic appearance of ovarian lymphoma is similar to that seen in extraovarian sites (fig. 18-62) except that there is a greater tendency for the tumor cells to grow in cords (fig. 18-63), islands, and trabeculae (fig. 18-64); occasionally form follicle-like spaces or alveoli (fig. 18-65); and have a sclerotic stroma. The tumor may spare ovarian follicles and their

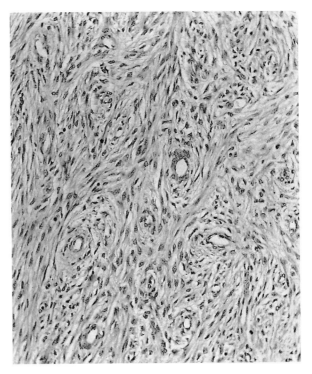

Figure 18-59
METASTATIC ENDOMETRIAL STROMAL SARCOMA
Characteristic arterioles are evident. The cells are spindle shaped and are separated by collagen.

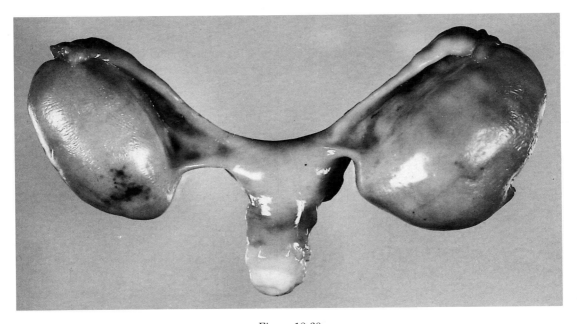

Figure 18-60
BURKITT'S LYMPHOMA
These bilateral ovarian tumors were from a 4-year-old girl. (Courtesy of Dr. Ronald Dorfman, Stanford, CA.)

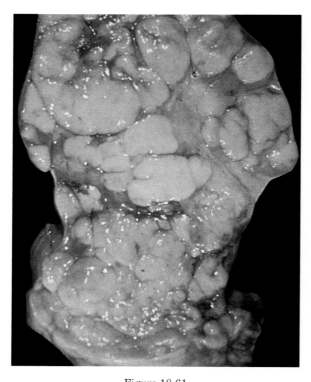

Figure 18-61
MALIGNANT LYMPHOMA
The lobulation and cream color of the sectioned surface resemble those of a dysgerminoma (see figure 13-1).

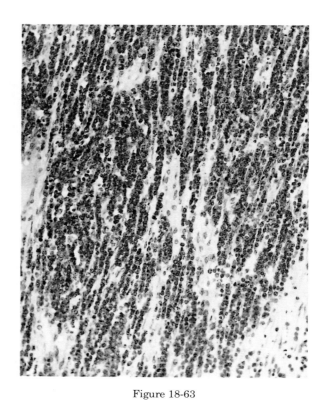

Figure 18-63
MALIGNANT LYMPHOMA
The arrangement of the tumor cells in cords simulates a metastatic breast carcinoma.

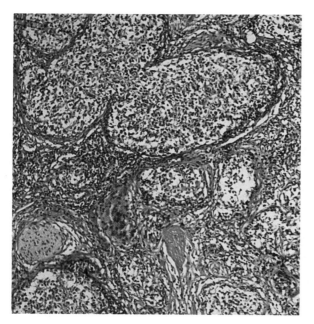

Figure 18-62
MALIGNANT LYMPHOMA
The tumor has a follicular pattern.

derivatives or obliterate all the underlying tissue. The cytologic features are similar to those seen in lymphoma involving lymph nodes (fig. 18-66). Lymphoma presenting in the ovary is very rarely accompanied by stromal luteinization; in one case the occurrence of amenorrhea suggested steroid hormone production by the luteinized cells (154).

Patients with many types of lymphoma present with ovarian involvement. In one series, 59 percent of lymphomas were of the diffuse large cell type, 27 percent of the small noncleaved (Burkitt or non-Burkitt) cell type, and 15 percent follicular (small cleaved, mixed small cleaved and large cell, and large cell types) (160). Most diffuse large cell lymphomas were immunoblastic. The 39 cases in another series included 21 of the small noncleaved cell type (54 percent); 12 of the diffuse large cell type (31 percent), 3 of which had follicular areas; 2 of the immunoblastic type (5 percent); 3 of the diffuse mixed small and large cell type (8 percent); and 1 of follicular and diffuse small cleaved cell type (2 percent) (155). In a third series, poorly

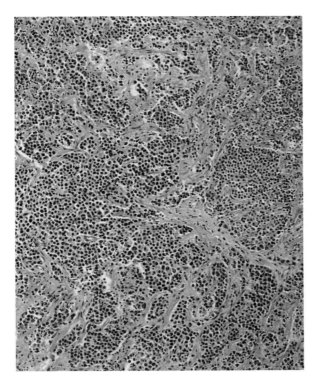

Figure 18-64
MALIGNANT LYMPHOMA
The arrangement of the tumor cells in nests and trabeculae simulates that of a carcinoma.

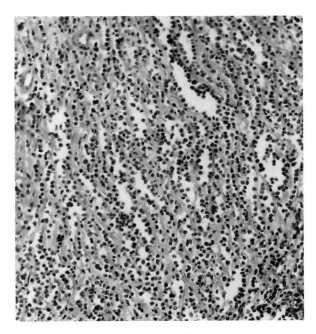

Figure 18-65
MALIGNANT LYMPHOMA
An alveolar pattern is present focally. (Fig. 7 from Young RH, Scully RE. Alveolar rhabdomyosarcoma metastatic to the ovary. A report of two cases and discussion of the differential diagnosis of small cell malignant tumors of the ovary. Cancer 1989;64:899–904.)

differentiated or small cleaved cell lymphomas (not specified whether follicular or diffuse) were the most common type, accounting for 36 percent of the total, with large cell and small noncleaved cell lymphomas slightly less frequent (161). In patients in the first two decades, the small non-cleaved cell type is the most common. In one series, 10 of 14 patients under 20 years of age had this subtype and 4 had immunoblastic lymphoma (160). In another series, 9 of 12 patients in this age group had small noncleaved cell lymphoma (155). In contrast to adults in whom lymphomas of many types, both follicular and diffuse, are encountered, children in general almost always have aggressive diffuse lymphomas (high grade in the working formulation) (157). Most ovarian lymphomas are of B-cell type (152): in one series, 25 of 26 were of B-cell type, and 1 of T-cell type (155). Involvement of the ovary by Hodgkin's disease is unusual, even at autopsy (151), and presentation of Hodgkin's disease as ovarian enlargement is exceedingly rare (133,150,153).

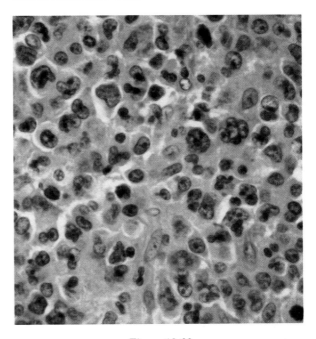

Figure 18-66
LARGE CELL LYMPHOMA
Large lymphoid cells have irregular, focally reniform, malignant-appearing nuclei.

Differential Diagnosis. The most common error in the pathologic evaluation of ovarian lymphomas, particularly those of the large cell type, is their misinterpretation as dysgerminoma, which they may mimic both grossly and microscopically. The differential diagnosis is discussed on page 244.

Ovarian lymphomas also must be differentiated from undifferentiated carcinomas, small cell carcinomas of hypercalcemic type (165), and metastatic breast carcinomas (pages 166, 319, and 350); other tumors in the differential diagnosis are listed in Table 5-4. Malignant lymphoma of the large cell type must also be distinguished from granulocytic sarcoma of the ovary (see below).

Prognosis. Patients with malignant lymphoma who present with ovarian involvement have a poor prognosis. Only 4 of 55 patients (7 percent) in one series treated by oophorectomy, radiation, or both, survived longer than 5 years (163). In another study, 9 of 37 patients (24 percent) survived for 5 years, but 2 of these patients eventually died of lymphoma (160). Overall, the average length of survival is less than 3 years. In contrast to the above figures, however, 47 percent of the patients in a more recent series were alive at their last follow-up examination, with a median survival of 5 years (155). In one series, features associated with a good prognosis were unilateral ovarian involvement, focal involvement of the ovary, FIGO stage Ia, and a follicular pattern (160). In another series, features associated with a poor prognosis were a rapid onset of symptoms related to a mass, the presence of systemic symptoms, bilaterality of the ovarian tumors, and an advanced stage (143).

OTHER HEMATOLOGIC TUMORS

Plasmacytoma

Six females, 12 to 63 years of age, have had unilateral ovarian plasmacytomas. These tumors ranged up to 24 cm in diameter and were white, pale yellow, or gray (129,131,140,146, 164a). In two cases, immunohistochemical studies showed expression of monotypic immunoglobulin. Overt multiple myeloma developed in one woman 2 years after oophorectomy.

Leukemia

In an autopsy study of 1,206 patients with leukemia who died between 1958 and 1982 (132), there was ovarian involvement by acute myelogenous leukemia in 11 percent, chronic myelogenous leukemia in 9 percent, acute lymphoblastic leukemia in 21 percent, and chronic lymphocytic leukemia in 22 percent of the cases.

Rarely, a patient with acute myelogenous leukemia presents with an ovarian granulocytic sarcoma, with or without hematologic evidence of leukemia. One or the other of these presentations has been described in two infants, one 3-year-old child, and 11 women (128,138,141a, 153a,156,159a,160,161a). After chemotherapy 4 patients underwent remission; most of the remainder were either alive with or died of disease. The ovary can also be a clinically apparent, but usually not isolated, site of relapse after chemotherapy for acute myelogenous leukemia (130, 136,144). The ovarian tumors are unilateral or bilateral and have ranged up to 19 cm in diameter (mean, 12 to 14 cm). They are typically solid, soft, and white, yellow (fig. 18-67), or red-brown, but cystic degeneration, hemorrhage, or necrosis may be seen. A few ovarian granulocytic sarcomas have sufficient cytoplasmic myeloperoxidase to impart a green color to the gross specimen and be designated "chloroma" (142).

Microscopic examination shows patterns similar to those of malignant lymphoma (fig. 18-68), which is the most important tumor in the differential diagnosis. The granulocytic sarcoma is generally composed of cells with more finely dispersed nuclear chromatin and more abundant cytoplasm, which may be deeply eosinophilic, than lymphoma cells with nuclei of the same size. The identification of eosinophilic myelocytes may be helpful in making a diagnosis of granulocytic sarcoma. In the absence of known myelogenous leukemia, staining for chloroacetate esterase or immunohistochemical staining for lysozyme or myeloperoxidase almost always confirms the diagnosis.

We are unaware of documented cases of acute lymphoblastic or chronic lymphocytic leukemia presenting as an ovarian mass, but eight cases of acute lymphoblastic leukemia (five in children, two in teenagers, and one in an adult) that recurred in the ovaries during bone marrow remission have been reported (135,137,139,147,159,166).

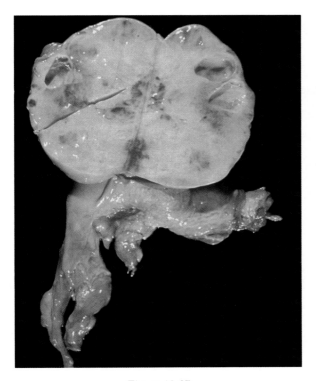

Figure 18-67
ACUTE LEUKEMIA INVOLVING OVARY
The sectioned surface of the tumor is yellow.

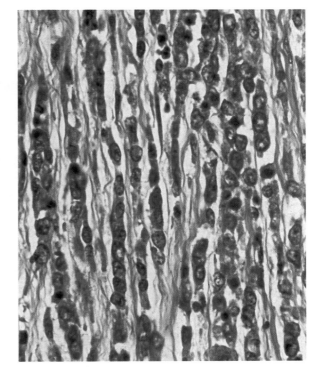

Figure 18-68
GRANULOCYTIC SARCOMA
The leukemic cells are arranged in thin cords, simulating metastatic breast carcinoma.

In one case, the ovary was the first site of relapse 5 years after treatment of the leukemia; the interval before relapse was shorter in the other cases. The ovaries are usually not the only site of relapse: additional involvement of the peritoneum, omentum, fallopian tubes, lymph nodes, and central nervous system is common. After relapse, three of the eight patients were treated successfully; the other five died of leukemia or complications of its treatment.

REFERENCES

General References

1. Abrams HL, Spiro R, Goldstein N. Metastases in carcinoma. Analysis of 1000 autopsied cases. Cancer 1950;3:74–85.
2. Demopoulos RI, Touger L, Dubin N. Secondary ovarian carcinoma: a clinical and pathological evaluation. Int J Gynecol Pathol 1987;6:166–75.
3. Israel SL, Helsel EV Jr, Hausman DH. The challenge of metastatic ovarian carcinoma. Am J Obstet Gynecol 1965;93:1094–101.
4. Johansson H. Clinical aspects of metastatic ovarian cancer of extragenital origin. Acta Obstet Gynecol Scand 1960;39:681–97.
5. Karsh J. Secondary malignant disease of the ovaries. A study of 72 autopsies. Am J Obstet Gynecol 1951;61:154–60.
6. Luisi A. Metastatic ovarian tumors. In Gentil F, Junqueira AC, eds. Ovarian cancer. UICC Monograph Series, Vol. 11, Berlin: Springer-Verlag, 1968:87–124.
7. Mazur MT, Hsueh S, Gersell DJ. Metastases to the female genital tract. Analysis of 325 cases. Cancer 1984;53:1978–84.
8. Petru E, Pickel H, Heydarfadai M, et al. Nongenital cancers metastatic to the ovary. Gynecol Oncol 1992;44:83–6.
9. Ulbright TM, Roth LM, Stehman FB. Secondary ovarian neoplasia. A clinicopathologic study of 35 cases. Cancer 1984;53:1164–74.
10. Webb MJ, Decker DG, Mussey E. Cancer metastatic to the ovary: factors influencing survival. Obstet Gynecol 1975;45:391–6.

11. Woodruff JD, Murthy YS, Bhaskar TN, Bordbar F, Tseng SS. Metastatic ovarian tumors. Am J Obstet Gynecol 1970;107:202–9.

12. Yazigi R, Sandstad J. Ovarian involvement in extragenital cancer. Gynecol Oncol 1989;34:84–7.

13. Young RH, Scully RE. Metastatic tumors in the ovary: a problem-oriented approach and review of the recent literature. Semin Diagn Pathol 1991;8:250–76.

Carcinoma of Stomach Including Krukenberg Tumor

14. Bullon A, Arseneau J, Prat J, Young RH, Scully RE. Tubular Krukenberg tumor. A problem in histopathologic diagnosis. Am J Surg Pathol 1981;5:225–32.

15. Diddle AW. Krukenberg tumors: diagnostic problem. Cancer 1955;8:1026–34.

16. Duarte I, Llanos O. Patterns of metastases in intestinal and diffuse types of carcinoma of the stomach. Hum Pathol 1981;12:237–42.

17. Hale RW. Krukenberg tumor of the ovaries. A review of 81 records. Obstet Gynecol 1968;32:221–5.

18. Hirschfield LS, Kahn LB, Winkler B, Bochner RZ, Gibstein AA. Adenocarcinoid of the appendix presenting as bilateral Krukenberg's tumor of the ovaries. Immunohistochemical and ultrastructural studies and literature review. Arch Pathol Lab Med 1985;109:930–3.

19. Holtz F, Hart WR. Krukenberg tumors of the ovary. A clinicopathologic analysis of 27 cases. Cancer 1982;50:2438–47.

20. Joshi VV. Primary Krukenberg tumor of ovary. Review of literature and case report. Cancer 1968;22:1199–207.

21. Leffel JM Jr, Masson JC, Dockerty MB. Krukenberg's tumors. A survey of forty-four cases. Ann Surg 1942;115:102–13.

22. Novak E, Gray LA. Krukenberg tumors of the ovary. Clinical and pathological study of 21 cases. Surg Gynecol Obstet 1938;66:157–67.

23. Saphir O. Signet-ring cell carcinoma. Mil Surg 1951;109:360–9.

24. Shiromizu K, Kawana T, Sugase M, Izumi R, Mizuno M. Experience with the treatment of metastatic ovarian carcinoma. Arch Gynecol Obstet 1988;243:111–4.

25. Wong PC, Ferenczy A, Fan LD, McCaughey WT. Krukenberg tumors of the ovary. Ultrastructural, histochemical, and immunohistochemical studies of 15 cases. Cancer 1986;57:751–60.

26. Woodruff JD, Novak ER. The Krukenberg tumor. Study of 48 cases from the Ovarian Tumor Registry. Obstet Gynecol 1960;15:351–60.

27. Yakushiji M, Tazaki T, Nishimura H, Kato T. Krukenberg tumors of the ovary: a clinicopathologic analysis of 112 cases. Acta Obstet Gynaec Jpn 1987;39:479–85.

Intestinal Carcinoma

27a. Abu-Rustum NR, Barakat RR, Curtin JP. Ovarian and uterine disease in women with colorectal cancer. Gynecol Oncol 1997;89:85–7.

28. Birnkrant A, Sampson J, Sugarbaker PH. Ovarian metastasis from colorectal cancer. Dis Col Rectum 1986;29:767–71.

29. Blamey SL, McDermott FT, Pihl E, Hughes ES. Resected ovarian recurrence from colorectal adenocarcinoma: a study of 13 cases. 1981;24:272–5.

30. Burt CA. Prophylactic oophorectomy with resection of the large bowel for cancer. Am J Surg 1951;82:572–7.

31. Charpin C, Bhan AK, Zurawski VE, Scully RE. Carcinoembryonic antigen (CEA) and carbohydrate determinant (19-9) localization in 121 primary ovarian tumors: an immunohistochemical study with use of monoclonal antibodies. Int J Gynecol Pathol 1982;1:231–45.

32. Cutait R, Lesser ML, Enker WE. Prophylactic oophorectomy in surgery for large-bowel cancer. Dis Col Rectum 1983;26:6–11.

32a. Dabbs DJ, Sturtz K, Zaino RJ. The immunohistochemical discrimination of endometrioid adenocarcinomas. Hum Pathol 1996;27:172–7.

33. Daya D, Nazerali L, Frank GL. Metastatic ovarian carcinoma of large intestinal origin simulating primary ovarian carcinoma. A clinicopathologic study of 25 cases. Am J Clin Pathol 1992;97:751–8.

33a. De Costanzo DC, Elias JM, Chumas JC. Necrosis in 84 ovarian carcinomas: a morphologic study of primary versus metastatic colonic carcinomas with a selective immunohistochemical analysis of cytokeratin subtypes and carcinoembryonic antigen. Int J Gynecol Pathol 1997;16:245–9.

33b. Fowler LJ, Maygarden SJ, Novotny DB. Human alveolar macrophage-56 and carcinoembryonic antigen monoclonal antibodies in the differential diagnosis between primary ovarian and metastatic gastrointestinal carcinomas. Hum Pathol 1994;25:666–70.

34. Graffner HO, Alm PO, Oscarson JE. Prophylactic oophorectomy in colorectal carcinoma. Am J Surg 1983;146:233–5.

35. Harcourt KF, Dennis DL. Laparotomy for ovarian tumors in unsuspected carcinoma of the colon. Cancer 1968;21:1244–6.

36. Herrera LO, Ledesma EJ, Natarajan N, Lopez GE, Tsukada Y, Mittelman A. Metachronous ovarian metastases from adenocarcinoma of the colon and rectum. Surg Gynecol Obstet 1982;154:531–3.

37. Herrera LO, Natarajan N, Tsukada Y, et al. Adenocarcinoma of the colon masquerading as primary ovarian neoplasia. An analysis of ten cases. Dis Col Rectum 1983;26:377–80.

37a. Jewell LD, Barr JR, Caughey WT, Nguyen GK, Owen DO. Clear-cell epithelial neoplasm of the large intestine. Arch Pathol Lab Med 1988;12:197–9.

38. Knoepp LF, Ray JE Jr, Overby I. Ovarian metastases from colorectal carcinoma. Dis Col Rectum 1973; 16:305–11.

39. Lash RH, Hart WR. Intestinal adenocarcinomas metastatic to the ovaries. A clinicopathological evaluation of 22 cases. Am J Surg Pathol 1987;11:114–21.

40. Loy TS, Abshier J. Immunostaining with HAM 56 in the diagnosis of adenocarcinomas. Mod Pathol 1993;6:473–5.

40a. Loy TS, Calaluce RD, Keeney GL. Cytokeratin immunostaining in differentiating primary ovarian carcinoma from metastatic colonic adenocarcinoma. Mod Pathol 1996;9:1040–4.

41. Loy TS, Quesenberry JT, Sharp SC. Distribution of CA 125 in adenocarcinomas: an immunohistochemical study of 481 cases. Am J Clin Pathol 1992;98:175–9.

42. MacKeigan JM, Ferguson JA. Prophylactic oophorectomy and colorectal cancer in premenopausal patients. Dis Col Rectum 1979;22:401–5.
43. Morrow M, Enker WE. Late ovarian metastases in carcinoma of the colon and rectum. Arch Surg 1984;119:1385–8.
44. Niemiec TR, Senekjian EK, Montag AG. Adenocarcinoma of the small intestine presenting as an ovarian mass. A case report. J Reproduct Med 1989;34:917–20.
45. O'Brien PH, Newton BB, Metcalf JS, Rittenbury MS. Oophorectomy in women with carcinoma of the colon and rectum. Surg Gynecol Obstet 1981;153:827–30.
46. Pavelic ZP, Pavelic L, Pavelic K, Peacock JS. Utility of anti-carcinoembryonic antigen monoclonal antibodies for differentiating ovarian adenocarcinomas from gastrointestinal metastasis to the ovary. Gynecol Oncol 1991;40:112–7.
47. Pitluk H, Poticha SM. Carcinoma of the colon and rectum in patients less than 40 years of age. Surg Gynecol Obstet 1983;157:335–7.
48. Saphir O. Signet-ring cell carcinoma. Mil Surg 1951;109:360–9.
49. Tsukamoto N, Uchino H, Matsukuma K, Kamura T. Carcinoma of the colon presenting as bilateral ovarian tumors during pregnancy. Gynecol Oncol 1986;24:386–91.
50. Tunca JC, Starling JR, Hafex GR, Buchler DA. Colon carcinoma metastatic to the ovary. J Surg Oncol 1983;23:269–72.
51. Wheelock MC, Putong P. Ovarian metastases from adenocarcinomas of colon and rectum. Obstet Gynecol 1959;14:291–5.
52. Younes M, Katikaneni PR, Lechago LV, Lechago J. HAM 56 antibody: a tool in the differential diagnosis between colorectal and gynecological malignancy. Mod Pathol 1994;7:396–400.
52a. Young RH, Hart WR. Metastatic intestinal carcinomas simulating primary ovarian clear cell carcinoma and secretory endometrioid carcinoma. A clinicopathologic and immunohistochemical study of five cases. Am J Surg Pathol 1998;22:805–15.

Appendiceal Tumors and Carcinoid Tumors

53. Chen KT. Appendiceal adenocarcinoid with ovarian metastasis. Gynecol Oncol 1990;38:286–8.
54. Hirschfield LS, Kahn LB, Winkler B, Bochner RZ, Gibstein AA. Adenocarcinoid of the appendix presenting as bilateral Krukenberg's tumor of the ovaries. Immunohistochemical and ultrastructural studies and literature review. Arch Pathol Lab Med 1985;109:930–3.
55. Ikeda E, Tsutsumi Y, Yoshida H, Yanagi K. Goblet cell carcinoid of the vermiform appendix with ovarian metastasis mimicking mucinous cystadenocarcinoma. Acta Pathol Jpn 1991;41:455–60.
56. Merino MJ, Edmonds P, LiVolsi V. Appendiceal carcinoma metastatic to the ovaries and mimicking primary ovarian tumors. Int J Gynecol Pathol 1985;4:110–20.
57. Paone JF, Bixler TJ II, Imbembo AL. Primary mucinous adenocarcinoma of the appendix with bilateral Krukenberg ovarian tumors. Johns Hopkins Med J 1978;143:43–7.
58. Prayson RA, Hart WR, Petras RE. Pseudomyxoma peritonei. A clinicopathologic study of 19 cases with emphasis on site of origin and nature of associated ovarian tumors. Am J Surg Pathol 1994;18:591–603.
59. Robboy SJ, Scully RE, Norris HJ. Carcinoid metastatic to the ovary. A clinicopathologic analysis of 35 cases. Cancer 1974;33:798–811.
59a. Ronnett BM, Kurman RJ, Shmookler BM, Sugarbaker PH, Young RH. The morphologic spectrum of ovarian metastases of appendiceal adenocarcinomas: a clinicopathologic and immunohistochemical analysis of tumors often misinterpreted as primary ovarian tumors or metastatic tumors from other gastrointestinal sites. Am J Surg Pathol 1997;21:1144–55.
59b. Ronnett BM, Kurman RJ, Zahn CM, et al. Pseudomyxoma peritonei in women. A clinicopathologic analysis of 30 cases with emphasis on site of origin, prognosis, and relationship to ovarian mucinous tumors of low malignant potential. Hum Pathol 1995;26:509–24.
60. Seidman JD, Elsayed AM, Sobin LH, Tavassoli FA. Association of mucinous tumors of the ovary and appendix. A clinicopathologic study of 25 cases. Am J Surg Pathol 1993;17:22–34.
61. Thorsen P, Dybdahl H, Søgaard H, Møller BR. Ovarian tumors caused by metastatic tumors of the appendix: two case reports. Europ J Obstet Gynecol Reproduc Biol 1991;40:67–71.
62. Young RH, Gilks CB, Scully RE. Mucinous tumors of the appendix associated with mucinous tumors of the ovary and pseudomyxoma peritonei. A clinicopathological analysis of 22 cases supporting an origin in the appendix. Am J Surg Pathol 1991;15:415–29.

Tumors of the Pancreas, Biliary Tract, and Liver

63. Green LK, Silva EG. Hepatoblastoma in an adult with metastasis to the ovaries. Am J Clin Pathol 1989;92:110–5.
64. Lashgari M, Behmaram B, Hoffman JS, Garcia J. Primary biliary carcinoma with metastasis to the ovaries. Gynecol Oncol 1992;47:272–4.
65. Leffel JM, Masson JC, Dockerty MB. Krukenberg's tumors. Ann Surg 1942;115:102–13.
65a. Lonardo F, Cubilla AL, Klimstra DS. Microadenocarcinoma of the pancreas—morphologic pattern or pathologic entity? A reevaluation of the original series. Am J Surg Pathol 1996;20:1385–93.
66. Oortman EH, Elliott JP. Hepatocellular carcinoma metastatic to the ovary: a case report. Am J Obstet Gynecol 1983;146:715–7.
66a. Petru E, Pickel H, Heydarfadai M et al. Nongenital cancers metastatic to the ovary. Gynecol Oncol 1992;44:83–6.
66b. Yakushiji M, Tazaki T, Nishimura H, Kato T. Krukenberg tumors of the ovary: a clinicopathologic analysis of 112 cases. Acta Obstet Gynaec Jpn 1987;39:479–85.
66c. Yazigi R, Sandstad J. Ovarian involvement in extragenital cancer. Gynecol Oncol 1989;34:84–7.
67. Young RH, Gersell DJ, Clement PB, Scully RE. Hepatocellular carcinoma metastatic to the ovary: a report of three cases discovered during life with discussion of the differential diagnosis of hepatoid tumors of the ovary. Hum Pathol 1992;23:574–80.
68. Young RH, Hart WR. Metastases from carcinomas of the pancreas simulating primary mucinous tumors of the ovary: a report of seven cases. Am J Surg Pathol 1989;13:748–56.
69. Young RH, Scully RE. Ovarian metastases from carcinoma of the gallbladder and extrahepatic bile ducts simulating primary tumors of the ovary: a report of six cases. Int J Gynecol Pathol 1990;9:60–72.

Breast Carcinoma

70. Brickman M, Ferreira B. Metastasis of breast carcinoma to the ovaries—incidence, significance, and relationship to survival. A preliminary study. Grace Hosp Bull 1967;45:44–9.

71. Curtin JP, Barakat RR, Hoskins WJ. Ovarian disease in women with breast cancer. Obstet Gynecol 1994;84:449–52.

72. Fleischhacker DS, Young RH, Scully RE. Breast carcinoma metastatic to the ovary: a study of 76 cases [Abstract]. Mod Pathol 1994;7:88A.

73. Gagnon Y, Tetu B. Ovarian metastases of breast carcinoma. A clinicopathologic study of 59 cases. Cancer 1989;64:892–8.

74. Harris M, Howell A, Chrissohou M, Swindell RI, Hudson M, Sellwood RA. A comparison of the metastatic pattern of infiltrating lobular carcinoma and infiltrating duct carcinoma of the breast. Br J Cancer 1984;50:23–30.

75. Kasilag FB Jr, Rutledge FN. Metastatic breast carcinoma in ovary. Am J Obstet Gynecol 1957;74:989–92.

76. Lecca U, Medda F, Marcello C, et al. Ovarian metastasis in breast carcinoma. Eur J Gynaecol Oncol 1980;1:168–74.

77. Lee YN, Hori JM. Significance of ovarian metastases in therapeutic oophorectomy for advanced breast cancer. Cancer 1971;27:1374–8.

78. Lumb G, Mackenzie DH. The incidence of metastases in adrenal glands and ovaries removed for carcinoma of the breast. Cancer 1959;12:521–6.

79. Monteagudo C, Merino MJ, Laporte N, Neumann RD. Value of gross cystic disease fluid protein-15 in distinguishing metastatic breast carcinomas among poorly differentiated neoplasms involving the ovary. Hum Pathol 1991;22:368–72.

80. Osborne MP, Pitts RM. Therapeutic oophorectomy for advanced breast cancer. The significance of metastases to the ovary and of ovarian cortical stromal hyperplasia. Cancer 1961;14:126–30.

81. Puga FJ, Gibbs CP, Williams TJ. Castrating operations associated with metastatic lesions of the breast. Obstet Gynecol 1973;41:713–9.

82. Saphir O. Signet-ring cell carcinoma. Mil Surg 1951;109:360–9.

83. Turksoy N. Ovarian metastasis of breast carcinoma. A surgical surprise. Obstet Gynecol 1960;15:573–8.

84. Viadana E, Bross ID, Pickren JW. An autopsy study of some routes of dissemination of cancer of the breast. Br J Cancer 1973;27:336–40.

85. Warren S, Witham EM. Studies on tumor formation. 2. The distribution of metastases in cancer of the breast. Surg Gynecol Obstet 1953;57:81–5.

86. Wick MR, Lillemo TJ, Copland GT, Swanson PE, Manivel JC, Kiang DT. Gross cystic disease fluid protein-15 as a marker for breast cancer: immunohistochemical analysis of 690 human neoplasms and comparison with alpha-lactalbumin. Hum Pathol 1989;20:281–7.

87. Young, RH, Carey RW, Robboy SJ. Breast carcinoma masquerading as a primary ovarian neoplasm. Cancer 1981;48:210–2.

87a. Young RH, Scully RE. Metastatic tumors in the ovary: a problem-oriented approach and review of the recent literature. Semin Diagn Pathol 1991;8:250–76.

Renal Tumors

88. Hsiu JG, Kemp GM, Singer GA, Rawls WH, Siddiky MA. Transitional cell carcinoma of the renal pelvis with ovarian metastasis. Gynecol Oncol 1991;41:178–81.

89. Oliva E, Musulen E, Prat J, Young RH. Transitional cell carcinoma of the renal pelvis with symptomatic ovarian metastases. Int J Surg Pathol 1995;2:231–6.

90. Spencer JR, Eriksen B, Garnett JE. Metastatic renal tumor presenting as ovarian clear cell carcinoma. Urology 1993;41:582–4.

91. Young RH, Hart WR. Renal cell carcinoma metastatic to the ovary: a report of three cases emphasizing possible confusion with ovarian clear cell adenocarcinoma. Int J Gynecol Pathol 1992;11:96–104.

92. Young RH, Kozakewich HP, Scully RE. Metastatic ovarian tumors in children: a report of 14 cases and review of the literature. Int J Gynecol Pathol 1993;12:8–19.

Pulmonary and Mediastinal Tumors

93. Eichhorn JH, Young RH, Scully RE. Non-pulmonary small cell carcinomas of extragenital origin metastatic to the ovary. Cancer 1993;71:177–86.

94. Eichhorn JH, Young RH, Scully RE. Primary ovarian small cell carcinoma of pulmonary type. A clinicopathologic, immunohistologic, and flow cytometric analysis of 11 cases. Am J Surg Pathol 1992;16:926–38.

95. Yoshida A, Shigematsu T, Mori H, Yoshida H, Fukunishi R. Non-invasive thymoma with widespread blood-borne metastasis. Virch Arch [A] 1981;390:121–6.

96. Young RH, Kozakewich HP, Scully RE. Metastatic ovarian tumors in children: a report of 14 cases and review of the literature. Int J Gynecol Pathol 1993;12:8–19.

97. Young RH, Scully RE. Ovarian metastases from cancer of the lung: problems in interpretation—a report of seven cases. Gynecol Oncol 1985;21:337–50.

Metastatic Malignant Melanoma

98. Das Gupta T, Brasfield R. Metastatic melanoma. A clinicopathological study. Cancer 1964;17:1323–39.

99. Fitzgibbons PL, Martin SE, Simmons TJ. Malignant melanoma metastatic to the ovary. Am J Surg Pathol 1987;11:959–64.

100. Young RH, Scully RE. Malignant melanoma metastatic to the ovary: a clinicopathologic analysis of 20 cases. Am J Surg Pathol 1991;15:849–60.

Miscellaneous Nongenital Tract Primaries

101. Clement PB, Young RH, Scully RE. Malignant mesotheliomas presenting as ovarian masses: a report of nine cases, including two primary ovarian mesotheliomas. Am J Surg Pathol 1996;20:1067–80.
102. Eichhorn JH, Young RH, Scully RE. Non-pulmonary small cell carcinomas of extragenital origin metastatic to the ovary. Cancer 1993;71:177–86.
103. Goldblum J, Hart WR. Localized and diffuse mesotheliomas of the genital tract and peritoneum in women. A clinicopathologic study of nineteen true mesothelial neoplasms, other than adenomatoid tumors, multicystic mesotheliomas, and localized fibrous tumors. Am J Surg Pathol 1995;19:1124–37.
104. Longacre TA, O'Hanlan K, Hendrickson MR. Adenoid cystic carcinoma of the submandibular gland with symptomatic ovarian metastases. Int J Gynecol Pathol 1996;15:349–55.
105. Rainwater LM, Martin JK, Gaffey TA, Van Heerden JA. Angiosarcoma of the breast. Arch Surg 1986;121:669–72.
106. Sedgely MG, Östör AG, Fortune DW. Angiosarcoma of breast metastatic to the ovary and placenta. Aust NZ J Obstet Gynaecol 1985;25:299–302.
107. Soslow RA, Rouse RV, Hendrickson MR, Silva EG, Longacre TA. Transitional cell neoplasms of the ovary and urinary bladder: a comparative immunohistochemical analysis. Int J Gynecol Pathol 1996;15:257–65.
107a. Young RH. Urachal adenocarcinoma metastatic to the ovary simulating primary mucinous cystadenocarcinoma of the ovary: report of a case. Virchows Arch 1995; 426:529–32.
108. Young RH, Eichhorn JH, Dickersin GR, Scully RE. Ovarian involvement by the intra-abdominal desmoplastic small round cell tumor with divergent differentiation: a report of three cases. Hum Pathol 1992;23:454–64.
109. Young RH, Jackson A, Wells M. Ovarian metastasis from thyroid carcinoma twelve years after partial thyroidectomy mimicking struma ovarii: report of case. Int J Gynecol Pathol 1994;13:181–5.
110. Young RH, Kozakewich HP, Scully RE. Metastatic ovarian tumors in children: a report of 14 cases and review of the literature. Int J Gynecol Pathol 1993;12:8–19.
111. Young RH, Scully RE. Alveolar rhabdomyosarcoma metastatic to the ovary. A report of two cases and discussion of the differential diagnosis of small cell malignant tumors of the ovary. Cancer 1989;64:899–904.
112. Young RH, Scully RE. Sarcomas metastatic to the ovary: a report of 21 cases. Int J Gynecol Pathol 1990;9:231–52.
113. Young RH, Scully RE. Urothelial and ovarian carcinomas of identical cell types: problems in interpretation. A report of three cases and review of the literature. Int J Gynecol Pathol 1988;7:197–211.
114. Zukerberg LR, Young RH. Chordoma metastatic to the ovary. Arch Pathol Lab Med 1990;114:208–10.

Genital Tract Tumors

115. Beck RP, Latour JP. Necropsy reports on 36 cases of endometrial carcinoma. Am J Obstet Gynecol 1963;85:307–11.
116. Bunker ML. The terminal findings in endometrial carcinoma. Am J Obstet Gynecol 1959;77:530–8.
117. Eifel P, Hendrickson M, Ross J, Ballon S, Martinez A, Kempson R. Simultaneous presentation of carcinoma involving the ovary and uterine corpus. Cancer 1982;50:163–70.
118. Kaminski PF, Norris HJ. Coexistence of ovarian neoplasm and endocervical adenocarcinoma. Obstet Gynecol 1984;64:553–6.
119. Kim KR, Scully RE. Peritoneal keratin granulomas with carcinomas of endometrium and ovary and atypical polypoid adenomyoma of endometrium. A clinicopathological analysis of 22 cases. Am J Surg Pathol 1990;14:925–32.
120. LiVolsi VA, Merino MJ, Schwartz PE. Coexistent endocervical adenocarcinoma and mucinous adenocarcinoma of ovary: a clinicopathological study of four cases. Int J Gynecol Pathol 1983;1:391–402.
120a. Pins MR, Young RH, Crum CP, Leach IH, Scully RE. Cervical squamous carcinoma in situ with superficial extension to corpus and tubes and invasion of tubes and ovaries. Int J Gynecol Pathol 1997;16:272–8.
121. Russell P. Bannatyne PM, Solomon HJ, Stoddard LD, Tattersall MH. Multifocal tumorigenesis in the upper female genital tract—implications for staging and management. Int J Gynecol Pathol 1985;4:192–210.
122. Tabata M, Ichinoe K, Sakuragi N, Shina Y, Yamaguchi T, Mabuchi Y. Incidence of ovarian metastasis in patients with cancer of the uterine cervix. Gynecol Oncol 1987;28:255–61.
123. Toki N, Tsukamoto N, Kaku T, et al. Microscopic ovarian metastasis of the uterine cervical cancer. Gynecol Oncol 1991;41:46–51.
124. Ulbright TM, Roth LM. Metastatic and independent cancers of the endometrium and ovary: a clinicopathologic study of 34 cases. Hum Pathol 1985;16:28–34.
125. Young RH, Gersell DJ, Roth LM, Scully RE. Ovarian metastases from cervical carcinomas other than pure adenocarcinomas. A report of 12 cases. Cancer 1993;71:407–18.
126. Young RH, Scully RE. Mucinous tumors of the ovary associated with mucinous adenocarcinomas of the cervix. A clinicopathological analysis of 16 cases. Int J Gynecol Pathol 1988;7:99–111.
127. Young RH, Scully RE. Sarcomas metastatic to the ovary. A report of 21 cases. Int J Gynecol Pathol 1990; 9:231–52.

Malignant Lymphoma, Plasmacytoma, and Leukemia

128. Aguiar RC, Pozzi DH, Chamone DA. Granulocytic sarcoma of the ovary in a non-leukemic patient. Haematologica 1993;78:53–5.
129. Andze G, Pagbe JJ, Tchokoteu PF, et al. Solitary extra-osseous ovarian plasmacytoma. Apropos of an unusual case in a 12-year-old child. J Chir (Paris) 1993;130:137–40.
130. Ballon SC, Donaldson RC, Berman ML, Swanson GA, Byron RL. Myeloblastoma (granulocytic sarcoma) of the ovary. Arch Pathol Lab Med 1978;102:474–6.
131. Bambirra EA, Miranda D, Mugalhaes GM. Plasma cell myeloma simulating Krukenberg's tumor. South Med J 1982;75:511–2.

132. Barcos M, Lane W, Gomez GA, et al. An autopsy study of 1206 acute and chronic leukemias (1958-1982). Cancer 1987;60:827–37.

133. Bare WW, McCloskey JF. Primary Hodgkin's disease of the ovary. Report of a case. Obstet Gynecol 1961;17:477–80.

134. Barzilay J, Rakowsky E, Rahima M, Yanai-Inbar I. Malignant lymphoma of the ovary: report of a case and review of the literature. Obstet Gynecol 1984;64:93S–4S.

135. Case Records of the Massachusetts General Hospital (Case 45-1981). N Engl J Med 1981;305:1135–46.

136. Castaldo TW, Ballon SC, Lagasse LD, Petrilli ES. Reticuloendothelial neoplasia of the female genital tract. Obstet Gynecol 1979;54:167–70.

137. Cecalupo AJ, Frankel LS, Sullivan MP. Pelvic and ovarian extramedullary leukemic relapse in young girls: a report of four cases and review of the literature. Cancer 1982;50:587–93.

138. Chorlton I, Norris HJ, King FM. Malignant reticuloendothelial disease involving the ovary as a primary manifestation: a series of 19 lymphomas and 1 granulocytic sarcoma. Cancer 1974;34:397–407.

139. Chu JY, Craddock TV, Danis RK, Tennant NE. Ovarian tumor as manifestation of relapse in acute lymphoblastic leukemia. Cancer 1981;48:377–9.

140. Cook HT, Boylston AW. Plasmacytoma of the ovary. Gynecol Oncol 1988;29:378–81.

141. Dorfman RF. Diagnosis of Burkitt's tumor in the United States. Cancer 1968;21:563–74.

141a. Drinkard LC, Waggoner S, Stein RN, et al. Acute myelomonocytic leukemia with abnormal eosinophils presenting as an ovarian mass: a report of two cases and a review of the literature. Gynecol Oncol 1995;56:307–11.

142. Finkle HI, Goldman RL. Burkitt's lymphoma: gynecologic considerations. Obstet Gynecol 1974;43:281–4.

143. Fox H, Langley FA, Govan AD, Hill AS, Bennett MH. Malignant lymphoma presenting as an ovarian tumour: a clinicopathological analysis of 34 cases. Br J Obstet Gynaecol 1988;95:386–90.

144. Gralnick HR, Dittmar K. Development of myeloblastoma with massive breast and ovarian involvement during remission in acute leukemia. Cancer 1969;24:746–9.

145. Halpin TF. Gynecologic implications of Burkitt's tumor. Obstet Gynecol Surv 1975;30:351–8.

146. Hautzer NW. Primary plasmacytoma of the ovary. Gynecol Oncol 1984;18:115–4.

147. Heaton DC, Duff GB. Ovarian relapse in a young woman with acute lymphoblastic leukemia. Am J Hematol 1989;30:42–3.

148. Hinkamp JF, Szanto PB. Chloroma of the ovary. Am J Obstet Gynecol 1959;78:812–6.

149. Iliya FA, Muggia FM, O'Leary JA, King TM. Gynecologic manifestations of reticulum cell sarcoma. Obstet Gynecol 1968;31:266–9.

150. Khan MA, Dahill SW, Stewart SK. Primary Hodgkin's disease of the ovary. Case report. Br J Obstet Gynaecol 1986;93:1300–1.

151. Lathrop JC. Malignant pelvic lymphomas. Obstet Gynecol 1967;30:137–45.

152. Linden MD, Tubbs RR, Fishleder AJ, Hart WR. Immunotypic and genotypic characterization of non-Hodgkin's lymphoma of the ovary. Am J Clin Pathol 1988;89:156–62.

153. Long JP, Patchefsky AS. Primary Hodgkin's disease of the ovary. A case report. Obstet Gynecol 1971;38:680–2.

153a. Magliocco AM, Demetrick DR, Jones AR, Kossakowska AE. Granulocytic sarcoma of the ovary. An unusual case presentation. Arch Pathol Lab Med 1991;115:830–4.

154. Mittal KR, Blechman A, Greco MA, Alfonso F, Demopoulos R. Lymphoma of the ovary with stromal luteinization, presenting as secondary amenorrhea. Gynecol Oncol 1992;45:69–75

155. Monterroso V, Jaffe ES, Merino MJ, Medeiros LJ. Malignant lymphomas involving the ovary. A clinicopathologic analysis of 39 cases. Am J Surg Pathol 1993;17:154–70.

156. Morgan ER, Labotka RJ, Gonzalez-Crussi F, et al. Ovarian granulocytic sarcoma as the primary manifestation of acute infantile myelomonocytic leukemia. Cancer 1981;48:1819–24.

157. National Cancer Institute sponsored study of classifications of non-Hodgkin's lymphomas: summary and description for a working formulation for clinical usage. Cancer 1982;49:2112–35.

158. Norris HJ, Jensen RD. Relative frequency of ovarian neoplasms in children and adolescents. Cancer 1972;30:713–9.

159. Obeid D, Cotter P, Sturdee DW. Acute leukaemia relapse presenting as ovarian tumour. Br J Obstet Gynaecol 1979;86:578–80.

159a. Oliva E, Ferry JA, Young RH, Prat J, Srigley JR, Scully RE. Granulocytic sarcoma of the female genital tract: a clinicopathologic study of 11 cases. Am J Surg Pathol 1997;21:1156–65.

160. Osborne BM, Robboy SJ. Lymphomas or leukemia presenting as ovarian tumors. An analysis of 42 cases. Cancer 1983;52:1933–43.

161. Paladugu RR, Bearman RM, Rappaport H. Malignant lymphoma with primary manifestation in the gonad: a clinicopathologic study of 38 patients. Cancer 1980;45:561–71.

161a. Pressler H, Horny HP, Wolf A, Kaiserling E. Isolated granulocytic sarcoma of the ovary: histologic, electron microscopic and immunohistochemical findings. Int J Gynecol Pathol 1992;11:68–74.

162. Rosenberg SA, Diamond HD, Jaslowitz B, Craver LF. Lymphosarcoma: a review of 1269 cases. Medicine 1961;40:31–84.

163. Rotmensch J, Woodruff JD. Lymphoma of the ovary: report of twenty new cases and update of previous series. Am J Obstet Gynecol 1982;143:870–5.

164. Skodras G, Fields V, Kragel PJ. Ovarian lymphoma and serous carcinoma of low malignant arising in the same ovary. A case report with literature review of 14 primary ovarian lymphomas. Arch Pathol Lab Med 1994;118:647–50.

164a. Voegt H. Extramedulläre plasmacytome. Virchows Arch J Path Anat 1938;302:497–508.

165. Young RH, Oliva E, Scully RE. Small cell carcinoma of the ovary, hypercalcemic type. A clinicopathological analysis of 150 cases. Am J Surg Pathol. 1994;18:1102–16.

166. Wyld PJ, Lilleyman JS. Ovarian disease in childhood lymphoblastic leukemia. Acta Haematol 1983;69:278–80.

19

TUMORS WITH FUNCTIONING STROMA

Definition. These are tumors other than those in the sex cord–stromal and steroid cell categories that are characterized by: 1) a stroma that is morphologically compatible with steroid hormone secretion and 2) clinical, biochemical, or pathologic evidence of endocrine function (12). Almost all types of ovarian tumor, both benign and malignant, primary and metastatic, have been reported to be associated with endocrine abnormalities of estrogenic, androgenic, or rarely, progestagenic type, or combinations thereof. It is possible in some of these cases that the neoplastic cells themselves also have a role in the hormone production.

Frequency and Age Distribution. It is impossible to ascertain the frequency of tumors in this category because steroid hormone levels are rarely measured in patients with ovarian tumors unless there is an obvious endocrine abnormality, usually androgenic. Several lines of evidence, however, suggest that ovarian tumors with functioning stroma (OTFSs) are common, at least at a laboratory level. For example, a number of investigators have found estrogenic changes in vaginal smears (15,22) or endometrial hyperplasia (14) in a significantly higher percentage of patients with ovarian tumors exclusive of sex cord–stromal and steroid cell tumors than in age-matched controls. Also, approximately 50 percent of postmenopausal women with benign and malignant surface epithelial–stromal tumors or carcinomas metastatic to the ovary have elevated urinary estrogen levels (14). Patients with OTFSs accompanied by overt endocrine manifestations are much rarer than those with only laboratory evidence of increased steroid hormone secretion and are mostly the subject of individual case reports. Nevertheless, there are numerous descriptions in the literature of postmenopausal women with these tumors who have bled from a proliferative or hyperplastic endometrium and occasionally, have experienced swelling or tenderness of the breasts. Few, if any, estrogenic tumors of this type have been reported in women in the reproductive age group, possibly because of the greater difficulty in establishing a cause and effect relationship between an ovarian tumor and estrogenic manifestations in that age category. The only reported OTFS that caused isosexual pseudoprecocity was a dysgerminoma containing syncytiotrophoblastic cells (20). There are over 60 reported examples of virilizing ovarian tumors with functioning stroma, slightly over one third of which occurred in pregnant women. Some of these women had virilized female offspring as well (18). Rare tumors with functioning stroma have been associated with progestational changes manifested by a decidual reaction (1,13) or an Arias-Stella change in the endometrium (24).

Mechanisms of Hormone Secretion. Because the stromal cells of OTFSs characteristically resemble known steroid hormone–secreting cells to varying degrees, it is most logical to conclude that such cells are the major source of the excess steroid hormones. In the rare cases in which syncytiotrophoblastic cells are a component of the neoplasm, their secretion of chorionic gonadotropin (hCG) most probably stimulates the stromal cells to luteinize and produce hormones (fig. 19-1). There is abundant morphologic, clinical, and biochemical evidence that the high circulating level of hCG during pregnancy is responsible for its relatively frequent association with virilizing OTFSs (fig. 19-2) (3,4). The explanation for the stromal stimulation is not so clear, however, in patients with similar neoplasms who are not pregnant and whose tumors do not contain syncytiotrophoblast. On the basis of immunohistochemical evidence, several authors have suggested that ectopic production of hCG by neoplastic epithelial cells is responsible for the stromal stimulation in some of these patients (10). The high level of circulating luteinizing hormone may be an additional factor in postmenopausal women. A nonhormonal theory to explain stromal stimulation in cases of OTFS is mechanical, purporting that progressive expansion of aggregates of tumor cells or cysts lined by tumor cells, simulating expansion of a graafian follicle, exerts mechanical pressure on the stroma, stimulating it to transform into hormone-producing

373

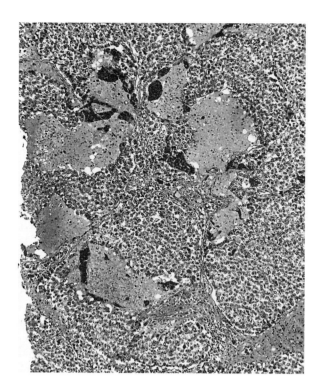 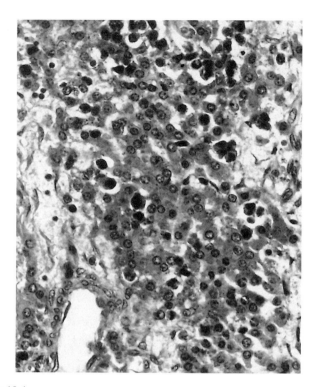

Figure 19-1

DYSGERMINOMA WITH SYNCYTIOTROPHOBLAST CELLS AND FUNCTIONING STROMA

Left: The syncytiotrophoblast cells are arranged around pools of blood. (Fig. 3 from Case Records of the Massachusetts General Hospital. Case 11-1972. N Eng J Med 1972;286:594–600.)

Right: Small groups of large, degenerating dysgerminoma cells and single cells of similar type are surrounded by smaller cells with small round nuclei and abundant cytoplasm, which was eosinophilic, within the peripheral portion of the tumor. The smaller cells resemble lutein cells and apparently secreted the androgens that virilized the patient. (Fig. 5 from Case Records of the Massachusetts General Hospital. Case 11-1972. N Eng J Med 1972;286:594–600.)

Figure 19-2

MUCINOUS CYSTADENOMA WITH LUTEINIZATION OF STROMA RESULTING IN VIRILIZATION DURING PREGNANCY

The mucinous glands are separated by diffuse masses of lutein cells.

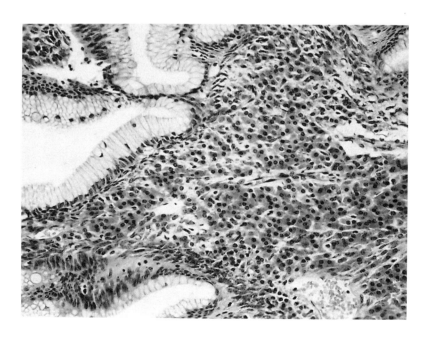

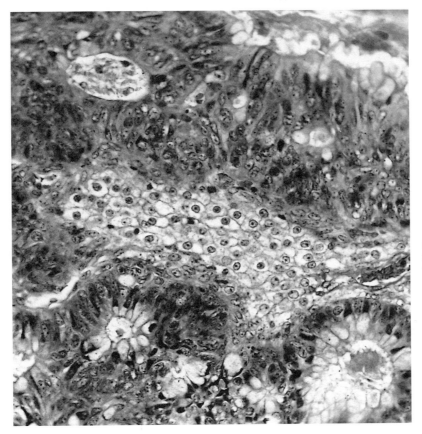

Figure 19-3
ADENOCARCINOMA,
METASTATIC FROM COLON,
WITH LUTEINIZATION
OF STROMA
The luteinized stromal cells have central nuclei with prominent nucleoli and abundant cytoplasm filled with (lipid) vacuoles.

tissue. While this mechanism may have a role it is much more probable that the phenomenon of functioning stroma has a biochemical basis.

It has been known for some time that carcinoma cells may have aromatase activity, and therefore, a capacity to convert androgens to estrogens (19). More recently, hormonal studies of patients with ovarian cancer have shown that abnormal amounts of a variety of steroid hormones are secreted, with the highest levels in patients with extensive tumor spread (6,9). These findings suggest that ovarian cancer growing outside the ovary is capable of secreting hormones. The demonstration that cultures of carcinoma cells from omental metastases of ovarian carcinoma are capable of estrogen and progesterone production in vitro (21) provides evidence that these cells may also secrete steroid hormones in vivo. It is also possible that the stromal cells of ovarian carcinomas growing outside the ovary can aromatize steroids and possibly perform other steroid interconversions. This

mechanism is suggested by the immunohistochemical demonstration of aromatase in the stroma of breast carcinomas (17).

Microscopic Findings. The functioning stroma of the tumor may be its intrinsic stroma, which is derived from ovarian stroma, the stroma adjacent to the tumor, or a combination of the two. The involved stroma resembles, to varying degrees, ovarian stromal derivatives that are responsible for hormone formation in both the normal and hyperactive ovary (stromal hyperthecosis). Accordingly, the stromal cells transform into plump spindle cells resembling theca externa cells, theca lutein cells, stromal lutein cells, or a combination of these cell types (fig. 19-3). Rarely, the stromal cells differentiate into Leydig cells, identified by their content of Reinke crystals (5). In some patients with clinical or laboratory evidence of an increased production of estrogens one may find only "condensation" of spindle-shaped stromal cells adjacent to the neoplastic cells. That these spindle cells may be capable of steroid hormone formation is suggested by the finding that spindle cells at the margins of lutein cell nests in stromal hyperthecosis, although indistinguishable from other ovarian stromal cells with ordinary staining, may be positive immunohistochemically for enzymes that participate in steroid hormone interconversions (7).

Most OTFSs exhibit evidence of stromal stimulation within the tumor, but some neoplasms, particularly those with little intrinsic stroma, may be associated with similar evidence that predominates along their margins (16). These changes include stromal luteinization, stromal Leydig cell differentiation, and hilar Leydig cell hyperplasia restricted to the hilar margin of the tumor (figs. 19-4; 19-5, left). In some cases the peripheral steroid cells contain large amounts of intracytoplasmic lipid, and a thin layer of yellow tissue is visible grossly on the outer surface of the tumor (fig. 19-5, right).

Regardless of the specific type of intrinsic or extrinsic stromal change (condensed spindle cells, lutein cells, or Leydig cells) OTFSs may be associated with estrogenic, androgenic, or progestagenic changes, or a combination of them. The rare tumors associated with the formation of Leydig cells or hyperplasia of adjacent hilus cells, however, appear to be virilizing more often than tumors that contain lutein cells in their intrinsic or marginal stroma (16). Also, since the ovarian stroma is generally considered a primarily androgenic component of the ovary it is not surprising that in some of the "estrogenic" OTFSs the neoplasm itself produces androgens, which are converted peripherally to estrogens (8).

Types of Tumor with Functioning Stroma. A wide variety of ovarian neoplasms, even including lymphoma (11), have been associated with a functioning stroma, with malignant forms in this category more common than benign tumors. Although it is difficult to establish the frequency of various types of tumor accompanied by estrogenic manifestations, laboratory studies suggest that the most common are the surface epithelial–stromal carcinomas, particularly those in the mucinous and endometrioid categories, and metastatic carcinomas, especially from the large intestine (14). Of the over 60 reported ovarian tumors with an androgenic stroma, one third have been Krukenberg tumors, mostly of gastric origin, and one fifth have been primary mucinous

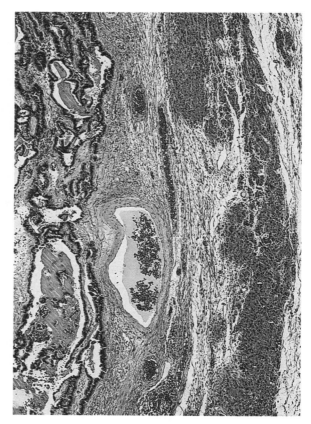

Figure 19-4
STRUMAL CARCINOID TUMOR WITH
FORMATION OF LAYER OF STEROID CELLS
IN ADJACENT OVARIAN STROMA
Some of these cells contained crystals of Reinke, identifying them as Leydig cells.

cystic tumors, mostly benign; less common have been rete cystadenomas, metastatic carcinomas from the large intestine, dermoid cysts, strumal carcinoid tumors, and miscellaneous others (18).

Differential Diagnosis. It is important not to be misled by the presence of endocrine manifestations into making an erroneous diagnosis of a sex cord–stromal tumor. Tumors that are particularly likely to create confusion are Krukenberg tumors with a prominent tubular pattern (2) and surface epithelial–stromal tumors with luteinized stroma. Tubular Krukenberg tumors (page 216), unlike Sertoli-Leydig cell tumors, have tubules lined by glandular cells, at least some of which contain large amounts of mucin. Endometrioid carcinomas, as discussed on pages 116 and 120, may simulate sex cord–stromal

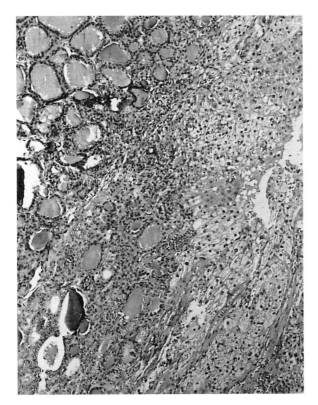 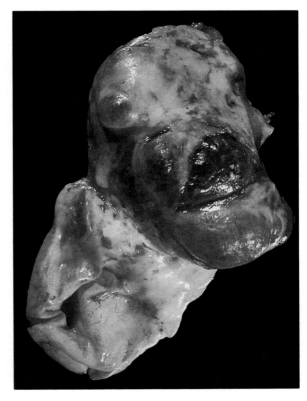

Figure 19-5
STRUMA OVARII WITH PERIPHERAL FORMATION OF LUTEIN CELLS
Left: The lutein cells are filled with (lipid) vacuoles. This tumor was associated with elevated estrogen levels and endometrial hyperplasia.
Right: The lipid-filled lutein cells illustrated on the left produced patchy yellow discoloration of the outer surface of the tumor.

tumors, particularly Sertoli cell tumors, and if there is luteinization of the stroma, Sertoli-Leydig cell tumors (23). Mucinous cysts may be a prominent feature of Sertoli-Leydig cell tumors (page 213); therefore, any virilizing tumor with a mucinous component must be searched carefully for Sertoli-Leydig cell elements before making a diagnosis of a virilizing mucinous cystic tumor.

REFERENCES

1. Bruno MS, Ober WB. Clinicopathologic conference. N Y State J Med 1959;59:4001–7.
2. Bullon A Jr, Arseneau J, Prat J, Young RH, Scully RE. Tubular Krukenberg tumor. A problem in histopathologic diagnosis. Am J Surg Pathol 1981;5:225–32.
3. Connor TB, Ganis FM, Levin HS, Migeon CJ, Martin LG. Gonadotropin-dependent Krukenberg tumor causing virilization during pregnancy. J Clin Endocrinol Metab 1968;28:198–214.
4. DePalma P, Wronski M, Bifernino V, Bovani I. Krukenberg tumor in pregnancy with virilization. A case report. Eur J Gynaec Oncol 1995;16:59–64.
5. Hameed K. Brenner tumor of the ovary with Leydig cell hyperplasia. A histologic and ultrastructural study. Cancer 1972;30:945–52.
6. Heinonen PK, Koivula T, Rajaniemi H, Pystynen P. Peripheral and ovarian venous concentrations of steroid and gonadotropin hormones in postmenopausal women with epithelial ovarian tumors. Gynecol Oncol 1986;25:1–10.
7. Hirakawa T, Thor A, Osawa Y, Mason JI, Scully RE. Stromal hyperthecosis of the ovary: immunohistochemical distribution of steroidogenic enzymes [Abstract]. Mod Pathol 1992;5:65A.

7a. López-Beltrán A, Calañas AS, Jimena P, et al. Virilizing mature ovarian cystic teratomas. Virchows Arch 1997;431:149–51.

8. MacDonald PC, Grodin JM, Edman CD, Vellios F, Siiteri PK. Origin of estrogen in a postmenopausal woman with a nonendocrine tumor of the ovary and endometrial hyperplasia. Obstet Gynecol 1976;47:644–50.

9. Mahlck CG, Backstrom T, Kjellgren O. Androstenedione production by malignant epithelial ovarian tumors. Gynecol Oncol 1986;25:217–22.

10. Matias-Guiu X, Prat J. Ovarian tumors with functioning stroma. An immunohistochemical study of 100 cases with human chorionic gonadotropin monoclonal and polyclonal antibodies. Cancer 1990;65:2001–5.

11. Mittal KR, Blechman A, Greco MA, Alfonso F, Demopoulos R. Case report. Lymphoma of ovary with stromal luteinization, presenting as secondary amenorrhea. Gynecol Oncol 1992;45:69–75.

12. Morris JM, Scully RE. Endocrine pathology of the ovary. St. Louis: Mosby, 1958.

13. Ober WB, Pollak A, Gerstmann KE, Kupperman HS. Krukenberg tumor with androgenic and progestational activity. Am J Obstet Gynecol 84:739–44.

14. Rome RM, Fortune DW, Quinn MA, Brown JB. Functioning ovarian tumors in postmenopausal women. Obstet Gynecol 1981;57:705–10.

15. Rubin DK, Frost JK. The cytologic detection of ovarian cancer. Acta Cytologica 1963;7:191–5.

16. Rutgers JL, Scully RE. Functioning ovarian tumors with peripheral steroid cell proliferation: a report of twenty-four cases. Int J Gynecol Pathol 1986;5:319–37.

17. Sasano H, Nagura H, Harada N, Goukon Y, Kimura M. Immunolocalization of aromatase and other steroidogenic enzymes in human breast disorders. Hum Pathol 1994;25:530–5.

18. Scully RE. Ovarian tumours with functioning stroma. In: Fox H, ed. Haines and Taylor obstetrical and gynaecological pathology, Vol. 2, 4th ed. Edinburgh: Churchill Livingstone, 1995.

19. Thompson MA, Adelson MD, Kaufaran LM, Marshall LD, Cable DA. Aromatization of testosterone by epithelial tumor cells cultured from patients with ovarian carcinoma. Cancer Res 1988;48:6491–7.

20. Ueda G, Hamanaka N, Hayakawa K, et al. Clinical, histochemical, and biochemical studies of an ovarian dysgerminoma with trophoblasts and Leydig cells. Am J Obstet Gynecol 1972;114:748–54.

21. Wimalasena J, Dostal R, Meehan D. Gonadotropins, estradiol and growth factors regulate epithelial ovarian cancer cell growth. Gynecol Oncol 1992;26:1–6.

22. Wren BG, Frampton J. Oestrogenic activity associated with nonfeminizing ovarian tumours after the menopause. Brit Med J 1963;2:842–4.

23. Young RH, Prat J, Scully RE. Ovarian endometrioid carcinomas resembling sex cord-stromal tumors. A clinicopathological analysis of 13 cases. Am J Surg Pathol 1982;6:513–22.

24. Zaloudek CJ, Tavassoli FA, Norris HJ. Dysgerminoma with syncytiotrophoblastic giant cells. A histologically and clinically distinctive subtype of dysgerminoma. Am J Surg Pathol 1981;5:361–7.

❖❖❖

20
PARAENDOCRINE, PARANEOPLASTIC, AND OTHER SYNDROMES ASSOCIATED WITH OVARIAN TUMORS

A variety of unusual endocrine syndromes and paraendocrine and paraneoplastic phenomena may be associated with ovarian tumors. Other ovarian tumors are components of heritable or nonheritable disorders that may have a variety of extraovarian manifestations. The carcinoid syndrome associated with ovarian carcinoid tumors and the hyperthyroidism that is occasionally associated with struma ovarii are discussed on pages 291 and 285, respectively.

UNUSUAL ENDOCRINE AND PARAENDOCRINE SYNDROMES

Chorionic Gonadotropin Production

Clinical evidence of chorionic gonadotropin (hCG) secretion by ovarian tumors is most commonly associated with germ cell tumors containing syncytiotrophoblastic cells. In such cases, the production of steroid hormones is attributed to the presence of luteinized cells within the stroma of the tumor or in the adjacent ovarian stroma (see chapter 19), or to stimulation of the follicular apparatus of uninvolved ovarian tissue by the high hCG levels.

Clinically evident hCG production by ovarian tumors other than those of germ cell origin is rare. Ectopic hCG production was reported by Civantos and Rywlin (2) in three women with serous papillary or mucinous adenocarcinoma of the ovary. Each of the tumors contained syncytiotrophoblast-like cells that were shown to contain hCG by an immunofluorescence technique (fig. 20-1). In one patient, who had postmenopausal bleeding, the stroma of the contralateral ovary contained numerous lutein cells, and a decidual reaction was present in the endometrium. No endocrine effects were observed in the other two patients. Oliva et al. (8) described two poorly differentiated ovarian carcinomas of surface epithelial type that had a choriocarcinomatous component; this appeared as a necrotic, hemorrhagic, circumscribed, brown nodule on gross examination. The stroma of each tumor was luteinized. Both tumors were associated with extra-abdominal metastases, elevated serum hCG levels, and a fatal outcome. Additionally, Kobayashi et al. (5) reported a case of ovarian clear cell carcinoma immunoreactive for hCG in a patient who presented with postmenopausal bleeding and elevated serum concentrations of hCG and estradiol; no trophoblastic elements were identified within the tumor.

Vaitukaitis (10) reported that 10 of 28 ovarian tumors of various types were associated with the presence of immunoreactive hCG in the serum, and Samaan et al. (9) found the beta-subunit of hCG in the serum of 41 percent of women with carcinomas of surface epithelial type. Surface epithelial tumors, including benign, borderline, and invasive types, have been immunoreactive for hCG in 10 to 40 percent of the cases (1,3,4,6,7). Metastatic carcinomas to the ovary may also contain immunoreactive hCG, a feature found in five of nine metastatic gastrointestinal adenocarcinomas in one series (6). In that series, the authors found a correlation between hCG immunoreactivity and a "morphologically active stroma," defined as the presence of luteinized stromal cells or stromal condensation (a concentration of spindle cells arranged in a storiform pattern). Forty percent of the hCG-positive tumors had "active" stroma, in contrast to only 20 percent of the hCG-negative tumors. The results of these studies indicate that hCG or hCG-like substances may play a role in activating the stroma of both primary and secondary ovarian tumors.

Hypercalcemia

In addition to small cell carcinomas of hypercalcemic type (page 316), a variety of ovarian tumors have been associated with paraendocrine hypercalcemia (Table 20-1) (11–21). The pathologic features of these tumors are similar to those of tumors unassociated with hypercalcemia. The tumors are only rarely accompanied by hypercalcemia-related clinical manifestations, but when

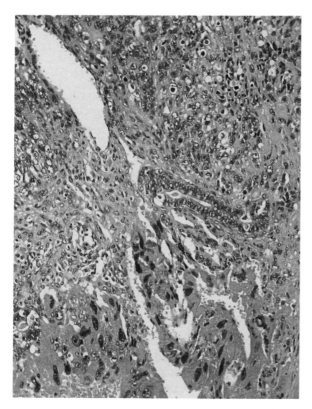 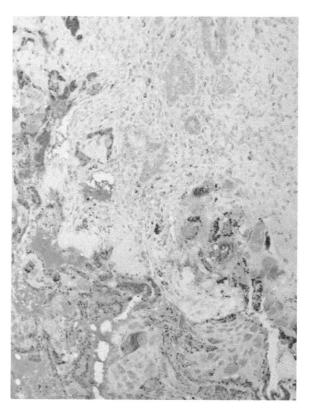

Figure 20-1
OVARIAN CARCINOMA WITH TROPHOBLASTIC DIFFERENTIATION
Left: Poorly differentiated carcinoma (top) in a 59-year-old woman contains syncytiotrophoblastic giant cells (bottom).
Right: The syncytiotrophoblastic cells are immunoreactive for hCG.

Table 20-1

OVARIAN TUMORS OTHER THAN SMALL CELL CARCINOMA ASSOCIATED WITH HYPERCALCEMIA*

Tumor Type	Number of Cases	Percent
Clear cell carcinoma	19	43
Serous carcinoma	6	14
Dysgerminoma	6	14
Squamous cell carcinoma arising in dermoid cyst	6	14
Mucinous carcinoma	3	7
Undifferentiated carcinoma	1	2
Mixed clear cell/endometrioid carcinoma	1	2
Steroid cell tumor	1	2
Dermoid cyst	1	2

*Modified from reference 13.

present, they are sometimes dramatic and life-threatening (11).

The mechanism of the hypercalcemia is unknown. Attempts to demonstrate parathormone (PTH) within the tumor cells have been unsuccessful, with rare exceptions, and in several cases in which PTH has been measured in the plasma, the level was normal. Roles for osteoclast-activating factor, prostaglandins, and a vitamin D–like steroid have also been proposed (17,18). Some hypercalcemic ovarian tumors have been associated with elevated serum levels of parathyroid hormone–related protein (PTHrP), have been immunoreactive for it, or both (12,14,15,18a,19). Although almost all of the ovarian tumors associated with hypercalcemia have been malignant, one was a dermoid cyst in which PTHrP was demonstrated immunohistochemically within squamous epithelium, neural elements, and colonic type mucosa (18a).

Cushing's Syndrome

Five cases of biochemically documented, clinically typical Cushing's syndrome have been caused by cortisol production by a steroid cell tumor (22,26,30,38). Four of the tumors occurred in adults, had metastasized within the abdomen at the time of presentation, and were eventually fatal (26,30,38). In contrast to clinically benign steroid cell tumors, these tumors were focally necrotic, exhibited at least moderate nuclear atypia, and had a high mitotic rate. The fifth tumor occurred in a 2-year-old girl who presented with Cushing's syndrome and isosexual precocity, both of which regressed during a 6-week postoperative follow-up period (22). The clinical and biochemical findings in these cases suggest a possible origin from adrenal cortical rests, which have been identified in the broad ligament and less commonly in the hilus of the ovary in over 25 percent of hysterectomy specimens (27). Such rests are rare in the ovary itself, however (34,35,37), suggesting that cortisol production by these tumors probably results from ectopic secretion of the hormone by steroid cells of ovarian origin.

Rarely, other ovarian tumors have been associated with Cushing's syndrome, probably due in most cases to ectopic production of adrenocorticotropic hormone (ACTH) or corticotropin-releasing factor. These neoplasms include bilateral endometrioid adenocarcinoma (25), a poorly differentiated adenocarcinoma (33), a "malignant Sertoli cell tumor" (31), a bilateral Sertoli-Leydig cell tumor (28), a trabecular carcinoid (in which the tumor cells were immunoreactive for ACTH) (36), and a tumor that resembled an atypical carcinoid and small cell carcinoma of the lung (24). The last tumor was also associated with the carcinoid syndrome. Another tumor associated with Cushing's syndrome was interpreted originally as an "arrhenoblastoma" but was more likely a metastatic small cell carcinoma from the lung or thymus (32). Finally, two cases have been described in which anterior pituitary tissue within a dermoid cyst caused clinically and biochemically typical Cushing's syndrome, including an elevated plasma level of ACTH (23,29). In one of these cases, it was not clear whether the pituitary tissue was truly neoplastic (29), but in the other case it had given rise to a chromophobe adenoma in which the neoplastic cells were immunoreactive for ACTH (23).

Zollinger-Ellison and Inappropriate Antidiuresis Syndromes

Eleven ovarian mucinous tumors (2 cystadenomas, 5 borderline tumors [fig. 20-2, left], and 4 cystadenocarcinomas) have caused the Zollinger-Ellison syndrome (40–43,45–47,49,51–53). Gastrin-containing cells were identified immunohistochemically within the cyst lining in all 10 of the cases in which staining was performed (fig. 20-2, right); in 6 cases, gastrin was demonstrated within the cyst fluid. The clinical manifestations of the syndrome, including elevated plasma gastrin levels, disappeared after removal of the ovarian tumor in each case.

The association between ovarian mucinous tumors and the Zollinger-Ellison syndrome is consistent with the frequent finding of neuroendocrine intestinal-type cells within mucinous tumors removed from asymptomatic patients (39,44,48, 50,54–56). A number of studies have shown that all categories of mucinous tumors (benign, borderline, and malignant) commonly contain argyrophil, argentaffin, and hormone-immunoreactive cells, although in most of the studies, these cells were most frequent in borderline tumors. The argyrophil cells are often immunoreactive for serotonin and a variety of polypeptide hormones. The lack of clinical manifestations in these cases may be related to the production of only small quantities of biologically active peptides, their intermittent release or rapid degradation, the production of only biologically inactive peptides, or a failure of recognition of subtle clinical signs and symptoms (39). Possibly, if blood levels of the various hormones had been measured preoperatively, the results might have uncovered laboratory evidence of function in some of the patients.

In one case a serous carcinoma with a component of small call carcinoma of pulmonary type (page 320) was associated with the inappropriate antidiuresis syndrome. Neuroendocrine granules were found on electron microscopic examination of the tumor cells, which were also positive immunohistochemically for antidiuretic hormone (56a).

Hypoglycemia

Six ovarian tumors associated with hypoglycemia have been reported: a serous cystadenocarcinoma (60), a dysgerminoma (62), a fibroma (58), a malignant schwannoma (61), a strumal

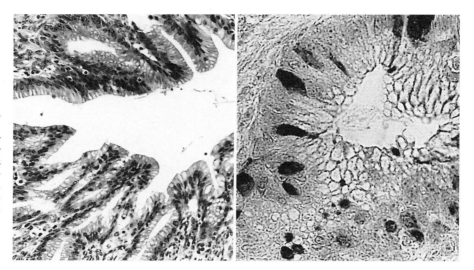

Figure 20-2
OVARIAN MUCINOUS
TUMOR ASSOCIATED
WITH THE ZOLLINGER-
ELLISON SYNDROME
Left: The tumor is of borderline malignancy, intestinal type.
Right: Some of the tumor
cells are immunoreactive for
gastrin. (Fig. 3 from Clement
PB, Young RH, Scully RE. Clinical syndromes associated with
tumors of the female genital
tract. Semin Diagn Pathol
1991;8:204–33.)

carcinoid tumor (57), and a carcinoid tumor with a mixed insular and trabecular pattern (59). Insulin and proinsulin were recovered from the tumor tissue of the malignant schwannoma (61), and the cells of the carcinoid tumors were immunoreactive for insulin (57,59). At least two of the six tumors contained dense core granules on ultrastructural examination (59,61). The patient with the strumal carcinoid also had cutaneous melanosis and tumor cells immunoreactive for alpha-melanocyte–stimulating hormone, and the patient with the insular-trabecular carcinoid tumor also had a parathyroid adenoma and pituitary hyperplasia, suggesting a variant of the type I multiple endocrine neoplasia syndrome.

Renin and Aldosterone Production

Thirteen cases of hypertension related to hormone secretion by an ovarian tumor have been reported (63,66–74,76–78); two of the patients also had Gorlin's syndrome (69,78) (page 387). In 8 cases, the hypertension was associated with a renin-secreting tumor, hyperreninism, and secondary hyperaldosteronism (63,66,67,69,70,72, 76,78). In 3 cases (71,73,77), an aldosterone-secreting ovarian tumor resulted in primary hyperaldosteronism and low or normal plasma renin levels. Elevated aldosterone levels were present in a 12th case but plasma renin levels were not measured (68) and in the 13th case, reported in 1966, neither renin nor aldosterone levels were determined (74). In 4 cases the tumor also produced steroid hormones, as manifested by isosexual pseudoprecocity in 2 cases (68,74) and elevated plasma levels of estradiol, testosterone, or both in 2 others (77,78).

Of the 12 cases in which the microscopic features of the tumor were described, 8 were sex cord–stromal tumors (fig. 20-3), 2 were steroid cell tumors, 1 was a leiomyosarcoma (66), and 1 was a mucinous adenocarcinoma (67). Three tumors in the sex cord–stromal group were well differentiated Sertoli cell tumors (63,68,72), 1 was a fibromatous tumor in a patient with Gorlin's syndrome (69), and the other 4 had an appearance that was too nonspecific or poorly differentiated to subclassify (fig. 20-3) (70, 71,76,77). One of the last group of tumors occurred in a woman with the Peutz-Jeghers syndrome and was benign, whereas the other 3 were clinically malignant, and 2 were fatal. One of the "steroid cell" tumors occurred in a 7-year-old girl and had a prominent follicular pattern more consistent with a diagnosis of juvenile granulosa cell tumor (74). Immunohistochemical staining in 5 of the sex cord–stromal tumors and the leiomyosarcoma revealed cells containing immunoreactive renin or prorenin (63,66,69,72,76,78). One other steroid cell tumor, which occurred in a 53-year-old normotensive virilized woman with elevated plasma levels of prorenin and testosterone, was immunoreactive with an antibody that recognizes both prorenin and renin (64). The prorenin and testosterone levels became normal postoperatively.

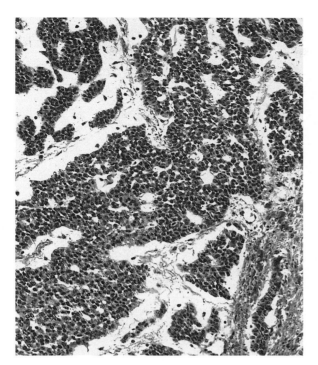

Figure 20-3
OVARIAN TUMOR ASSOCIATED
WITH HYPERTENSION

Sex cord–stromal tumor associated with elevated plasma levels of renin and aldosterone. The neoplastic cells were immunoreactive for renin. (Fig. 9 from Clement PB, Young RH, Scully RE. Clinical syndromes associated with tumors of the female genital tract. Semin Diagn Pathol 1991;8:204–33.)

In contrast to the rarity of ovarian tumors associated with clinical evidence of renin production, recent evidence suggests that subclinical secretion of renin by some ovarian tumors may be relatively common. Anderson et al. (65), in a retrospective study of eight ovarian sex cord–stromal tumors, found that four of them were immunoreactive for renin. None of the patients had documented hypertension or hypokalemia. The occurrence of renin-secreting ovarian tumors is consistent with recent observations that a complete renin-angiotensin system exists in the follicular apparatus of the normal ovary (75) (page 19).

Hyperprolactinemia

Two cases of ovarian dermoid cyst associated with the production of prolactin have been described (80,81). One patient, a 41-year-old woman with amenorrhea and hyperprolactinemia, had a dermoid cyst that contained a tumor

2.5 cm in length and 0.25 cm in greatest width, subjacent to squamous epithelium (fig. 20-4A). The tumor was composed of small rounded nests of epithelial cells, some of which surrounded lumens filled with colloid-like material; the cells had scanty cytoplasm and small, round, uniform, mitotically inactive nuclei (fig. 20-4B). Most of the tumor cells were strongly immunoreactive for prolactin, establishing a diagnosis of prolactinoma (fig. 20-4C). The prolactin level became normal postoperatively.

In the other case, a 25-year-old woman presented with amenorrhea, galactorrhea, and hyperprolactinemia (80). A right adnexal mass was detected, and a dermoid cyst was excised from the right ovary. The serum level of prolactin returned to normal. Pathologic examination revealed an otherwise typical dermoid cyst that also contained a 1-mm focus of large polygonal cells with abundant eosinophilic cytoplasm immunoreactive for prolactin; a few cells also stained for growth hormone.

The only other ovarian tumor with documented prolactin secretion was a gonadoblastoma (79). The patient did not have hyperprolactinemia but a prolactin gradient was present between the vein draining the tumor and peripheral veins. Cells within the gonadoblastoma that resembled Sertoli cells were immunoreactive for prolactin.

PARANEOPLASTIC SYNDROMES

Nervous System and Muscular Disorders

Ovarian cancer is one of the malignant tumors that is most often associated with paraneoplastic disorders of the nervous system. A disorder of this type was present in 16 percent of patients with ovarian carcinoma in one study (83). A variety of lesions affecting both the gray matter and white matter of the cerebrum, cerebellum, and spinal cord; the peripheral nerves; and the neuromuscular junction (accompanied by myasthenia gravis) have been encountered in patients with ovarian cancer (82,83,87,90), although only one nervous system disorder, subacute cerebellar degeneration (SCD), has a strong association.

Ovarian cancer accounted for 12, 37, and 47 percent of the cases of paraneoplastic SCD in three series (86,87,89a). The ovarian tumors have usually been poorly differentiated adenocarcinomas of

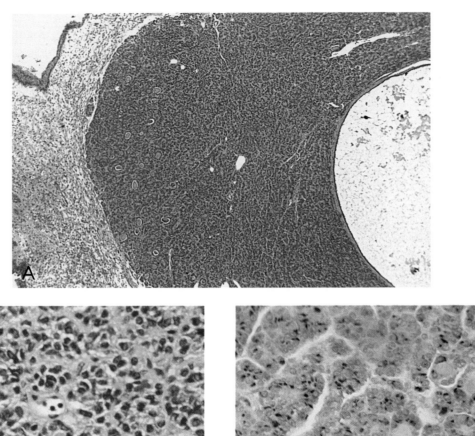

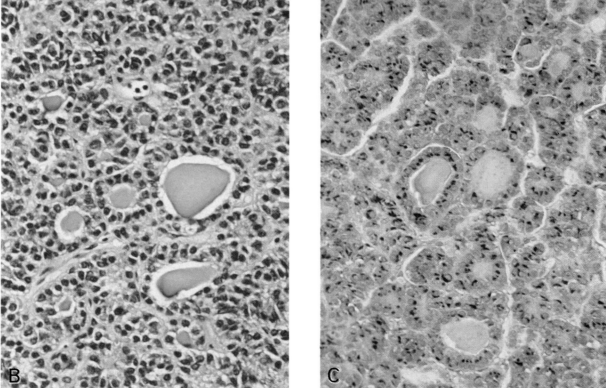

Figure 20-4
PROLACTINOMA IN DERMOID CYST

A: A nodule of tumor is present beneath the squamous epithelial lining of the dermoid cyst.

B: The tumor is composed of epithelial cells with scanty cytoplasm and small, round, uniform nuclei, some of which surround lumens filled with colloid-like material.

C: The tumor cells are strongly immunoreactive for prolactin. (Figs. 1 and 2 from Palmer PE, Bogojavlensky S, Bhan AK, Scully RE. Prolactinoma in wall of ovarian dermoid cyst with hyperprolactinemia. Obstet Gynecol 1990;75:540–2.)

surface epithelial type, and when a subtype has been specifically noted, it has usually been serous (88); occasionally it has been clinically occult (86a,89a). The cerebellar manifestations antedated, sometimes by several years, or coincided with the initial recognition of the cancer in over 75 percent of the cases in one series; they preceded the diagnosis of recurrent cancer in the remainder (88). The cardinal finding on neuropathologic examination is a diffuse pronounced loss in the numbers of cerebellar Purkinje cells (87). A subset of patients also have a prominent inflammatory reaction, which may be confined to the cerebellum or also involve other parts of the brain (87). The pathogenesis of SCD in these cases appears to be related to the presence of circulating anti-Purkinje cell antibodies that also react with antigens in the tumor (84–86,89,89a).

Connective Tissue Disorders

The risk of ovarian as well as other types of cancer appears to be increased in patients with dermatomyositis or polymyositis (91,93,94,99–101,103,106,108,109a). Malignant tumors were found in 5 of 25 women with dermatomyositis in one series; 3 of the tumors were ovarian carcinomas (101). In two studies of patients with dermatomyositis or polymyositis and a gynecologic cancer (a total of 15 cases), the primary site was ovary in six of the cases (94,108). In another study (109), two of six women with dermatomyositis and breast cancer were also found to have an ovarian carcinoma. Mordel et al. (99), in a review of 30 literature cases of ovarian tumors associated with dermatomyositis, found that all of the histologically verified tumors were adenocarcinomas (most commonly high-grade serous carcinomas), and except for one, were stage III or IV. One dysgerminoma (104) and 1 ovarian leiomyoma (107) were also associated with dermatomyositis. The onset of the dermatomyositis usually precedes recognition of the tumor, which becomes evident within 2 years in most cases (108). The dermatologic and, to a lesser extent, the myopathic symptoms typically regress after removal of the tumor, and return if it recurs (109a).

In seven patients, rheumatoid-like polyarthritis and palmar fasciitis have preceded a high-stage ovarian carcinoma by 1 to 25 months (98,102). Four of the ovarian tumors were endometrioid carcinomas, two were serous carcinomas, and one was an undifferentiated carcinoma. Other connective tissue disorders that have been associated rarely with ovarian cancer include hypertrophic pulmonary osteoarthropathy (96,97), rheumatoid or rheumatoid-like arthritis (92), scleroderma (95,110), and the shoulder-hand syndrome (105).

Hematologic Disorders

Approximately 30 ovarian tumors have been reported to be associated with autoimmune hemolytic anemia, which is usually Coombs-positive (113). Most of these tumors were dermoid cysts (113,129), but some were carcinomas (113) and one, a granulosa cell tumor (118). In the last case, the patient also had splenic angiomas. For many patients, corticosteroid therapy, splenectomy, or both resulted in little or no improvement, but removal of the ovarian tumor produced a rapid remission of the hemolytic disorder. Payne et al. (129) have listed several potential mechanisms to explain the relation of a dermoid cyst to the anemia: 1) the tumor elaborates a substance that alters the surfaces of red blood cells, making them antigenic to the host; 2) an antigen in the wall or lumen of the cyst stimulates production of an antibody that cross reacts with red blood cells; and 3) the tumor directly produces a red blood cell antibody. Support for the last theory is provided by the finding of immunoglobulin in the cyst fluid in several cases (129).

Ovarian tumors are commonly associated with laboratory evidence of disseminated intravascular coagulation (DIC), but clinical manifestations of this disorder are uncommon. In one study (112), 72 percent, and in another (111), 94 percent of women with ovarian cancer had fibrin degradation products in the serum. In a review of 231 cases of clinically evident DIC in women with tumors, however, Sack et al. (131) found only 7 that were associated with ovarian cancer. Additional cases have been reported (114,119,130,132), some of which have been accompanied by nonbacterial thrombotic endocarditis (114,119) or microangiopathic hemolytic anemia (130). Ovarian carcinomas have also been associated with migratory thrombophlebitis (Trousseau's syndrome), a manifestation of chronic DIC (119a,122,131). A wide variety of pathogenetic mechanisms have been proposed, although most tumors probably initiate DIC by expressing tissue factor on their cell surfaces, potentially initiating both the intrinsic and extrinsic pathways (116). Additional pathogenetic factors proposed in cases of ovarian cancer have included elevations in serum viscosity, erythrocyte aggregation, fibrinogen, beta-thromboglobulin, and platelet factor 4 (123,125).

Except in cases of androgenic ovarian tumors, erythrocytosis is only rarely associated with gynecologic tumors. In a series of 340 reported cases of paraneoplastic erythrocytosis, ovarian tumors accounted for only 2 percent; the histologic types of the tumors were not specified (121). The erythrocytosis appeared to be related to the secretion of erythropoietin by the ovarian tumors in cases of a dermoid cyst (120) and a steroid cell tumor (127).

Other hematologic abnormalities occasionally associated with ovarian tumors include nonthrombocytopenic purpura (mucinous cystadenoma) (117), granulocytosis (clear cell carcinoma) (133), thrombocytopenia (hemangiomas, carcinoma, adenofibroma) (124,126,134,135), pancytopenia (granulosa cell tumor) (128), systemic mastocytosis (page 388), and thrombocytosis (115,116, 136), which was present in 56 percent of patients with ovarian carcinoma in one study (115).

Cutaneous Disorders

In addition to the cutaneous manifestations of dermatomyositis, scleroderma (page 385), and the Peutz-Jeghers and nevoid basal cell carcinoma syndromes (page 387), a variety of cutaneous lesions have been described in association with ovarian tumors or tumor-like lesions. Acanthosis nigricans occurs in some, typically young women with polycystic ovarian disease, stromal hyperthecosis, or combinations thereof, becoming a component of the HAIR-AN syndrome (hyperandrogenemia, insulin resistance, and acanthosis nigricans) (page 413). In these cases (so-called benign acanthosis nigricans), the cutaneous lesions diminish or disappear with normalization of the blood androgen levels. In contrast, so-called malignant acanthosis nigricans typically occurs in older women in association with a malignant tumor, usually an adenocarcinoma, which in most cases has metastasized by the time of its discovery (138). The cutaneous lesions may precede, coincide with, or follow the

detection of the neoplasm. This type of acanthosis nigricans has been associated with four ovarian carcinomas, at least two of which were serous papillary carcinomas (138,139). Some authors consider the sign of Leser-Trelat (sudden onset and rapid enlargement of numerous seborrheic keratoses in association with an occult cancer) a variant of "malignant" acanthosis nigricans (142). One such case was reported in a 76-year-old woman 9 months before the discovery of a stage III ovarian adenocarcinoma (142).

The Torre-Muir syndrome is an autosomal dominant disorder characterized by the occurrence of solitary or multiple sebaceous tumors in patients with internal cancer (137,141). Ovarian tumors associated with the syndrome have included four carcinomas and a granulosa cell tumor (137,141). Eruptive keratoacanthomas in the absence of sebaceous tumors (144) and a case of an aggressive keratoacanthoma (140) have also been reported in patients with ovarian carcinomas. Acute neutrophilic dermatosis (Sweet's syndrome) is characterized by tender erythematous plaques with a distinctive microscopic appearance, fever, and leukocytosis (145). The disorder may occur in patients with an underlying cancer, usually leukemia, but also in occasional patients with carcinoma, including one with a clear cell carcinoma of the ovary (143). A case of cutaneous melanosis due to a strumal carcinoid tumor has been referred to on page 295.

Nephrotic Syndrome

In 1966, Lee et al. (146) documented the nephrotic syndrome and membranous glomerulopathy in three patients with gynecologic tumors, one of which was an ovarian "adenocarcinoma" and another, an ovarian dermoid cyst. It was not established, however, whether the two lesions were other than coincidental. A 65-year-old woman had the nephrotic syndrome 8 months prior to the detection of a stage IV poorly differentiated serous carcinoma of the ovary (147). A renal biopsy revealed membranous glomerulopathy. The proteinuria diminished greatly after debulking of the tumor. After combination chemotherapy for 10 months, the proteinuria disappeared and there was no evidence of tumor at a second-look laparotomy.

HERITABLE AND OTHER CONGENITAL SYNDROMES

Peutz-Jeghers Syndrome

The Peutz-Jeghers syndrome (PJS) is a rare autosomal dominant disorder characterized by hamartomatous gastrointestinal polyps, mucocutaneous melanin pigmentation, and predisposition to a wide variety of neoplasms, including those of the intestine, pancreas, breast, and female genital tract. The ovarian tumor associated most commonly with the PJS is the sex cord tumor with annular tubules (page 219), but two other distinctive sex cord–stromal tumors also occur in these patients, suggesting a possible association (pages 203 and 224). A number of other ovarian tumors have been described in patients with the PJS, although the great variety of types encountered suggests that most of them are coincidental. A possible exception is the mucinous cystic tumor, which may be benign, borderline, or malignant, and has been described in nine patients with the syndrome (148–150,152,154–157); in two cases, the tumors were bilateral (149,155). That such mucinous tumors may be a manifestation of the PJS is also suggested by the occurrence of other mucinous lesions in patients with this disorder, specifically adenoma malignum of the cervix and mucinous metaplasia of the fallopian tube (149,151,153).

Nevoid Basal Cell Carcinoma Syndrome

The nevoid basal cell carcinoma syndrome (NBCS), also referred to as the *basal cell nevus syndrome* and *Gorlin's syndrome,* is an autosomal dominant disorder with high penetrance and variable expressivity (160). Its most common features, which gradually appear with increasing patient age, include: multiple nevoid basal cell carcinomas; multiple jaw keratocysts; developmental defects of the skeletal system, especially rib, vertebral, and craniofacial abnormalities; palmar and plantar pits secondary to defective keratin production; epidermal inclusion cysts (including milia); ectopic calcification (falx cerebri, diaphragma sellae); and extracutaneous neoplasms of the ovary, and less often the brain (medulloblastoma, meningioma), heart (fibroma), and other sites. A wide variety of other lesions are seen less commonly (160). As approximately 10 percent of individuals with the NBCS

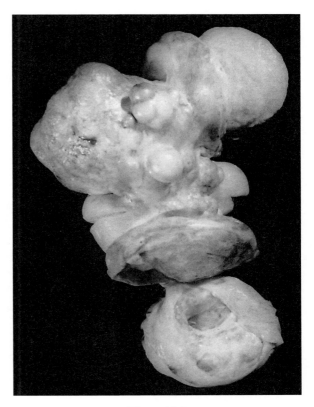

Figure 20-5
OVARIAN FIBROMA FROM PATIENT WITH
NEVOID BASAL CELL CARCINOMA SYNDROME
The tumor is multinodular and was calcified. (Fig. 7 from Case records of the Massachusetts General Hospital, Case 14. N Engl J Med 1976;294:772–7.) (Figures 20-5 and 20-6 are from the same patient.)

never have basal cell carcinomas, the diagnosis may be overlooked in patients without skin lesions (160).

Approximately 75 percent of females with the NBCS who are referred to gynecologists are found to have ovarian fibromas (160) (page 194). In contrast to fibromas in patients without the syndrome, the syndrome-related tumors are bilateral in approximately 75 percent of the cases, are frequently multinodular (fig. 20-5) or multifocal (as many as 10 in one ovary), and are almost always calcified, sometimes massively so (fig. 20-6) (158). They also tend to occur at a younger age than in patients without the syndrome, and are usually diagnosed in young adults, adolescents, or even children; the youngest affected patient described in the literature was 3 years of age (162). Additional tumors may arise years after local

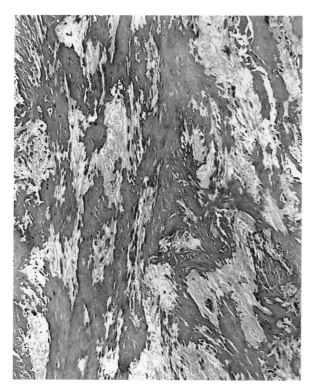

Figure 20-6
OVARIAN FIBROMA IN PATIENT WITH
NEVOID BASAL CELL CARCINOMA SYNDROME
The tumor is massively calcified.

excision (164). In two cases, an ovarian tumor in a patient with NBCS was associated with renin production and hypertension (page 382). Ovarian fibrosarcomas have also been encountered in two patients with NBCS, but only one such case was reported in detail (163). A pregnant patient with NBCS had a virilizing sclerosing stromal tumor (161); a relation to the syndrome was suggested by the bilaterality of the tumor, a feature that had not been previously described in cases of sclerosing stromal tumor.

Ovarian fibromas with clinicopathologic features similar to those occurring in the NBCS may be found in the absence of other stigmata of the disorder. Dumont-Herskowitz et al. (159) recently described a kindred in which female members in four successive generations had ovarian fibromas: they were usually diagnosed at a young age (as young as 3 years), were often calcified and multinodular or multiple, and were occasionally bilateral.

Ollier's, Maffucci's, and Other Disorders

Ollier's disease is a rare nonhereditary congenital syndrome characterized by multiple enchondromas; when the latter are associated with multiple hemangiomas, the designation Maffucci's syndrome is used. The juvenile granulosa cell tumor (JGCT) is a rare component of these syndromes: eight such tumors have been described in patients with Ollier's disease (167,170,174,175,177–180) and three in patients with Maffucci's syndrome (168,169,176). Single examples of ovarian fibroma (173) and fibrosarcoma (165) have also been reported in patients in Maffucci's syndrome.

JGCTs, especially when bilateral, may occur in association with other congenital syndromes or abnormalities. Pysher et al. (171) described a 4-month-old infant with bilateral JGCTs and multiple craniofacial and skeletal abnormalities suggestive of Goldenhar's syndrome. Also, bilateral JGCTs have been reported in a newborn with Potter's syndrome (172), and occasional phenotypically normal patients with a unilateral JGCT have had bone or soft tissue tumors (180). Systemic mastocytosis appeared in a 21-year-old woman following surgery and chemotherapy for a mixed malignant germ cell tumor of the ovary (166).

Sertoli-Leydig Cell Tumors and Thyroid Abnormalities

In 1974, Jensen et al. (183) described a kindred in which a number of female members from four consecutive generations were found to have Sertoli-Leydig cell tumors (SLCTs), thyroid adenomas, or both. These authors found reports of five similarly affected families in the literature, and since their report, at least three more families have been described (181,184,186). In some families, male members have also had thyroid lesions (181,184). It has been suggested that this syndrome is transmitted in an autosomal dominant fashion with a variable degree of expressivity (183,184). Jensen et al. (183) also found that 29 percent of patients under 20 years of age with sporadic SLCTs in the files of the Armed Forces Institute of Pathology had thyroid abnormalities. In contrast, only 2 percent of 207 patients with SLCTs in another series had thyroid masses (187).

The thyroid abnormalities associated with both familial and sporadic SLCTs have usually been interpreted as solitary or multiple adenomas or nodular goiter, but examples of Graves' disease (186) and carcinoma (186,187) have also been reported. The clinical and pathologic features of the SLCTs have not differed from those of tumors occurring in the absence of thyroid abnormalities, although in several familial cases, the SLCT was associated with an ipsilateral or contralateral ovarian mucinous tumor (cystadenoma or cystadenocarcinoma) or there was a mucinous ovarian tumor in a family member. Some of these "mucinous tumors" might have resulted from overgrowth of heterologous mucinous epithelium within a SLCT (183,187).

The only other association between ovarian tumors and thyroid abnormalities are two reported cases of a masculinizing steroid cell tumor and multiple endocrine adenomatosis, including thyroid and parathyroid adenomas (182,185).

Ataxia-Telangiectasia

Ataxia-telangiectasia is an autosomal recessive disorder characterized by progressive cerebellar ataxia, oculocutaneous telangiectasias, and immune deficiency, with recurrent sinopulmonary infections and a high frequency of malignant neoplasms. Although most of the tumors have been leukemias and lymphomas, a wide variety of other cancers have also been encountered. Ovarian tumors in patients with this disorder have included a yolk sac tumor (191) and three dysgerminomas (188–190), one of which was bilateral (188) and another of which was associated with a contralateral gonadoblastoma (189).

OTHER SYNDROMES

Lymphangioleiomyomatosis

Lymphangioleiomyomatosis is a rare disorder occurring almost exclusively in premenopausal women that is characterized by hamartomatous proliferations of smooth muscle around pulmonary airways, vessels, and lymphatics, and extrapulmonary lymphatics (192–195). As patients with tuberous sclerosis can have pulmonary lesions identical to those of lymphangioleiomyomatosis, the latter may be a forme fruste of the tuberous sclerosis complex. Lack et al. (194) reported the case of a 33-year-old mentally retarded woman with pulmonary and widespread extrapulmonary lymphangioleiomyomatosis, which included involvement of the uterus and ovaries. The smooth muscle cells of the lesion are immunoreactive for HMB-45 (193), and in some cases, estrogen and progesterone receptors (192). Progestin therapy has resulted in symptomatic improvement in a number of patients (195).

Meigs' Syndrome

In 1954, 17 years after his initial report (201), Meigs redefined the syndrome that bears his name as an association of an ovarian fibroma or a "predominantly fibrous tumor" (including thecoma, granulosa cell tumor, and Brenner tumor), ascites, and unilateral or bilateral pleural effusion, with disappearance of the ascitic fluid and effusion(s) after removal of the ovarian tumor (199,200). Subsequently, the term Meigs' syndrome has been applied to the same constellation of findings associated with any benign pelvic tumor or tumor-like process, while the term "pseudo-Meigs" syndrome has been used for cases in which the features of the syndrome are associated with a primary or secondary ovarian cancer, and in which the fluid has not been shown to contain malignant cells. The ascitic and pleural fluids in Meigs' and pseudo-Meigs' syndromes are usually serous, but may be serosanguinous (199).

The wide variety of ovarian tumors that have been associated with Meigs' and pseudo-Meigs' syndromes include benign, borderline, and malignant surface epithelial tumors; germ cell tumors (dermoid cyst, dysgerminoma, struma ovarii); rare other primary tumors (fibrosarcoma, lymphoma); and metastatic ovarian tumors (Krukenberg tumor, metastatic colon carcinoma) (197,199,202,205). A non-neoplastic lesion, massive ovarian edema, has also occasionally caused Meigs' syndrome (198). Nonovarian tumors have included uterine leiomyomas and a fallopian tube papilloma (200).

The ascitic fluid in Meigs' and pseudo-Meigs' syndromes appears to be due to transudation of fluid from the surface of the tumor, with the pleural fluid being a result of passage of the fluid through diaphragmatic fenestrations, lymphatics, or both. The predominance of right-sided pleural space involvement in the syndrome is consistent with the greater number of diaphragmatic fenestrations and lymphatics in the right hemidiaphragm. The likelihood of an ovarian stromal tumor being associated with ascites increases with the size of the tumor and the amount of edema fluid it contains. In their study of 70 fibromas and thecomas, Samanth and Black (204) found that tumors less than 10 cm in diameter and larger tumors that lacked edema were not accompanied by ascites; in contrast, 40 percent of the tumors 10 cm or larger in diameter were associated with ascites and the corresponding figure for tumors that were both large and edematous was 67 percent. There appeared to be no correlation, however, between these two features and the amount of ascitic fluid.

Many of the tumors that have been associated with Meigs' and pseudo-Meigs' syndromes, are much more commonly accompanied by ascites alone. For example, in two large series of ovarian fibromas totaling 78 cases (196,203), 30 percent of the tumors were associated with ascites but only 4 percent with Meigs' syndrome.

The syndrome of ovarian luteinized thecomas and sclerosing peritonitis has been discussed on page 192.

Amylase Secretion

Surface epithelial tumors, especially of the serous and, less often, of the endometrioid type, may produce amylase that is detectable immunohistochemically within the tumor cells or biochemically in cystic, ascitic, and pleural fluid; urine; and serum (206–217). Occasionally, fluid aspirated from ovarian tumors has been misinterpreted as ascitic fluid (206), or the clinical presentation has mimicked that of a pancreatic pseudocyst (211) or acute pancreatitis (210,212). The amylase produced by genital tract neoplasms, however, is similar to that of salivary gland origin, and can be distinguished electrophoretically from pancreatic amylase (212).

Approximately 15 patients with ovarian tumors associated with hyperamylasemia have been reported (206,209,210,212,214,217). Most of the tumors were high-stage serous carcinomas, but two were stage I endometrioid carcinomas (212,217). A serous carcinoma of peritoneal origin was also accompanied by hyperamylasemia (213). The serum amylase level may be a useful marker of tumor progression and therapeutic response in such patients.

Cramer and Bruns (208) described an unusual example of pseudo-Meigs' syndrome in a patient with a pleural effusion rich in amylase; hyperamylasemia was not present. The effusion disappeared after removal of a serous tumor of borderline malignancy, which had ruptured preoperatively.

Uveal Melanocytic Lesions

Diffuse bilateral uveal melanocytic lesions have been associated with visceral cancers. Three examples occurred in women with ovarian carcinoma (218–220); two women, 77 and 89 years of age, suffered gradual loss of vision during the 18 to 24 months before their deaths from poorly differentiated ovarian carcinoma (218,219); the third patient, a 60-year-old woman, complained of bilateral eye pain and blurring of vision almost immediately after oophorectomy for bilateral ovarian serous carcinoma. The visual loss progressed, and she died 1 year later of the ovarian tumor (220). Microscopic examination of the eyes from each patient revealed a bilateral diffuse proliferation of melanocytes throughout the uveal tracts; the sclerae were also involved in two cases. All or most of the polygonal and spindle-shaped cells appeared benign in two cases; foci of atypical cells were seen in one of them, and in the third case, most of the cells had malignant features.

Pyrexia

Two cases in which pyrexia was the presenting manifestation of an ovarian carcinoma have been reported: one was a poorly differentiated clear cell carcinoma (222) and the other, a "cystadenocarcinoma" (221).

REFERENCES

Tumors Associated with hCG Production

1. Casper S, van Nagell JR Jr, Powell DF, et al. Immunohistochemical localization of tumor markers in epithelial ovarian cancer. Am J Obstet Gynecol 1981;149:154–8.
2. Civantos F, Rywlin AM. Carcinomas with trophoblastic differentiation and secretion of chorionic gonadotrophins. Cancer 1972;29:789–98.
3. Hayata T, Fenoglio CM, Crum CP, Richart RM. The simultaneous expression of human chorionic gonadotropin and carcinoembryonic antigen in the female genital tract. Localization by immunocytochemistry. Diagn Gynecol Obstet 1981;3:309–14.
4. Khalifa MA, Sesterhenn IA. Tumor markers of epithelial ovarian neoplasms. Int J Gynecol Pathol 1990;9:217–30.
5. Kobayashi M, Hamada H, Yamoto M, Nakano R. Ovarian clear-cell carcinoma producing estradiol and human chorionic gonadotropin. Acta Obstet Gynecol Scand 1990;69:183–5.
6. Matias-Guiu X, Prat J. Ovarian tumors with functioning stroma. An immunohistochemical study of 100 cases with human chorionic gonadotropin monoclonal and polyclonal antibodies. Cancer 1990;65:2001–5.
7. Mohabeer J, Buckley CH, Fox H. An immunohistochemical study of the incidence and significance of human chorionic gonadotrophin synthesis by epithelial ovarian neoplasms. Gynecol Oncol 1983;16:78–84.
8. Oliva E, Andrada E, Pezzica E, Prat J. Ovarian carcinomas with choriocarcinomatous differentiation. Cancer 1993;72:2441–6.
9. Samaan NA, Smith JP, Rutledge FN, Schultz PN. The significance of measurement of human placental lactogen, human chorionic gonadotropin, and carcinoembryonic antigen in patients with ovarian carcinoma. Am J Obstet Gynecol 1976;126:186–9.
10. Vaitukaitis JL. Human chorionic gonadotropin as a tumor marker. Ann Clin Lab Sci 1974;4:276–80.

Tumors Associated with Hypercalcemia

11. Allan SG, Lockhart SP, Leonard RC, Smyth JF. Paraneoplastic hypercalcaemia in ovarian carcinoma. Br Med J 1984;288:1714–5.
12. Burton PB, Knight DE, Quirke P, Smith R, Moniz C. Parathyroid hormone related peptide in ovarian carcinoma. J Clin Pathol 1990;43:784.
13. Fleischhacker DS, Young RH. Dysgerminoma of the ovary associated with hypercalcemia. Gynecol Oncol 1994;52:87–90.
14. Fujino T, Watanabe T, Yamaguchi K, et al. The development of hypercalcemia in a patient with an ovarian tumor producing parathyroid hormone-related protein. Cancer 1992;70:2845–50.
15. Hoekman K, Tjandra YI, Papapoulos SE. The role of 1, 15-dihydroxyvitamin D in the maintenance of hypercalcemia in a patient with an ovarian carcinoma producing parathyroid hormone-related protein. Cancer 1991;68:642–7.
16. Holtz G. Paraneoplastic hypercalcemia in gynecologic malignancy. Obstet Gynecol Surv 1980;35:129–36.
17. Josse RG, Wilson DR, Heersche JN, Mills JR, Murray TM. Hypercalcemia with ovarian carcinoma: evidence of a pathogenetic role for prostaglandins. Cancer 1981;48:1233–41.
18. Kim W, Bockman R, Lemos L, Lewis JL Jr. Hypercalcemia associated with epidermoid carcinoma in ovarian cystic teratoma. Obstet Gynecol 1981;57:81S–5S.
18a. Knecht TP, Behling CA, Burton DW, Glass CK, Deftos LJ. The humoral hypercalcemia of benignancy. A newly appreciated syndrome. Am J Clin Pathol 1996;105:487–92.
19. Nussbaum SR, Gaz RD, Arnold A. Hypercalcemia and ectopic secretion of parathyroid hormone by an ovarian carcinoma with rearrangement of the gene for parathyroid hormone. N Engl J Med 1990;323:1324–8.
20. Ribeiro G, Hughesdon P, Wiltshaw E. Squamous carcinoma arising in dermoid cysts and associated with hypercalcemia: a clinicopathologic study of six cases. Gynecol Oncol 1988;29:222–30.
21. Stewart AF, Romero R, Schwartz PE, Kohorn EI, Broadus AE. Hypercalcemia associated with gynecologic malignancies: biochemical characterization. Cancer 1982;49:2389–94.

Tumors Associated with Cushing's Syndrome

22. Adeyemi SD, Grange AO, Giwa-Osagie OF, Elesha SO. Adrenal rest tumour of the ovary associated with isosexual precocious pseudopuberty and cushingoid features. Eur J Pediatr 1986;145:236–8.
23. Axiotis CA, Lippes HA, Merino MJ, deLanerolle NC, Stewart AF, Kinder B. Corticotroph cell pituitary adenoma within an ovarian teratoma. A new cause of Cushing's syndrome. Am J Surg Pathol 1987;11:218–24.
24. Brown H, Lane M. Cushing's and malignant carcinoid syndromes from ovarian neoplasm. Arch Intern Med 1965;115:490–4.
25. Crawford SM, Pyrah RD, Ismail SM. Cushing's syndrome associated with recurrent endometrioid adenocarcinoma of the ovary. J Clin Pathol 1994;47:766–8.
26. Donovan JT, Otis CN, Powell JL, Cathcart HK. Cushing's syndrome secondary to malignant lipoid cell tumor of the ovary. Gynecol Oncol 1993;50:249–53.
27. Falls JL. Accessory adrenal cortex in the broad ligament. Incidence and functional significance. Cancer 1955;8:143–50.
28. Kasperlik-Zaluska AA, Sikorowa L, Ploch E, et al. Ectopic ACTH syndrome due to ovarian androblastoma with double, gynandroblastic differentiation in one ovary. Eur J Obstet Gynecol Reprod Biol 1993;52:223–8.

29. Kronke E, Parade GW. Morbus Cushing bei ovarial teratoma. Z Klin Med 1938;134:698–718.
30. Marieb NJ, Spangler S, Kashgarian M, Heimann A, Schwartz ML, Schwartz PE. Cushing's syndrome secondary to ectopic cortisol production by an ovarian carcinoma. J Clin Endocrinol Metab 1983;57:737–40.
31. Nichols J, Warren JC, Mantz FA. ACTH-like secretion from carcinoma of the ovary. JAMA 1962;182:713–8.
32. Norris EH. Arrhenoblastoma. A malignant ovarian tumor associated with endocrinological effects. Am J Cancer 1938;32:1–29.
33. Parsons V, Rigby B. Cushing's syndrome associated with adenocarcinoma of the ovary. Lancet 1958;2:992–4.
34. Reis RA, Saphir O. Masculinizing elements in the ovary. Am J Obstet Gynecol 1938;35:954–60.
35. Sauramo H. Development, occurrence and pathology of aberrant adrenocortical tissue in the region of the ovary. Acta Obstet Gynecol Scand (Suppl) 1953;33:4–58.
36. Schlaghecke R, Kreuzpaintner G, Burrig KF, Juli E, Kley HK. Cushing's syndrome due to ACTH-production of an ovarian carcinoid. Klin Wochenschr 1989;67:640–4.
37. Symonds DA, Driscoll SG. An adrenal cortical rest within the fetal ovary: report of a case. Am J Clin Pathol 1973;60:562–4.
38. Young RH, Scully RE. Ovarian steroid cell tumors associated with Cushing's syndrome: a report of three cases. Int J Gynecol Pathol 1987;6:40–8.

Tumors Associated with Zollinger-Ellison and Inappropriate Antidiuresis Syndromes

39. Aguirre P, Scully RE, Dayal Y, DeLellis RA. Mucinous tumors of the ovary with argyrophil cells. An immunohistochemical analysis. Am J Surg Pathol 1984;8:345–56.
40. Boixeda D, Roman AL, Pascasio JM, et al. Zollinger-Ellison syndrome due to gastrin-secreting ovarian cystadenocarcinoma. Case report. Acta Chir Scand 1990;156:409–10.
41. Bollen EC, Lamers CB, Jansen JM, Larsson LI, Joosten HJ. Zollinger-Ellison syndrome due to a gastrin-producing ovarian cystadenocarcinoma. Br J Surg 1981;68:776–7.
42. Cocco AE, Conway SJ. Zollinger-Ellison syndrome associated with ovarian mucinous cystadenocarcinoma. N Engl J Med 1975;293:485–6.
43. Connell WR, Newell Price JD, Lowe DG, Shepherd JH, Farthing MJ. Zollinger-Ellison syndrome caused by a mucinous cystadenocarcinoma of the ovary [Letter]. Aust NZ J Med 1993;23:520–1.
44. Fox H, Kazzaz B, Langley FA. Argyrophil and argentaffin cells in the female genital tract and in ovarian mucinous cysts. J Pathol Bacteriol 1964;88:479–88.
45. Garcia-Villanueva M, Figuerola NB, del Arbol LR, Ortiz MJ. Zollinger-Ellison syndrome due to a borderline mucinous cystadenoma of the ovary. Obstet Gynecol 1990;75:549–52.
46. Heyd J, Livni N, Herbert D, Mor-Yosef S, Glaser B. Gastrin-producing ovarian cystadenocarcinoma: sensitivity to secretin and SMS 201-995. Gastroenterology 1989;97:464–7.
47. Julkunen R, Partanen S, Salaspuro M. Gastrin-producing ovarian mucinous cystadenoma. J Clin Gastroenterol 1983;5:67–70.
48. Klemi PJ. Pathology of mucinous ovarian cystadenomas. I. Argyrophil and argentaffin cells and epithelial mucosubstances. Acta Pathol Microbiol Scand A 1978;86:465–70.
49. Long TT III, Barton TK, Draffin R, Reeves WJ, McCarty KS Jr. Conservative management of the Zollinger-Ellison syndrome. Ectopic gastrin production by an ovarian cystadenoma. JAMA 1980;243:1837–9.
50. Louwerens JK, Schaberg A, Bosman FT. Neuroendocrine cells in cystic mucinous tumours of the ovary. Histopathology 1983;7:389–98.
51. Maton PN, Mackem SM, Norton JA, Gardner JD, O'Dorisio TM, Jensen RT. Ovarian carcinoma as a cause of Zollinger-Ellison syndrome. Natural history, secretory products, and response to provocative tests. Gastroenterology 1989;97:468–71.
52. Morgan DR, Wells M, MacDonald RC, Johnston D. Zollinger-Ellison syndrome due to a gastrin secreting ovarian mucinous cystadenoma. Case report. Br J Obstet Gynaecol 1985;92:867–9.
53. Primrose JN, Maloney M, Wells M, Bulgim O, Johnston D. Gastrin-producing ovarian mucinous cystadenomas: a cause of the Zollinger-Ellison syndrome. Surgery 1988;104:830–3.
54. Sasaki E, Sasano N, Kimura N, Andoh N, Yajima A. Demonstration of neuroendocrine cells in ovarian mucinous tumors. Int J Gynecol Pathol 1989;8:189–200.
55. Sporrong B, Alumets J, Clase L, et al. Neurohormonal peptide immunoreactive cells in mucinous cystadenomas and cystadenocarcinomas of the ovary. Virch Arch [A] 1981;392:27–180.
56. Takeda A, Matsuyama M, Chihara T, Suchi T, Sato T, Tomoda Y. Ultrastructure and immunohistochemistry of gastro-entero-pancreatic (GEP) endocrine cells in mucinous tumors of the ovary. Acta Path Jpn 1982;32:1003–5.
56a. Taskin M, Barker B, Calanog A, Jormark S. Syndrome of inappropriate antidiuresis in ovarian serous carcinoma with neuroendocrine differentiation. Gynecol Oncol 1996;62:400–4.

Tumors Associated with Hypoglycemia

57. Ashton MA. Strumal carcinoid of the ovary associated with hyperinsulinemic hypoglycemia and cutaneous melanosis. Histopathology 1995;27:463–7.
58. Michael CA. Pelvic fibroma causing recurrent attacks of hypoglycemia. J Obstet Gynaecol Br Commonw 1967;74:301–3.
59. Morgello S, Schwartz E, Horwith M, King ME, Gorden P, Alonso DR. Ectopic insulin production by a primary ovarian carcinoid. Cancer 1988;61:800–5.
60. O'Neill RT, Mikuta JJ. Hypoglycemia associated with serous cystadenocarcinoma of the ovary. Obstet Gynecol 1970;35:287–9.
61. Shetty MR, Boghossian HM, Duffell D, Freel R, Gonzalez JC. Tumor-induced hypoglycemia: a result of ectopic insulin production. Cancer 1982;49:1920–3.
62. Srivastava KP. Hypoglycemia associated with non-pancreatic mesenchymal tumors. Int Surg 1976;61:282–6.

Tumors Associated with Renin and Aldosterone Production

63. Aiba M, Hirayama A, Sakurada M, Naruse K, Ishikawa C, Aiba S. Spironolactone bodylike structure in renin-producing Sertoli cell tumor of the ovary. Surg Pathol 1990;3:143–9.

64. Anderson PW, d'Ablaing G, Penny R, Sherrod A, Do YS. Secretion of prorenin by a virilizing ovarian tumor. Gynecol Oncol 1992;45:58–61.

65. Anderson PW, d'Ablaing G, Sherrod G, Bullock T, Hsueh WA. Immunohistochemical localization of renin in ovarian stromal tumors [Abstract]. Program of Endocrine Society, 1989;1764.

66. Anderson PW, Macaulay L, Do YS, et al. Extrarenal renin-secreting tumors: insights into hypertension and ovarian renin production. Medicine 1989;68:257–68.

67. Atlas SA, Sherman RL, Pasmantier MW, Taufield P, Sealey JE, Laragh JH. Response of active and inactive renins, aldosterone and blood pressure to chemotherapy in a patient with a possible renin-secreting ovarian carcinoma. Clin Research 1982;30:333A.

68. Ehrlich EN, Dominguez OV, Samuels LT, Lynch D, Oberhelman H, Warner NE. Aldosteronism and precocious puberty due to an ovarian androblastoma (Sertoli cell tumor). J Clin Endocrinol Metab 1963;23:358–67.

69. Fox R, Eckford S, Hirschowitz L, Browning J, Lindop G. Refractory gestational hypertension due to a renin-secreting ovarian fibrothecoma associated with Gorlin's syndrome. Br J Obstet Gynaecol 1994;101:1015–7.

70. Herve JP, Leroy JP, Gentric-Tilly A, et al. Hypertension arterielle secondaire a une tumeur a renine d'origine ovarienne. La Presse Med 1989;18:2021–2.

71. Jackson B, Valentine R, Wagner G. Primary aldosteronism due to a malignant ovarian tumour. Aust NZ J Med 1986;16:69–71.

72. Korzets A, Nouriel H, Steiner Z, et al. Resistant hypertension associated with a renin-producing ovarian Sertoli cell tumor. Am J Clin Pathol 1986;85:242–7.

73. Kulkarni JN, Mistry RC, Kamat MR, Chinoy R, Lotlikar RG. Autonomous aldosterone-secreting ovarian tumor. Gynecol Oncol 1990;37:284–9.

74. Motlik K. An estrogen-producing yellow tumour of the ovary associated with arterial hypertension. A case report contributing to the problem of classification of functioning ovarian neoplasms. Endokrynol Polska 1966;17:525–39.

75. Sealey JE, Glorioso N, Itskovitz J, Laragh JH. Prorenin as a reproductive hormone. New form of the renin system. Am J Med 1986;81:1041–6.

76. Tetu B, Lebel M, Camilleri J. Renin-producing ovarian tumor. A case report with immunohistochemical and electron-microscopic study. Am J Surg Pathol 1988;12:634–40.

77. Todesco S, Terribile V, Borsatti A, Mantero F. Primary aldosteronism due to a malignant ovarian tumor. J Clin Endocrinol Metab 1975;41:809–19.

78. Yoshizumi J, Vaughan RS, Jasani B. Pregnancy associated with Gorlin's syndrome. Anaesthesia 1990;45:1046–8.

Tumors Associated with Prolactin Secretion

79. Hoffman WH, Gala RR, Kovacs K, Subramanian MG. Ectopic prolactin secretion from a gonadoblastoma. Cancer 1987;60:2690–5.

80. Kallenberg GA, Pesce CM, Norman B, Ratner RE, Silverberg SG. Ectopic hyperprolactinemia resulting from an ovarian teratoma. JAMA 1990;262:2472–4.

81. Palmer PE, Bogojavlensky S, Bhan AK, Scully RE. Prolactinoma in wall of ovarian dermoid cyst with hyperprolactinemia. Obstet Gynecol 1990;75:540–2.

Tumors Associated with Nervous System Disorders

82. Cavaletti G, Bogliun G, Marzorati L, Marzola M, Pittelli MR, Tredici G. The incidence and course of paraneoplastic neuropathy in women with epithelial ovarian cancer. J Neurol 1991;238:371–4.

83. Croft PB, Wilkinson M. The incidence of carcinomatous neuromyopathy in patients with various types of carcinoma. Brain 1965;88:427–34.

84. Furneaux HM, Rosenblum MK, Dalmau J, et al. Selective expression of Purkinje-cell antigens in tumor tissue from patients with paraneoplastic cerebellar degeneration. N Engl J Med 1990;322:1844–51.

85. Greenlee JE, Brashear HR. Antibodies to cerebellar Purkinje cells in patients with paraneoplastic cerebellar degeneration and ovarian carcinoma. Ann Neurol 1983;14:609–13.

86. Hammack JE, Kimmel DW, O'Neill BP, Lennon VA. Paraneoplastic cerebellar degeneration: A clinical comparison of patients with and without Purkinje cell cytoplasmic antibodies. Mayo Clin Proc 1990;65:1423–31.

87. Henson RA, Urich H. Cancer and the nervous system: the neurological manifestations of systemic malignant disease. Boston: Blackwell Scientific, 1982:346-67

88. Hetzel DJ, Stanhope R, O'Neill BP, Lennon VA. Gynecologic cancer in patients with subacute cerebellar degeneration predicted by anti-Purkinje cell antibodies and limited in metastatic volume. Mayo Clin Proc 1990;65:1558–63.

88a. Mason WP, Dalman J, Curtin JP, Posner JB. Normalization of the tumor marker CA-125 after oophorectomy in a patient with paraneoplastic cerebellar degeneration without detectable cancer. Gynecol Oncol 1997;65:173–6.

89. McLellan R, Currie JL, Royal W, Rosenshein NB. Ovarian carcinoma and paraneoplastic cerebellar degeneration. Obstet Gynecol 1988;72:922–4.

89a. Peterson K, Rosenblum MK, Kotanides H, Posner JB. Paraneoplastic cerebellar degeneration. I. A clinical analysis of 55 anti-Yo antibody-positive patients. Neurology 1992;42:1931–7.

90. Tyler HR. Paraneoplastic syndromes of nerve, muscle, and neuromuscular junction. Ann NY Acad Sci 1974;230:348–57.

Tumors Associated with Connective Tissue Disorders

91. Barnes BE. Dermatomyositis and malignancy. A review of the literature. Ann Intern Med 1976;84:68-76.

92. Bennett RM, Ginsberg MH, Thomsen S. Carcinomatous polyarthritis. Arthritis Rheum 1976;19:953–8.

93. Calabro JJ. Cancer and arthritis. Arthritis Rheum 1967;10:553–67.

94. Callen JP. Dermatomyositis and female malignancy. J Surg Oncol 1986;32:121–4.

95. Duncan SC, Winkelmann RK. Cancer and scleroderma. Arch Dermatol 1979;115:950–5.

96. Lester WM, Robertson DI. Hypertrophic osteoarthropathy complicating metastatic ovarian adenocarcinoma. Can J Surg 1981;24:520–3.

97. MacKenzie AH, Scherbel AL. Connective tissue syndromes associated with carcinoma. Geriatrics 1963;18:745–53.

98. Medsger TA Jr, Dixon JA, Garwood VF. Palmar fasciitis and polyarthritis associated with ovarian carcinoma. Ann Intern Med 1982;96:424–31.

99. Mordel N, Margalioth EJ, Harats N, Ben-Baruch N, Schenker JG. Concurrence of ovarian cancer and dermatomyositis. A report of two cases and literature review. J Reprod Med 1988;33:649–55.

100. Peters WA III, Andersen WA, Thornton WN Jr. Dermatomyositis and coexistent ovarian cancer: a review of the compounding clinical problems. Gynecol Oncol 1983;15:440–6.

101. Scaling ST, Kaufman RH, Patten BM. Dermatomyositis and female malignancy. Obstet Gynecol 1979;54:474–7.

102. Shiel WC Jr, Prete PE, Jason M, Andrews BS. Palmar fasciitis and arthritis with ovarian and non-ovarian carcinomas. New syndrome. Am J Med 1985;79:640–4.

103. Sigurgeirsson B, Lindelof B, Edhag O, Allander E. Risk of cancer in patients with dermatomyositis or polymyositis. A population-based study. N Engl J Med 1992;326:363–7.

104. Solomon SD, Maurer KH. Association of dermatomyositis and dysgerminoma in a 16-year-old patient [Letter]. Arthritis Rheumatol 1983;26:572–3.

105. Taggart AJ, Iveson JM, Wright V. Shoulder-hand syndrome and symmetrical arthralgia in patients with tubo-ovarian carcinoma. Ann Rheumat Dis 1984;43:391–3.

106. Talbott JH. Acute dermatomyositis-polymyositis and malignancy. Semin Arthritis Rheum 1977;6:305–60.

107. Van Winter JT, Stanhope CR. Giant ovarian leiomyoma associated with ascites and polymyositis. Obstet Gynecol 1992;80:560–3.

108. Verducci MA, Malkasian GD Jr, Friedman SJ, Winkelmann RK. Gynecologic carcinoma associated with dermatomyositis-polymyositis. Obstet Gynecol 1984;64:695–8.

109. Voravud N, Dimopoulos M, Hortobagyi G, Ross M, Theriault R. Breast cancer and second primary ovarian cancer in dermatomyositis. Gynecol Oncol 1991;43:286–90.

109a. Whitmore SE, Rosenshein NB, Provost TT. Ovarian cancer in patients with dermatomyositis. Medicine 1994;73:153–60.

110. Young R, Towbin B, Isern R. Scleroderma and ovarian carcinoma [Letter]. Br J Rheumatol 1990;29:314.

Tumors Associated with Hematologic Disorders

111. Anstey JT, Blythe JG. Fibrin degradation products and the diagnosis of ovarian carcinoma. Obstet Gynecol 1978;52:605–8.

112. Astedt B, Svanberg L, Nilsson IM. Fibrin degradation products and ovarian tumours. Br Med J 1971;4:458–9.

113. Carreras Vescio LA, Toblli JE, Rey JA, Assaf ME, De Maria HE, Marletta J. Autoimmune hemolytic anemia associated with an ovarian neoplasm. Medicina 1983;45:415–24.

114. Case records of the Massachusetts General Hospital, Case 13-1978. N Engl J Med 1978;298:786–92.

115. Chalas E, Welshinger M, Engellener W, Chumas J, Barbieri R, Mann WJ. The clinical significance of thrombocytosis in women presenting with a pelvic mass. Am J Obstet Gynecol 1992;166:974–7.

116. Colman RW, Rubin RN. Disseminated intravascular coagulation due to malignancy. Semin Oncol 1990;17:172–86.

117. Dales M. Purpura associated with ovarian tumour. Br Med J 1965;1:127.

118. Dawson MA, Talbert W, Yarbro JW. Hemolytic anemia associated with an ovarian tumor. Am J Med 1971;50:552–6.

119. Delgado G, Smith JP. Gynecological malignancy associated with nonbacterial thrombotic endocarditis (NBTE). Gynecol Oncol 1975;3:205–9.

119a. Evans TR, Mansi JL, Bevan DH. Trousseau's syndrome in association with ovarian carcinoma. Cancer 1996;77:2544–9.

120. Ghio R, Haupt E, Ratti M, Boccaccio P. Erythrocytosis associated with a dermoid cyst of the ovary and erythropoietic activity of the tumour fluid. Scand J Haematol 1981;27:70–4.

121. Hammond D, Winnick S. Paraneoplastic erythrocytosis and ectopic erythropoietins. Ann NY Acad Sci 1974;230:219–27.

122. Henderson PH. Multiple migratory thrombophlebitis associated with ovarian carcinoma. Am J Obstet Gynecol 1955;70:452–3.

123. Landolfi R, Storti S, Sacco F, Scribano D, Cudillo L, Leone G. Platelet activation in patients with benign and malignant ovarian diseases. Tumori 1984;70:459–62.

124. Lawhead RA, Copeland LJ, Edwards CL. Bilateral ovarian hemangiomas associated with diffuse abdominopelvic hemangiomatosis. Obstet Gynecol 1985;65:597–9.

125. Miller B, Heilmann L. Hemorheological parameters in patients with gynecologic malignancies. Gynecol Oncol 1989;33:177–81.

126. Miyauchi J, Yamazaki K, Kiso I, Higashi S, Hori S. Bilateral ovarian hemangiomas associated with diffuse hemangioendotheliomatosis: a case report. Acta Pathol Jpn 1987;37:1347–55.

127. Montag TW, Murphy RE, Belinson JL. Virilizing malignant lipid cell tumor producing erythropoietin. Gynecol Oncol 1984;19:98–103.

128. Napoli VM, Wallach H. Pancytopenia associated with a granulosa cell tumor of the ovary. Report of a case. Am J Clin Pathol 1976;65:344–50.

129. Payne D, Muss HB, Homesley HD, Jobson VW, Baird FG. Autoimmune hemolytic anemia and ovarian dermoid cysts: case report and review of the literature. Cancer 1981;48:721–4.

130. Pogliani EM, Fowst C, Maffe P, Marozzi A, Stefani M, Polli E. CNS metastasis in ovarian cancer with microangiopathic hemolytic anemia associated with diffuse intravascular coagulation. Tumori 1988;74:731–6.

131. Sack GH Jr, Levin J, Bell WR. Trousseau's syndrome and other manifestations of chronic disseminated coagulopathy in patients with neoplasms: clinical, pathophysiologic and therapeutic features. Medicine 1977;56:1–37.

132. Siegman-Igra Y, Flatau E, Deligdish L. Chronic diffuse intravascular coagulation (DIC) in nonmetastatic ovarian cancer: report of a case and review of the literature. Gynecol Oncol 1977;5:92–100.

133. Takeda A, Suzumori K, Sugimoto Y, et al. Clear cell carcinoma of the ovary with colony-stimulating-factor production. Occurrence of marked granulocytosis in a patient and nude mice. Cancer 1984;54:1019–23.

134. Tarraza HM, Carroll R, De Cain M, Jones M. Recurrent ovarian carcinoma: presentation as idiopathic thrombocytopenic purpura and a splenic mass. Eur J Gynaecol Oncol 1991;12:439–43.

135. von dem Borne AE, van Oers RH, Wiersinga WM, van der Tweel JG. Complete remission of autoimmune thrombocytopenia after extirpation of a benign adenofibroma of the ovary. Br J Rheumatol 1990;74:119–20.

136. Zeimet AG, Marth C, Muller-Holzner E, Daxenbichler G, Dapunt O. Significance of thrombocytosis in patients with epithelial ovarian cancer. Am J Obstet Gynecol 1994;170:549–54.

Tumors Associated with Cutaneous Disorders

137. Cohen PR, Kohn SR, Kurzrock R. Association of sebaceous gland tumors and internal malignancy: the Muir-Torre syndrome. Am J Med 1991;90:606–13.

138. Curth HO, Hilberg AW, Machacek GF. The site and histology of the cancer associated with malignant acanthosis nigricans. Cancer 1962;15:364–82.

139. Dingley ER, Marten RH. Adenocarcinoma of the ovary presenting as acanthosis nigricans. J Obstet Gynaecol Brit Commonw 1957;64:898–900.

140. Fathizadeh A, Medenica MM, Soltani K, Lorincz AL, Griem ML. Aggressive keratoacanthoma and internal malignant neoplasm. Arch Dermatol 1982;118:112–4.

141. Graham R, McKee P, McGibbon D, Heyderman E. Torre-Muir syndrome. An association with isolated sebaceous carcinoma. Cancer 1985;55:2868–73.

142. Holguin T, Padilla RS, Ampuero F. Ovarian adenocarcinoma presenting with the sign of Leser-Trelat. Gynecol Oncol 1986;25:128–32.

143. Nguyen KQ, Hurst CG, Pierson DL, Rodman OG. Sweet's syndrome and ovarian carcinoma. Cutis 1983;32:152–4.

144. Snider BL, Benjamin DR. Eruptive keratoacanthoma with an internal malignant neoplasm. Arch Dermatol 1981;117:788–90.

145. Sweet RD. An acute febrile neutrophilic dermatosis. Br J Dermatol 1964;76:349–56.

Tumors Associated with the Nephrotic Syndrome

146. Lee JC, Yamauchi H, Hopper J Jr. The association of cancer and the nephrotic syndrome. Ann Intern Med 1966;64:41–51.

147. Hoyt RE, Hamilton JF. Ovarian cancer associated with the nephrotic syndrome. Obstet Gynecol 1987;70:513–4.

Peutz-Jeghers Syndrome

148. Burdick D, Prior JT. Peutz-Jeghers syndrome. A clinicopathologic study of a large family with a 27-year follow-up. Cancer 1982;50:2139–46.

149. Chen KT. Female genital tract tumors in Peutz-Jeghers syndrome. Hum Pathol 1986;17:858–61.

150. Choi CG, Kim SH, Kim J, Song ES, Han MC. Adenoma malignum of uterine cervix in Peutz-Jeghers syndrome: CT and US features. J Comput Assist Tomogr 1993;17:819–21.

151. Costa J. Peutz-Jeghers syndrome. Case presentation. Obstet Gynecol 1977;50:15S–7S.

152. Dozois RR, Judd ES, Dahlin DC, Bartholomew LG. The Peutz-Jeghers syndrome. Is there a predisposition to the development of intestinal malignancy? Arch Surg 1969;98:509–17.

153. Fetissof F, Berger G, Dubois MP, Philippe A, Lansax J, Jobard P. Female genital tract and Peutz-Jeghers syndrome: an immunohistochemical study. Int J Gynecol Pathol 1985;4:219–29.

154. Humphries AL, Shepherd MH, Peters HJ. Peutz-Jeghers syndrome with colonic adenocarcinoma and ovarian tumor. JAMA 1966;197:296–8.

155. McGowan L, Young RH, Scully RE. Peutz-Jeghers syndrome with adenoma malignum of the cervix. A report of two cases. Gynecol Oncol 1980;10:125–33.

156. Steenstrup EK. Ovarian tumours and Peutz-Jeghers syndrome. A sex cord tumour with annular tubules. Acta Obstet Gynecol Scand 1972;51:237–40.

157. Vignali M, Zannini M. Melanosi di Peutz-Jeghers associata a tumore ovarico. Ann Ost Ginecol Med Perinat 1977;98:169–75.

Nevoid Basal Cell Carcinoma Syndrome

158. Case records of the Massachusetts General Hospital. Case 14-1976. N Engl J Med 1976;294:772–7.

159. Dumont-Herskowitz RA, Safaii HS, Senior B. Ovarian fibromata in four successive generations. Am J Obstet Gynecol 1978;93:621–4.

160. Gorlin RJ. Nevoid basal-cell carcinoma syndrome. Medicine 1987;66:98–113.

161. Ismail SM, Walker SM. Bilateral virilizing sclerosing stromal tumours of the ovary in a pregnant patient with Gorlin's syndrome: implications for pathogenesis of ovarian stromal neoplasms. Histopathology 1990;17:159–63.

162. Johnson AD, Hebert AA, Esterly NB. Nevoid basal cell carcinoma syndrome: bilateral ovarian fibromas in a 3 1/2-year-old girl. J Am Acad Derm 1986;14:371–4.

163. Kraemer BB, Silva EG, Sneige N. Fibrosarcoma of ovary. A new component in the nevoid basal-cell carcinoma syndrome. Am J Surg Pathol 1984;8:231–6.

164. Raggio M, Kaplan AL, Harberg JF. Recurrent ovarian fibromas with basal cell nevus syndrome (Gorlin syndrome). Obstet Gynecol 1983;61:95S–6.

Ollier's, Maffucci's, and Other Disorders

165. Christman JE, Ballon SC. Ovarian fibrosarcoma associated with Maffucci's syndrome. Gynecol Oncol 1990;37:290–1.

166. Delacrétaz F, Stalder M, Meugé-Moraw C, et al. Systemic mastocytosis following a malignant ovarian germ cell tumour. Histopathology 1997;30:582–4.

167. Grenet P, Badoual J, Gallet JP, Lange C. Dyschondroplasie et tumeur de l'ovaire. Ann Pediatr (Paris) 1972;19:759–64.

168. Kuzma JF, King JM. Dyschondroplasia with hemangiomatosis (Maffucci's syndrome) and teratoid tumor of the ovary. Arch Pathol 1948;46:74–82.

169. Lewis RJ, Ketcham AS. Maffucci's syndrome: functional and neoplastic significance. J Bone Joint Surg 1973;55A:1465–79.

170. Pounder DJ, Iyer PV, Davy ML. Bilateral juvenile granulosa cell tumours associated with skeletal enchondromas. Aust NZ J Obstet Gynaecol 1985;25:123–6.

171. Pysher TJ, Hitch DC, Krous HF. Bilateral juvenile granulosa cell tumors in a 4-month-old dysmorphic infant. A clinical, histologic, and ultrastructural study. Am J Surg Pathol 1981;5:789–94.

172. Roth LM, Nicholas TR, Ehrlich CE. Juvenile granulosa cell tumor: a clinicopathologic study of three cases with ultrastructural observations. Cancer 1979;44:2194–205.

173. Strang C, Rannie I. Dyschondroplasia with hemangiomata (Maffucci's syndrome). J Bone Joint Surg 1950;32B:376–83.

174. Sugiyama M, Kohmoto Y, Miyoshi T, Ogawa S. In vivo and vitro steroid biosynthesis by ovarian juvenile granulosa cell tumor of a girl with Ollier's disease. Acta Obstet Gynaecol Jpn 1983;35:2185.

175. Tamimi HK, Bolen JW. Enchondromatosis (Ollier's disease) and ovarian juvenile granulosa cell tumor. A case report and review of the literature. Cancer 1984;53:1605–8.

176. Tanaka Y, Sasaki Y, Nishihira H, Izawa T, Nishi T. Ovarian juvenile granulosa cell tumor associated with Maffucci's syndrome. Am J Clin Pathol 1992;97:523–7.

177. Vassal G, Flamant F, Caillaud JM, Demeocq F, Nihoul-Fekete C, Lemerle J. Juvenile granulosa cell tumor of the ovary in children: a clinical study of 15 cases. J Clin Oncol 1988;6:990–5.

178. Vaz RM, Turner C. Ollier disease (enchondromatosis) associated with ovarian juvenile granulosa cell tumor and precocious puberty. J Pediatr 1986;108:945–7.

179. Velasco-Oses A, Alonso-Alvaro A, Blanco-Pozo A, Nogales FF Jr. Ollier's disease associated with ovarian juvenile granulosa cell tumor. Cancer 1988;62:222–5.

180. Young RH, Dickersin GR, Scully RE. Juvenile granulosa cell tumor of the ovary. A clinicopathological analysis of 125 cases. Am J Surg Pathol 1984;8:575–96.

Sertoli-Leydig Cell Tumors and Thyroid Abnormalities

181. Benfield GF, Tapper-Jones L, Stout TV. Androblastoma and raised serum alpha-fetoprotein with familial multinodular goitre. Case report. Br J Obstet Gynaecol 1982;89:323–6.

182. Griffin PE Jr. Multiple endocrine adenomatosis. Rocky Mt Med J 1972;69:64–5.

183. Jensen RD, Norris HJ, Fraumeni JF Jr. Familial arrhenoblastoma and thyroid adenoma. Cancer 1974;33:218–23.

184. O'Brien PK, Wilansky DL. Familial thyroid nodulation and arrhenoblastoma. Am J Clin Pathol 1981;75:578–81.

185. Szeplaki F, Halmy L, Feher T, Korenyi-Both A. Polyadenomatosis associated ovarian hilar cell tumor. Orv Hetil 1968;109:2431–3.

186. Whitcomb RW, Calkins JW, Lukert BP, Kyner JL, Schimke RN. Androblastomas and thyroid disease in postmenopausal sisters. Obstet Gynecol 1986;67:89S–91S.

187. Young RH, Scully RE. Ovarian Sertoli-Leydig cell tumors. A clinicopathological analysis of 207 cases. Am J Surg Pathol 1985;9:543–69.

Ataxia-Telangiectasia

188. Dunn HG, Meuwissen H, Livingstone CS, Pump KK. Ataxia-telangiectasia. Can Med Assoc J 1964;91:1106–18.

189. Goldsmith CI, Hart WR. Ataxia-telangiectasia with ovarian gonadoblastoma and contralateral dysgerminoma. Cancer 1975;36:1838–42.

190. Narita T, Takagi K. Ataxia-telangiectasia with dysgerminoma of right ovary, papillary carcinoma of thyroid, and adenocarcinoma of pancreas. Cancer 1984;54:1113–6.

191. Pecorelli S, Sartori E, Favalli G, Ugazio AG, Gastaldi A. Ataxia-telangiectasia and endodermal sinus tumor of the ovary: report of a case. Gynecol Oncol 1988;29:240–4.

Lymphangioleiomyomatosis

192. Colley MH, Geppert E, Franklin WA. Immunohistochemical detection of steroid receptors in a case of pulmonary lymphangioleiomyomatosis. Am J Surg Pathol 1989;13:803–7.

193. Gyure KA, Hart WR, Kennedy AW. Lymphangioleiomyomatosis of the uterus associated with tuberous sclerosis and malignant neoplasia of the female genital tract: a report of two cases. Int J Gynecol Pathol 1995;14:344–51.

194. Lack EE, Dolan MF, Finisio J, Grover G, Singh M, Triche TJ. Pulmonary and extrapulmonary lymphangio-leiomyomatosis. Am J Surg Pathol 1986;10:650–7.

195. Taylor JR, Ryu J, Colby TV, Raffin TA. Lymphangio-leiomyomatosis: clinical course in 32 patients. N Engl J Med 1990;323:1254–60.

Meigs' Syndrome

196. Hoon MR. Fibromata of the ovary. Surg Gynecol Obstet 1923;36:247–51.

197. Kempers RD, Dockerty MB, Hoffman DL, Bartholomew LG. Struma ovarii—ascitic, hyperthyroid, and asymptomatic syndromes. Ann Intern Med 1970;72:883–93.

198. Lacson AG, Alrabeeah A, Gillis DA, Salisbury S, Grantmyre EB. Secondary massive ovarian edema with Meigs' syndrome. Am J Clin Pathol 1989;91:597–603.

199. Meigs JV. Fibroma of the ovary with ascites and hydrothorax—Meigs' syndrome. Am J Obstet Gynecol 1954;67:962–87.

200. Meigs JV. Pelvic tumors other than fibromas of the ovary with ascites and hydrothorax. Obstet Gynecol 1954;3:471–86.

201. Meigs JV, Cass J. Fibroma of the ovary with ascites and hydrothorax. Am J Obstet Gynecol 1937;33:249–67.

202. Mueller-Heubach E, Reisfield DR. Pseudo-Meigs' syndrome resulting from ovarian malignancy. Review of the literature and report of a case with sanguinous pleural effusion. Obstet Gynecol Surv 1970;25:815–24.

203. Rubin IC, Novak J, Squire JJ. Ovarian fibromas and theca-cell tumors: report of 78 cases with special reference to production of ascites and hydrothorax (Meigs' syndrome). Am J Obstet Gynecol 1944;48:601–16.

204. Samanth KK, Black WC III. Benign ovarian stromal tumors associated with free peritoneal fluid. Am J Obstet Gynecol 1970;107:538–45.

205. Yutani C, Maeda H, Nakajima T, Takeuchi N, Kimura M, Kitamura H. Primary ovarian lymphoma associated with Meigs' syndrome. A case report. Acta Cytol 1982;26:44–8.

Hyperamylasemia

206. Brophy CM, Morris J, Sussman J, Modlin IM. "Pseudoascites" secondary to an amylase-producing serous ovarian cystadenoma. A case study. J Clin Gastroenterol 1989;11:703–6.

207. Bruns DE, Mills SE, Savory J. Amylase in fallopian tube and serous ovarian neoplasms. Arch Pathol Lab Med 1982;106:17–20.

208. Cramer SF, Bruns DE. Amylase-producing ovarian neoplasm with pseudo-Meigs' syndrome and elevated pleural amylase. Cancer 1979;44:1715–21.

209. Hayakawa T, Kameya A, Mizuno R, Noda A, Kondo T, Hirabayashi N. Hyperamylasemia with papillary serous cystadenocarcinoma of the ovary. Cancer 1984;54:1662–5.

210. Hodes ME, Sisk CJ, Karn RC, et al. An amylase-producing serous cystadenocarcinoma of the ovary. Oncology 1985;42:242–7.

211. Joseph RR, Frey CF, Michaels R, McCann DS. Amylase-containing ovarian cystadenocarcinoma simulating a pancreatic pseudocyst. Am J Obstet Gynecol 1976;126:515–6.

212. Norwood SH, Torma MJ, Fontanelle LJ. Hyperamylasemia due to poorly differentiated adenosquamous carcinoma of the ovary. Arch Surg 1981;116:225–6.

213. O'Riordan T, Gaffney E, Tormey V, Daly P. Hyperamylasemia associated with progression of a serous surface papillary carcinoma. Gynecol Oncol 1990;36:432–4.

214. Shapiro R, Dropkin R, Finkelstein J, Aledort D, Greenstein AJ. Ovarian carcinomatosis presenting with hyperamylasemia and pleural effusion. Am J Gastroenterol 1981;76:365–8.

215. Ueda G, Yamasaki M, Inoue M, Tanaka Y, Abe Y, Ogawa M. Immunohistochemical study of amylase in common epithelial tumors of the ovary. Int J Gynecol Pathol 1985;4:240–4.

216. Van Kley H, Cramer S, Bruns DE. Serous ovarian neoplastic amylase (SONA): a potentially useful marker for serous ovarian tumors. Cancer 1981;48:1444–9.

217. Yagi C, Miyata K, Hanai J, Ogawa M, Ueda G. Hyperamylasemia associated with endometrioid carcinoma of the ovary: case report and immunohistochemical study. Gynecol Oncol 1986;25:250–5.

Uveal Melanocytic Lesions

218. Barr CC, Zimmerman LE, Curtin VT, Font RL. Bilateral diffuse melanocytic uveal tumors associated with systemic malignant neoplasms. A recently recognized syndrome. Arch Ophthalmol 1982;100:249–55.

219. Margo CE, Pavan PR, Gendelman D, Gragoudas E. Bilateral melanocytic uveal tumors associated with systemic non-ocular malignancy. Malignant melanomas or benign paraneoplastic syndrome? Retina 1987;7:137–41.

220. Mullaney J, Mooney D, O'Connor M, McDonald GS. Bilateral ovarian carcinoma with bilateral uveal melanoma. Br J Ophthalmol 1984;68:261–7.

Pyrexia

221. Maestu RP, Buzon LM, Fraile I, et al. Carcinoma de ovario como causa de fiebre de origen desconocido. Revista Clinica Espanola 1979;153:65–7.

222. Schofield PM, Kirsop BA, Reginald P, Harington M. Ovarian carcinoma presenting as pyrexia of unknown origin. Postgrad Med J 1985;61:177–8.

21

TUMORS AND TUMOR-LIKE LESIONS ASSOCIATED WITH ABNORMAL SEXUAL DEVELOPMENT

Gonadal tumors of several types are frequent in patients with certain forms of abnormal gonadal development. The gonadoblastoma is one of the most common of these tumors, originating almost exclusively in a dysgenetic gonad; it has been discussed in detail in chapter 16. Since most other tumors that arise in abnormal gonads belong in the germ cell category and also have been described earlier, this chapter will be devoted to a description of the most common disorders of gonadal development in phenotypic females and a brief consideration of the tumors and tumor-like conditions associated with them.

GONADAL DYSGENESIS

The types of gonadal dysgenesis and their associated gonads are listed in Table 21-1. The gonadal streak is an elongated structure with the gross appearance of an infantile ovary. Early in fetal life, it may be indistinguishable on microscopic examination from a normal ovary but subsequently, the ova gradually disappear so that typically none are detectable at the time of puberty; exceptionally, a few remain, and graafian follicles and even corpora lutea may develop, usually within the first few postpubertal years. The typical streak in the adult is composed almost exclusively of ovarian stroma,

Table 21-1

TYPES OF GONADAL DYSGENESIS AND THEIR ASSOCIATED GONADS*

Turner's syndrome	Bilateral streak gonads (most cases)
Pure gonadal dysgenesis	Bilateral streak gonads
Mixed gonadal dysgenesis	1. Streak and testis 2. Streak-testis, bilateral 3. Streak-testis and streak 4. Streak-testis and testis 5. Dysgenetic testis, bilateral

*From references 5,6,7.

but rete ovarii, wolffian remnants, and hilus cells can be found in the hilus (fig. 21-1). The testis of mixed gonadal dysgenesis varies greatly in its degree of structural and functional abnormality. It is almost always undescended. Microscopic examination may show only the changes of cryptorchidism; if the testis is descended, spermatogenesis may occur. Much more frequently, the testis is small; may contain abnormally shaped, branching tubules devoid of germ cells; and may exhibit varying degrees of interstitial fibrosis. When streak tissue is additionally present, typically in the cortical portion of the gonad, the term streak-testis is appropriate (fig. 21-2).

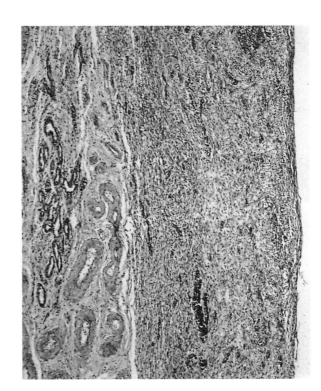

Figure 21-1
GONADAL STREAK
A thin strip of ovarian stroma devoid of follicles (right) lies adjacent to the hilus, which contains rete (left center). (Fig. 9.14 from Scully RE. Gonadal pathology of genetically determined diseases. In: Kraus FT, Damjanov I, eds. Pathology of reproductive failure. Baltimore: Williams & Wilkins, 1991:257–85.)

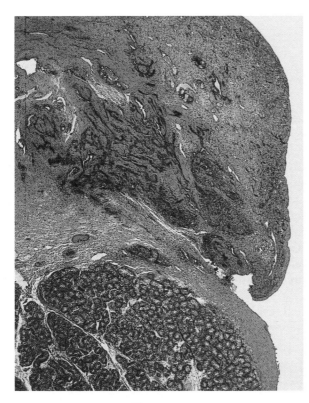

Figure 21-2
GONAD OF MIXED GONADAL DYSGENESIS
Streak tissue and rete (top) are separated by tunica albuginea from testis (bottom).

The disorder characterized by bilateral dysgenetic testes and initially designated "dysgenetic male pseudohermaphroditism" is now considered a variant of mixed gonadal dysgenesis because of pathologic and clinical overlap in the two disorders (2,4).

Pure gonadal dysgenesis with bilateral streaks is characterized by a failure of development of the secondary sex organs and characteristics at puberty, but patient height is normal and other congenital anomalies are absent. In Turner's syndrome, in contrast, the patient is not only sexually immature but is almost always less than 150 cm in height and has one or more congenital anomalies, including neonatal lymphedema, webbed neck, prognathous, shield-shaped chest, widely spaced nipples, cubitus valgus, congenital nevi, coarctation of the aorta, renal anomalies, short 5th metacarpal bones, and others. Patients with mixed gonadal dysgenesis are usually phenotypic females with varying degrees of male develop-

ment of the external genitalia; the internal secondary sex organs can vary but a uterus is almost always present. Rarely, the patient is a phenotypically normal male or female. Approximately one third of patients with mixed gonadal dysgenesis also have Turner's syndrome.

Gonadoblastoma and Germ Cell Tumors

Gonadoblastomas and pure germ cell tumors, most of which are germinomas (dysgerminomas-seminomas), are the most common forms of tumor in cases of gonadal dysgenesis, but their occurrence is almost entirely confined to patients who have a Y chromosome or Y-chromosome material in their karyotype (5–7) (page 307). Those patients with a 46,XX karyotype, which is sometimes associated with pure gonadal dysgenesis, or a 45,X karyotype, the most frequent finding in patients with Turner's syndrome, rarely have tumors of these types. Other ovarian tumors, such as those in the surface epithelial–stromal category and hilus cell tumors, may occur, however. In contrast, gonadoblastomas and pure germ cell tumors often complicate gonadal dysgenesis associated with a 46,XY karyotype, a common finding in cases of pure gonadal dysgenesis; a 45,X/ 46,XY karyotype, the characteristic finding in cases of mixed gonadal dysgenesis; or a variety of other mosaic karyotypes that include a Y chromosome. About three fourths of the gonadal tumors occurring in patients with gonadal dysgenesis and Y-chromosome material are gonadoblastomas, which may be mixed with various types of pure germ cell neoplasia; most of the remaining tumors are pure germinomas. Because of a calculated risk of malignancy of 28 percent by the age of 20 years for patients with pure gonadal dysgenesis and a Y chromosome, and a 19 percent risk by the same age for patients with mixed gonadal dysgenesis, prophylactic removal of the gonads is advisable in both groups of patients at an early age (1a).

Juvenile Granulosa Cell Tumor

Juvenile granulosa cell tumors have been reported in six infants with gonadal dysgenesis, ambiguous genitalia, and an abnormal karyotype that included a Y chromosome. The tumors arose in a testis in five of these cases; the gonad of origin of the sixth tumor could not be determined (1,3,8,9).

TRUE HERMAPHRODITISM

This disorder is characterized by the coexistence of well-developed ovarian and testicular tissue in the form of an ovary and a contralateral testis, or unilateral or bilateral ovotestes (fig. 21-3) (10,12). The testicular tissue is typically more normal structurally and functionally than that of mixed gonadal dysgenesis, and the ovarian tissue characteristically maintains a normal or close to normal appearance throughout life. The phenotype of the patient ranges from normal female to normal male, but most patients show varying degrees of sexual ambiguity. The most common karyotype is 46,XX, but a number of other karyotypes, including 46,XY and mosaic forms, have been reported. Eight phenotypically female true hermaphrodites with a 46,XX or mosaic karyotype have borne children. The most common tumor occurring in true hermaphrodites is the dysgerminoma-seminoma; a few gonadoblastomas have also occurred (13) as well as a variety of epithelial-stromal tumors in addition to endometriosis (10–12,14). Malignant gonadal tumors occur in less than 3 percent of the cases.

MALE PSEUDOHERMAPHRODITISM

This complex and incompletely understood category of disorders includes all cases in which the presence of testes is associated with varying degrees of female development, which range from slight to almost complete; lack of male development; or both (17,18). The primary abnormality may be at the testicular level and involve either structure or function (enzyme defects in the biosynthesis of testosterone; hernia uteri inguinale due to mullerian-inhibiting substance deficiency), at the end-organ level (androgen-insensitivity syndrome and 5 α-reductase deficiency), and rarely, at the hypothalamus-pituitary level. Since many of the cases in the literature have not been sorted out clearly, and subtypes of male pseudohermaphroditism are relatively rare, it is difficult to determine the frequency of development of malignant tumors in most forms of this disorder. It has already been mentioned that so-called dysgenetic male pseudohermaphroditism is associated with an increased frequency of gonadoblastoma and seminoma but that condition is now generally included in the

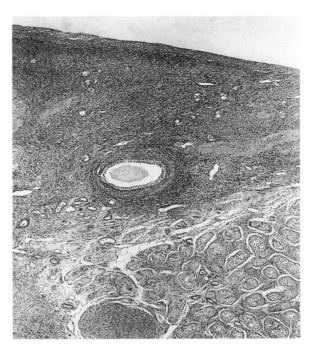

Figure 21-3
OVOTESTIS

An ovarian component containing follicles, including an antral follicle, overlies a testicular component containing sclerotic tubules and prominent Leydig cells, which form a small nodule in the lower center. (Fig. 4 from Rutgers JL, Scully RE. Pathology of the testis in intersex syndromes. Semin Diagn Pathol 1987;4:275–91.)

category of mixed gonadal dysgenesis (15,16). The form of male pseudohermaphroditism that has been recognized for many years to have an association with the development of a variety of gonadal tumors and tumor-like lesions is the complete form of the androgen-insensitivity syndrome (testicular feminization).

Androgen-Insensitivity Syndrome

General Features. The androgen-insensitivity syndrome (AIS), which may be familial and transmitted through the female, or sporadic, is characterized by a 46,XY karyotype, bilateral testes, and varying degrees of insensitivity of end-organs, including the testes, to androgens, resulting in varying degrees of deficient virilization (24–26).

The complete form of AIS (testicular feminization) (20) is characterized by testes that are usually abdominal, but may be inguinal or labial or rarely scrotal, and at least initially, produce normal quantities of androgens; a failure of development of the male internal and external secondary sex organs; an absence or scantiness of pubic and axillary hair; and breast development. Because the testes typically secrete a normal amount of mullerian-inhibiting substance the uterus and fallopian tubes are usually absent, but, enigmatically, one or both tubes develop in 10 percent of the patients (25). The disorder is caused by an abnormality in the androgen receptor gene in the long arm of the X chromosome, or in cases in which the receptor mechanism appears to be normal, to a postreceptor cellular defect (receptor-positive androgen resistance).

The diagnosis of testicular feminization may be suggested by the existence of the disorder in a sister or maternal aunt of the patient, by the finding of a testis in an inguinal hernia sac in a prepubertal phenotypic female, by the failure of the menarche to occur at the time of puberty, or by the development of symptoms or signs caused by a gonadal tumor or adnexal cyst. The diagnosis has been made as late as the ninth decade. The testes are normal histologically in early life but begin to lose their germ cells in late childhood (21). The Leydig cells secrete normal amounts of androgens initially, but because of end-organ insensitivity, virilization does not occur and the development of the external genitalia is female. Because of lack of sensitivity of the hypothalamus to androgens, the luteinizing hormone (LH) level becomes elevated, with increased stimulation of the Leydig cells to produce abnormal quantities of both androgens and estrogens. At the time of puberty estrogens stimulate the secondary sex organs, including the breasts, the development of which has not been inhibited by androgens in the fetus because of end-organ insensitivity. Menstruation does not appear because of absence of a uterus. The testicular tubules fail to develop at the time of puberty due to androgen insensitivity although there may be some enlargement of the Sertoli cells. Spermatogonia are present but may be difficult to find and exhibit no evidence of maturation. The interstitial tissue is composed of Leydig cells, which usually appear hyperplastic as a result of the increased LH level, and stroma that closely resembles ovarian stroma. The Leydig cells rarely contain crystals of Reinke. The three major components of the testis in the adult patient (the tubules, ovarian-type stroma, and Leydig cells) vary

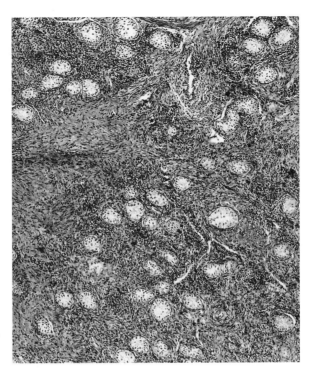

Figure 21-4
TESTIS OF ANDROGEN-INSENSITIVITY
SYNDROME (TESTICULAR FEMINIZATION)
Immature solid tubules containing Sertoli cells are widely separated by stroma resembling ovarian stroma. (Fig. 9.1 from Scully RE. Gonadal pathology of genetically determined diseases. In: Kraus FT, Damjanov I, eds. Pathology of reproductive failure. Baltimore: Williams & Wilkins, 1991:257–85.)

widely in amount from case to case (figs. 21-4–21-7). Although in most specimens all three components are readily recognized, the appearance of the gonads may range from a uniform distribution of tubules and Leydig cells to a predominance of ovarian-type stroma with only a few clusters of Leydig cells, tubules, or both. The latter structures may be easily overlooked, with resultant misinterpretation of the gonad as an ovary (fig. 21-7).

Hamartomas. Beginning after puberty, hamartomas and neoplasms, both benign and malignant, may alter the appearance of the gonads (figs. 21-8–21-14) (24–27). The most common of these lesions are hamartomas composed of varying combinations of Sertoli cells, Leydig cells, stromal cells, fibromatous tissue, and spermatogonia. The hamartomas are typically multiple, and in most of the cases, bilateral, ranging up to 4 cm in diameter. Immature tubules resembling

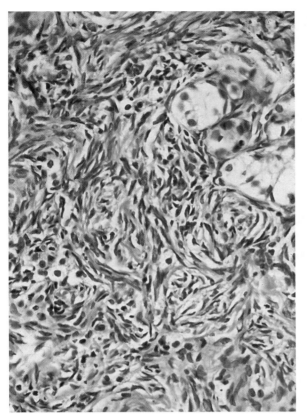

Figure 21-5
TESTIS OF ANDROGEN-INSENSITIVITY
SYNDROME (TESTICULAR FEMINIZATION)
Ovarian-type stroma with a storiform pattern containing a few lutein-like cells envelops two small solid tubules containing Sertoli cells.

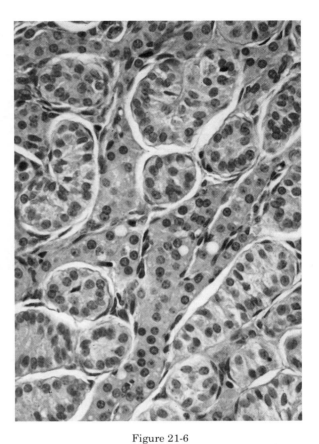

Figure 21-6
TESTIS OF ANDROGEN-INSENSITIVITY
SYNDROME (TESTICULAR FEMINIZATION)
Tubules containing immature Sertoli cells are separated by cells resembling Leydig cells.

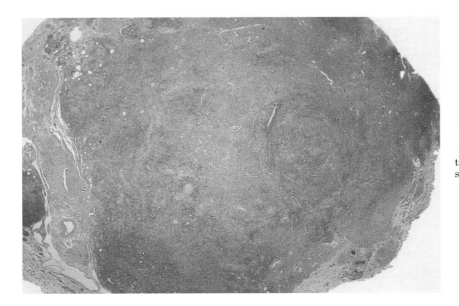

Figure 21-7
TESTIS OF ANDROGEN-
INSENSITIVITY SYNDROME
(TESTICULAR FEMINIZATION)
The testis is composed almost entirely of stroma resembling ovarian stroma.

Figure 21-8
TESTES OF ANDROGEN-
INSENSITIVITY SYNDROME
(TESTICULAR FEMINIZATION)

The sectioned surfaces reveal multiple hamartomas on a background of brown parenchyma. The nodule at each upper (medial) pole is a mass of smooth muscle; the small white nodule at the lower (lateral) pole of the left testis was composed largely of fibromatous tissue and resembles an ovarian fibroma. The remaining hamartomas contained Sertoli and Leydig cells and stroma. A small adnexal cyst is present at the lower (lateral) pole of the left testis.

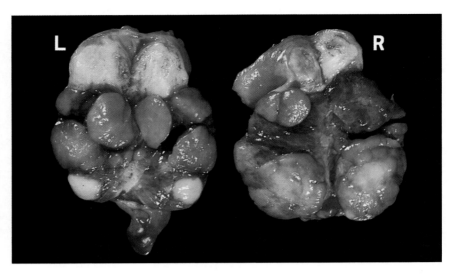

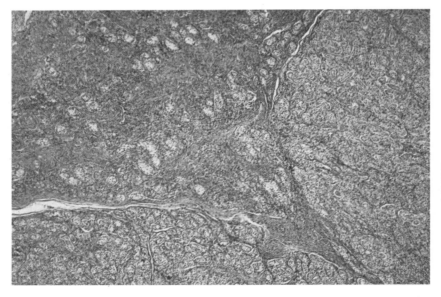

Figure 21-9
HAMARTOMAS IN
ANDROGEN-INSENSITIVITY
SYNDROME (TESTICULAR
FEMINIZATION)

The hamartomas are composed of Sertoli and Leydig cells and lie in the lower and right portions of the field; testicular parenchyma is present in the upper left portion of the field.

those in the testicular parenchyma are the most common constituents of hamartomas, but Leydig cells are present in almost all the cases as well; a rare hamartoma is composed predominantly of fibromatous tissue, resembling an ovarian fibroma (fig. 21-8).

Sex Cord–Stromal Tumors. Sertoli cell adenomas, which are composed entirely or almost entirely of uniform, solid tubules filled with immature, cytologically benign Sertoli cells, are less common than hamartomas. They are typically larger than the latter and may attain a considerable size, sometimes obliterating the underlying testicular tissue. An incorrect diagnosis of Sertoli cell tumor of the ovary often results if the diagnosis of AIS has not been made preoperatively (figs. 21-10, 21-11). Rare Sertoli cell tumors have the features of a large cell, calcifying Sertoli cell tumor of the testis and a sex cord tumor with annular tubules. Exceptionally, unclassified malignant tumors of sex cord type and granulosa cell tumors appear to arise within Sertoli cell adenomas (fig. 21-12). Small Leydig cell tumors are occasionally seen as well.

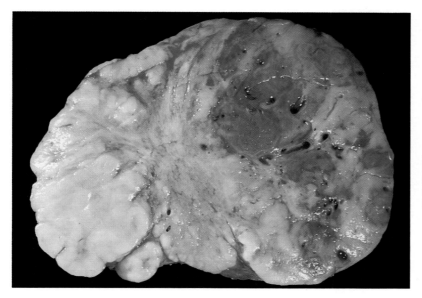

Figure 21-10
SERTOLI CELL ADENOMA
IN PATIENT WITH
ANDROGEN-INSENSITIVITY
SYNDROME (TESTICULAR
FEMINIZATION)

The sectioned surface is composed of pale, yellow-white, lobulated tissue with large areas of hemorrhagic infarction. (Fig. 2 from Case Records of the Massachusetts General Hospital. Case 11-1972. N Eng J Med 1972;286:594–600.)

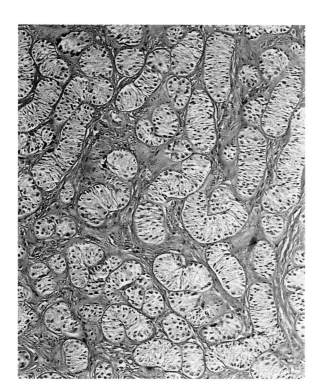

Figure 21-11
SERTOLI CELL ADENOMA IN PATIENT WITH
ANDROGEN-INSENSITIVITY SYNDROME
(TESTICULAR FEMINIZATION)

The tumor is composed of solid tubules containing immature Sertoli cells separated by hyalinized stroma. (Fig. 9.5 from Scully RE. Gonadal pathology of genetically determined diseases. In: Kraus FT, Damjanov I, eds. Pathology of reproductive failure. Baltimore: Williams & Wilkins, 1991:257–85.)

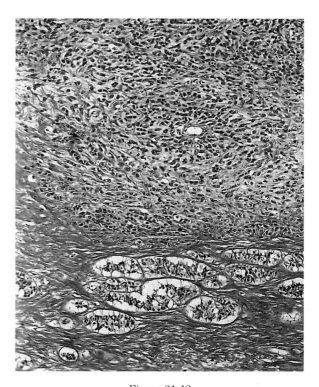

Figure 21-12
MALIGNANT SEX CORD TUMOR ARISING IN
SERTOLI CELL ADENOMA IN CASE OF
ANDROGEN-INSENSITIVITY SYNDROME
(TESTICULAR FEMINIZATION)

The tumor is composed of a diffuse arrangement of sex cord–type cells within a variable amount of fibrous stroma. The residual Sertoli cell adenoma is visible below.

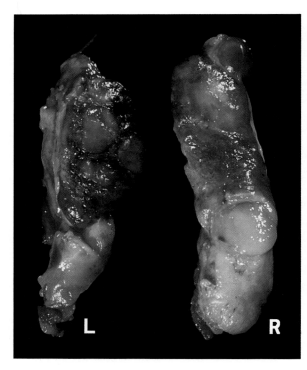

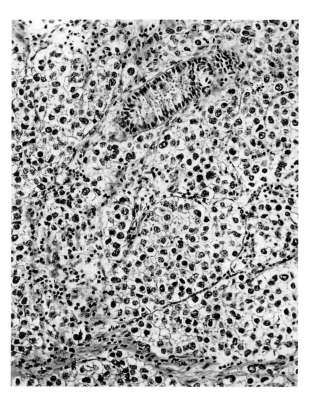

Figure 21-13
SEMINOMA ARISING IN RIGHT TESTIS OF
PATIENT WITH ANDROGEN-INSENSITIVITY
SYNDROME (TESTICULAR FEMINIZATION)

The seminoma is the round, cream-colored nodule in the
lower (medial) pole of the right testis, lying just above the
characteristic smooth muscle nodule.

Figure 21-14
SEMINOMA ARISING IN TESTIS OF PATIENT
WITH ANDROGEN-INSENSITIVITY SYNDROME
(TESTICULAR FEMINIZATION)

A tubule containing peripheral Sertoli cells is surrounded
by the tumor.

Figure 21-15
INTRATUBULAR GERM CELL
NEOPLASIA, UNCLASSIFIED
("CARCINOMA IN SITU")
IN TESTIS OF PATIENT WITH
ANDROGEN-INSENSITIVITY
SYNDROME (TESTICULAR
FEMINIZATION)

The tumor cells are large and rounded
with clear cytoplasm, resembling the
cells of seminoma-dysgerminoma and enlarging the tubules in the right portion of
the field.

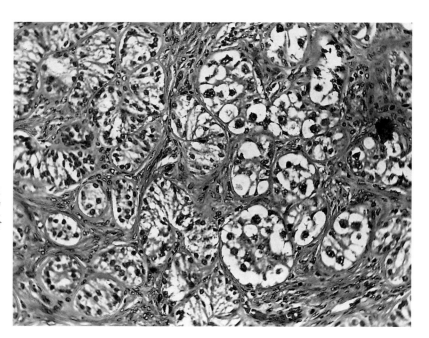

Germ Cell Tumors. Germ cell tumors develop in approximately 8 percent of adults with testicular feminization (19). They are almost always seminomas (figs. 21-13, 21-14), but other types of germ cell tumor may be seen as well. Intratubular germ cell neoplasia, unclassified (carcinoma in situ), with or without early stromal infiltration, has also been reported (fig. 21-15) (22).

Patients with incomplete forms of androgen insensitivity show varying degrees of virilization, and in the mildest form of the disorder impaired spermatogenesis with infertility, gynecomastia, or both may be the only manifestation in an otherwise normal male. It is not clear how often neoplasms develop in these rarer forms of AIS.

REFERENCES

Gonadal Dysgenesis

1. Manivel JC, Sibley RK, Dehner LP. Complete and incomplete Drash syndrome. A clinicopathologic study of five cases of a dysontogenetic-neoplastic complex. Hum Pathol 1987;18:80–9.

1a. Manuel M, Katayama KP, Jones HW Jr. The age of occurrence of gonadal tumors in intersex patients with a Y chromosome. Am J Obstet Gynecol 1976;124:293–300.

2. Rajfer J, Walsh PC. Mixed gonadal dysgenesis-dysgenetic male pseudohermaphroditism. Pediatr Adolesc Endocrinol 1981;8:105–15.

3. Raju U, Fine G, Warrier R, et al. Congenital testicular juvenile granulosa cell tumor in a neonate with X/XY mosaicism. Am J Surg Pathol 1986;10:577–83.

4. Robboy SJ, Miller T, Donahoe PK, et al. Dysgenesis of testicular and streak gonads in the syndrome of mixed gonadal dysgenesis: perspective derived from a clinicopathologic analysis of twenty-one cases. Hum Pathol 1982;13:700–16.

5. Rutgers JL. Advances in the pathology of intersex conditions. Hum Pathol 1991;22:884–91.

6. Scully RE. Gonadal pathology of genetically determined diseases. In: Kraus FT, Damjanov I, eds. The pathology of reproductive failure. (International Academy of Pathology Monograph No. 33). Baltimore: Williams & Wilkins, 1991:257–85.

7. Scully RE. Neoplasia associated with anomalous sexual development and abnormal sex chromosomes. Pediatr Adolesc Endocrinol 1981;8:203–17.

8. Tanaka Y, Sasaki Y, Tachibana K, Suwa S, Terashima K, Nakatani Y. Testicular juvenile granulosa cell tumor in an infant with X/XY mosaicism clinically diagnosed as true hermaphroditism. Am J Surg Pathol 1994;18:316–22.

9. Young RH, Lawrence WD, Scully RE. Juvenile granulosa cell tumor: another neoplasm associated with abnormal chromosomes and ambiguous genitalia. A report of three cases. Am J Surg Pathol 1985;9:737–43.

True Hermaphroditism

10. Rutgers JL. Advances in the pathology of intercex conditions. Hum Pathol 1991;22:884–91.

11. Scully RE. Gonadal pathology of genetically determined diseases. In: Kraus FT, Damjanov I, eds. The pathology of reproductive failure. (International Academy of Pathology Monograph No. 33). Baltimore: Williams & Wilkins, 1991:257–85.

12. Scully RE. Neoplasia associated with anomalous sexual development and abnormal sex chromosomes. Pediatr Adolesc Endocrinol 1981;8:203–17.

13. Talerman A, Verp MS, Senekjian E, Gilewski T, Vogelzang N. True hermaphrodite with bilateral ovotestes, gonadoblastoma and dysgerminomas, 46,XX/46,XY karyotype and a successful pregnancy. Cancer 1990;66:2668–72.

14. Young RE, Scully RE. Tumors and tumor like lesions in intersexual disorders. In: Testicular tumors. Chicago: ASCP Press, 1990:137–50.

Male Pseudohermaphroditism

15. Rajfer J, Walsh PC. Mixed gonadal dysgenesis-dysgenetic male pseudohermaphroditism. Pediatr Adolesc Endocrinol 1981;8:105–15.

16. Robboy SJ, Miller T, Donahoe PK, et al. Dysgenesis of testicular and streak gonads in the syndrome of mixed gonadal dysgenesis: perspective derived from a clinicopathologic analysis of twenty-one cases. Hum Pathol 1982;13:700–16.

17. Rutgers JL. Advances in the pathology of intersex conditions. Hum Pathol 1991;22:884–91.

18. Scully RE. Gonadal pathology of genetically determined diseases. In: Kraus FT, Damjanov I, eds. The pathology of reproductive failure. (International Academy of Pathology Monograph No. 33). Baltimore: Williams & Wilkins, 1991:257–85.

Androgen-Insensitivity Syndrome

19. Manuel M, Katayama KP, Jones HW Jr. The age of occurrence of gonadal tumors in intersex patients with a Y chromosome. Am J Obstet Gynecol 1976;124:293–300.

20. Morris JM, Scully RE. Endocrine pathology of the ovary. St. Louis: CV Mosby, 1958:58–9.

21. Müller J. Morphometry and histology of gonads from twelve children and adolescents with the androgen insensitivity (testicular feminization) syndrome. J Clin Endocrinol Metab 1984;59:785–9.

22. Müller J, Skakkebaek NE. Testicular carcinoma in situ in children with the androgen insensitivity (testicular feminisation) syndrome. Br Med J 1984;288:1419–20.

23. O'Dowd J, Gaffney EF, Young RH. Malignant sex cord-stromal tumor in a patient with the androgen insensitivity syndrome. Histopathology 1990;16:279–82.

24. Rutgers JL. Advances in the pathology of intersex conditions. Hum Pathol 1991;22:884–91.

25. Rutgers JL, Scully RE. The androgen insensitivity syndrome (testicular feminization): a clinicopathological study of 43 cases. Int J Gynecol Pathol 1991;10:126–45.

26. Scully RE. Gonadal pathology of genetically determined diseases. In: Kraus FT, Damjanov I, eds. The pathology of reproductive failure. (International Academy of Pathology Monograph No. 33). Baltimore: Williams & Wilkins, 1991:257–85.

27. Scully RE. Neoplasia associated with anomalous sexual development and abnormal sex chromosomes. Pediatr Adolesc Endocrinol 1981;8:203–17.

22
TUMOR-LIKE LESIONS

FOLLICLE CYST

Definition. A follicle cyst is one lined by granulosa cells, theca cells, or both.

General Features. Solitary follicle cysts are assumed to be caused by an absence of the normal preovulatory luteinizing hormone (LH) surge that triggers ovulation. These cysts are most common in nonpregnant women of reproductive age, particularly around the times of the menarche and menopause. They may be associated with menstrual irregularities; or may rupture and cause acute abdominal pain with hemoperitoneum and, exceptionally, exsanguination (4,8,9). Occasionally, a solitary follicle cyst forms several years after the onset of menopausal symptoms and amenorrhea; in such cases it may result in uterine bleeding or breast tenderness due to estrogen production by the cells in its wall (12,13).

Follicle cysts, although rare in children, are a relatively common cause of isosexual pseudoprecocity, which regresses after removal or puncture of the cyst (1,7), or occasionally, spontaneously (10). These cysts are thought to be autonomous because they are not associated with elevated gonadotropin levels at the time of diagnosis. In addition to being isolated lesions, they may be a component of the McCune-Albright syndrome (polyostotic fibrous dysplasia, cutaneous melanin pigmentation, and endocrine organ hyperactivity). In such cases there may be either one or a small number of cysts, which may be bilateral (5). An enlarging follicle in the McCune-Albright syndrome progresses rarely to ovulation, with corpus luteum formation and the possibility of pregnancy. In contrast to isolated follicle cysts, those associated with the syndrome may recur after removal, with a return of the precocity (5). Rarely, follicle cysts develop in utero or during the neonatal period (2,3,6,11,14). Such cysts may be complicated by torsion, hemorrhage, or rupture; they almost always regress within the first 4 months of life.

Gross Findings. Solitary follicle cysts rarely exceed 8 cm in diameter except during pregnancy or the puerperium (page 426). Typically, they have smooth surfaces and thin walls (fig. 22-1), and contain watery fluid or occasionally, blood.

Microscopic Findings. The cysts are lined by granulosa cells, theca cells, or both types of cells, which are characteristically luteinized (fig. 22-2). The granulosa cells may be denuded to varying extents, with underlying reactive changes and fibrosis; some simple cysts in women of reproductive age are probably end-stage follicle cysts.

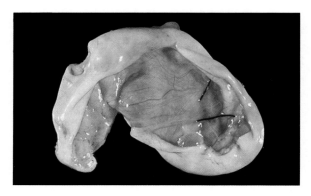

Figure 22-1
FOLLICLE CYST
A unilocular cyst has a smooth lining.

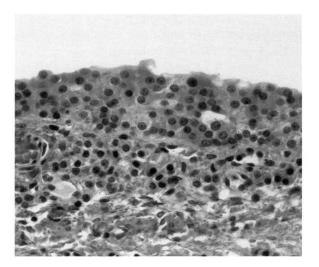

Figure 22-2
FOLLICLE CYST
The cyst is lined by luteinized granulosa cells, beneath which are luteinized theca cells.

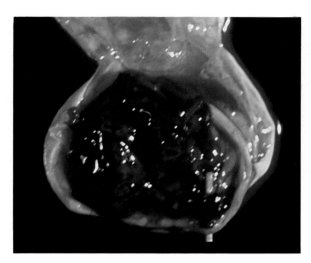

Figure 22-3
CORPUS LUTEUM CYST, RUPTURED
The cyst is full of blood; a probe indicates the point of rupture.

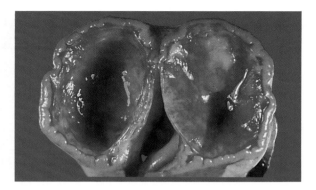

Figure 22-4
CORPUS LUTEUM CYST
The wall is thick and yellow; the lining is smooth.

Differential Diagnosis. Because the solitary follicle cyst is often palpable it can be confused clinically with a neoplasm, and when it also has endocrine manifestations, it may be mistaken for a functioning tumor. The pathologist encounters a problem in differential diagnosis only rarely when a unilocular granulosa cell tumor has an orderly arrangement of granulosa cells and theca cells in its wall. Almost always, however, such a tumor is much larger than a follicle cyst and the two cell types have a disorderly pattern, with obviously neoplastic aggregates of granulosa cells in the cyst wall.

CORPUS LUTEUM CYST

General Features. When a cystic corpus luteum reaches a diameter of over 3 cm the designation corpus luteum cyst is appropriate (19). Corpus luteum cysts may be associated with menstrual irregularities and sometimes amenorrhea (19). Like follicle cysts, they may rupture and cause intra-abdominal hemorrhage (fig. 22-3) (16, 17,20,21). Rarely, corpora lutea and cysts derived from them are found in neonates (15,18).

Gross Findings. The lumen is typically distended with blood, and focal or circumferential yellow coloration of the cyst wall is frequent (figs. 22-3, 22-4). The lining may be smooth or roughened by adherent blood.

Microscopic Findings. The wall is composed, at least in part, of a thick, often convoluted layer of large luteinized granulosa cells interrupted at its periphery by wedges of much smaller theca lutein cells (fig. 22-5).

OVARIAN REMNANT SYNDROME

Patients with this syndrome have had a presumably total oophorectomy but present with symptoms related to the presence of residual ovarian tissue (23,24). The preceding operation was often difficult because of involvement of one or both ovaries in dense fibrous adhesions, which are usually a complication of either pelvic inflammatory disease or endometriosis. The patient may present weeks to years postoperatively with pelvic pain, which may be cyclical; a mass is palpated in about half the cases (24). Rarely, patients have ureteral or small intestinal obstruction (22,25). At reoperation corpus luteum cysts or ill-defined masses of fibrous tissue with focal hemorrhage may be found. Microscopic examination discloses ovarian tissue, which may contain cystic follicles or corpora lutea surrounded by fibrous tissue with chronic inflammatory cells; endometriosis may also be present.

POLYCYSTIC OVARIAN DISEASE

Definition. Polycystic ovarian disease (PCOD) is a disorder characterized by anovulation or infrequent ovulation and numerous follicle cysts in both ovaries, which are usually enlarged.

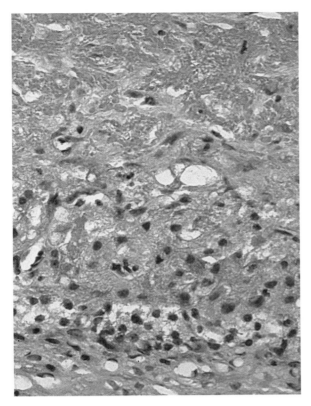

Figure 22-5
CORPUS LUTEUM CYST
A layer of luteinized granulosa cells with abundant cyto-plasm lines the blood-filled cyst. Small theca cells underlie the granulosa cells.

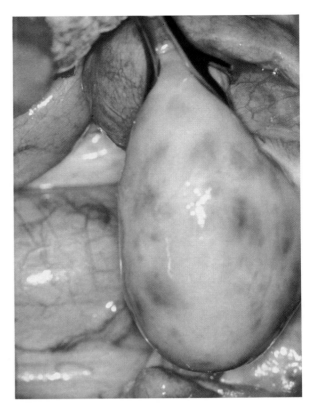

Figure 22-6
POLYCYSTIC OVARIAN DISEASE
The external surface of the enlarged ovary is pearly white. Multiple cysts are visible beneath the surface.

General Features. The typical patient is a young woman who does not ovulate, is infertile, and has menstrual disturbances, which range from amenorrhea to oligomenorrhea (Stein-Leventhal syndrome) to menometrorrhagia; hirsutism and obesity are common. Some patients have hyperprolactinemia, and others have late-onset congenital adrenal hyperplasia (31, 33,34,38). There is usually slight elevation of one or more androgens in the plasma, and often the estrone level is high due to peripheral conversion of excessive androstenedione, with a reversal of the estradiol-estrone ratio. Other features include low to normal follicle-stimulating hormone (FSH), a high level of LH, and an exaggerated response of LH to gonadotropin-releasing hormone (28). Ultrasonographic studies have revealed that ovulating women with minor evidence of hyperandrogenism, but without menstrual irreg-

ularity, may have polycystic ovaries similar to those of patients with overt clinical manifestations except that the ovaries contain corpora lutea and albicantia as well as multiple follicle cysts (26,36). Thus, the boundary between the clinical syndromes associated with PCOD and normalcy is not clear-cut. Examination of the endometrium in patients with PCOD may reveal hypoactivity, cystic hyperplasia, atypical hyperplasia, or in less than 5 percent of the cases, adenocarcinoma, which is almost always low grade.

Gross Findings. Both ovaries are typically enlarged and rounded, with multiple small follicle cysts visible beneath their surfaces (fig. 22-6); occasionally the ovaries are of normal size (37). The superficial cortex is thick and white giving the appearance of a true capsule (fig. 22-6). Sectioning reveals multiple cysts of approximately equal size, typically situated superficially beneath the thickened outer cortex, while the central portion

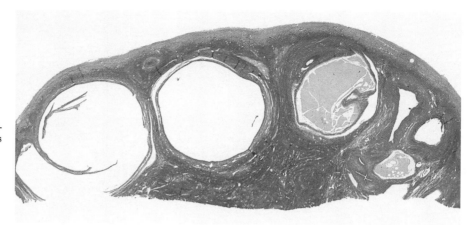

Figure 22-7
POLYCYSTIC
OVARIAN DISEASE
The outer cortex is collagenized; several follicle cysts are arrayed beneath it.

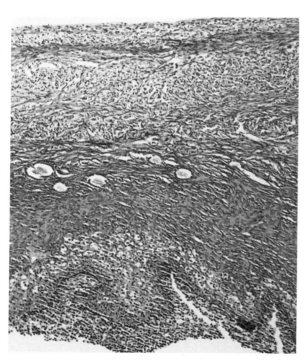

Figure 22-8
POLYCYSTIC OVARIAN DISEASE

The outer cortex is collagenized and a follicle cyst (bottom) is lined by granulosa cells with a prominent underlying layer of theca cells. (Fig. 11 from Young RH, Clement PB, Scully RE. Pathology of the ovary. In: Sternberg SS, ed. Diagnostic surgical pathology, Vol 2, 2nd ed. New York: Raven Press, 1994:2201.)

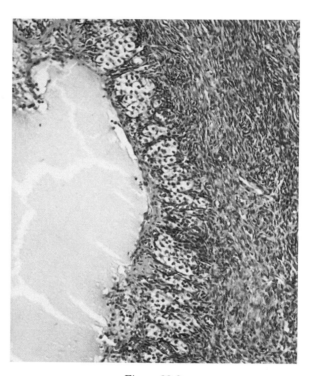

Figure 22-9
POLYCYSTIC OVARIAN DISEASE

A prominent band of luteinized theca cells surrounds the cavity of an atretic follicle (follicular hyperthecosis).

of the ovary consists of homogeneous stroma with only rare or no evidence of ovulation (corpora lutea or corpora albicantia).

Microscopic Findings. The outer cortex is typically hypocellular and contains an increased amount of collagen and often thick-walled blood vessels (figs. 22-7, 22-8) (29,37). The cysts, as well as atretic follicles, are usually, but not always, lined predominantly by hyperplastic, enlarged, lipid-laden theca interna cells, giving rise to the term follicular hyperthecosis (fig. 22-9). Granulosa cells are less conspicuous than in normal follicles and are not luteinized. Examination

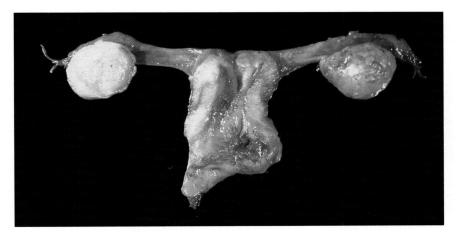

Figure 22-10
STROMAL HYPERTHECOSIS
Both ovaries are enlarged. The sectioned surface of the left ovary is composed of white tissue, which was firm, and simulated that of a neoplasm.

of only a few sections of wedge resection specimens of the ovaries generally fails to reveal the presence of luteinized cells in the stroma. If numerous sections are examined, however, such cells have been seen in small numbers in up to 80 percent of the cases (32).

Differential Diagnosis. PCOD is a clinicopathologic syndrome, and the finding of polycystic ovaries with little or no evidence of prior ovulation in wedge biopsy specimens does not per se warrant the diagnosis. Polycystic ovaries that resemble those of PCOD are seen occasionally in prepubertal children, in otherwise normal girls during the first few years after the onset of puberty, and in girls in the second decade with primary hypothyroidism (28,35). Although PCOD is usually not confused with a neoplasm, the clinical manifestations may suggest the possibility of an androgenic or estrogenic ovarian tumor, particularly in the exceptional cases in which the disease coexists with a nonfunctioning ovarian neoplasm (27). If the associated ovarian tumor is capable of function, such as a Sertoli-Leydig cell tumor, it may be difficult to determine which lesion was responsible for the endocrine manifestations (30).

STROMAL HYPERTHECOSIS

Definition. This is a disorder in which luteinized cells are scattered singly and in small nests or nodules throughout a typically hyperplastic ovarian stroma.

General Features. The clinical manifestations may be identical to those of PCOD but in many of the reported cases the findings include marked virilization, obesity, hypertension, and decreased glucose tolerance (43,44,49). The latter three abnormalities were present respectively in 33, 27, and 20 percent of the patients in one series (51). The clinical picture typically evolves gradually, but occasionally there is an abrupt onset and a rapid course, simulating that of an androgenic tumor. The resemblance to a virilizing tumor has been greatest in very rare (unreported) cases in which the stromal hyperthecosis was unilateral and caused tumor-like ovarian enlargement.

Generally, a plasma testosterone level over 200 ng/dl is considered to favor a virilizing tumor, and a lower level, stromal hyperthecosis, but numerous exceptions to this differential feature have been reported. Almost all the women who present with virilization are premenopausal (43). When hormonal manifestations are present in postmenopausal patients, they are usually estrogenic (42). The disorder is occasionally familial (47). Insulin resistance, sometimes accompanied by diabetes, acanthosis nigricans, and hyperandrogenism (HAIR-AN syndrome) has been described in a small subset of women considered to have stromal hyperthecosis or PCOD on clinical grounds (page 386) (39,53). Hyperplasia and carcinoma of the endometrium occasionally develop in cases of stromal hyperthecosis (42,51).

Gross Findings. Both ovaries may be enlarged up to 7 cm in greatest diameter and are replaced to a variable extent by solid white to yellow stroma, sometimes simulating bilateral solid tumors (fig. 22-10). In premenopausal women the external ovarian surface may appear white and opaque, and multiple superficial follicle cysts

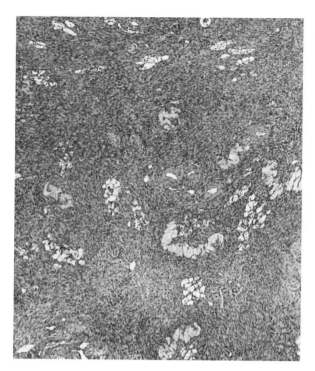

Figure 22-11
STROMAL HYPERTHECOSIS
Numerous nests of vacuolated luteinized cells are present in the ovarian stroma.

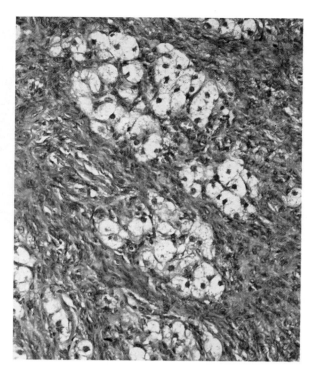

Figure 22-12
STROMAL HYPERTHECOSIS
Luteinized cells contain abundant vacuolated cytoplasm. (Fig. 13 from Young RH, Clement PB, Scully RE. Pathology of the ovary. In: Sternberg SS, ed. Diagnostic surgical pathology, Vol 2, 2nd ed. New York: Raven Press, 1994:2201.)

may be visible. Exceptionally, only a single ovary is involved. Stromal hyperthecosis rarely coexists with a neoplasm, usually a stromal luteoma, which may also have a hormone-secreting potential.

Microscopic Findings. Microscopic examination reveals nests of lutein cells (figs. 22-11, 22-12) or scattered single lutein cells, which contain no visible lipid or variable amounts of it in their cytoplasm (figs. 22-13, 22-14); typically there is a background of stromal hyperplasia. In premenopausal women follicular hyperthecosis and sclerosis of the outer cortex, characteristic of PCOD, are also commonly present. Usually, the luteinized stromal cells are conspicuously larger than the follicular theca lutein cells. Rarely, the former cells proliferate to form grossly visible nodular aggregates 1 cm or less in diameter (nodular hyperthecosis) (fig. 22-15) (50) or a stromal luteoma (over 1 cm in diameter) (45). Hilus cell hyperplasia or a hilus cell tumor may be present additionally in one or both ovaries (45,48). When both ovaries are thoroughly examined microscopically, hyperthecosis is almost always bilateral but routine sectioning occasionally documents its presence in only one ovary (51). In one study of the ovaries from 11 patients with the HAIR-AN syndrome, stromal hyperthecosis with multiple follicle cysts was found in all the specimens; sclerosis of the outer cortex and edema and fibrosis of the underlying stroma were also observed (41).

In cases of stromal hyperthecosis immunohistochemical staining for various enzymes involved in the conversion of cholesterol to steroid hormones has been consistent with androgen synthesis, not only in the luteinized stromal cells characteristic of the disorder but also in the adjacent spindle-shaped stromal cells. Also, the more frequent demonstration of aromatase in the theca lutein cells of cystic follicles in young women with stromal hyperthecosis than in the stromal lutein cells suggests a predominant role of the latter cells in the androgen overproduction that usually characterizes this disorder (46).

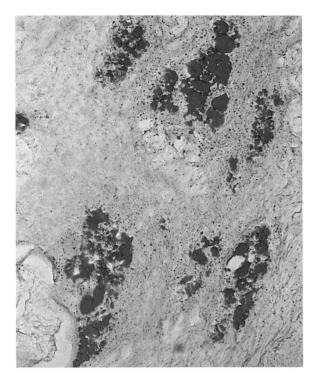

Figure 22-13
STROMAL HYPERTHECOSIS
The lutein cells contain abundant lipid. (Oil red-O stain)

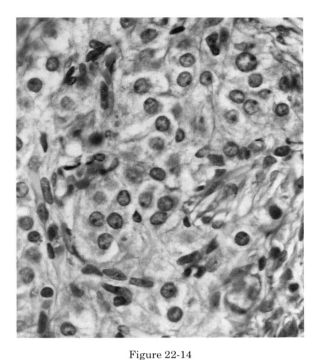

Figure 22-14
STROMAL HYPERTHECOSIS
The luteinized cells have eosinophilic, nonvacuolated cytoplasm and regular, round nuclei with prominent nucleoli.

Differential Diagnosis. The differential diagnosis of stromal hyperthecosis and luteinized thecoma is discussed on page 192.

STROMAL HYPERPLASIA

Definition. This is an abnormal proliferation of ovarian stroma without the additional presence of lutein cells.

General Features. Stromal hyperplasia is typically found during the menopause or in the early postmenopausal years. It is occasionally associated with androgenic or estrogenic manifestations as well as obesity, hypertension, and disorders of glucose metabolism (40) although much less frequently and less obtrusively than in cases of stromal hyperthecosis.

Gross Findings. The medulla, cortex, or both regions of the ovary are occupied by ill-defined, white or pale yellow nodules, which may coalesce (fig. 22-16). Marked stromal hyperplasia, like stromal hyperthecosis, can extensively replace and enlarge the ovaries.

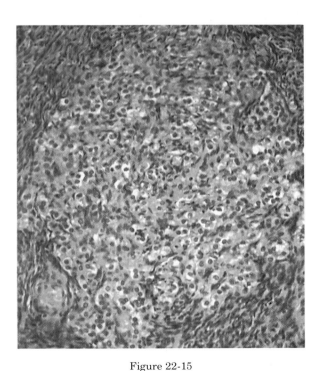

Figure 22-15
STROMAL HYPERTHECOSIS
A large nodule of luteinized cells is present within the ovarian stroma (nodular hyperthecosis).

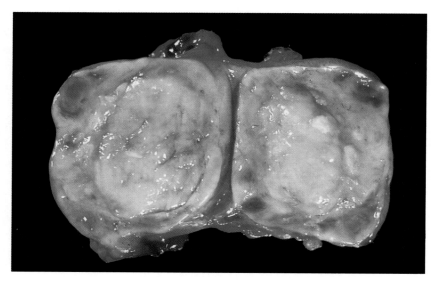

Figure 22-16
STROMAL HYPERPLASIA
Ill-defined, pale yellow tissue occupies the center of the ovary.

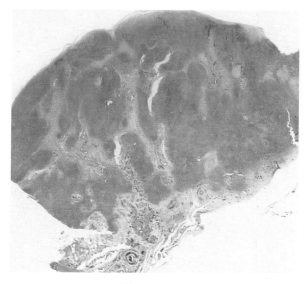

Figure 22-17
STROMAL HYPERPLASIA
The ovarian medulla and cortex of an elderly woman are replaced by cellular stroma.

Microscopic Findings. The medulla, and to a lesser extent, the cortex, are replaced by a nodular or diffuse, densely cellular proliferation of small stromal cells (figs. 22-17, 22-18). Follicular derivatives may lie within the hyperplastic stroma, but may be rare or absent in advanced cases.

That hyperplastic stroma apparently free of lutein cells is capable of steroid hormone secretion is supported by the finding that some of the hyperplastic cells contain oxidative enzymes that are important in steroid hormone production (52). Also, in cases of stromal hyperthecosis spindle-shaped cells that are transitional morphologically between typical stromal cells and lutein cells can be identified on careful examination of routine sections after they have been localized by immunohistochemical staining for steroidogenic enzymes (46). It is possible that transitional cells of this type produce steroid hormones in cases of stromal hyperplasia without hyperthecosis; an alternative explanation is that focally distributed lutein cells may be missed by incomplete sampling.

Differential Diagnosis. In contrast to a fibroma, stromal hyperplasia is characterized by cells with smaller nuclei, scanty collagen formation, and nodules that commonly coalesce. The lesion is distinguished from a low-grade endometrioid stromal sarcoma by the spindle shape of its cells, and by an absence of mitotic figures and regularly distributed arterioles.

MASSIVE EDEMA

Definition. This process causes a tumor-like enlargement of one or both ovaries by edema fluid.

General Features. Patients with this lesion range in age from 6 to 33 years, with an average of 21 years (55–59). Three quarters of them present with abdominal pain, which may be acute and accompanied by abdominal swelling. In the remaining patients the clinical manifestations are usually disorders of menstruation, evidence of androgen

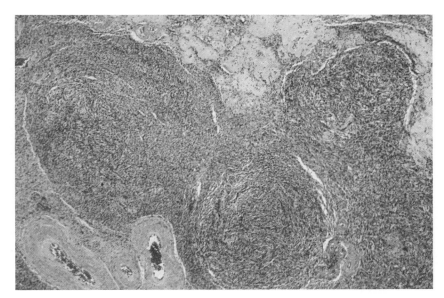

Figure 22-18
STROMAL HYPERPLASIA
Confluent nodules of hyperplastic stroma occupy the medulla.

Figure 22-19
MASSIVE EDEMA
The sectioned surface of the enlarged ovary is occupied by gelatinous tissue. (Fig. 14 from Young RH, Clement PB, Scully RE. Pathology of the ovary. In: Sternberg SS, ed. Diagnostic surgical pathology, Vol 2, 2nd ed. New York: Raven Press, 1994:2202.)

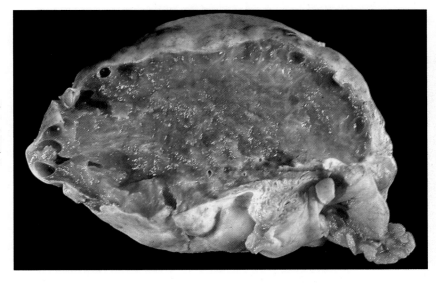

excess, or both. Abdominal exploration reveals that the ovarian enlargement is unilateral in about 90 percent of the cases. Partial or complete torsion of the ovarian pedicle is reported in approximately half the cases (59) and intermittent torsion has been implicated in the causation of the lesion (56).

Gross Findings. The ovaries range from 5.5 to 35 (average, 11.5) cm in diameter. Their outer surfaces are usually opaque and white; small follicle cysts may be seen beneath them. Abundant watery fluid typically exudes from the sectioned surfaces, which appear edematous or gelatinous (fig. 22-19).

Microscopic Findings. Microscopic examination reveals edematous, hypocellular stroma surrounding rather than displacing follicles and their derivatives (fig. 22-20). The presence of stromal cells around collections of edema fluid may impart a microcystic appearance. Minor foci of a fibromatous stromal proliferation may be seen. The peripheral cortex is typically composed of dense collagenous tissue and does not participate in the edema. Lutein cells are identified in the edematous areas in 40 percent of the cases (fig. 22-21) and in the thickened outer cortex in occasional cases.

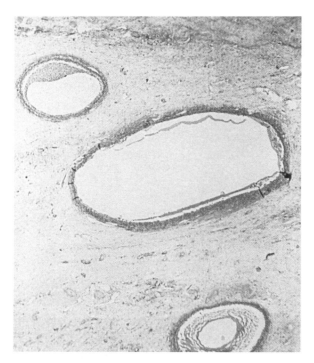

Figure 22-20
MASSIVE EDEMA
Pale edematous stroma surrounds several cystic follicles beneath an outer cortex thickened by collagen. (Fig. 15 from Young RH, Clement PB, Scully RE. Pathology of the ovary. In: Sternberg SS, ed. Diagnostic surgical pathology, Vol 2, 2nd ed. New York: Raven Press, 1994:2203.)

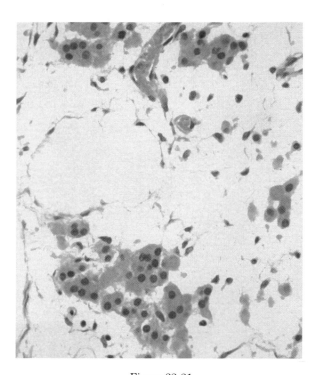

Figure 22-21
MASSIVE EDEMA
Clusters of lutein cells lie in the edematous stroma.

Differential Diagnosis. The gross appearance of massive edema may simulate closely that of any edematous neoplasm, most typically an edematous fibroma or a Krukenberg tumor. Recognition of massive edema is therefore of great importance to prevent unnecessary oophorectomy in a young female. Distinction from an edematous fibroma depends largely on the inclusion of follicular derivatives within massive edema. Distinction from a Krukenberg tumor depends on the absence of signet-ring cells in the edematous tissue. The rare luteinized thecoma associated with sclerosing peritonitis (page 192) may also be misinterpreted as massive edema.

FIBROMATOSIS

Definition. Fibromatosis is a tumor-like enlargement of one or both ovaries resulting from a non-neoplastic fibromatoid proliferation of ovarian stroma. The designation does not apply to microscopic foci of fibromatoid change that do not result in ovarian enlargement.

General Features. The patients range from 13 to 39 (average, 25) years of age (54,59). The presenting manifestations are usually menstrual irregularities or amenorrhea, and rarely virilization. The process is unilateral in 80 percent of the cases; occasional involved ovaries have twisted on their pedicles.

Gross Findings. The enlarged ovaries are 8 to 14 cm in diameter, with smooth or lobulated external surfaces. The sectioned surfaces are typically firm and white or grey; small cysts may be visible (fig. 22-22).

Microscopic Findings. Proliferating spindle cells producing variable but usually large amounts of collagen surround follicular derivatives (fig. 22-23). Luteinized stromal cells may be seen as well as foci of stromal edema. In some cases nests of cells of sex cord type are present in small numbers (fig. 22-24). In most cases of fibromatosis the process is diffuse, but it may be localized; occasionally, it is confined to or predominantly involves the cortex (cortical fibromatosis) (fig. 22-25).

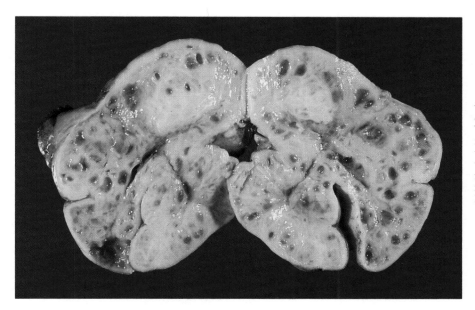

Figure 22-22
FIBROMATOSIS
Yellow-white tissue, which was firm, envelops numerous cystic follicles. (Fig. 1 from Young RH, Scully RE. Fibromatosis and massive edema of the ovary, possibly related entities: a report of 14 cases of fibromatosis and 11 cases of massive edema. Int J Gynecol Pathol 1984;3:153–78.)

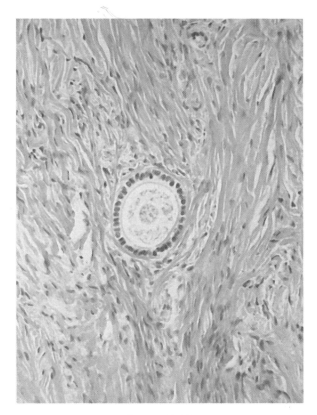

Figure 22-23
FIBROMATOSIS
Dense collagenous tissue envelops a primary follicle. (Fig. 17 from Young RH, Clement PB, Scully RE. Pathology of the ovary. In: Sternberg SS, ed. Diagnostic surgical pathology, Vol 2, 2nd ed. New York: Raven Press, 1994:2203.)

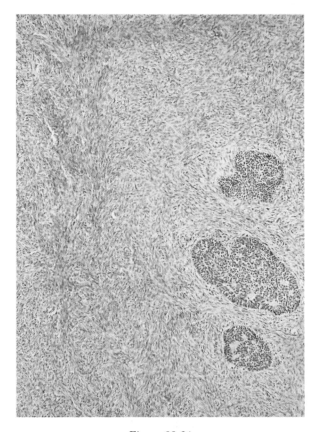

Figure 22-24
FIBROMATOSIS
Several nests of cells of sex cord type are present within dense fibromatous stroma.

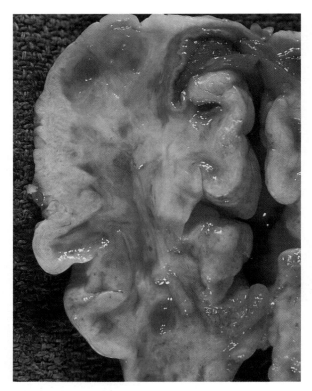

Figure 22-25
FIBROMATOSIS, CORTICAL
The cortex is thickened and yellow-white.

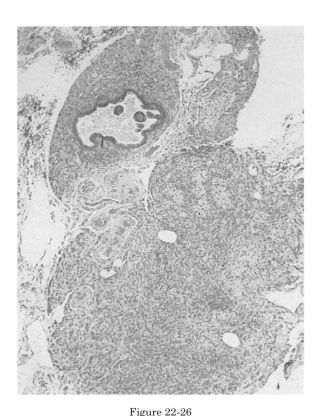

Figure 22-26
HILUS CELL HYPERPLASIA
Large nodular masses of hilus cells are present, one surrounding the rete ovarii.

Differential Diagnosis. The tumor that enters the differential diagnosis most often is the fibroma (page 194). Entrapment of follicular derivatives by fibromatosis, however, strongly favors its diagnosis. The lesion may resemble a Brenner tumor if the sex cord–like nests are prominent. The nests in fibromatosis, however, are easily distinguishable from those of a Brenner tumor in their number, shapes, and cell types. Ovarian fibromatosis lacks the extraovarian involvement seen with fibromatosis of the soft tissue type involving the ovary (page 316).

HILUS (LEYDIG) CELL HYPERPLASIA

Hilus cell hyperplasia (fig. 22-26) is difficult to define because hilus cell nests are typically widely separated and cannot be quantitated adequately without sectioning both ovaries extensively. Also, hilus cell proliferation can occur physiologically as a result of elevated chorionic gonadotropin (hCG) or LH levels, such as occur during pregnancy (page

428) or after the menopause, respectively. In an autopsy study in which both ovaries were sectioned extensively (60), hilus cells were found in 83 percent of the cases. Their quantity was graded 0 to 4; grade 3 or 4 hilus cells were not found in 24 women under 55 years of age, but were present in 21 percent of 33 women 56 to 70 years of age and 42 percent of 33 women 71 years of age or older. Grade 3 or 4 cells were not present in 20 nulliparous patients in contrast to 31 percent of 45 parous patients. Hyperplasia is typically nodular, and may be characterized by cellular enlargement, nuclear pleomorphism (fig. 22-27) and hyperchromasia, and multinucleation. The lesion has been reported to be associated with androgenic or estrogenic manifestations and elevated plasma testosterone levels (62).

Hilus cell hyperplasia is commonly accompanied by other ovarian lesions, including stromal hyperplasia, stromal hyperthecosis, and hilus cell tumor (60a,63). It is seen occasionally along the hilar border of an ovarian tumor or cyst (see

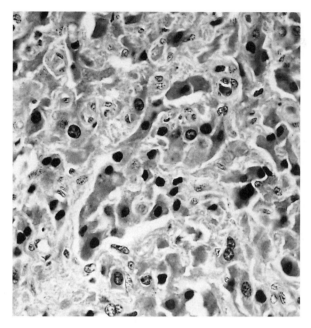

Figure 22-27
HILUS CELL HYPERPLASIA
IN A POSTMENOPAUSAL WOMAN
The hilus cells have bizarre shapes and abundant cyto-
plasm, which was eosinophilic. Some nuclei are enlarged
and hyperchromatic.

chapter 19). One case of hilus cell hyperplasia
was associated with the resistant ovary syndrome (62), and other cases have been reported
in association with gonadal dysgenesis (61); in
both disorders, LH levels are elevated.

From a pathologic viewpoint the distinction between a large hyperplastic nodule of hilus cells and
a hilus cell tumor is arbitrary; we diagnose neoplasia
when the nodule is over 1 cm in diameter.

SIMPLE CYST

This type of cyst is of unknown origin because
its lining has disappeared or has been destroyed
by rubbing it or allowing it to dry after removal,
or because the lining consists of a thin layer of
indifferent-appearing cells resembling epithelial
cells. The wall is composed of fibrous tissue. The
identification of theca lutein cells in the cyst wall
or a serous, endometrioid, or other epithelial
lining on additional sampling may lead to a more
specific diagnosis. Even a rare cystic struma ovarii
may be misdiagnosed as a simple cyst if inconspicuous follicles in the wall are overlooked.

IDIOPATHIC CALCIFICATION

In one case, extensive idiopathic calcification
resulted in a stony hard consistency of both
ovaries, which were of normal size (64). Microscopic examination showed numerous spherical,
laminated, calcific foci without accompanying
epithelial cells. This process must be distinguished from a serous borderline tumor or carcinoma with confluent psammoma bodies, in
which at least occasional neoplastic epithelial
cells should be identified, and from a "burned-
out" gonadoblastoma replaced by laminated calcified masses. Patients with gonadoblastoma almost always have evidence of abnormal gonadal
development and Y-chromosome material in their
karyotypes, as well as residual typical gonadoblastoma in the same or contralateral gonad.

UTERUS-LIKE ADNEXAL MASS

The three reported examples have been characterized by a central cavity lined by endometrium
surrounded by a thick wall composed of smooth
muscle at the site of an ovary (65–67). A congenital
malformation of the mullerian duct has been suggested as the cause in two of the reported cases
because of the presence of a congenital abnormality of the ipsilateral upper urinary tract (66,68). In
the third case, however, residual ovarian parenchyma was identified at the periphery of the mass
and no urinary tract anomaly was evident, suggesting a possible origin in ovarian endometriosis,
with smooth muscle metaplasia of the endometriotic or adjacent ovarian stroma (67).

SPLENIC-GONADAL FUSION

Splenic-gonadal fusion is a rare anomaly resulting from fusion of the anlage of both organs
during embryonic development (fig. 22-28) (69–
71). The male to female ratio is 9 to 1. Three
examples have been described in newborn females, two of whom had partially undescended
ovaries as well as multiple other congenital
anomalies (71). In all three cases the lesion was
of the continuous type in which a cord-like structure connected the spleen to the left ovary. In one
of these cases, several intraovarian splenic nodules were found. An additional case has been
described in an adult female, who was found to
have a septate uterus and a cluster of splenic

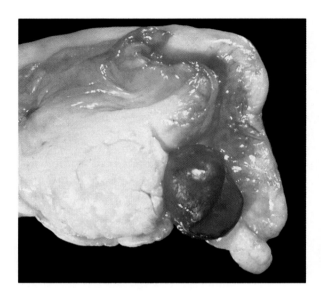

Figure 22-28
SPLENIC-OVARIAN FUSION
A nodule of brown-red splenic tissue abuts the ovary.

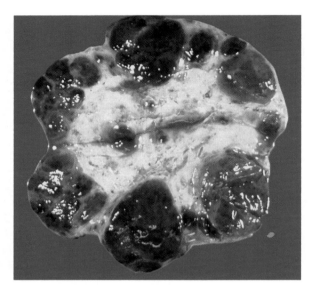

Figure 22-29
PREGNANCY LUTEOMA
Many brown to red nodules are present. (Fig. 2 from Malinak LR, Miller GV. Bilateral multicentric ovarian luteomas of pregnancy associated with masculinization of a female infant. Am J Obstet Gynecol 1965;91:251–9.)

nodules surrounding an otherwise normal left ovary (69). The differential diagnosis in the last case would include traumatic splenosis, but in such cases there is usually a history of trauma and the nodules of splenic tissue are more widely dispersed throughout the peritoneal cavity.

PREGNANCY LUTEOMA

Definition. These single or multiple hyperplastic nodules of large lutein cells develop during pregnancy and involute during the puerperium; the nodules probably arise from ovarian stromal cells.

General Features. The patients are typically in their third or fourth decade; 80 percent are multiparous and a similar proportion are black (73,76,77,78). Most of the patients are asymptomatic, and the ovarian enlargement is usually an incidental finding at term during cesarean section or postpartum tubal ligation. Rarely, however, a pelvic mass is palpable or obstructs the birth canal. In approximately 25 percent of the cases, hirsutism or virilization appears during the latter half of pregnancy (79). Seventy percent of female infants born to masculinized mothers are also virilized (72,74). Plasma testosterone and other androgens may reach levels 70 times normal in the virilized patients; increased values

have also been demonstrated in nonvirilized women. The levels in the infants may be elevated but are usually lower than the maternal levels and may be normal. Pregnancy luteomas begin to regress within days after delivery, and the ovaries become normal in size within several weeks (75). Simultaneously, elevated androgen levels decrease rapidly, usually becoming normal within 2 weeks postpartum.

Gross Findings. Pregnancy luteomas vary in size from microscopic to over 20 cm in diameter; a median diameter of 6.6 cm was found in one study (76). The cut surfaces are solid, fleshy, circumscribed, and red to brown (fig. 22-29); hemorrhagic foci are common. The lesions form multiple nodules in almost half of the cases and are bilateral in at least one third. Examination of affected ovaries days to weeks postpartum reveals brown puckered scars (fig. 22-30).

Microscopic Findings. Low-power examination discloses masses of cells (fig. 22-31), which occasionally contain follicles filled with pale fluid or colloid-like material (fig. 22-32). The cells are intermediate in size between the luteinized granulosa cells and luteinized theca cells of adjacent follicles, and have abundant eosinophilic cytoplasm,

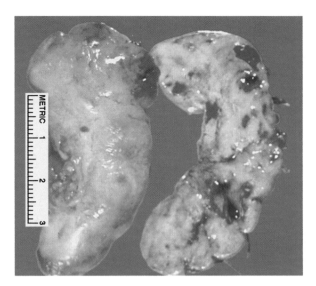

Figure 22-30
PREGNANCY LUTEOMA, POSTPARTUM

This previously conserved ovary was contralateral to the one shown in figure 22-29. The luteomas have regressed, appearing as small, dark brown, puckered foci; a fresh corpus luteum is also visible at the upper right of the external and sectioned surfaces. (Fig. 4 from Malinak LR, Miller GV. Bilateral multicentric ovarian luteomas of pregnancy associated with masculinization of a female infant. Am J Obstet Gynecol 1965;91:251–9.)

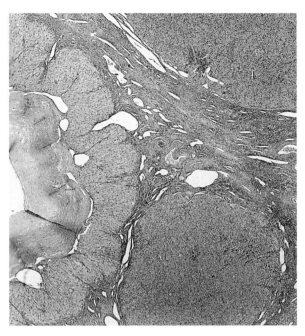

Figure 22-31
PREGNANCY LUTEOMA

Two luteomas are present adjacent to a cystic corpus luteum. (Fig. 125 from Serov SF, Scully RE, Sobin LH. Histological typing of ovarian tumours. International Histological Classification of Tumours No. 9. Geneva: World Health Organization, 1973.)

which contains little or no stainable lipid, and central nuclei. The nuclei may vary slightly in size and are hyperchromatic; nucleoli are usually prominent (fig. 22-33). Mitotic figures, which range up to 7 per 10 high-power fields, with an average of 2 or 3, are usually present (fig. 22-34); occasional mitotic figures may be atypical (76). Less common features include focal balloon-like degeneration of the cytoplasm and intracellular colloid droplets similar to those seen in the corpus luteum of pregnancy. The stroma is scanty and reticulin fibrils surround groups of cells. Examination of lesions removed postpartum shows shrunken aggregates of degenerating lipid-filled luteoma cells with pyknotic nuclei, infiltration by lymphocytes, and fibrosis (fig. 22-35).

Differential Diagnosis. When pregnancy luteomas are multiple, intraoperative inspection may suggest nodules of metastatic tumor. Such a diagnosis can usually be excluded by frozen section examination of one of the nodules but the distinction may be difficult if the patient has a history or clinical evidence of an oxyphilic malignant tumor

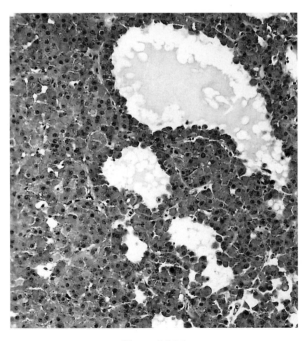

Figure 22-32
PREGNANCY LUTEOMA
Several follicle-like spaces are present.

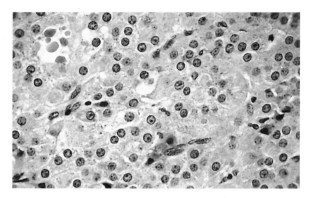

Figure 22-33
PREGNANCY LUTEOMA
The lesional cells have abundant cytoplasm, which was eosinophilic, and regular, round nuclei with prominent nucleoli.

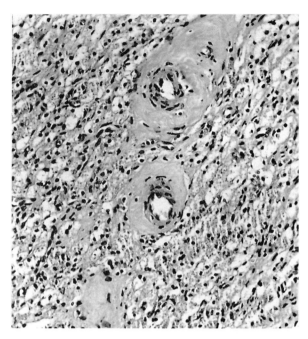

Figure 22-35
PREGNANCY LUTEOMA, POSTPARTUM
The luteoma cells have degenerated and contain pale cytoplasm and pyknotic nuclei. This illustration corresponds to a nodule shown in figure 22-30. (Fig. 125 from Serov SF, Scully RE, Sobin LH. Histological typing of ovarian tumours. International Histological Classification of Tumours No. 9. Geneva: World Health Organization, 1973.)

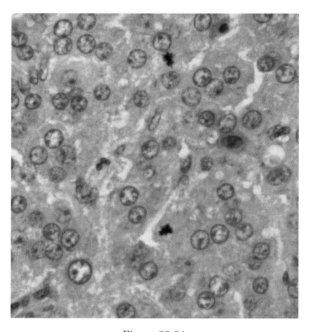

Figure 22-34
PREGNANCY LUTEOMA
The lesional cells have abundant eosinophilic cytoplasm. Two mitotic figures are visible.

such as a malignant melanoma. When the luteoma is a single nodule, the microscopic differential diagnosis also includes an extensively luteinized thecoma (page 192), a lipid-poor or lipid-free steroid cell tumor (page 237), and other tumors listed in Table 6-1. An ovarian mass composed entirely of lipid-free steroid-type cells from a pregnant woman in the third trimester

should be considered a pregnancy luteoma unless there is convincing evidence to the contrary.

HYPERREACTIO LUTEINALIS

Definition. This lesion is characterized by bilateral ovarian enlargement due to the presence of numerous luteinized follicle cysts that develop during pregnancy or ovulation induction (ovarian hyperstimulation syndrome).

General Features. Hyperreactio luteinalis most frequently accompanies disorders associated with elevated hCG levels, such as hydatidiform mole, choriocarcinoma, fetal hydrops, and multigestation (82,84,86,89). The frequency of hyperreactio luteinalis in women with gestational trophoblastic disease (GTD) ranges from 10 to almost 40 percent, depending on whether the method of detection is clinical examination or ultrasonography. Sixty percent of the lesions unassociated with GTD have occurred during a normal singleton pregnancy (85,92).

Hyperreactio luteinalis may be detected as a pelvic mass during any trimester of pregnancy, at the time of cesarean section, or rarely, during the puerperium (80). Symptoms are usually absent, but hemorrhage into the cysts may cause abdominal pain. Rarely, the involved ovary undergoes torsion or rupture, with intra-abdominal bleeding, which is exceptionally fatal. In patients with hyperreactio luteinalis secondary to GTD, ovarian enlargement may be detected at the time of diagnostic dilatation and curettage or during the postoperative follow-up period. In approximately 15 percent of the cases unassociated with trophoblastic disease, there has been virilization of the patient but not the female infant (81). Elevated plasma testosterone levels have been demonstrated in these patients as well as in nonvirilized patients with trophoblastic disease, with the levels paralleling the degree of ovarian enlargement. Regression of hyperreactio luteinalis typically occurs during the puerperium, but may be incomplete until 6 months postpartum (80). In exceptional cases the cysts regress spontaneously during pregnancy (88). In cases associated with trophoblastic disease, gradual regression typically occurs 2 to 12 weeks after uterine evacuation (84); occasionally, however, the cysts may persist for long periods after the hCG level has returned to normal (89).

The ovarian hyperstimulation syndrome develops in women undergoing ovulation induction, typically after the administration of an FSH preparation followed by hCG, and less often after the administration of clomiphene alone (83,87,90,91). The syndrome occurs only after ovulation and is more severe in patients who conceive. The disorder is particularly prone to occur if the ovaries were polycystic before the institution of therapy. In severe cases, the ovaries can become massively enlarged, and ascites, sometimes with hydrothorax (acute Meigs' syndrome), can develop due to increased serosal permeability. Hemoconcentration associated with oliguria and thromboembolic phenomena is a life-threatening complication. Elevation of plasma estrogens, progesterone, and testosterone typically occurs. High plasma levels of renin, aldosterone, and antidiuretic hormone have been reported (87). Careful selection of patients for ovulation induction and regulation of drug dosage by monitoring estrogen levels and ovarian size have reduced the frequency of the syndrome. Pa-

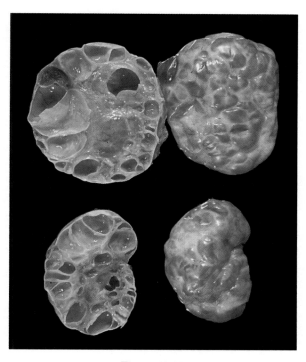

Figure 22-36
HYPERREACTIO LUTEINALIS
Both ovaries are enlarged by multiple thin-walled cysts.

tients with the ovarian hyperstimulation syndrome usually respond to conservative therapy, such as cyst aspiration under ultrasonographic guidance, and the cysts typically regress within 6 weeks. Surgical intervention in cases of hyperreactio luteinalis and the ovarian hyperstimulation syndrome is needed only to remove infarcted tissue, control hemorrhage, or diminish androgen production in virilized patients.

Gross Findings. Multiple, almost always bilateral, thin-walled cysts result in moderate to massive enlargement of the ovaries (fig. 22-36), which may be over 35 cm in diameter. The cysts are filled with clear or hemorrhagic fluid.

Microscopic Findings. Microscopic examination reveals multiple, large follicle cysts, in which the theca interna cells and, to a lesser degree, the granulosa cells lining the cysts are hyperplastic, enlarged, and luteinized (fig. 22-37); occasionally, the luteinized granulosa cells have bizarre nuclei. Marked edema of the luteinized theca layer and the intervening stroma (figs. 22-38, 22-39) is common; the stroma may contain luteinized cells. Examination of the ovaries in the

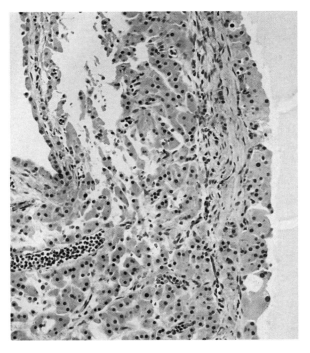

Figure 22-37
HYPERREACTIO LUTEINALIS
Two cysts are lined by luteinized granulosa cells, beneath which are luteinized theca cells.

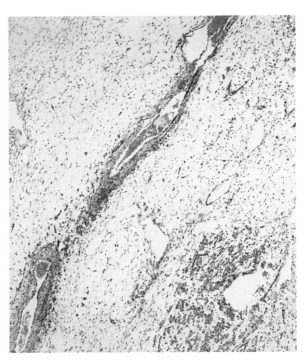

Figure 22-39
HYPERREACTIO LUTEINALIS
The ovarian stroma is markedly edematous.

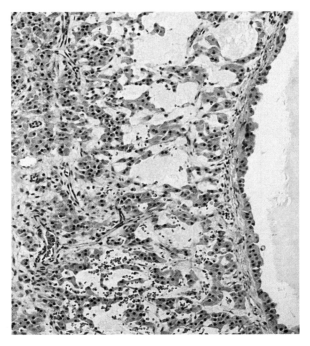

Figure 22-38
HYPERREACTIO LUTEINALIS
There is prominent edema in the luteinized theca cell layer.

hyperstimulation syndrome shows one or more corpora lutea in addition to the above changes.

Differential Diagnosis. Misinterpretation of the gross appearance of the enlarged ovaries of hyperreactio luteinalis as cystic ovarian tumors occasionally leads to an unwarranted bilateral oophorectomy. If doubt exists about the diagnosis, a frozen section examination of the cyst wall should solve the problem. Rarely, pregnancy luteomas coexist with hyperreactio luteinalis, heightening the suspicion of a neoplasm at operation.

LARGE SOLITARY LUTEINIZED FOLLICLE CYST OF PREGNANCY AND PUERPERIUM

Definition. This unilateral cyst appears during pregnancy or the puerperium and is characterized by an unusually large size and a lining composed of luteinized cells, some of which contain bizarre nuclei.

General Features. The cyst may cause abdominal swelling, but it is usually an incidental finding at the time of cesarean section or on

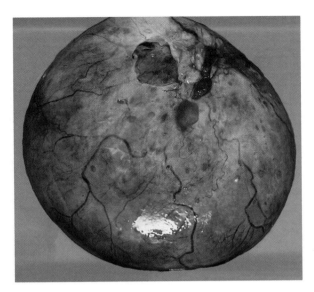

Figure 22-40
LARGE SOLITARY LUTEINIZED FOLLICLE
CYST OF PREGNANCY AND PUERPERIUM
This unilocular cyst was 25 cm in diameter.

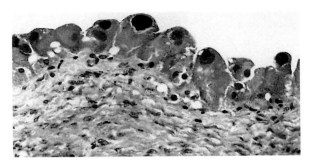

Figure 22-41
LARGE SOLITARY LUTEINIZED FOLLICLE
CYST OF PREGNANCY AND PUERPERIUM
A cyst is lined by cells with large bizarre nuclei and abundant cytoplasm, which was eosinophilic. (Fig. 6-2 from Clement PB. Tumor-like conditions of the ovary. In: Roth LM, Czernobilsky B, eds. Tumors and tumor-like conditions of the ovary. New York: Churchill-Livingstone, 1995:111.)

routine physical examination during the first postpartum visit (93). No endocrine disturbance has been reported to date.

Gross Findings. The cyst is unilocular and thin-walled, and contains watery fluid (fig. 22-40). The diameter ranged from 8 to 26 (median, 25) cm in one series (93).

Microscopic Findings. The cyst lining is composed of one to several layers of luteinized granulosa and theca cells, which frequently appear indistinguishable. Nests of luteinized cells may be embedded within fibrous tissue in the cyst wall. The cells have abundant eosinophilic to vacuolated cytoplasm, vary considerably in size and shape, and in all the reported cases have exhibited focal marked nuclear pleomorphism and hyperchromasia; mitotic figures have been absent (fig. 22-41). All the patients have had an uneventful postoperative course.

Differential Diagnosis. The major differential diagnosis involves unilocular cystic granulosa cell tumors of either the adult or juvenile type, both of which may be indistinguishable from the luteinized cyst on gross inspection, but rarely have bizarre nuclei and typically have foci of obvious tumor in the cyst wall (pages 177 and 180).

GRANULOSA CELL PROLIFERATIONS OF PREGNANCY

General and Pathologic Features. Granulosa cell proliferations that simulate or possibly are small neoplasms have been encountered as incidental findings in the ovaries of pregnant women (94). The older literature documented the presence of similar lesions in the ovaries of nonpregnant women (95), and we have seen them in a newborn ovary that also contained a corpus luteum. The lesions in the pregnant patients are usually multiple and lie within atretic follicles enveloped by a thick layer of luteinized theca cells. The granulosa cells may be arranged in solid, insular, microfollicular (fig. 22-42), or trabecular patterns, mimicking similar patterns in clinically evident granulosa cell tumors. In one case, a solid tubular pattern was identical to that seen in some Sertoli cell tumors (fig. 22-43). The granulosa cells typically have scanty cytoplasm and grooved nuclei, resembling the cells of the adult-type granulosa cell tumor. In the case with the sertoliform pattern, the cells contained moderate amounts of finely vacuolated cytoplasm suggesting the presence of lipid (94). In one case, there were large nodules of luteinized granulosa cells with variably sized, round, nongrooved nuclei, resembling pregnancy luteomas except for their obvious origin in granulosa cells and the larger size of their cells (94).

Differential Diagnosis. The differential diagnosis in most of the cases is with a small

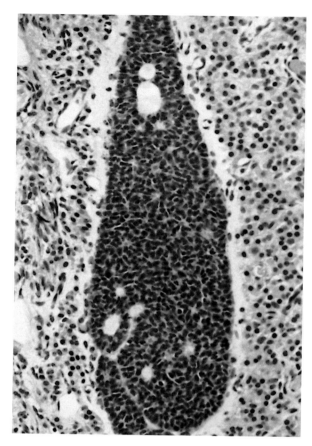

Figure 22-42
GRANULOSA CELL PROLIFERATION
IN PREGNANCY
An atretic follicle from a pregnant patient is filled with
a proliferation of granulosa cells growing in a pattern sim-
ulating that of a microfollicular granulosa cell tumor.

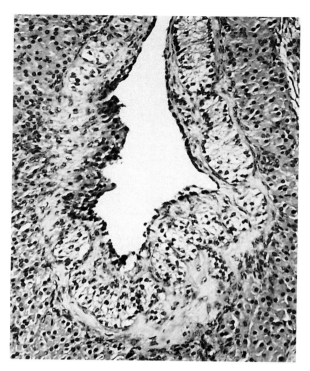

Figure 22-43
GRANULOSA CELL PROLIFERATION
IN PREGNANCY
The granulosa cell layer of a cystic atretic follicle is replaced
by solid tubules simulating those of a Sertoli cell tumor. The
tubules are surrounded by a layer of theca lutein cells.

granulosa cell or Sertoli cell tumor. Although
similar proliferations have been previously interpreted as small tumors, the frequency of the
lesions during pregnancy suggests an unusual
non-neoplastic hormonal response, possibly to
an intrinsic FSH-like function of hCG. The microscopic size of the lesions, their multifocality,
and their confinement to atretic follicles support
this interpretation.

HILUS (LEYDIG) CELL
PROLIFERATION OF PREGNANCY

A proliferation of hilus cells is occasionally
striking during pregnancy (fig. 22-44), consistent with their sensitivity to endogenous as well

as exogenous hCG stimulation (96). Hilus cell
proliferation may account for at least some of the
hirsutism that is frequently observed during the
pregnant state.

ECTOPIC DECIDUA

A decidual reaction in the ovary is most commonly a response to the hormonal milieu of pregnancy (97–105). Ectopic decidua may be seen as
early as the ninth week of gestation, and is present
in almost all ovaries at term. Although ovarian
decidua is not associated with clinical manifestations, it is accompanied rarely by masses of extraovarian intra-abdominal decidua, which may
result in massive, sometimes fatal, bleeding (104).

Gross examination may be unrevealing or disclose variably sized tan, often hemorrhagic nodules on the ovarian surface. On microscopic examination, the decidual cells typically occur in the
superficial cortical stroma and on the ovarian

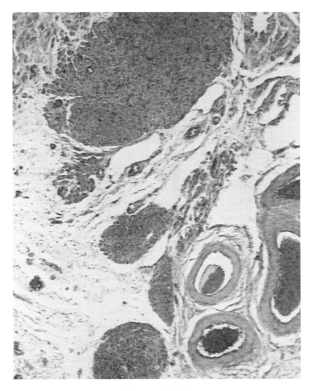

Figure 22-44
HILUS CELL PROLIFERATION,
NODULAR, DURING PREGNANCY

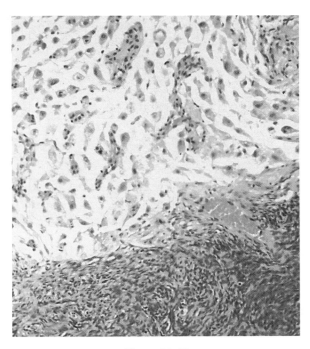

Figure 22-45
ECTOPIC DECIDUA ON OVARIAN SURFACE
One cell is vacuolated, somewhat resembling a signet-ring cell.

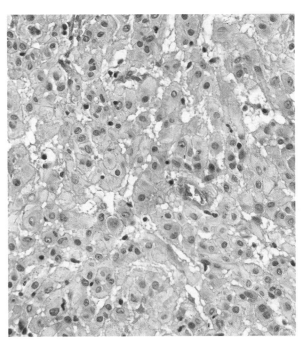

Figure 22-46
ECTOPIC DECIDUA FROM PREGNANT PATIENT

Large nodules were present on the ovarian and perito-neal surfaces. The cells have central, pale, round nuclei and abundant cytoplasm.

surface, often within periovarian adhesions, and are usually indistinguishable from eutopic decidual cells on light microscopic (figs. 22-45, 22-46) and ultrastructural examination (100). Prominent distended capillaries and a sprinkling of lymphocytes are typically found within the decidual foci. Smooth muscle cells, probably derived from submesothelial myofibroblasts (101) or ovarian stroma, may be admixed. Focal mild nuclear pleomorphism and hyperchromasia, sometimes in association with hemorrhagic necrosis, should not be misinterpreted as evidence of a malignant tumor. Occasionally, ectopic decidual cells contain vacuoles and eccentric nuclei, simulating signet-ring cells (fig. 22-45) (99). The bland appearance of most of the nuclei, the absence of mitotic figures, the periodic acid–Schiff (PAS) negativity of the vacuoles, and the association with pregnancy should facilitate the correct diagnosis. Ectopic decidua in postpartum patients may undergo hyalinization.

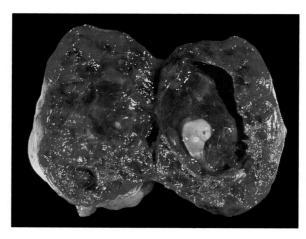

Figure 22-47
ECTOPIC PREGNANCY
The ovary is replaced by a hemorrhagic mass within which a small, pale yellow fetus is identifiable.

Less commonly, ovarian decidua is associated with trophoblastic disease; or occurs after progestin therapy, in the vicinity of a corpus luteum, in association with hormonally active neoplastic and non-neoplastic lesions of the ovary or adrenal gland, or following pelvic irradiation (98). It may, however, be idiopathic in both premenopausal and postmenopausal women (98,103). In these various settings, ectopic decidua rarely, if ever, simulates a neoplasm.

OVARIAN PREGNANCY

In some series, up to 1 percent of all ectopic pregnancies have been ovarian (107). The diagnosis of ovarian pregnancy should be restricted to cases in which there is no involvement of the fallopian tube. There is an increased frequency of ovarian pregnancy in patients with an intrauterine contraceptive device (106). The typical clinical presentation is severe pain with hemoperitoneum, and at laparotomy and on gross examination the enlarged hemorrhagic ovary may mimic a hemorrhagic neoplasm. In a minority of the cases, an embryo can be identified grossly (fig. 22-47); in other cases microscopic examination is diagnostic. An ovarian pregnancy is distinguished from very rare examples of primary ovarian gestational trophoblastic disease (page 331) by applying criteria similar to those used in the uterus.

ENDOMETRIOSIS

Definition. This is the presence of tissue resembling endometrium outside the endometrium and myometrium. Usually both epithelium and stroma are seen, but occasionally the diagnosis can be made when only one component is present. Tumors and preneoplastic lesions arising from endometriosis are discussed in chapter 5.

General Features. Ovarian endometriosis is typically encountered in women in the reproductive age group, but is occasionally seen in postmenopausal women. As ovarian endometriosis is often associated with extraovarian pelvic endometriosis, the symptoms include, to varying degrees, dysmenorrhea; lower abdominal, pelvic, and back pain; dyspareunia; irregular bleeding; and infertility, which is present in up to 30 percent of the cases (109). Some patients are asymptomatic and have a palpable adnexal mass on pelvic examination. Rare complications of ovarian endometriosis include rupture with acute abdominal symptoms, usually during pregnancy (121), and ascites, which may be serosanguineous; the presence of ascites, particularly in the setting of an ovarian mass, may suggest an ovarian neoplasm (117).

Gross Findings. Depending on their duration and their superficial or deep location in the ovary, endometriotic foci may appear as punctate, red, blue, brown, or white spots or patches with either a slightly raised or a puckered surface (figs. 22-48, 22-49) (114,119). Brown areas have sometimes been described as "powder burns" (109). The endometriotic foci are frequently associated with adhesions.

Endometriotic cysts (endometriomas), which rarely exceed 15 cm in diameter, may partially or completely replace normal ovarian tissue and are commonly covered by dense fibrous adhesions, which can result in fixation to adjacent structures. The cysts are bilateral in one third to half of the cases (115,116). They usually have a thick, fibrotic wall and a shaggy, brown to yellow lining (fig. 22-50), although in some cases much of the cyst lining is smooth and pale (fig. 22-51). The cyst contents typically consist of semi-fluid or inspissated, chocolate-colored material (fig. 22-50); rarely, the cyst is filled with watery fluid. Any solid areas in the cyst wall or intraluminal polypoid projections should be sampled microscopically as

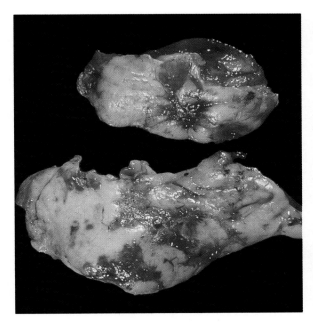

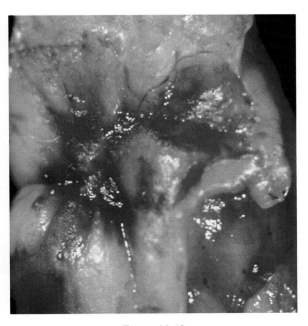

Figure 22-48
ENDOMETRIOSIS
The external surfaces of ovarian wedges show red, blue, and brown areas, several of which are associated with fibrotic puckering.

Figure 22-49
ENDOMETRIOSIS
The red to brown, puckered area in figure 22-48 is shown at a higher magnification.

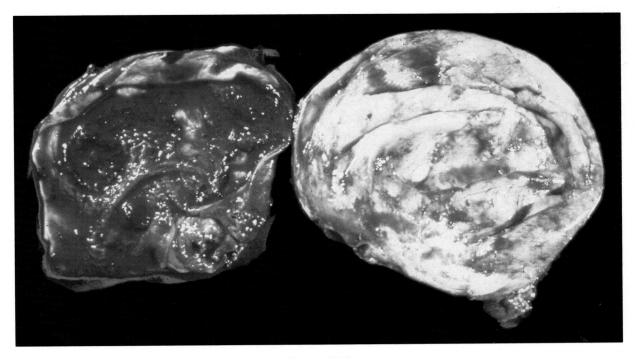

Figure 22-50
ENDOMETRIOTIC CYST
The outer surface has many foci of red-brown discoloration and adhesions. The lumen contains chocolate-colored fluid.

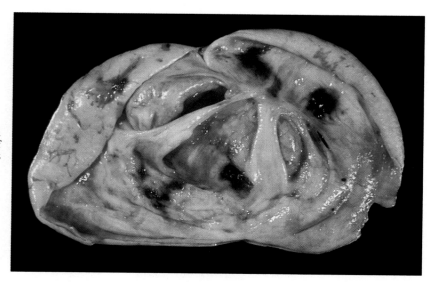

Figure 22-51
ENDOMETRIOTIC CYST
Although most of the lining is pale and smooth, the presence of several foci of dark brown discoloration is consistent with endometriosis.

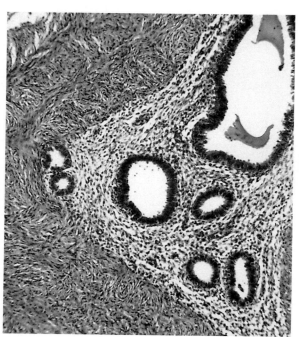

Figure 22-52
ENDOMETRIOSIS
Endometrioid glands that vary in size lie in cellular endometrial-type stroma within denser ovarian stroma.

they may be malignant tumors of epithelial or occasionally stromal origin (see chapter 5). Rarely, an adenomyoma forms a discrete nodule in the cyst wall.

Microscopic Findings. Noncystic ovarian endometriosis is characterized by endometrioid glands surrounded by endometrial-type stroma (fig. 22-52). The lesions may be seen anywhere in the ovary, but are often most conspicuous superficially and may be incorporated into fibrous adhesions. The glands may be proliferative (fig. 22-53) or secretory (108,120), or exhibit atypical hyperplasia (113) (page 107) or some type of endometrial metaplasia; an Arias-Stella reaction may occur during pregnancy (fig. 22-54). The stroma most often resembles typical endometrial stroma, but its appearance may be altered, to varying degrees, by hemorrhage and a frequently striking, occasionally exclusive component of histiocytes containing hemofuscin (fig. 22-53), hemosiderin, or both (so called pseudoxanthoma cells) (111). Rarely, prominent cholesterol clefts or so-called Liesegang rings are present (fig. 22-55) (110). In pregnant patients and women taking progestational agents, a decidual change, which may be striking, is sometimes present (fig. 22-56).

The epithelial lining and underlying stroma of an endometriotic cyst frequently become attenuated, and the former may be reduced to a single layer of cuboidal cells that may appear nonspecific. In such circumstances, recognition of the cyst as endometriotic may be possible only if a rim of subjacent endometrioid stroma persists. Commonly, the stroma is replaced by dense fibrous tissue containing fibroblasts with distinctive small spindle-shaped nuclei (fig. 22-57) and variable numbers of pseudoxanthoma cells. The epithelial cells lining an endometriotic cyst

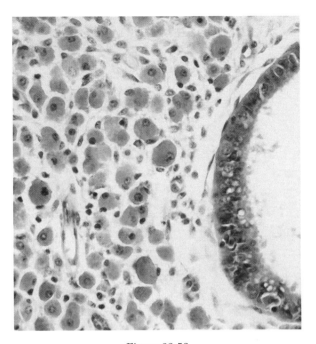

Figure 22-53
ENDOMETRIOSIS
The wall of an endometriotic cyst contains pseudo-xanthoma cells filled with hemofuscin pigment.

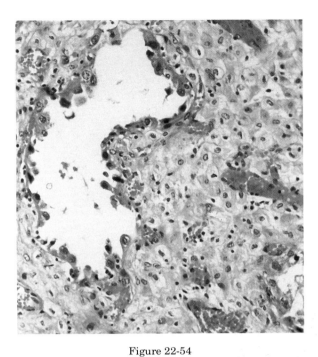

Figure 22-54
ENDOMETRIOSIS (DURING PREGNANCY)
A gland is lined by cells with hyperchromatic, smudgy nuclei of the type seen in the Arias-Stella reaction. The adjacent stroma shows decidual change.

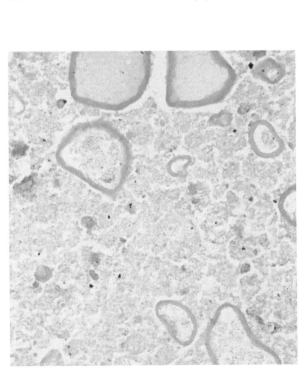

Figure 22-55
ENDOMETRIOSIS
Liesegang rings are scattered in debris.

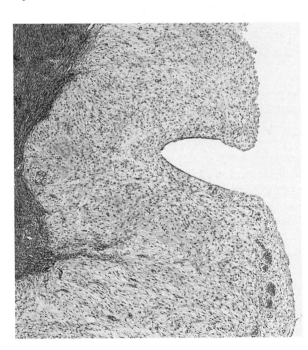

Figure 22-56
ENDOMETRIOSIS (IN PATIENT TAKING NORETHYNODREL WITH MESTRANOL)
There is marked decidual change of the stroma.

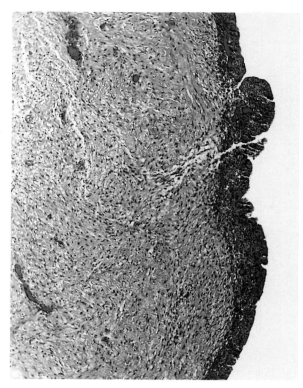

Figure 22-57
ENDOMETRIOSIS
The deeper portion of the wall of an endometriotic cyst is fibrotic. The subepithelial layer is composed of hemorrhagic cellular stroma.

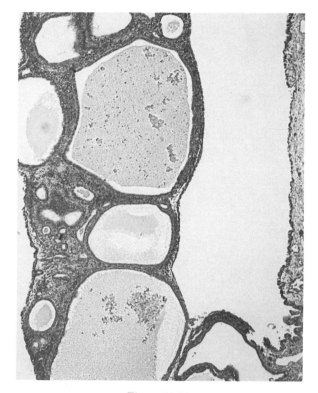

Figure 22-58
POLYPOID ENDOMETRIOSIS
A polyp composed mainly of cystic glands projects into the lumen of an endometriotic cyst.

may become large and cuboidal, with abundant eosinophilic cytoplasm and large atypical nuclei (113,122). The malignant potential of these cells is uncertain (page 107). Some endometriotic cysts contain variable amounts of smooth muscle bundles in their walls.

Both ovarian and extraovarian endometriosis may resemble an endometrial polyp (polypoid endometriosis) (fig. 22-58), or form granuloma-like lesions, so-called necrotic pseudoxanthomatous nodules. These lesions are characterized by a central zone of necrosis surrounded by pseudoxanthoma cells, often in a palisaded arrangement; hyalinized fibrous tissue; or both (figs. 22-59, 22-60) (111); typical endometriotic glands with stroma may be absent. Rare cases of ovarian endometriosis are characterized by an absence of glands, so-called stromal endometriosis (112, 118). Such foci are almost always microscopic and are usually unassociated with endometriosis

elsewhere. They probably result from focal metaplasia of the ovarian stroma (118).

In most postmenopausal patients with endometriosis, the endometriotic tissue is atrophic, resembling simple or cystic atrophy of the endometrium. In a minority of cases, however, the endometriotic tissue appears active, with or without metaplastic and hyperplastic changes, as seen more commonly in premenopausal women.

Differential Diagnosis. Endometriotic cysts may simulate cystic ovarian tumors clinically and at operation. Because of the occasional origin of tumors in them, they must be examined grossly and sampled microscopically with great care. Differentiation from an endometrioid cystadenoma is discussed on page 109. The necrotic pseudoxanthomatous nodules of endometriosis, particularly when situated on the peritoneum and associated with an ovarian endometriotic cyst, may be mistaken at operation for metastatic tumor.

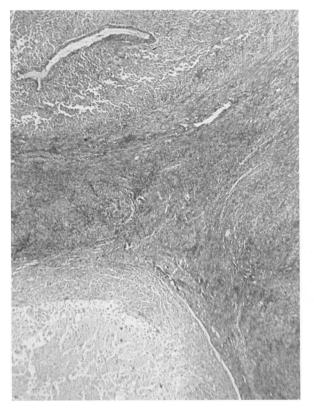

Figure 22-59
ENDOMETRIOSIS
Two pseudoxanthomatous necrotic nodules are seen at the top and bottom. An endometriotic gland is seen in the upper nodule.

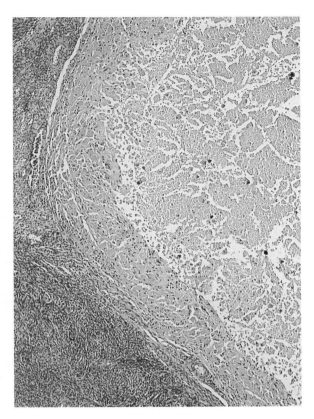

Figure 22-60
ENDOMETRIOSIS
A pseudoxanthomatous nodule is centrally necrotic with a surrounding granulomatous reaction.

INFECTIOUS DISEASES

Due to Miscellaneous Bacteria

Ovarian involvement in pelvic inflammatory disease (PID) is almost always secondary to salpingitis, and generally takes the form of a tubo-ovarian abscess (fig. 22-61), which is usually bilateral. The typical clinical manifestations are abdominal or pelvic pain, and less often, fever, vaginal discharge or bleeding, and urinary symptoms (142). An adnexal mass is palpable, demonstrable with imaging techniques, or visible at laparoscopy. A history of an acute infectious episode is present in only one third to half of the cases, suggesting that subclinical infections are common (142). A mixed flora with a preponderance of anaerobic organisms is typically recovered from the contents of the abscess (131,142). With resolution, the only sequelae may be tubo-ovarian fibrous adhesions, but occasionally a healed abscess becomes a cyst.

A unilateral or bilateral ovarian abscess without tubal involvement (fig. 22-62) is much rarer than a tubo-ovarian abscess. The former is usually secondary to direct or lymphatic spread of organisms from a nongynecologic pelvic inflammatory process, such as diverticulitis, appendicitis, inflammatory bowel disease, or postoperative pelvic infection. Rarely, an ovarian abscess is the result of blood-borne infection (158,159).

The external surface of an ovarian abscess is often unremarkable, and the process may not be apparent until the organ is sectioned. Uncommonly, rupture of an ovarian or tubo-ovarian abscess leads to secondary peritonitis (151) or rarely, fistulas involving the colon (156), urinary bladder (144), or vagina (130).

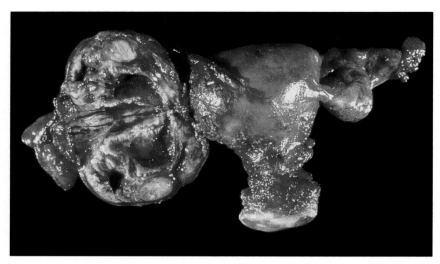

Figure 22-61
TUBO-OVARIAN ABSCESS
(COMPLICATING COLONIC
DIVERTICULITIS)
The left ovary and tube have been
transformed into a multicystic mass
with a yellow lining.

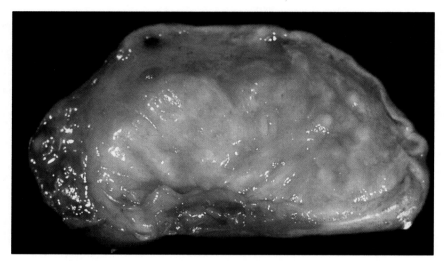

Figure 22-62
OVARIAN ABSCESS
ASSOCIATED WITH
CROHN'S DISEASE
The sectioned surface is exten-
sively replaced by yellow tissue,
which was soft.

Milder, chronic or recurrent forms of ovarian involvement by PID may take the form of a chronic perioophoritis, with tubo-ovarian and peri-ovarian adhesions. Polycystic ovarian changes have been described in such cases (153). Rarely, a chronic abscess results in a solid tumor-like mass, variably designated xanthogranuloma, xanthogranulomatous oophoritis, or inflammatory pseudotumor (150) and characterized microscopically by admixtures of foamy histiocytes, multinucleated giant cells, plasma cells, neutrophils, foci of necrosis, and fibrosis (fig. 22-63). Several examples of pseudotumorous xanthogranuloma with more diffuse involvement of the adnexa have been described (140,141,155).

Actinomycosis

Pelvic actinomycosis is usually a complication of an intrauterine device (IUD), although most cases of IUD-related PID are nonactinomycotic (127,128,135,136,147,154). Almost 85 percent of the cases have occurred in women who have had an IUD in place for 3 or more years. The adnexal involvement is usually unilateral, with abscesses, which are often multiple, involving the ovary and fallopian tube (fig. 22-64). Rarely, the characteristic actinomycotic (sulfur) granules may be grossly visible within the abscess cavities.

Microscopic examination reveals a characteristic but nonspecific inflammatory infiltrate composed predominantly of neutrophils and

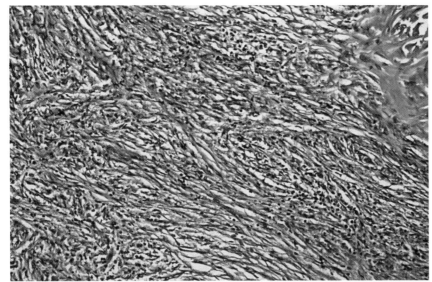

Figure 22-63
XANTHOGRANULOMA
The ovarian stroma is replaced by collagenous tissue containing numerous chronic inflammatory cells.

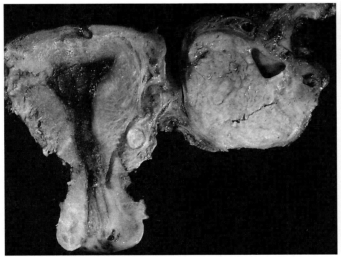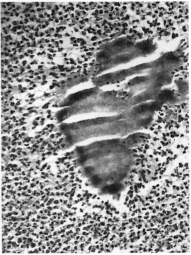

Figure 22-64
ACTINOMYCOSIS
The ovary is replaced by tissue that was soft and yellow. A characteristic sulfur granule surrounded by polymorphonuclear leukocytes is seen on the right.

foamy histiocytes, sometimes admixed with lymphocytes and plasma cells. A specific histologic diagnosis can be made only by finding the sulfur granules within the inflammatory exudate (fig. 22-64), but numerous blocks may be necessary to demonstrate them. The granules are composed of circumscribed rounded collections of basophilic, gram-positive bacteria growing as branching filaments, with a characteristic radial or palisading pattern at the periphery. A fluorescent antibody stain may facilitate their detection (152). A diagnosis of actinomycosis may be made prior to salpingo-oophorectomy in some cases by finding the granules within endometrial curettings or cervicovaginal smears. Almost 90 percent of patients with actinomyces demonstrated in the latter specimens have a tubo-ovarian abscess (128,136).

Tuberculosis

Tuberculous oophoritis is uncommon and usually secondary to tuberculous salpingitis. The tubes are almost always involved in tuberculosis of the female genital tract, but the ovary is affected in only 10 percent of the cases (149). On gross inspection, the ovaries are typically adherent to the tubal ampullae. Grossly visible caseation is rare. On histologic examination, the tuberculosis is typically confined to the cortex. In cases in which the ovary is enlarged, granulomas on the adjacent peritoneum may simulate metastatic ovarian cancer at operation (149,157).

Malacoplakia

Of approximately 25 reported cases of gynecological malacoplakia, only 3 have involved the ovary (123,138). Friable, yellow, focally hemorrhagic and necrotic masses occupy one or both ovaries and the adjacent fallopian tubes. In one case, the process also involved contiguous portions of small and large bowel, simulating a malignant ovarian tumor (138). Histologic examination revealed the typical features of malacoplakia.

Parasitic Infections

Parasitic infections of the ovary are extremely rare in most parts of the world. Ovarian schistosomiasis, however, is common in endemic areas; the fallopian tube is typically also involved (124, 126,145). Patients usually have lower abdominal pain and a pelvic mass, and occasionally, irregular menses and infertility. The typical operative findings are enlargement of the tube or ovary, or both, numerous adhesions, and scattered peritoneal nodules, which may simulate the implants of a malignant tumor. On histologic examination, granulomas, often containing eosinophils, surround schistosoma ova. Dense fibrosis is frequently seen in the later stages of the disease.

Ovarian involvement by *Enterobius vermicularis* is usually an incidental finding on the external surface, or rarely, within the ovary (137, 143). In several cases, there has been simultaneous involvement of the pelvic peritoneum, simulating metastatic tumor (133). Granulomas, which may undergo caseation and may contain eosinophils, surround the adult female worms and ova (146). The worms probably reach the perito-

neal cavity by migrating from the perineum through the lumen of the female genital tract.

Rare cases of ovarian echinococcosis have been described (125,134). In one of them, a typical hydatid cyst enlarged an ovary to 12 cm in diameter.

Fungal Infections

Fungal infections of the ovary are extremely rare, even in patients with disseminated disease. Three examples of tubo-ovarian abscess, caused by *Blastomyces dermatitidis,* have been reported (132,148). In one case the abscesses were bilateral and associated with miliary nodules involving the pelvic peritoneum. In two of the cases the abscesses were probably secondary to hematogenous spread from the lungs, while in the third case the infection was sexually transmitted.

Seven of 11 patients with coccidioidomycosis of the upper female genital tract had tubo-ovarian and peritoneal involvement (129). One case of tubo-ovarian abscess caused by *Aspergillus* has been reported in an IUD user (139); rupture of the abscess led to generalized peritonitis.

GRANULOMAS

Foreign Body Granulomas

A variety of foreign materials may evoke a granulomatous reaction on the ovarian and extraovarian peritoneal surfaces, mimicking a malignant tumor at operation. Examples include lipid material used in hysterosalpingographic examinations (168), talc (164), starch granules from surgical gloves (165,166), douche fluid (163), and lubricants (167). Rarely, the starch granulomas are of the tuberculoid type, with or without caseous necrosis, and mimic tuberculosis on microscopic examination (165). Granulomatous oophoritis is occasionally secondary to bowel contents that entered the ovary via a colo-ovarian fistula (160–162). Finally, sebaceous material or keratin from a ruptured dermoid cyst or keratin or necrotic squamous cells from an endometrioid tumor with squamous differentiation of the endometrium or ovary may result in granulomas on peritoneal surfaces (page 127).

Isolated Palisading Granulomas

Isolated palisading granulomas of uncertain pathogenesis have been encountered in the

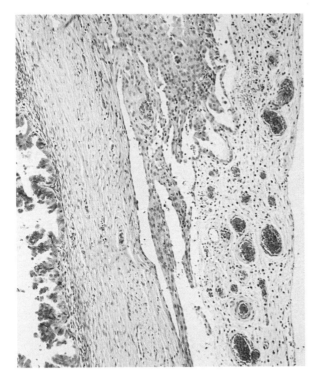

Figure 22-65
MESOTHELIAL HYPERPLASIA
Mesothelial cell hyperplasia (center) is evident between the vascular adhesion (right) and the outer surface of an ovarian serous borderline tumor (left).

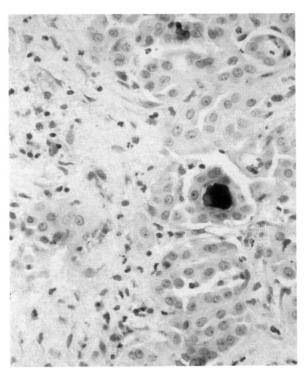

Figure 22-66
MESOTHELIAL HYPERPLASIA
The mesothelial cells have conspicuous, pale, eosinophilic cytoplasm. A small focus of calcification is evident. (High-power view of figure 22-65.)

ovary, usually as incidental microscopic findings (169–172). In five of eight reported cases, an operation had been performed on the involved ovary 6 months to 12 years earlier. The granulomas are typically multiple and occasionally bilateral. Central zones of fibrinoid necrosis or hyalinization are usually surrounded by palisading, sometimes multinucleated, histiocytes and variable numbers of other inflammatory cells including lymphocytes, plasma cells, and eosinophils; a fibrous pseudocapsule forms in some of the cases. In one series the granulomas contained carbon pigment produced by previous operative fulguration or laser therapy. The differential diagnosis of these granulomas includes other ovarian granulomas, including the necrotic pseudoxanthomatous nodules of endometriosis (page 434).

Granulomas Secondary to Systemic Disease

Four cases of ovarian involvement by sarcoidosis have been reported (174,176–178). The granulomas were incidental microscopic findings in each case. In the three cases reported in detail, the patients had systemic sarcoidosis with involvement of other gynecologic sites or para-aortic lymph nodes. The finding of sarcoid-like granulomas in the ovary should alert the pathologist to the possibility of a rare dysgerminoma with a granulomatous reaction sufficiently extensive to obscure the malignant tumor cells. Crohn's disease is another rare cause of granulomatous oophoritis, usually by direct extension of the inflammatory process from the bowel (173,175,179); the ipsilateral fallopian tube is also involved in most cases.

MESOTHELIAL PROLIFERATION

Proliferation of mesothelial cells within periovarian fibrous adhesions (figs. 22-65, 22-66) on the ovarian surface or elsewhere on the pelvic peritoneum is usually a response to pelvic inflammation, but also occurs overlying ovarian tumors

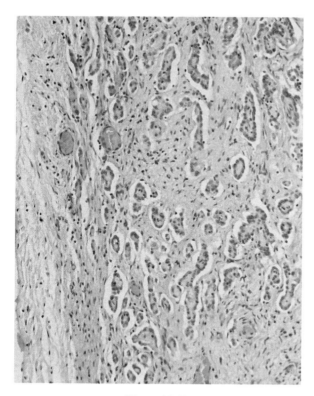

Figure 22-67
MESOTHELIAL HYPERPLASIA
Numerous small tubular structures and cords composed of
mesothelial cells are growing in parallel array.

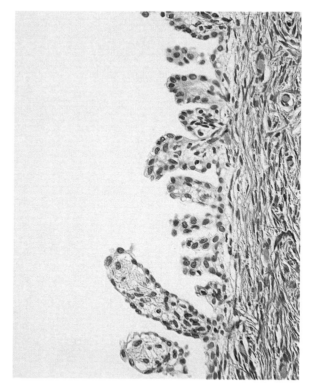

Figure 22-68
SURFACE EPITHELIAL-STROMAL PROLIFERATION

(181). Florid examples may be characterized by tubules, papillae, which may be complex, or both, lined by mildly to moderately atypical cells, sometimes with psammoma bodies. This combination of findings can simulate stromal invasion by a serous borderline tumor or peritoneal involvement by a carcinoma. The architectural features of mesothelial cell proliferation associated with adhesions, such as a linear arrangement of the cells more or less parallel to the surface (fig. 22-67), as well as cytologic and immunohistochemical differences between mesothelial cells and neoplastic epithelial cells are helpful in the differential diagnosis (page 73).

Rarely, multilocular or unilocular peritoneal inclusion cysts (see fig. 27-18) involve the ovarian surfaces extensively, suggesting at operation a primary ovarian cyst or cystic neoplasm (183). These cysts have also been reported to encase ovaries harboring metastatic colon carcinoma (182). Microscopic examination reveals cysts

with fibrous walls and a mesothelial lining; in some cases parallel arrays of mesothelial cells in the cyst walls may lead to an erroneous diagnosis of malignancy. The pathology of peritoneal inclusion cysts is discussed in detail elsewhere (180).

SURFACE EPITHELIAL-STROMAL PROLIFERATION

Polypoid stromal proliferations on the ovarian surface may be visible as warty excrescences on gross examination and are a common incidental microscopic finding in women of late reproductive and postmenopausal ages (fig. 22-68). These projections are composed mainly of ovarian stroma, which may be hyalinized, covered by a single layer of surface epithelium. The lesions are typically 1 to 3 mm in diameter and do not exceed 1 cm, the dividing line between this type of proliferation and a serous surface papillary adenofibroma.

AUTOIMMUNE OOPHORITIS

Approximately 25 cases of autoimmune oophoritis, a subtype of primary ovarian failure, have been documented pathologically (184–187). The patients, who have ranged in age from 17 to 48 (mean, 31) years, typically present with oligomenorrhea or amenorrhea, or manifestations related to multiple follicle cysts, including pelvic pain and adnexal torsion. Most patients have antibodies against steroid cells of various types in their sera; Addison's disease, Hashimoto's thyroiditis, or both; and a variety of other autoimmune disorders in some cases.

On gross examination, the ovaries may be small or normal in size, but in one third of the cases one or both are enlarged by multiple follicle cysts and may simulate cystic neoplasms (185–187). The cysts are more common in the earlier phases of the disease, and are probably due to elevated gonadotropin levels (185).

The cardinal feature on microscopic examination is a round cell infiltration of developing follicles. The intensity of the inflammatory infiltrate increases with the degree of follicular maturation. The theca interna layer is typically more intensely infiltrated than the granulosa layer and may be focally destroyed; the granulosa layer is usually disrupted focally, with sloughing of its cells into the follicular lumens. The inflammatory infiltrate consists predominantly of lymphocytes and plasma cells, but eosinophils, histiocytes, and occasionally, sarcoid-like granulomas are also present, and may predominate (187). In some cases, hilus cells are infiltrated by the inflammatory process.

TORSION AND INFARCTION

Ovarian or adnexal torsion is most frequently a complication of an ovarian or paraovarian lesion, usually a non-neoplastic cyst or benign tumor, but occasionally a malignant neoplasm (page 31) (188,191). Torsion of a normal ovary occurs rarely, especially in infants and children (193,194,196) but also in adults (195). Bilateral adnexal torsion, synchronous or asynchronous, has been reported (192).

The patients present with clinical findings similar to those of acute appendicitis or because of recurrent episodes of abdominal pain; occa-

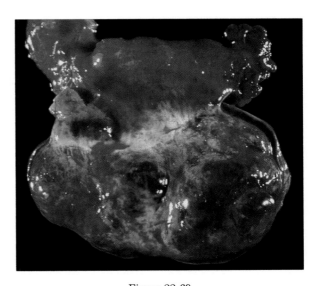

Figure 22-69
HEMORRHAGIC INFARCTION
The external surface of the ovary and fallopian tube is dusky red.

sionally, an adnexal mass is palpable. Laparotomy reveals a swollen hemorrhagic and, in some cases, infarcted tubo-ovarian mass twisted on its pedicle (fig. 22-69). In rare cases the torsion and infarction may be asymptomatic (188–190), and autoamputation may result in a mass, which is occasionally calcified, lying free in the peritoneal cavity or attached to adjacent structures. The possible role of intermittent torsion of the ovary in the development of massive edema has been mentioned on page 417.

It is crucial to examine thoroughly any hemorrhagic infarcted ovarian mass to exclude a neoplasm. A search should be made for viable foci at the periphery of the lesion and the necrotic tissue should be scrutinized for shadows of neoplastic cells. Oil-immersion magnification may be helpful in identifying the nature of the necrotic material.

CHANGES SECONDARY TO METABOLIC DISEASE

Amyloidosis occasionally involves the ovaries, typically as an incidental histologic finding in patients with systemic disease (197). There has been a single case of tumor-like amyloidosis confined to the ovary (199). Rare cases of ovarian enlargement secondary to involvement by systemic storage disorders have been reported (198,200). In

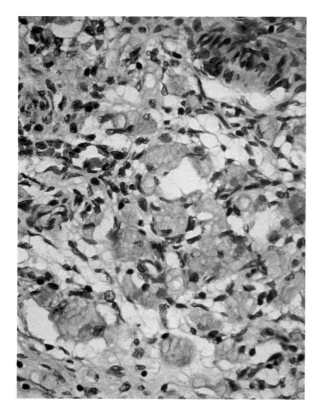

Figure 22-70
MUCICARMINOPHILIC HISTIOCYTOSIS
Histiocytes with abundant bubbly, gray-pink cytoplasm simulate signet-ring cells.

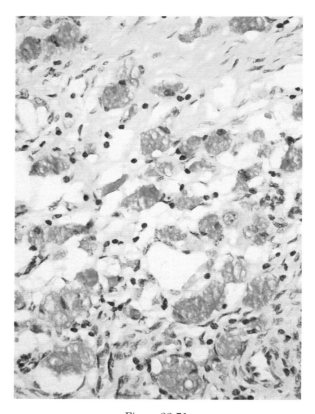

Figure 22-71
MUCICARMINOPHILIC HISTIOCYTOSIS
The histiocytes are mucicarminophilic; PAS staining was negative.

such cases, the stored material is typically within histiocytes, allowing histologic distinction from a steroid cell tumor.

MUCICARMINOPHILIC HISTIOCYTOSIS

A variety of tissues and organs from patients who have received polyvinylpyrrolidone (PVP), a blood substitute or "tonic," intravenously may accumulate mucicarminophilic histiocytes with eccentric nuclei and bubbly to basophilic cytoplasm, which simulate neoplastic signet-ring cells (figs. 22-70, 22-71) (202). In one series of cases the cells appeared within the ovary in 3 of 12 affected women. Similar cells often accumulate in lymph nodes, enhancing the resemblance to carcinoma. Features that distinguish this rare process from signet-ring cell carcinoma include absence of a mass, bland appearance of the nuclei, Congo red and Masson-Fontana positivity, and absence of

PAS staining. Similar mucicarminophilic histiocytes can accumulate beneath the peritoneal lining after topical administration of oxidized regenerated cellulose, a hemostatic agent (201). The cytoplasm of these cells is PAS positive diastase resistant, CD-68 positive, and S-100 and cytokeratin negative.

MISCELLANEOUS LESIONS

Rarely, a twisted, infarcted appendix epiploica becomes attached to the ovarian surface, simulating a small tumor. The finding of focal calcification on microscopic examination may cause confusion with a calcified epithelial neoplasm (fig. 22-72) but the presence of shadows of the necrotic lipocytes establishes the diagnosis.

A rare pseudoneoplastic alteration that we have seen in ovarian surface epithelial inclusion glands is characterized by a striking hydropic swelling of

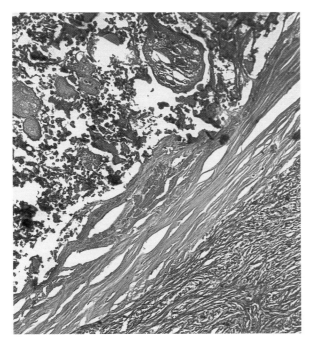

Figure 22-72
APPENDIX EPIPLOICA, INFARCTED,
ATTACHED TO SURFACE OF OVARY
The lesion (above) is focally calcified.

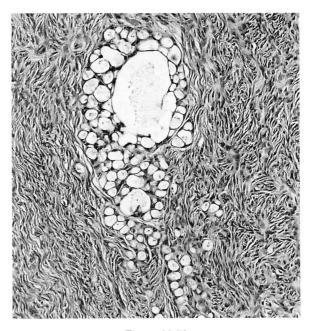

Figure 22-73
VACUOLAR CHANGE WITHIN SURFACE
EPITHELIAL INCLUSION GLANDS
The lining cells exhibit an hydropic change, simulating signet-ring cells.

the cytoplasm of the lining cells, which displaces the nucleus (fig. 22-73), mimicking signet-ring cell carcinoma, especially when the cells proliferate to form solid nests. Awareness of this phenomenon, additional sectioning, if necessary, to demonstrate a relation to inclusion glands, and negative staining for mucin facilitate the diagnosis.

The granulosa cells of normal follicles can be artifactually introduced into tissue spaces or vascular channels during sectioning (figs. 22-74, 22-75). This finding, especially when the displaced cells are shrunken or crushed, is occasionally misinterpreted as a small cell carcinoma. Awareness of this artifact, the bland nuclear features of the cells, and their similarity to cells lining nearby follicles are helpful clues to the correct diagnosis. Granulosa cells that appear to be deposited on the surface of the ovary secondary to follicle rupture also may be misinterpreted as mesothelial cells, and when numerous, may even suggest the diagnosis of mesothelioma. Immunohistochemical staining for granulosa cells, which are positive for vimentin and α-inhibin and may be positive for cytokeratin in a punctate pattern, may confirm their identity in difficult cases.

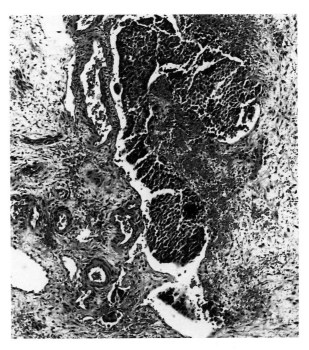

Figure 22-74
ARTIFACTUAL PRESENCE OF GRANULOSA
CELLS IN BLOOD VESSEL LUMEN

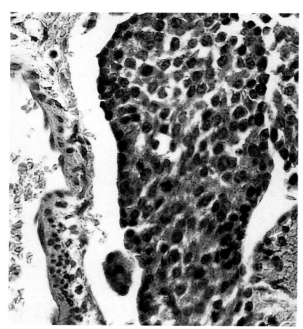

Figure 22-75
ARTIFACTUAL PRESENCE OF GRANULOSA
CELLS IN BLOOD VESSEL
The cells appeared identical to those lining a nearby graafian follicle.

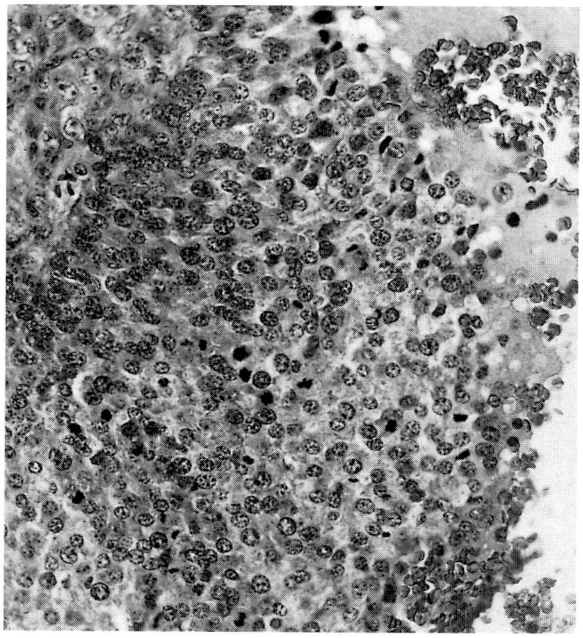

Figure 22-76
GRANULOSA CELLS OF PROLIFERATING
FOLLICLE EXHIBITING
MARKED MITOTIC ACTIVITY

Granulosa cells of the normal follicle typically exhibit brisk mitotic activity (fig. 22-76), and we have seen one case in which 27 mitotic figures were present in a single high-power field. Similarly, the theca externa cells of the normal developing follicle may contain numerous mitotic figures, occasionally misinterpreted as evidence of an incipient sarcoma (see fig. 1-17). Finally, the corpus luteum of late pregnancy and the puerperium may contain numerous round calcific deposits; we have seen one case in which their presence in a patient with a history of a serous borderline tumor was misinterpreted as recurrent tumor.

REFERENCES

Follicle Cyst

1. Adelman S, Benson CD, Hertzler JH. Surgical lesions of the ovary in infancy and childhood. Surg Gynecol Obstet 1975;141:219–26.
2. Ahmed S. Neonatal and childhood ovarian cysts. J Pediatr Surg 1971;6:702–8.
3. Brune WH, Pulaski EJ, Shuey HE. Giant ovarian cyst. Report of a case in a premature infant. N Engl J Med 1957;257:876–8.
4. Claman AD. Bleeding from ovary: graafian follicle and corpus luteum. Can Med Assn J 1957;76:1036–40.
5. Danon M, Robboy SJ, Kim S, Scully R, Crawford JD. Cushing's syndrome, sexual precocity and polyostotic fibrous dysplasia (Albright's syndrome) in infancy. J Pediatr 1975;87:917–21.
6. De Sa DJ. Follicular ovarian cysts in stillbirths and neonates. Arch Dis Child 1975;50:45–50.
7. Eberlein WR, Bongiovanni AM, Jones IT, Yakovac WC. Ovarian tumors and cysts associated with sexual precocity. J Pediatr 1960;57:484–97.
8. Fitzgerald JA, Berrigan MW. Accurate diagnosis of ovarian vascular accidents. Obstet Gynecol 1959;13:175–80.
9. Hoyt WF, Meigs JV. Rupture of graafian follicle and corpus luteum. Surg Gynecol Obstet 1936;62:114–7.

10. Liapi C, Evain-Brion D. Diagnosis of ovarian follicular cysts from birth to puberty: a report of twenty cases. Acta Pediatr Scand 1987;76:91–6.
11. Nussbaum AR, Sanders RC, Hartman DS, Dudgeon DL, Parmley TH. Neonatal ovarian cysts: sonographic-pathologic correlation. Radiology 1988;168:817–21.
12. Stevens ML, Plotka ED. Functional lutein cyst in a postmenopausal woman. Obstet Gynecol 1977;50:27s–9s.

13. Strickler RC, Kelly RW, Askin FB. Postmenopausal ovarian follicle cyst: an unusual cause of estrogen excess. Int J Gynecol Pathol 1984;3:318–22.
14. Widdowson DJ, Pilling DW, Cook RC. Neonatal ovarian cysts: therapeutic dilemma. Arch Dis Child 1988;63:737–42.

Corpus Luteum Cyst

15. Boles ET, Hardacre JM, Newton WA. Ovarian tumors and cysts in infants and children. Arch Surg 1961;83:112–24.
16. Dacus RM. Massive intraperitoneal hemorrhage from a ruptured corpus luteum hematoma in women taking anticoagulants. Report of 2 cases. Obstet Gynecol 1968;31:471–4.
17. Hallatt JG, Steele CH Jr, Snyder M. Ruptured corpus luteum with hemoperitoneum: a study of 173 surgical cases. Am J Obstet Gynecol 1984;149:5–9.

18. Miles PA, Penney LL. Corpus luteum formation in the fetus. Obstet Gynecol 1983;61:525–9.
19. Piver MS, Williams LJ, Marcuse PM. Influence of luteal cysts on menstrual function. Obstet Gynecol 1970;35:740–51.
20. Rosenthal AH. Rupture of the corpus luteum including four cases of massive intraperitoneal hemorrhage. Am J Obstet Gynecol 1960;79:1008–11.
21. Taniguchi T, Kilkenny GS. Rupture of corpus luteum with production of hemoperitoneum: report of nineteen cases. JAMA 1951;147:1420–4.

Ovarian Remnant Syndrome

22. Shah MS, Pellman C. Ureteral obstruction caused by hemorrhagic corpus luteum cyst. Urology 1974;3:770–3.
23. Shemwell RE, Weed JC. Ovarian remnant syndrome. Obstet Gynecol 1970;36:299–303.

24. Symmonds RE, Pettit PD. Ovarian remnant syndrome. Obstet Gynecol 1979;54:174–7.
25. Wilder JR, Barnes WA. Obstruction of the small intestine by corpus luteum cyst: report of a case. JAMA 1953;151:730–2.

Polycystic Ovarian Disease

26. Adams J, Polson DW, Franks S. Prevalence of polycystic ovaries in women with anovulation and idiopathic hirsutism. Brit Med J 1986;293:355–8.
27. Babaknia A, Calfopoulos P, Jones HW. The Stein-Leventhal syndrome and coincidental ovarian tumors. Obstet Gynecol 1976;47:223–4.
28. Barnes R, Rosenfield RL. The polycystic ovary syndrome: pathogenesis and treatment. Ann Int Med 1989;110:386–99.
29. Benedict PH, Cohen R, Cope O, Scully RE. Ovarian and adrenal morphology in cases of hirsutism or virilism and Stein-Leventhal syndrome. Fertil Steril 1962;13:380–95.
30. Case Records of the Massachusetts General Hospital (Case 40072). N Engl J Med 1954;250:296–300.
31. Chrousos GP, Loriaux L, Mann DL, Cutler GB. Late onset 21-hydroxylase deficiency mimicking idiopathic hirsutism or polycystic ovarian disease. Ann Int Med 1982;96:143–8.

32. Hughesdon PE. Morphology and morphogenesis of the Stein-Leventhal ovary and of so-called hyperthecosis. Obstet Gynecol Surv 1982;37:59–77.
33. Givens JR. Hirsutism and hyperandrogenism. Adv Inter Med 1976;21:221–47.
34. Goldzieher JW. Polycystic ovarian disease. Fertil Steril 1981;35:371–94.
35. Lindsay AN, Voorhess ML, Macgillivray MH. Multicystic ovaries detected by sonography in children with hypothyroidism. Am J Dis Child 1980;134:588–92.
36. Polson DW, Wadsworth J, Adams J, Franks S. Polycystic ovaries—a common finding in normal women. Lancet 1988;1:870–2.
37. Smith KD, Steinberger E, Perloff WH. Polycystic ovarian disease. A report of 301 patients. Am J Obstet Gynecol 1965;93:994–1001.
38. Yen SS. The polycystic ovary syndrome. Clin Endocrinol 1980;12:177–207.

Stromal Hyperthecosis and Hyperplasia

39. Barbieri RL, Ryan KJ. Hyperandrogenism, insulin resistance, and acanthosis nigricans syndrome: a common endocrinopathy with distinct pathophysiologic features. Am J Obstet Gynecol 1983;147:90–101.
40. Boss JH, Scully RE, Wegner KH, Cohen RB. Structural variations in the adult ovary—clinical significance. Obstet Gynecol 1965;25:747–64.
41. Dunaif A, Hoffman AR, Scully RE, et al. Clinical, biochemical, and ovarian morphologic features in women with acanthosis nigricans and masculinization. Obstet Gynecol 1985;66:545–52.
42. Fienberg R. The stromal theca cell and postmenopausal endometrial adenocarcinoma. Cancer 1969;24:32–8.

43. Fienberg R. Thecosis. In: Sommers SC, Rosen PP, eds. Pathology annual, vol 16. Appleton Century Crofts, 1981.
44. Geist SH, Gaines JA. Diffuse luteinization of the ovaries associated with the masculinization syndrome. Am J Obstet Gynecol 1942;43:975–83.
45. Givens JR, Kerber IJ, Wiser WL, Andersen RN, Coleman SA, Fish SA. Remission of acanthosis nigricans associated with polycystic ovarian disease and a stromal luteoma. J Clin Endocrinol Metabol 1974;38:347–55.
46. Hirakawa T, Thor AD, Osawa Y, Mason JI, Scully RE. Stromal hyperthecosis of the ovary: immunohistochemical distribution of steroidogenic enzymes [Abstract]. Mod Pathol 1992;5:65a.

445

47. Judd HL, Scully RE, Herbst AL, Yen SS, Ingersoll FM, Kliman B. Familial hyperthecosis: comparison of endocrinologic and histologic findings with polycystic ovarian disease. Am J Obstet Gynecol 1973;117:976–82.

48. Katz M, Hamilton SM, Albertyn L, Pimstone BL, Cohen BL, Tiltman AJ. Virilization with diffuse involvement of ovarian androgen secreting cells. Obstet Gynecol 1977;50–5:623–7.

49. Koss LG, Pierce V, Brunschwig A. Pseudothecomas of ovaries. A syndrome of bilateral ovarian hypertrophy with diffuse luteinization, endometrial carcinoma, obesity, hirsutism and diabetes mellitus—report of 2 cases. Cancer 1964;17:76–85.

50. Leedman PJ, Bierre AR, Martin FI. Virilizing nodular ovarian stromal hyperthecosis, diabetes mellitus and insulin resistance in a postmenopausal woman. Brit J Obstet Gynecol 1989;96:1095–8.

51. Sasano H, Fukunaga M, Rojas M, Silverberg SG. Hyperthecosis of the ovary. Clinicopathologic study of 19 cases with immunohistochemical analysis of steroidogenic enzymes. Int J Gynecol Pathol 1989;8:311–20.

52. Scully RE, Cohen RB. Oxidative enzyme activity in normal and pathologic human ovaries. Obstet Gynecol 1964;24:667–81.

53. Taylor SI, Dons RF, Hernandez E, Roth J, Gorden P. Insulin resistance associated with androgen excess in women with autoantibodies to the insulin receptor. Ann Intern Med 1982;97:851–5.

Massive Edema and Fibromatosis

54. Byrne P, Vella EJ, Rollason T, Frampton J. Ovarian fibromatosis with minor sex cord elements. Case report. Brit J Obstet Gynaecol 1989;96:245–8.

55. Chervenak FA, Castadot MJ, Wiederman J, Sedlis A. Massive ovarian edema: review of world literature and report of two cases. Obstet Gynecol Surv 1980;35:677–84.

56. Kalstone CE, Jaffe RB, Abell MR. Massive edema of the ovary simulating fibroma. Obstet Gynecol 1969;34:564–71.

57. Roth LM, Deaton RL, Sternberg WH. Massive ovarian edema. A clinicopathologic study of five cases including ultrastructural observations and review of the literature. Am J Surg Pathol 1979;3:11–21.

58. Spinas GA, Heitz PH, Oberholzer M, Torhorst J, Stahl M, Girard J. Massive ovarian edema with production of testosterone. Virch Arch [A] 1981;390:365–71.

59. Young RH, Scully RE. Fibromatosis and massive edema of the ovary, possibly related entities: a report of 14 cases of fibromatosis and 11 cases of massive edema. Int J Gynecol Pathol 1984;3:153–78.

Hilus (Leydig) Cell Hyperplasia

60. Boss JH, Scully RE, Wegner KH, Cohen RB. Structural variation in the adult ovary—clinical significance. Obstet Gynecol 1965;25:747–64.

60a. Davidson BJ, Waisman J, Judd HL. Long-standing virilism in a woman with hyperplasia and neoplasia of ovarian lipidic cells. Obstet Gynecol 1981;58:753–9.

61. Judd HL, Scully RE, Atkins L, Neer RM, Kliman B. Pure gonadal dysgenesis with progressive hirsutism. Demonstration of testosterone production by gonadal streaks. N Eng J Med 1970;282:881–5.

62. Meldrum DR, Frumar AM, Shamonki IM, et al. Ovarian and adrenal steroidogenesis in a virilized patient with gonadotropin-resistant ovaries and hilus cell hyperplasia. Obstet Gynecol 1980;56:216–21.

63. Sternberg WH. The morphology, androgenic function, hyperplasia, and tumors of the human ovarian hilus cells. Am J Pathol 1949;25:493–521.

Idiopathic Calcification

64. Clement PB, Cooney TP. Idiopathic multifocal calcification of the ovarian stroma. Arch Pathol Lab Med 1992;116:204–5.

Uterus-Like Ovarian Mass

65. Cozzutto C. Uterus-like mass replacing ovary: report of a new entity. Arch Pathol Lab Med 1981;105:508–11.

66. Pueblitz-Peredo S, Luevano-Flores E, Rincon-Taracena R, Ochoa-Carrillo FJ. Uterus like mass of the ovary: endomyometriosis or congenital malformation? A case with a discussion of histogenesis. Arch Pathol Lab Med 1985;109:361–4.

67. Rahilly MA, Al-Nafussi A. Uterus-like mass of the ovary associated with endometrioid carcinoma. Histopathology 1991;18:549–51.

68. Rosai J. Uterus-like mass replacing ovary [Letter]. Arch Pathol Lab Med 1982;106:364–5.

Splenic-Gonadal Fusion

69. Almenoff IA. Splenic-gonadal fusion. NY State J Med 1966;66:1679–81.

70. Meneses MF, Ostrowski ML. Female splenic-gonadal fusion of the discontinuous type. Hum Pathol 1989;20:486–8.

71. Putschar WG, Manion WC. Splenic-gonadal fusion. Am J Pathol 1956;32:15–33.

Pregnancy Luteoma

72. Cohen DA, Daughaday WH, Weldon VV. Fetal and maternal virilization associated with pregnancy. A case report and review of the literature. Am J Dis Child 1982;136:353–6.

73. Garcia-Bunuel R, Berek JS, Woodruff JD. Luteomas of pregnancy. Obstet Gynecol 1975;45:407–14.

74. Hensleigh PA, Woodruff JD. Differential maternal-fetal response to androgenizing luteoma or hyperreactio luteinalis. Obstet Gynecol Surv 1978;33:262–71.

75. Malinak LR, Miller GV. Bilateral multicentric luteomas of pregnancy associated with masculinization of a female infant. Am J Obstet Gynecol 1965;91:251–9.

76. Norris HJ, Taylor HB. Nodular theca-lutein hyperplasia of pregnancy (so-called "pregnancy luteoma"). A clinical and pathological study of 15 cases. Am J Clin Pathol 1967;47:557–66.

77. Rice BF, Barclay DL, Sternberg WH. Luteoma of pregnancy: steroidogenic and morphologic considerations. Am J Obstet Gynecol 1969;104:871–8.

78. Sternberg WH, Barclay DL. Luteoma of pregnancy. Am J Obstet Gynecol 1966;95:165–84.

79. Thomas E, Mestman J, Henneman C, Anderson G, Hoffman R. Bilateral luteomas of pregnancy with virilization. A case report. Obstet Gynecol 1972;39:577–84.

Hyperreactio Luteinalis

80. Barclay DL, Leverich EB, Kemmerly JR. Hyperreactio luteinalis: postpartum persistence. Am J Obstet Gynecol 1969;105:642–4.

81. Berger NG, Repke JT, Woodruff JD. Markedly elevated serum testosterone in pregnancy without fetal virilization. Obstet Gynecol 1984;63:260–2.

82. Caspi E, Schreyer P, Bukovsky J. Ovarian lutein cysts in pregnancy. Obstet Gynecol 1973;42:388–98.

83. Chow KK, Choo HT. Ovarian hyperstimulation syndrome with clomiphene citrate. Case report. Br J Obstet Gynaecol 1984;91:1051–2.

84. Curry SL, Hammond CB, Tyrey L, Creasman WT, Parker RT. Hydatidiform mole: diagnosis, management, and long-term followup of 347 patients. Obstet Gynecol 1975;45:1–8.

85. Dick JS. Bilateral theca lutein cysts associated with apparently normal pregnancy. J Obstet Gynaecol Br Comm 1972;79:852–4.

86. Girouard DP, Barclay DL, Collins CG. Hyperreactio luteinalis. Review of the literature and report of 2 cases. Obstet Gynecol 1964;23:513–25.

87. Haning RV Jr, Strawn EY, Nolten WE. Pathophysiology of the ovarian hyperstimulation syndrome. Obstet Gynecol 1985;66:220–4.

88. Levine SC, Huffaker J, Jacobson JB, Brodey PA, Fisch AE. Second- trimester spontaneous regression of theca lutein cysts. Obstet Gynecol 1982; 60:124–6.

89. Montz FJ, Schlaerth JB, Morrow CP. The natural history of theca lutein cysts. Obstet Gynecol 1988;72:247–51.

90. Schenker JG, Weinstein D. Ovarian hyperstimulation syndrome: a current survey. Fertil Steril 1978;30:255–68.

91. Tulandi T, McInnes RA, Arronet GH. Ovarian hyperstimulation syndrome following ovulation induction with human menopausal gonadotropin. Int J Fertil 1984;29:113–7.

92. Wajda KJ, Lucas JG, Marsh WL Jr. Hyperreactio luteinalis. Benign disorder masquerading as an ovarian neoplasm. Arch Pathol Lab Med 1989;113:921–5.

Large Solitary Luteinized Follicle Cyst of Pregnancy and Puerperium

93. Clement PB, Scully RE. Large solitary luteinized follicle cyst of pregnancy and puerperium: a clinicopathological analysis of eight cases. Am J Surg Pathol 1980;4:431–8.

Granulosa Cell Proliferations

94. Clement PB, Young RH, Scully RE. Ovarian granulosa cell proliferations of pregnancy. A report of nine cases. Hum Pathol 1988;19:657–62.

95. McKay DG, Hertig AT, Hickey WF. The histogenesis of granulosa and theca cell tumors of the human ovary. Obstet Gynecol 1953;1:125–36.

Hilus (Leydig) Cell Proliferation During Pregnancy

96. Sternberg WH, Segaloff A, Gaskill CJ. Influence of chorionic gonadotropin on human ovarian hilus cells (Leydig-like cells). J Clin Endocrinol Metab 1953;13:139–53.

Ectopic Decidua

97. Bassis ML. Pseudodeciduosis. Am J Obstet Gynecol 1956;72:1029–37.

98. Bersch W, Alexy E, Heuser HP, Staemmler HJ. Ectopic decidua formation in the ovary (so-called deciduoma). Virch Arch [A] 1973;360:173–7.

99. Clement PB, Young RH, Scully RE. Nontrophoblastic pathology of the female genital tract and peritoneum associated with pregnancy. Semin Diagn Pathol 1989;6:372–406.

100. Herr JC, Heidger PM Jr, Scott JR, Anderson JW, Curet LB, Mossman HW. Decidual cells in the human ovary at term. I. Incidence, gross anatomy and ultrastructural features of merocrine secretion. Am J Anat 1978;152:7–27.

101. Herr JC, Platz CE, Heidiger PM Jr, Curet LB. Smooth muscle with ovarian decidual nodules: a link to leiomyomatosis peritonealis disseminata? Obstet Gynecol 1979;53:451-6.

102. Israel SL, Rubenstone A, Meranze DR. The ovary at term. I. Decidua-like reaction and surface cell proliferation. Obstet Gynecol 1954;3:399–407.

103. Ober WB, Grady HG, Schoenbucher AK. Ectopic ovarian decidua without pregnancy. Am J Pathol 1957;33:199–217.

104. Rogers WS, Seckinger DL. Decidual tissue as a cause of intra-abdominal hemorrhage during labor. Obstet Gynecol 1965;25:391–7.

105. Starup J, Visfeldt J. Ovarian morphology in early and late human pregnancy. Acta Obstet Gynecol Scand 1974;53:211–8.

Ovarian Pregnancy

106. Gray CL, Ruffolo EH. Ovarian pregnancy associated with intrauterine contraceptive devices. Am J Obstet Gynecol 1978;132:134–9.

107. Hallatt JG. Primary ovarian pregnancy: a report of twenty-five cases. Am J Obstet Gynecol 1982;143:55–60.

Endometriosis

108. Bergqvist A, Ljungberg O, Myhre E. Human endometrium and endometriotic tissue obtained simultaneously: a comparative histological study. Int J Gynecol Pathol 1984;3:135–45.

109. Clement PB. Pathology of endometriosis. Path Annual 1990;25:245-95.

110. Clement PB, Young RH, Scully RE. Liesegang rings in the female genital tract. A report of three cases. Int J Gynecol Pathol 1989;8:271-6.

111. Clement PB, Young RH, Scully RE. Necrotic pseudoxanthomatous nodules of the ovary and peritoneum in endometriosis. Am J Surg Pathol 1988;12:390–7.

112. Clement PB, Young RH, Scully RE. Stromal endometriosis of the uterine cervix. A variant of endometriosis that may simulate a sarcoma. Am J Surg Pathol 1990;14:449–55.

113. Czernobilsky B, Morris WJ. A histologic study of ovarian endometriosis with emphasis on hyperplastic and atypical changes. Obstet Gynecol 1979;53:318–23.

114. Dmowski WP. Pitfalls in clinical laparoscopic and histologic diagnosis of endometriosis. Acta Obstet Gynecol Scand 1984;123(Suppl);61–6.

115. Dmowski WP, Radwanska E. Current concepts on pathology, histogenesis and etiology of endometriosis. Acta Obstet Gynecol Scand 1984;123(Suppl):29–33.

116. Egger H, Weigmann P. Clinical and surgical aspects of ovarian endometriotic cysts. Arch Gynecol 1982;233:37–45.

117. Halme J, Chafe W, Currie JL. Endometriosis with massive ascites. Obstet Gynecol 1985;65:591–2.

118. Hughesdon PE. The endometrial identity of benign stromatosis of the ovary and its relation to other forms of endometriosis. J Pathol 1976;119:201–9.

119. Jansen RP, Russell P. Nonpigmented endometriosis: clinical, laparoscopic, and pathologic definition. Am J Obstet Gynecol 1986;155:1154–9.

120. Metzger DA, Olive DL, Haney AF. Limited hormonal responsiveness of ectopic endometrium: histologic correlation with intrauterine endometrium. Hum Pathol 1988;19:1417–24.

121. Rossman F, D'Ablaing G III, Marrs RP. Pregnancy complicated by ruptured endometrioma. Obstet Gynecol 1983;62:519–21.

122. Schuger L, Simon A, Okon E. Cytomegaly in benign ovarian cysts. Arch Pathol Lab Med 1986;110:928–9.

Inflammatory Disorders

123. Aikat BK, Radhakrishnan VV, Rao MS. Malakoplakia—a report of two cases with review of the literature. Ind J Path Bact 1973;16:64–70.

124. Arean VM. Manson's schistosomiasis of the female genital tract. Am J Obstet Gynecol 1956;72:1038–53.

125. Azhar H. Primary echinococcal infection of the ovary. Br J Obstet Gynecol 1977;84:633.

126. Bahary CM, Ovadia Y, Neri A. Schistosoma mansoni of the ovary. Am J Obstet Gynecol 1967;98:290–2.

127. Bhagavan BS, Gupta PK. Genital actinomycosis and intrauterine contraceptive devices. Cytopathologic diagnosis and clinical significance. Hum Pathol 1978;9:567–78.

128. Burkman R, Schlesselman S, McCaffrey L, Gupta PK, Spence M. The relationship of genital tract actinomycetes and the development of pelvic inflammatory disease. Am J Obstet Gynecol 1982;143:585–9.

129. Bylund DJ, Nanfro JJ, Marsh WL Jr. Coccidioidomycosis of the female genital tract. Arch Pathol Lab Med 1986;110:232–5.

130. Claman P, Dover M, Saginur R, et al. Spontaneous ovarian-to-vaginal fistula: a case report. Am J Obstet Gynecol 1991;164:71–2.

131. Eschenbach DA. Epidemiology and diagnosis of acute pelvic inflammatory disease. Obstet Gynecol 1980;55:142S–53S.

132. Farber ER, Leahy MS, Meadows TR. Endometrial blastomycosis acquired by sexual contact. Obstet Gynecol 1968;32:195–9.

133. Fitzgerald TB, Mainwaring AR, Ahmed A. Pelvic peritoneal oxyuriasis simulating metastatic carcinoma. A case report. Br J Obstet Gynaecol 1974;81:248–50.

134. Hangval H, Habibi H, Moshref A, Rahimi A. Case report of an ovarian hydatid cyst. J Trop Med Hyg 1979;82:34–5.

135. Kaufman DW, Shapiro S, Rosenberg L, et al. Intrauterine contraceptive device use and pelvic inflammatory disease. Am J Obstet Gynecol 1980;136:159–62.

136. Keebler C, Chatwani A, Schwartz R. Actinomycosis infection associated with intrauterine contraceptive devices. Am J Obstet Gynecol 1983;145:596–9.

137. Khan JS, Stelle RJ, Stewart D. Enterobius vermicularis infestation of the female genital tract causing generalized peritonitis. Case report. Br J Obstet Gynaecol 1981;88:681–3.

138. Klempner LB, Giglio PG, Niebles A. Malacoplakia of the ovary. Obstet Gynecol 1987;69:537–40.

139. Kostelnik FV, Fremount HN. Mycotic tubo-ovarian abscess associated with the intrauterine device. Am J Obstet Gynecol 1976;125:272–4.

140. Kunakemakorn P, Ontai G, Balin H. Pelvic inflammatory pseudotumor: a case report. Am J Obstet Gynecol 1976;126:286–7.
141. Ladefoged C, Lorentzen M. Xanthogranulomatous inflammation of the female genital tract. Histopathology 1988;13:541–51.
142. Landers DV, Sweet RL. Current trends in the diagnosis and treatment of tubo-ovarian abscess. Am J Obstet Gynecol 1985;151:1098–110.
143. Lansman HH, Lapin A, Blaustein A. Pelvic oxyuris granuloma associated with endometriosis. Am J Obstet Gynecol 1960;79:1178–80.
144. London AM, Burkman RT. Tubo-ovarian abscess with associated rupture with fistula formation into the urinary bladder: a report of two cases. Am J Obstet Gynecol 1979;135:1113–4.
145. Mahmood K. Granulomatous oophoritis due to Schistosoma mansoni. Am J Obstet Gynecol 1975;123:919–20.
146. McMahon JN, Connolly CE, Long SV, Meehan FB. Enterobius granulomas of the uterus, ovary and pelvic peritoneum. Two case reports. Br J Obstet Gynaecol 1984;91:289–90.
147. Muller-Holzner E, Ruth NR, Abfalter E, et al. IUD-associated pelvic actinomycosis: a report of five cases. Int J Gynecol Path 1995;14:70–4.
148. Murray JJ, Clark CA, Lands RH, Heim CR, Burnett LS. Reactivation blastomycosis presenting as a tubo-ovarian abscess. Obstet Gynecol 1985;64:828–30.
149. Nogales-Ortiz F, Taracon I, Nogales FF Jr. The pathology of female genital tract tuberculosis. A 31-year study of 1,436 cases. Obstet Gynecol 1979;53:422–8.

150. Pace EH, Voet EH, Melancon JT. Xanthogranulomatous oophoritis: an inflammatory pseudotumor of the ovary. Int J Gynecol Pathol 1984;3:398–402.
151. Pedowitz P, Bloomfield RD. Ruptured adnexal abscess (tubo-ovarian) with generalized peritonitis. Am J Obstet Gynecol 1964;88:721–9.
152. Pine L, Curtis EM, Brown JM. Actinomyces and the intrauterine contraceptive device: aspects of the fluorescent antibody stain. Am J Obstet Gynecol 1985:152:287–90.
153. Quan A, Charles D, Craig JM. Histologic and functional consequences of periovarian adhesions. Obstet Gynecol 1963;22:96–101.
154. Schmidt WA, Bedrossian CW, Ali V, et al. Actinomycosis and intrauterine contraceptive devices. Diag Gynecol Obstet 1980;2:165–77.
155. Shalev E, Zuckerman H, Rizescu I. Pelvic inflammatory pseudotumor (xanthogranuloma). Acta Obstet Gynecol Scand 1982;61:285–6.
156. Simstein NL. Colo-tubo-ovarian fistula as complication of pelvic inflammatory disease. South Med J 1981;74:512–3.
157. Sutherland AM. Postmenopausal tuberculosis of the female genital tract. Obstet Gynecol 1982;59:54S–7S.
158. Wetchler SJ, Dunn LJ. Ovarian abscess. Report of a case and a review of the literature. Obstet Gynecol Surv 1985;40:476–85.
159. Willson JB, Black JR III. Ovarian abscess. Am J Obstet Gynecol 1964;90:34–43.

Foreign Body Granulomas

160. Benirschke K, Bonin ML, Rost T. Plant material in ovary following barium enema [Letter]. Arch Pathol Lab Med 1984;108:359–60.
161. Case records of the Massachusetts General Hospital. (Case 13-1988). N Engl J Med 1988;318:835–42.
162. Gilks CB, Clement PB. Colo-ovarian fistula: a report of two cases. Obstet Gynecol 1987;69:533–7.
163. Hidvegi D, Hidvegi I, Barrett J. Douche-induced pelvic peritoneal starch granuloma. Obstet Gynecol 1978;52:15S–8S.
164. Mostafa SA, Bargeron CB, Flower RW, Rosenshein NB, Parmley TH, Woodruff JD. Foreign body granulomas in normal ovaries. Obstet Gynecol 1985;66:701–2.

165. Nissim F, Ashkenazy M, Borenstein R, Czernobilsky B. Tuberculoid cornstarch granulomas with caseous necrosis. A diagnostic challenge. Arch Pathol Lab Med 1981;105:86–8.
166. Paine CG, Smith P. Starch granulomata. J Clin Pathol 1957;10:51–5.
167. Saxen L, Kassinen A, Saxen E. Peritoneal foreign-body reaction caused by condom emulsion. Lancet 1963;1:1295–6.
168. Teilum G, Madsen V. Endometriosis ovarii et peritonaei caused by hysterosalpingography. Br J Obstet Gynaecol 1950;57:10–6.

Isolated Palisading Granulomas

169. Al Dawoud A, Yates R, Foulis AK. Postoperative necrotizing granulomas in the ovary. J Clin Pathol 1991;44:524-5.
170. Herbold DR, Frable WJ, Kraus FT. Isolated non-infectious granuloma of the ovary. Int J Gynecol Pathol 1984;2:380–91.
171. Kernohan NM, Best PV, Jandial V, Kitchener HC. Palisading granuloma of the ovary. Histopathology 1991;19:279–80.

171a. McCluggage WG, Allen DC. Ovarian granulomas: a report of 32 cases. J Clin Pathol 1997;50:324–7.
171b. Tatum ET, Beattie JF Jr, Bryson K. Postoperative carbon pigment granuloma. A report of eight cases involving the ovary. Hum Pathol 1996;27:1008–11.
172. Wilson GE, Haboubi NY, McWilliam LJ, Hirsch PJ. Postoperative necrotizing granulomata in the cervix and ovary [Letter]. J Clin Pathol 1990;43:1037–8.

Granulomas Secondary to Systemic Disease

173. Brooks JJ, Wheeler JE. Granulomatous salpingitis secondary to Crohn's disease. Obstet Gynecol 1977;49:31–3.
174. Chalvardjian A. Sarcoidosis of the female genital tract. Am J Obstet Gynecol 1978;132:78–80.

175. Honore LH. Combined suppurative and noncaseating granulomatous oophoritis associated with distal ileitis (Crohn's disease). Eur J Obstet Gynaecol Reprod Biol 1981;12:91–4.

176. Sommers SC. Female genital tract granulomas. In: Ioachim HL, ed. Pathology of granulomas. New York: Raven Press, 1983:395–409.
177. White A, Flaris N, Elmer D, et al. Coexistence of mucinous cystadenoma of the ovary and ovarian sarcoidosis. Am J Obstet Gynecol 1990;162:1284–5.

178. Winslow RC, Funkhouser JW. Sarcoidosis of the female reproductive organs. Report of a case. Obstet Gynecol 1968;32:285–9.
179. Wlodarski FM, Trainer TD. Granulomatous oophoritis and salpingitis associated with Crohn's disease of the appendix. Am J Obstet Gynecol 1975;122:527–8.

Mesothelial Proliferation

180. Battifora H, McCaughey WT. Tumors of the serosal membranes. Atlas of Tumor Pathology, 3rd Series, Fascicle 15. Washington, D.C.: Armed Forces Institute of Pathology, 1995.
181. Clement PB, Young RH. Florid mesothelial hyperplasia associated with ovarian tumors: a potential source of error in tumor diagnosis and staging. Int J Gynecol Pathol 1993;12:51–8.

182. Herrera LO, Lopez GE, Ledesma EJ, Englander L, Mittelman A. Mesothelial cysts associated with metastases to ovary from primary colonic carcinoma. Dis Colon Rectum 1982;25:139–42.
183. McFadden DE, Clement PB. Peritoneal inclusion cysts with mural mesothelial proliferation. A clinicopathological analysis of six cases. Am J Surg Pathol 1986; 10:844–54.

Autoimmune Oophoritis

184. Bannatyne P, Russell P, Shearman RP. Autoimmune oophoritis: a clinicopathologic assessment of 12 cases. Int J Gynecol Pathol 1990;9:191–207.
185. Biscotti CV, Hart WR, Lucas JG. Cystic ovarian enlargement resulting from autoimmune oophoritis. Obstet Gynecol 1989;74:492–5.

186. Lonsdale RN, Roberts PF, Trowell JE. Autoimmune oophoritis associated with polycystic ovaries. Histopathology 1991;19:77–81.
187. Sedmak DD, Hart WR, Tubbs RR. Autoimmune oophoritis: a histopathologic study of involved ovaries with immunologic characterization of the mononuclear cell infiltrate. Int J Gynecol Pathol 1987;6:73–81.

Vascular Lesions

188. Azoury RS, Chehab RM, Mufarrij IK. The twisted adnexa: a clinical pathological review. Diagn Gynecol Obstet 1980;2:185–91.
189. Best CL, Feldman DB, Sobenes JR, Sueldo CE. Unexplained displacement of ipsilateral ovary and fallopian tube. Obstet Gynecol 1991;78:558–60.
190. Beyth Y, Bar-On E. Tubo-ovarian autoamputation and infertility. Fertil Steril 1984;42:932–4.
191. Demopoulos RI, Bigelow B, Vasa U. Infarcted uterine adnexa. Associated pathology. N Y State J Med 1978;78:2027–9.

192. Dunnihoo DR, Wolff J. Bilateral torsion of the adnexa: a case report and a review of the world literature. Obstet Gynecol 1984;64:55S–9S.
193. Evans JP. Torsion of the normal uterine adnexa in premenarcheal girls. J Pediatr Surg 1978;13:195–6.
194. Grosfeld JL. Torsion of the normal ovary in the first two years of life. Am J Surg 1969;117:726–7.
195. Hibbard LT. Adnexal torsion. Am J Obstet Gynecol 1985;152:456–61.
196. Schultz LR, Newton WA Jr, Clatworthy HW Jr. Torsion of previously normal tube and ovary in children. N Engl J Med 1963;268:343–6.

Ovarian Changes Secondary to Metabolic Disease

197. Copeland W Jr, Hawley PC, Teteris NJ. Gynecologic amyloidosis. Am J Obstet Gynecol 1985;153:555–6.
198. Dincsoy HP, Rolfes DB, McGraw CA, Schubert WK. Cholesterol ester storage disease and mesenteric lipodystrophy. Am J Clin Pathol 1984;81:263–9.

199. Salomonowitz E. Tumorformige Amyloidose des Ovars. Geburtsh u Frauenheilk 1980;40:644–7.
200. Wassman ER, Johnson K, Shapiro LJ, et al. Postmortem findings in the Hurler-Scheie syndrome (mucopolyssacharidosis I-H/S). Birth defects: original article series. 1982;18(3B):13–8.

Mucicarminophilic Histiocytosis

201. Kershisnik MM, Ro JY, Cannon GH, Ordonez NG, Ayala AG, Silva EG. Histiocytic reaction in pelvic peritoneum associated with oxidized regenerated cellulose. Am J Clin Pathol 1994;103:27–31.

202. Kuo TT, Hsueh S. Mucicarminophilic histiocytosis. A polyvinylpyrrolidone (PVP) storage disease simulating signet-ring cell carcinoma. Am J Surg Pathol 1984;8:419–28.

23
EXTRAOVARIAN ABDOMINAL TUMORS
RESEMBLING OVARIAN TUMORS

A variety of extraovarian neoplasms resemble histologically and often clinically tumors of ovarian origin. These tumors include those that arise from the "secondary mullerian system," that is, the pelvic and lower abdominal mesothelium and subjacent mesenchyme (44). The mullerian potential of this tissue is consistent with its close embryonic relation to the mullerian ducts, which arise by invagination of the coelomic epithelium. Some of these tumors, typically those of serous type, can involve peritoneal surfaces extensively without forming a dominant mass, suggesting the possibility of a multifocal origin. Localized extraovarian tumors of ovarian type may also be of peritoneal origin, or may arise from remnants of the mullerian duct (e.g. within the broad ligament), from foci of endometriosis, from ectopic ovarian tissue (page 3), or in the case of germ cell tumors, from germ cells that have become arrested during their embryonic migration. Tumors that most commonly have an extraovarian origin but that occasionally also arise in the ovaries, such as malignant mesotheliomas and tumors of probable wolffian origin, are covered in chapter 17. Tumors resembling ovarian tumors that arise in the fallopian tube and the broad ligament are discussed in chapters 25, 26, and 27, and those that arise in the uterine corpus and lower genital tract, in other tumor Fascicles (43a,67a).

SEROUS TUMORS

The full spectrum of serous neoplasia encountered in the ovary may also be seen in primary tumors of the extraovarian peritoneum. Most resemble ovarian serous carcinomas (OSCs), and have been referred to as *papillary carcinomas of the peritoneum* or, as we prefer, *primary serous carcinomas of the peritoneum (PSCPs).* Approximately 350 tumors have been reported as such (2,5,12,19,27,28,33,41,42,47,49,53,62, 63,66,67,72,78,79). Many have occurred in women from whom ovaries apparently free of carcinoma had been removed, in some cases prophylactically, for familial ovarian cancer

(40,60,71,76). The age distribution and clinical presentation are similar to those of patients with high-stage ovarian serous cancers. The intraoperative appearance of PSCP, with widespread peritoneal tumor associated with ovaries of normal size, may mimic that of a diffuse malignant mesothelioma or peritoneal carcinomatosis associated with an unknown primary tumor. In many cases, the ovaries are also involved by small surface "implants," but retain their normal size and shape ("normal-sized ovary carcinoma syndrome") (25).

There is evidence that at least some PSCPs have a multifocal origin from the peritoneum. Rutledge et al. (67) found a high frequency of DNA heterogeneity among tumor samples from different sites in the same patient. Similarly, Muto et al. (54) found that, in contrast to the results in the metastases of ovarian serous carcinomas, the pattern of allelic loss and the mutational pattern of p53 varied at tumor sites within the same patient in three of six cases of PSCP.

Criteria for the diagnosis of PSCP have varied in the literature; those proposed by the Gynecologic Oncology Group (GOG) are as follows (12):

1. Both ovaries are either normal in size or enlarged by a benign process. In the judgement of the surgeon and the pathologist, the bulk of the tumor is in the peritoneum and the extent of tumor involvement at one or more extraovarian sites is greater than on the surface of either ovary.

2. Microscopic examination of the ovaries reveals: 1) no tumor; 2) tumor confined to the surface epithelium with no evidence of cortical invasion; 3) tumor involving the ovarian surface and the underlying cortical stroma but less than 5 by 5 mm in diameter; or 4) tumor less than 5 by 5 mm within the ovarian substance, with or without surface involvement.

3. The histologic and cytologic characteristics of the tumor are predominantly serous and similar or identical to those of ovarian serous papillary carcinomas of any grade.

451

4. Cases in which an oophorectomy had been performed before the diagnosis of PSCP must have one of the following: 1) a pathology report to document the absence of carcinoma in the specimen, with review of all the slides of the ovarian specimen if the oophorectomy had been performed within 5 years of the diagnosis of PSCP; 2) if the oophorectomy had been performed more than 5 years before the diagnosis of PSCP, the pathology report of the specimen is required, and an attempt to review the slides must be made.

Psammocarcinomas (page 67) and other low-grade serous carcinomas are included within this category of neoplasms (14,32,48,76a).

The clinical presentation and the pathologic features, including the immunoprofile, of PSCPs do not differ significantly from those of advanced stage OSCs. The comparative behavior of the two tumors is controversial. Some investigators have suggested that the former are more aggressive and are associated with a shorter survival period than the latter (42,49). In contrast, another study showed that the 4-year survival rate for patients with PSCP was significantly better than that for those with OSC (28 versus 9 percent) (53). The author of a GOG study found that when PSCPs are matched with OSCs for extent and distribution of disease, grade, age, and treatment, there are no differences in response to therapy, disease-free interval, and actuarial survival between the two tumors (12).

Occasional tumors resembling ovarian serous borderline tumors are characterized by widespread extraovarian peritoneal involvement and normal-sized ovaries that are either free of disease or have serosal involvement similar to that of the extraovarian peritoneum (9,11). The most common presenting features in patients with these tumors, who are typically under the age of 35 years (range, 16 to 67), are infertility and chronic pelvic or abdominal pain. Many tumors, however, are discovered incidentally at laparotomy for other conditions. At operation, focal or diffuse miliary granules, fibrous adhesions, or both involve the pelvic peritoneum and omentum, and less commonly, the extraomental abdominal peritoneum. Microscopic examination reveals superficial tumor that resembles noninvasive epithelial or desmoplastic implants of serous borderline tumors of ovarian origin (page

61). Coexistent endosalpingiosis has been found in 85 percent of the cases (9,11).

Both primary peritoneal serous borderline tumors and psammocarcinomas may be associated with clinical evidence of disease postoperatively, but are typically indolent, with prolonged survival. Visible lesions should be resected as completely as possible, with preservation of the uterus and ovaries in young patients. Postoperative chemotherapy has not been shown to be of value in the treatment of these tumors.

Rare extraovarian serous tumors occur as localized, typically cystic masses, usually within the broad ligament (see chapter 27) and less commonly, within the retroperitoneum. These have taken the form of serous papillary cystadenomas and adenofibromas, serous borderline tumors, and serous carcinomas (3,4,21,30,31,38,73).

MUCINOUS TUMORS

Mucinous neoplasms similar to those arising in the ovary have been described in extraovarian sites, usually the retroperitoneum, (6,44,52,58, 59,65,70) but also the pancreas and biliary tract (1a,43,68a) and the inguinal region (69), in the absence of a primary tumor within the ovary. These tumors form large cystic masses that resemble grossly and microscopically ovarian mucinous cystadenomas, borderline tumors, or cystadenocarcinomas. Some of them have ovarian-type stroma in their walls, suggesting the possibility of an origin from a supernumerary or an ectopic ovary. Other tumors may originate from misplaced endodermal tissue or possibly directly from the peritoneum.

ENDOMETRIOID, CLEAR CELL, AND BRENNER TUMORS

A variety of extraovarian pelvic or retroperitoneal neoplasms of endometrioid or clear cell type have been described (also see chapter 27). Most such tumors arise within foci of endometriosis (page 108); other tumors lacking this association may be of mullerian remnant or secondary mullerian origin. Endometrioid tumors in the latter category have included a cystadenofibroma (35), a cystadenocarcinoma (15), endometrioid stromal sarcomas (13), homologous and heterologous malignant mesodermal mixed tumors

(29,50), and mesodermal adenosarcomas (16,57, 64). Two clear cell carcinomas of apparent peritoneal origin unassociated with endometriosis have been reported, one as a localized mass within the sigmoid mesocolon (24) and the other diffusely involving the peritoneum (45).

In contrast to the common occurrence of nests of transitional (urothelial) epithelium (Walthard nests) on the pelvic peritoneum in women of all ages, extraovarian Brenner tumors are rare. They have been encountered most commonly in the broad ligament (see chapter 27), but one example has been reported within the uterus (36).

GERM CELL TUMORS

These tumors have been reported to arise in many sites within the abdomen.

Rare dermoid cysts have originated within the pelvis, including the cul-de-sac (46) and uterosacral ligament (37), in the absence of a similar tumor in the ovary. In addition, a number of omental dermoid cysts have coexisted with a similar ovarian tumor (68). Although some extraovarian dermoid cysts may be primary extraovarian germ cell tumors, others, especially those associated with a similar tumor in an ovary, may be "parasitic" tumors of ovarian origin. Two predominantly solid mature teratomas have apparently arisen within the cul-de-sac (77) and the paracervical region (22); the first tumor was associated with peritoneal gliomatosis and the second with an omental implant of mature thyroid tissue.

In addition to an origin in the sacrococcygeal area (32a) extraovarian yolk sac tumors occasionally arise elsewhere within the pelvis. Eight such tumors have been reported, and have been mostly situated in the uterus, the uterine serosa, or the broad ligament (18). The clinical and pathologic features of these tumors are similar to those of yolk sac tumors of ovarian origin.

Four extraovarian ependymomas, similar clinically and pathologically to those occurring within the ovary (see chapter 15), have been reported. Two of them arose within the broad ligament (10) (see chapter 27), one from the uterosacral ligament (23), and one from the omentum (20). These tumors, however, were not associated with indisputable teratomatous elements, and therefore may not have been of germ cell origin.

SEX CORD–STROMAL AND STEROID CELL TUMORS

Rare examples of extraovarian sex cord–stromal tumors have been reported. Most of them originated within the broad ligament (see chapter 27), but several arose in other sites, including the retroperitoneum (39) and adrenal gland (see below). Two extraovarian sex cord tumors with annular tubules (page 219) have been described (8, 34). Both of them were incidental findings in women without evidence of the Peutz-Jeghers syndrome or a similar tumor in the ovary. One tumor was intimately admixed with endometriosis on the serosa of a fallopian tube, and the other was found within an umbilical hernia. In the latter case the tumor was associated with microscopic foci of similar tumor within the omentum and evidence of persistent disease following chemotherapy (8).

Virilizing tumors or tumor-like nodules resembling ovarian steroid cell tumors have been occasionally seen within the broad ligament. The tumors are discussed in chapter 27. Three examples of virilizing hyperplastic nodules occurred in patients with Nelson's syndrome (the development of an adrenocorticotropic hormone [ACTH]-secreting pituitary tumor following bilateral adrenalectomy for pituitary-dependent Cushing's syndrome) (7, 75,80). The three patients presented with virilization and elevated testosterone levels at intervals of 8, 13, and 24 years after bilateral adrenalectomy. Operation revealed multiple dark brown to black nodules up to 2 cm in diameter involving the broad ligament in two cases and the tubal fimbriae in the third. The nodules were bilateral in two cases. On microscopic examination, the nodules and smaller, grossly invisible aggregates were well circumscribed and consisted of sheets of variably sized polygonal cells that contained abundant eosinophilic cytoplasm and lipochrome pigment (fig. 23-1). The rounded, variably sized nuclei contained single prominent nucleoli; occasional mitotic figures were present. The proliferations in these cases most likely involved ectopic parovarian adrenal cortical tissue but in one case, the hyperplastic nodules abutted what appeared to be unstimulated adrenal rests (7). Ectopic hilus cells are another possible origin, but Reinke crystals have not been identified within the lesional cells.

Tumors resembling ovarian sex cord–stromal tumors have also been encountered rarely in the

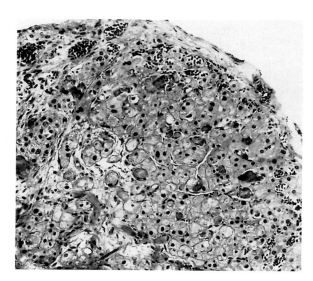 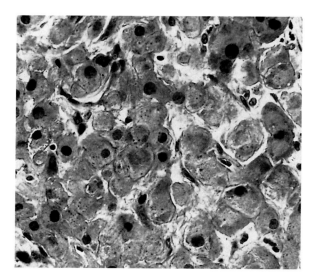

Figure 23-1
NELSON'S SYNDROME
Left: One of multiple nodules from the broad ligament of a virilized patient with Nelson's syndrome.
Right: The nodule is composed of cells resembling adrenocortical cells. Reinke crystals were not identified. (Fig. 8 from Clement PB, Young RH, Scully RE. Clinical syndromes associated with tumors of the female genital tract. Semin Diagn Pathol 1991;8:204–33.)

adrenal gland, a finding consistent with the close embryonic relationship between adrenal and gonadal anlagen. The tumors have included a granulosa cell tumor (56); testosterone-producing, virilizing Leydig cell adenomas (61,74); and a Leydig cell–containing, testosterone-secreting ganglioneuroma (1). Additionally, wedge-shaped subcapsular nodules of cells resembling ovarian stromal or thecal cells, so-called ovarian thecal metaplasia, have been encountered in as many as 4 percent of adrenalectomy specimens (26,81). These lesions, which occur almost exclusively in women, vary from microscopic to 2 mm in maximal diameter, are multiple in approximately half the cases, and are bilateral in approximately one third of the cases (26).

Finally, some extraovarian tumors of diverse origin have a variable microscopic resemblance to one or another type of ovarian sex cord–stromal tumor, but are otherwise unrelated. A heterogenous group of uterine tumors, referred to as "uterine tumors resembling ovarian sex cord tumors" or uterine "sex cord–like tumors," are of probable endometrial stromal, or occasionally, smooth muscle origin (17). Tumors reported in the older literature as "granulosa cell tumors" of the uterus almost certainly fall into this category (51). Similarly, peritoneal thecoma-like neoplasms, some of which have been associated with hypoglycemia (55), are now generally interpreted as solitary fibrous tumors ("fibrous mesotheliomas") (82).

REFERENCES

1. Aguirre P, Scully RE. Testosterone-secreting adrenal ganglioneuroma containing Leydig cells. Am J Surg Pathol 1983;7:699–705.
1a. Albores-Saavedra J, Henson DE. Tumors of the gallbladder and extrahepatic ducts. Atlas of Tumor Pathology. 2nd Series, Fascicle 22. Washington, D.C.: Armed Forces Institute of Pathology, 1986:155–7.
2. Altaras MM, Aviram R, Cohen I, et al. Primary peritoneal papillary serous adenocarcinoma: clinical and management aspects. Gynecol Oncol 1991;40:230–6.
3. Aslani M, Ahn GH, Scully RE. Serous papillary cystadenoma of borderline malignancy of broad ligament. A report of 25 cases. Int J Gynecol Pathol 1988;7:131–8.

4. Aslani M, Scully RE. Primary carcinoma of the broad ligament. Report of four cases and review of the literature. Cancer 1989;64:1540–5.
5. August CZ, Murad TM, Newton M. Multiple focal extraovarian serous carcinoma. Int J Gynecol Pathol 1985;4:11–23.
6. Banerjee R, Gough J. Cystic mucinous tumours of the mesentery and retroperitoneum: report of three cases. Histopathology 1988;12:527–32.
7. Baranetsky NG, Zipser RD, Goebelsmann U, et al: Adrenocorticotropin-dependent virilizing paraovarian tumors in Nelson's syndrome. J Clin Endocrinol Metab 1979;49:381–6.

8. Baron BW, Schraut WH, Azizi F, Talerman A. Extragonadal sex cord tumor with annular tubules in an umbilical hernia sac: a unique presentation with implications for histogenesis. Gynecol Oncol 1988;30:71–5.

9. Bell DA, Scully RE. Serous borderline tumors of the peritoneum. Am J Surg Pathol 1990;14:230–9.

10. Bell DA, Woodruff JM, Scully RE. Ependymoma of the broad ligament. A report of two cases. Am J Surg Pathol 1984;8:203–9.

11. Biscotti CV, Hart WR. Peritoneal serous micropapillomatosis of low malignant potential (serous borderline tumors of the peritoneum). A clinicopathologic study of 17 cases. Am J Surg Pathol 1992;16:467–75.

12. Bloss JD, Liao S, Buller RE, et al. Extraovarian peritoneal serous papillary carcinoma: a case-control retrospective comparison to papillary adenocarcinoma of the ovary. Gynecol Oncol 1993;50:347–51.

13. Chang KL, Crabtree GS, Lim-Tan SK, Kempson RL, Hendrickson MR. Primary extrauterine endometrial stromal neoplasms: a clinicopathologic study of 20 cases and a review of the literature. Int J Gynecol Pathol 1993;12:282–96.

14. Chen KT. Psammocarcinoma of the peritoneum. Diagn Cytol 1994;10:224–8.

15. Clark JE, Wood H, Jaffurs WJ, Fabro S. Endometrioid-type cystadenocarcinoma arising in the mesosalpinx. Obstet Gynecol 1979;54:656–8.

16. Clement PB, Scully RE. Extrauterine mesodermal (mullerian) adenosarcoma: a clinicopathologic analysis of five cases. Am J Clin Pathol 1978;69:276–83.

17. Clement PB, Scully RE. Uterine tumors resembling ovarian sex-cord tumors. A clinicopathologic analysis of fourteen cases. Am J Clin Pathol 1976;66:512–25.

18. Clement PB, Young RH, Scully RE. Extraovarian pelvic yolk sac tumors. Cancer 1988;62:620–6.

19. Dalrymple JC, Bannatyne P, Russell P, et al. Extraovarian peritoneal serous papillary carcinoma. A clinicopathologic study of 31 cases. Cancer 1989;64:110–5.

20. Dekmezian RH, Sneige N, Ordonez NG. Ovarian and omental ependymomas in peritoneal washings: cytologic and immunocytochemical features. Diagn Cytopathol 1986;2:62–8.

21. de Peralta MN, Delahoussaye PM, Tornos CS, Silva EG. Benign retroperitoneal cysts of mullerian type: a clinicopathologic study of three cases and review of the literature. Int J Gynecol Pathol 1994;13:273–8.

22. Deppe G, Malviya V, Jacobs AJ. Extragonadal mature, solid teratoma with omental implants. A case report. J Reprod Med 1988;33:792–4.

23. Duggan MA, Hugh J, Nation JG, Robertson DI, Stuart GC. Ependymoma of the uterosacral ligament. Cancer 1989;64:2565–71.

24. Evans H, Yates WA, Palmer WE, et al. Clear cell carcinoma of the sigmoid mesocolon: a tumor of the secondary mullerian system. Am J Obstet Gynecol 1990;162:161–3.

25. Feuer GA, Shevchuk M, Calanog A. Normal-sized ovary carcinoma syndrome. Obstet Gynecol 1989; 73:786–92.

26. Fidler WJ. Ovarian thecal metaplasia in adrenal glands. Am J Clin Pathol 1977;67:318–23.

27. Fowler JM, Nieberg RK, Schooler TA, Berek JS. Peritoneal adenocarcinoma (serous) of mullerian type: a subgroup of women presenting with peritoneal carcinomatosis. Int J Gynecol Cancer 1994;4:43–51.

28. Fromm G, Gershenson DM, Silva EG. Papillary serous carcinoma of the peritoneum. Obstet Gynecol 1990;75:89–95.

29. Garamvoelgyi E, Guillou L, Gebhard S, Salmeron M, Seematter RJ, Hadjii MH. Primary malignant mixed mullerian tumor (metaplastic carcinoma) of the female peritoneum. A clinical, pathologic, and immunohistochemical study of three cases and review of the literature. Cancer 1994;74:854–63.

30. Gardner GH, Greene RR, Peckham B. Tumors of the broad ligament. Am J Obstet Gynecol 1957;73:536–55.

31. Genadry R, Parmley T, Woodruff JD. The origin and clinical behavior of the parovarian tumor. Am J Obstet Gynecol 1977;129:873–80.

32. Gilks CB, Bell DA, Scully RE. Serous psammocarcinoma of the ovary and peritoneum. Int J Gynecol Pathol 1990;9:110–21.

32a. Gonzales-Crussi F. Extragonadal teratomas. Atlas of Tumor Pathology, 2nd Series, Fascicle 18. Washington, D.C.: Armed Forces Institute of Pathology, 1982.

33. Gooneratne S, Sassone M, Blaustein A, et al. Serous surface papillary carcinoma of the ovary: a clinicopathologic study of 16 cases. Int J Gyn Pathol 1982;1:258–69.

34. Griffith LM, Carcangiu ML. Sex cord tumor with annular tubules associated with endometriosis of the fallopian tube. Am J Clin Pathol 1991;96:259–62.

35. Hafiz MA, Toker C. Multicentric ovarian and extraovarian cystadenofibroma. Obstet Gynecol 1986;68:94S–8S.

36. Hampton HL, Huffman HT, Meeks GR. Extraovarian Brenner tumor. Obstet Gynecol 1992;79:844–6.

37. Heller DS, Keohane M, Bessim S, Jagirdar J, Deligdisch L. Pituitary-containing benign cystic teratoma arising from the uterosacral ligament. Arch Pathol Lab Med 1989;113:802–4.

38. Kanbour A, Salazar H, Stock R. Papillary cystadenoma originating in hydatid cyst of Morgagni: clinicopathologic study and observations on histogenesis [Abstract]. Lab Invest 1978;38:350.

39. Keitoku M, Konishi I, Nanbu K, et al. Extraovarian sex cord-stromal tumor: case report and review of the literature. Int J Gynecol Pathol 1997;16:180–5.

40. Kemp GM, Hsiu J, Andrews MC. Papillary peritoneal carcinomatosis after prophylactic oophorectomy. Gynecol Oncol 1992;47:395–7.

41. Khoury N, Raju U, Crissman JD, Zarbo RJ, Greenawald KA. A comparative immunohistochemical study of peritoneal and ovarian serous tumors, and mesotheliomas. Hum Pathol 1990;21:811–9.

42. Killackey MA, Davis AR. Papillary serous carcinoma of the peritoneal surface: matched-case comparison with papillary serous ovarian carcinoma. Gynecol Oncol 1993;51:171–4.

43. Kloppel G. Pancreatic, non-endocrine tumours. In: Kloppel G, Heitz PU, eds. Pancreatic pathology. New York: Churchill Livingstone, 1984:79–113.

43a. Kurman RJ, Norris HJ, Wilkinson E. Tumors of the cervix, vagina, and vulva. Atlas of Tumor Pathology. 3rd Series, Fascicle 4. Washington D.C.: Armed Forces Institute of Pathology, 1992.

44. Lauchlan SC. The secondary mullerian system. Obstet Gynecol Surv 1972;27:133–46.

45. Lee KR, Verma U, Belinson J. Primary clear cell carcinoma of the peritoneum. Gynecol Oncol 1991;41:259–62.

46. Lefkowitch JH, Fenoglio CM, Richart RM. Benign cystic teratoma of the retrouterine pouch of Douglas. Am J Obstet Gynecol 1978;131:818–20.

47. Lele SB, Piver MS, Matharu J, Tsukada Y. Peritoneal papillary carcinoma. Gynecol Oncol 1988;31:315–20.

48. McCaughey WT, Schryer MJ, Lin X, et al. Extraovarian pelvic serous tumor with marked calcification. Arch Pathol Lab Med 1986;110:78–80.

49. Mills SE, Andersen WA, Fechner RE, Austin MB. Serous surface papillary carcinoma. A clinicopathologic study of 10 cases and comparison with stage III-IV ovarian serous carcinoma. Am J Surg Pathol 1988;12:827–34.

50. Mira JL, Fenoglio-Preiser CM, Husseinzadeh N. Malignant mixed mullerian tumor of the extraovarian secondary mullerian system. Report of two cases and review of the English literature. Arch Pathol Lab Med 1995;119:1044–9.

51. Morehead RP, Bowman MC. Heterologous mesodermal tumors of the uterus: report of a neoplasm resembling a granulosa cell tumor. Am J Pathol 1945;21:53–61.

52. Motoyama T, Chida T, Fujiwara T, Watanabe H. Mucinous cystic tumor of the retroperitoneum. A report of two cases. Acta Cytol 1994;38:261–6.

53. Mulhollan TJ, Silva EG, Tornos C, Guerrieri C, Fromm GL, Gershenson D. Ovarian involvement by serous surface papillary carcinoma. Int J Gynecol Pathol 1994;13:120–6.

54. Muto MG, Welch WR, Mok SC, et al. Evidence for a multifocal origin of papillary serous carcinoma of the peritoneum [Abstract]. Gynecol Oncol 1994;52:127.

55. Nevius DB, Friedman NB. Mesotheliomas and extraovarian thecomas with hypoglycemic and nephrotic syndromes. Cancer 1959;12:1263–9.

56. Orselli RC, Bassler TJ. Theca granulosa cell tumor arising in adrenal. Cancer 1973;31:474–7.

57. Ostor AG, Nirenberg A, Ashdown ML, Murphy DJ. Extragenital adenosarcoma arising in the pouch of Douglas. Gynecol Oncol 1994;53:373–5.

58. Park U, Han KC, Chang HK, Huh MH. A primary mucinous cystadenocarcinoma of the retroperitoneum. Gynecol Oncol 1991;42:64–7.

59. Pennell TC, Gusdon JP Jr. Retroperitoneal mucinous cystadenoma. Am J Obstet Gynecol 1989;160:1229–31.

60. Piver MS, Jishi MF, Tsukuda Y, Nava G. Primary peritoneal carcinoma after prophylactic oophorectomy in women with a family history of ovarian cancer. A report of the Gilda Radner Familial Ovarian Cancer Registry. Cancer 1993;71:2751–5.

61. Pollock WJ, McConnell CF, Hilton C, Lavine RL. Virilizing Leydig cell adenoma of adrenal gland. Am J Surg Pathol 1986;10:816–22.

62. Raju U, Fine G, Greenawald KA, Ohorodnik JM. Primary papillary serous neoplasia of the peritoneum: a clinicopathologic and ultrastructural study of eight cases. Human Pathol 1989;20:426–36.

63. Ransom DT, Shreyaskumar RP, Keeney GL, Malkasian GD, Edmonson JH. Papillary serous carcinoma of the peritoneum. A review of 33 cases treated with platin-based chemotherapy. Cancer 1990;66:1091–4.

64. Roman LD, Mitchell MF, Tornos C, Glover A, Kavanagh JJ. Dedifferentiated extrauterine adenosarcoma responsive to chemotherapy. Gynecol Oncol 1993;49:389–94.

65. Rothacker D, Knolle J, Stiller D, Borchard F. Primary retroperitoneal mucinous cystadenomas with gastric epithelial differentiation. Path Res Pract 1993;189:1195–204.

66. Rothacker D, Mobius G. Varieties of serous surface papillary carcinoma of the peritoneum in Northern Germany: a thirty-year autopsy study. Int J Gynecol Pathol 1995;14:310–8.

67. Rutledge ML, Silva EG, McLemore D, El-Naggar A. Serous surface carcinoma of the ovary and peritoneum. A flow cytometric study. Pathol Annu 1989;24:227–35.

67a. Silverberg SG, Kurman RJ. Tumors of the uterine corpus and gestational trophoblastic disease. Atlas of Tumor Pathology. 3rd Series. Fascicle 3. Washington, D.C.: Armed Forces Insitute of Pathology, 1992.

68. Smith R, Deppe G, Selvaggi S, Lall C. Benign teratoma of the omentum and ovary coexistent with an ovarian neoplasm. Gynecol Oncol 1990;39:204–7.

68a. Subramony C, Herrera GA, Turbat-Herrera EA. Hepatobiliary cystadenoma. A study of five cases with reference to histogenesis. Arch Pathol Lab Med 1993;117:1036–42.

69. Sun CJ, Toker C, Masi JD, Elias EG. Primary low grade adenocarcinoma occurring in the inguinal region. Cancer 1979;44:340–5.

70. Tenti P, Carnevali L, Tateo S, Durola R. Primary mucinous cystadenocarcinoma of the retroperitoneum: two cases. Gynecol Oncol 1994;55:308–12.

71. Tobacman JK, Tucker MA, Kase R, Greene MH, Costa J, Fraumeni JF Jr. Intra-abdominal carcinomatosis after prophylactic oophorectomy in ovarian-cancer-prone families. Lancet 1982;2:795–7.

72. Truong LD, Maccato ML, Awalt H, et al. Serous surface carcinoma of the peritoneum: a clinicopathologic study of 22 cases. Hum Pathol 1990;21:99–110.

73. Ulbright TM, Morley DJ, Roth LM, et al. Papillary serous carcinoma of the retroperitoneum. Am J Clin Pathol 1983;79:633–7.

74. Vasiloff J, Chideckel EW, Boyd CB, Foshag LJ. Testosterone-secreting adrenal adenoma containing crystalloids characteristic of Leydig cells. Am J Med 1985;79:772–6.

75. Verdonk C, Guerin C, Lufkin E, Hodgson SF. Activation of virilizing adrenal rest tissues by excessive ACTH production. An unusual presentation of Nelson's syndrome. Am J Med 1982;73:455–9.

76. Weber AM, Hewett WJ, Gajewski WH, Curry SL. Serous carcinoma of the peritoneum after oophorectomy. Obstet Gynecol 1992;80:558–60.

76a. Weir MM, Bell DA, Young RH. Grade 1 peritoneal serous carcinomas: a report of 14 cases and comparison with 7 peritoneal serous psammocarcinomas and 19 peritoneal serous borderline tumors. Am J Surg Pathol 1998;22:849–62.

77. Wheeler JE. Extraovarian teratoma with peritoneal gliomatosis. Hum Pathol 1978;9:232–4.

78. White PF, Merino MJ, Barwick KW. Serous surface papillary carcinoma of the ovary: a clinical, pathologic, ultrastructural, and immunohistochemical study of 11 cases. Pathol Annu 1985;20(1):403–18.

79. Wick MR, Mills SE, Dehner LP, Bollinger DJ, Fechner RE. Serous papillary carcinomas arising from the peritoneum and ovaries. A clinicopathologic and immunohistochemical comparison. Int J Gynecol Pathol 1989; 8:179–88.

80. Wild RA, Albert RD, Zaino RJ, Abrams CS. Virilizing paraovarian tumors: a consequence of Nelson's syndrome? Obstet Gynecol 1988;71:1053–6.

81. Wong T, Warner NE. Ovarian theca metaplasia in the adrenal gland. Arch Pathol 1971;92:319–28.

82. Young RH, Clement PB, McCaughey WT. Solitary fibrous tumors ("fibrous mesotheliomas") of the peritoneum. A report of three cases and a review of the literature. Arch Pathol Lab Med 1990;114:493–5.

24
FALLOPIAN TUBE: EMBRYOLOGY AND ANATOMY

EMBRYOLOGY

The fallopian tubes are derived from the mullerian ducts, each of which begins as an invagination of the coelomic epithelium lateral to the cranial end of the mesonephric duct at 6 weeks of embryonic life. The blind caudal end of each mullerian duct grows downward into the mesonephric ridge, acquiring a lumen as it lengthens (8), and reaches the lower end of the mesonephros by 8 weeks. Each duct then turns medially, crosses ventral to the mesonephric duct, and near the midline grows caudally in close proximity to its contralateral counterpart. The two ducts reach the dorsal wall of the urogenital sinus during the third month. Their blind ends produce an elevation of the sinus, referred to as the mullerian tubercle (8).

The cranial portion of each mullerian duct becomes a fallopian tube, which opens into the coelomic cavity at the site of the original coelomic invagination (the abdominal ostium). At 7 to 8 weeks, the caudal vertical parts of each duct fuse to form the uterovaginal primordium, which becomes the uterus and upper vagina. In females, the mesonephric ducts atrophy almost completely, although remnants in the form of small tubules surrounded by a cuff of smooth muscle are common incidental microscopic findings within the broad ligament and ovarian hilus (see chapter 27) (3).

ANATOMY

Gross Anatomy

The tubes, which are 9 to 12 cm in length, extend laterally from the ipsilateral uterine cornu to the medial pole of the ovary, ascend along the mesovarian border, arch over the lateral pole of the ovary, and turn inferiorly to end close to its free border. Each tube consists of four segments, which, extending medially to laterally, are the intramural portion, the isthmus, the ampulla, and the infundibulum. The last three (or extrauterine) segments are attached by the mesosalpinx, a peritoneal fold at the superior margin of the broad ligament.

The lateral (fimbriated) end of the tube, which opens into the pelvic cavity, is composed of a variable number of irregular fringe-like extensions (fimbriae). The fimbriae are a continuation of the expanded, trumpet-shaped infundibulum, which is about 1 cm in length and diameter. The opening of the tube into the peritoneal cavity lies deep within the infundibulum, and is approximately 3 mm in diameter (8). The infundibulum is continuous with the somewhat tortuous, narrower, ampullary portion of the tube, which accounts for approximately half the tubal length. The ampullary portion is continuous with the isthmus, which is 2 to 3 cm in length. The isthmus joins the interstitial (intramural) segment of the tube, which is approximately 1 cm in length and enters the endometrial cavity at the tubal recess of the uterine fundus.

The fallopian tube has a dual blood supply, which originates from an anastomotic network of vessels in the mesosalpinx, supplied by a branch of the uterine artery and a branch of the ovarian artery. The venous drainage follows a similar course. Most of the efferent lymphatic channels draining the tube descend within the mesosalpinx behind the ovary where they form part of the subovarian plexus (6). Because lymph from the fallopian tubes, uterus, and ovary has a common drainage system, retrograde spread of tumor from one organ to another is possible, particularly if there is an obstruction to normal lymphatic flow. The lymph nodes into which the tubal lymphatics drain are discussed on page 471.

Microscopic Anatomy

The wall of the tube consists of mucosa and muscularis, and in its extrauterine parts, serosa composed of fibrovascular connective tissue covered by mesothelium (fig. 24-1). The myosalpinx contains an inner circular and outer longitudinal layer; the isthmic and intramural segments also contain an inner longitudinal layer. The mucosa consists of nonstratified epithelium and subjacent stroma composed of fibrovascular tissue (lamina propria); the two layers are separated by a basement membrane. Longitudinal branching

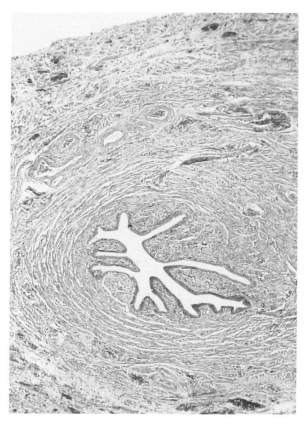

Figure 24-1
NORMAL FALLOPIAN TUBE
The lumen is surrounded by mucosa with plicae, muscularis, and serosa.

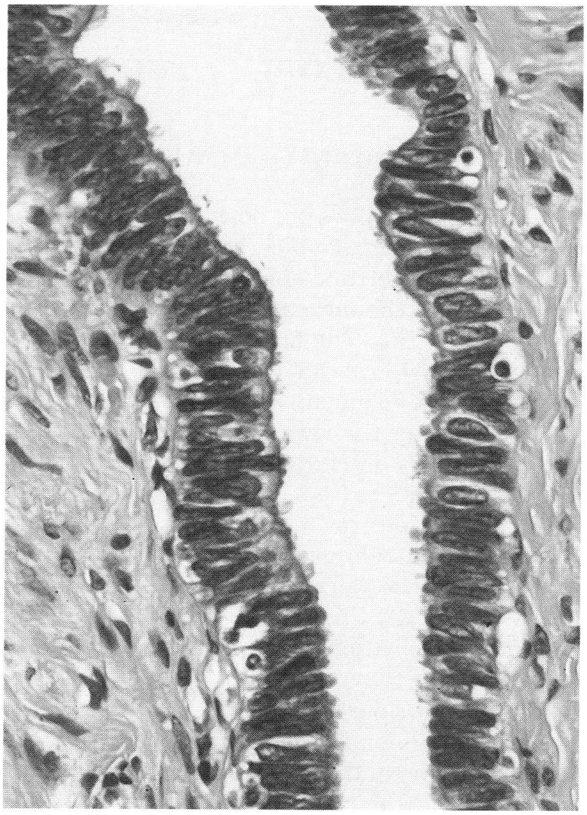

Figure 24-2
TUBAL EPITHELIUM
Ciliated and nonciliated secretory cells are seen.

folds of the mucosa, the plicae, increase in number, height, and complexity from the isthmus to the infundibulum, terminating in the fimbriae. The stroma of the plicae is often fibrotic and hypocellular in postmenopausal women.

During the reproductive era, the tubal epithelium is composed of three cell types: ciliated cells, secretory cells, and intercalated "peg" cells (fig. 24-2). The relative numbers of each cell type vary not only from one region of the tube to another, but also with the menstrual cycle (1,2). The secretory cells tend to be narrower than the ciliated cells and have a hyperchromatic compressed nucleus; an apical cytoplasmic vacuole may be present. Intercalated cells have a thin hyperchromatic nucleus and scanty cytoplasm; their nature

and function are not clear. Mitotic figures are occasionally seen in the lining cells in response to the normal estrogen levels in women of reproductive age; mitotic activity before puberty and after the menopause usually indicates endogenous or exogenous estrogenic stimulation.

"Physiological" salpingitis refers to the presence of luminal and mucosal neutrophils, sometimes accompanied by edema and lymphangiectasia of the plicae, during menstruation (5), during the puerperium (4), and, occasionally, to a lesser degree, throughout the menstrual cycle (7). The inflammation peaks at midmenses, only rarely involves the muscularis, is unaccompanied by necrosis or ulceration, and is not followed by a chronic inflammatory cell infiltrate.

REFERENCES

General References

Eddy CA, Pauerstein CJ. Anatomy and physiology of the fallopian tube. Clinical Obstet Gynecol 1980;23:1177–93.

Nicosia SV. Pathology of the oviducts and embryonal remnants. Obstet Gynecol Annu 1985;14:382–410.

Woodruff JD, Pauerstein CJ, eds. The fallopian tube. Structure, function, pathology, and management. Baltimore: Williams & Wilkins, 1969.

Embryology and Anatomy

1. Bonilla-Musoles F, Ferrer-Barriendos J, Pellicer A. Cyclical changes in the epithelium of the fallopian tube. Studies with scanner electron microscopy (SEM). Clin Exp Obstet Gynecol 1983;10:79–86.
2. Donnez J, Casanas-Roux F, Caprasse J, Ferin J, Thomas K. Cyclic changes in ciliation, cell height, and mitotic activity in human tubal epithelium during reproductive life. Fertil Steril 1985;43:554–9.
3. Gardner GH, Greene RR, Peckham BM. Normal and cystic structures of the broad ligament. Am J Obstet Gynecol 1948;55:917–39.
4. Hellman LM. The morphology of the human fallopian tube in the early puerperium. Am J Obstet Gynecol 1949;57:154–63.
5. Nassberg S, McKay DG, Hertig AT. Physiologic salpingitis. Am J Obstet Gynecol 1954;67:130–7.
6. Plentl AA, Friedman EA. Lymphatic system of the female genitalia: the morphologic basis of oncologic diagnosis and therapy. Philadelphia: WB Saunders, 1971.
7. Smith HA, Greene RR. Physiologic salpingitis? Am J Obstet Gynecol 1956;72:174–9.
8. Williams PL, Warwick R, Dyson M, Bannister LH, eds. Gray's anatomy. Edinburgh: Churchill Livingstone, 1989.

25

TUMORS OF THE FALLOPIAN TUBE:
HISTOLOGIC CLASSIFICATION AND CANCER STAGING
EPITHELIAL AND MIXED EPITHELIAL–MESENCHYMAL TUMORS

HISTOLOGIC CLASSIFICATION
AND CANCER STAGING

The World Health Organization (WHO) histologic typing of tumors of the fallopian tube is presented in Table 25-1 and the staging of tubal cancers by the International Federation of Gynecology and Obstetrics (FIGO) (52), in Table 25-2. In this staging system the term "mucosa" (which includes both the epithelium and lamina propria) is misused for "epithelium," and "submucosa" (which does not exist in the tube) is misused for "lamina propria." Also, no distinction is made between true (incidental) carcinoma in situ of the tube and intraluminal masses of carcinoma that are confined to the epithelium, but recur rarely and can be fatal (58,61). Finally, no provision is included for staging extraluminal

Table 25-1

**WORLD HEALTH ORGANIZATION HISTOLOGIC TYPING
OF TUMORS OF THE FALLOPIAN TUBE**

EPITHELIAL TUMORS
    Benign
        Endometrioid polyp
        Papilloma
        Metaplastic papillary tumor
    Malignant
        Carcinoma in situ
        Serous carcinoma
        Mucinous carcinoma
        Endometrioid carcinoma
        Clear cell carcinoma
        Transitional cell carcinoma
        Squamous cell carcinoma
        Glassy cell carcinoma
        Mixed carcinoma
        Undifferentiated carcinoma

MIXED EPITHELIAL–MESENCHYMAL TUMORS
    Benign
        Adenofibroma
    Malignant
        Adenosarcoma
        Malignant mullerian mixed tumor
          (carcinosarcoma)

SOFT TISSUE TYPE TUMORS
    Benign
        Leiomyoma
        Others
    Malignant
        Leiomyosarcoma
        Others

MESOTHELIAL TUMORS
    Solitary mesothelioma
    Adenomatoid tumor

GERM CELL TUMORS
    Teratoma
        Mature
          Dermoid cyst
          Solid
        Immature
        Struma
        Carcinoid
    Others

TROPHOBLASTIC DISEASE
    Hydatidiform mole
    Choriocarcinoma

SECONDARY TUMORS
    Carcinoma
        Squamous cell carcinoma in situ of cervix
        Carcinoma of cervix
        Carcinoma of endometrium
        Carcinoma of ovary
        Others
    Lymphoma and leukemia
    Others

TUMOR-LIKE LESIONS
    Atypical epithelial hyperplasia
    Endometrial colonization and endometriosis
    Salpingitis isthmica nodosa
    Tuberculous salpingitis
    Bacterial salpingitis
    Heat artifact
    Mesothelial hyperplasia
    Ectopic pregnancy
    Malakoplakia
    Others

Table 25-2

MODIFIED FIGO FALLOPIAN TUBE STAGING
(Based on Operative Findings Prior to Debulking and Pathologic Findings)

Stage 0	Carcinoma in situ* (limited to tubal mucosa).[†]
Stage I	Growth is limited to the fallopian tubes.
Stage IA	Growth is limited to one tube with extension into the submucosa[‡] and/or muscularis but not penetrating the serosal surface; no ascites.
Stage IB	Growth is limited to both tubes with extension into the submucosa[‡] and/or muscularis but not penetrating the serosal surface; no ascites.
Stage IC	Tumor either stage IA or IB but with tumor extension through or onto the tubal serosa; or with ascites present containing malignant cells or with positive peritoneal washings.
Stage II	Growth involving one or both fallopian tubes with pelvic extension.
Stage IIA	Extension and/or metastasis to the uterus and/or ovaries.
Stage IIB	Extension to other pelvic tissues.
Stage IIC	Tumor either stage IIA or IIB but with tumor extension through or onto the tubal serosa; or with ascites present containing malignant cells or with positive peritoneal washings.
Stage III	Tumor involves one or both fallopian tubes with peritoneal implants outside of the pelvis and/or positive retroperitoneal or inguinal nodes. Superficial liver metastases equals stage III. Tumor appears limited to the true pelvis but with histologically proven malignant extension to the small bowel or omentum.
Stage IIIA	Tumor is grossly limited to the true pelvis with negative nodes but with histologically confirmed microscopic seeding of abdominal peritoneal surfaces.
Stage IIIB	Tumor involving one or both tubes with histologically confirmed implants of abdominal peritoneal surfaces, none exceeding 2 cm in diameter. Lymph nodes are negative.
Stage IIIC	Abdominal implants greater than 2 cm in diameter and/or positive retroperitoneal or inguinal nodes.
Stage IV	Growth involving one or both fallopian tubes with distant metastases. If pleural effusion is present, there must be positive cytology to be stage IV. Parenchymal liver metastases equals stage IV.

Authors' footnotes:
*The staging system does not distinguish between microscopic foci of replacement of tubal epithelium by malignant epithelium and grossly evident masses in the tubal lumen that do not penetrate the wall beyond the epithelium. The former have not been reported to spread beyond the tube whereas the latter can extend beyond the tube, recur and be fatal.
[†]The "mucosa" presumably refers to the epithelium since involvement of the lamina propria component of the mucosa requires staging of the tumor as IA.
[‡]Since the fallopian tube has no "submucosa," this designation presumably refers to the lamina propria.

carcinomas originating in the fimbriae. In our combined consultation and hospital experience, 12 percent of tubal carcinomas do not invade the lamina propria (2) and 8 percent are fimbrial in origin (1). We stage the former tumors as Ia-0 and further divide stage Ia into Ia-1 (invasion only of lamina propria) and Ia-2 (deeper invasion of wall without serosal penetration) (2). We designate stage I fimbrial tumors as I(F); their cells are exposed directly to the peritoneal cavity, but unlike the cells of stage Ic tumors they do not invade the myosalpinx (1,2).

EPITHELIAL TUMORS

Benign Tumors

Endometrioid Polyp. The most common benign epithelial tumor is the endometrioid polyp, sometimes referred to as *adenomatous polyp*. Its frequency is difficult to determine since in a number of reported cases the diagnosis was based mostly on radiographic studies of infertile women, with infrequent pathologic confirmation. In two of these studies the prevalence

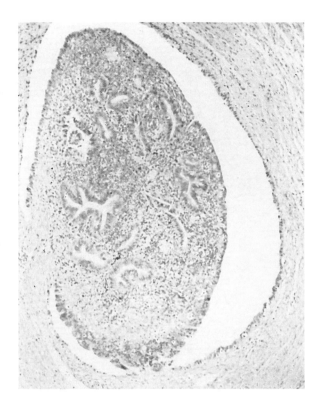

Figure 25-1
ENDOMETRIOID POLYP
The polyp protrudes into the lumen of the interstitial portion of the tube.

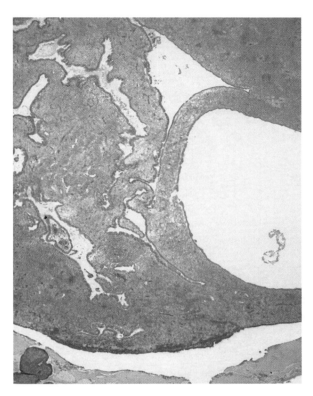

Figure 25-2
ENDOMETRIOID POLYP
A large polyp distends the lumen of the tube.

ranged from 1.2 to 2.5 percent (15,40). In the only large pathologic study, which was based on an examination of 300 hysterectomy specimens that included a fallopian tube, endometrioid polyps were found in the interstitial portion of the tube in 11 percent, and endometrial-type mucosa in 25 percent of the cases (page 490) (40). Ectopic endometrial mucosa elsewhere in the tube has been found occasionally as well (55). Polyps may obstruct the lumen of the tube and result in infertility or ectopic pregnancy. Although most of the lesions are not recognized grossly they can be as large as 1.3 cm in diameter. They are often attached to the tubal epithelium by a broad base and resemble intrauterine endometrial polyps (figs. 25-1, 25-2).

Papilloma and Cystadenoma. A few papillomas have been described in the fallopian tube (17,24,35,68). They range up to 3 cm in diameter, are loosely attached to the tubal mucosa, and consist of delicate, branching fibrovascular stalks lined by epithelial cells that may appear indifferent or resemble those of fallopian tube epithelium. One serous cystadenoma of fimbrial origin has been described (1).

Metaplastic Papillary Tumor. A few of these lesions have been reported (7,36,57), all of them incidental microscopic findings in segments of fallopian tube removed during the postpartum period. The lesions appear similar to serous borderline tumors of the ovary occurring during pregnancy, with proliferation of atypical epithelial cells, cellular budding, and the presence of abundant eosinophilic cytoplasm in most of the lesional cells (figs. 25-3, 25-4); some of the cells contain mucin, and extracellular mucin may be abundant. Rare mitotic figures may be present. It is uncertain whether these lesions are tiny serous borderline tumors with metaplastic changes related to pregnancy or are only proliferative and metaplastic (7,57). We have seen rare lesions of this type in the absence of pregnancy.

463

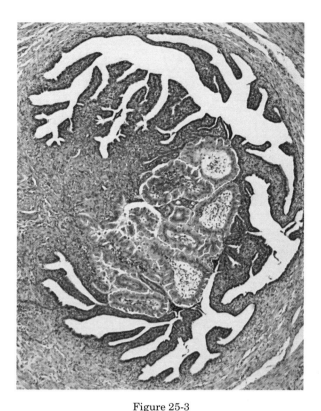

Figure 25-3
METAPLASTIC PAPILLARY TUMOR
This lesion from a pregnant patient is small and localized, and is characterized by papillary epithelial proliferation with cellular buds.

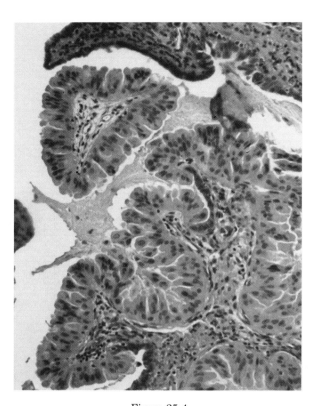

Figure 25-4
METAPLASTIC PAPILLARY TUMOR
The stratified epithelial cells contain abundant eosinophilic cytoplasm.

Borderline Tumors

A 6-cm serous borderline papillary tumor (70), a 1.7-cm serous borderline cystic tumor, and a 3-cm endometrioid borderline adenofibroma, all of them situated at the fimbrial end (1) have been reported. The first patient was well 6 years, and the second 2 years after salpingo-oophorectomy. Another serous tumor of the tube, designated carcinoma in a teenage girl, also had the features of a serous borderline tumor (23). Four tumors, three of which were associated with pseudomyxoma peritonei, have been reported as tubal "mucinous borderline tumors" (60). The existence of mucinous metaplasia of the tubal epithelium (fig. 25-5), of which 10 examples have been reported (3 associated with the Peutz-Jeghers syndrome, 3 with ovarian mucinous tumors [cystadenomas and carcinomas], and 3 with cervical mucinous tumors [carcinoma in situ and invasive

adenocarcinoma]), suggests a possible source of these tumors. In none of the four cases, however, was the appendix examined microscopically although in one case it was said to appear normal at operation. The possibility exists, therefore, that the tubal mucinous borderline tumors, at least in the three cases associated with pseudomyxoma peritonei, could have been implants of an undetected appendiceal tumor (page 99).

Malignant Tumors

General Features. Carcinomas of the fallopian tube are generally stated to account for approximately 0.3 percent of all gynecologic cancers (8), but this figure may be low because carcinomas of questionable origin involving both the tube and ovary are generally classified as carcinomas of the latter organ in view of their much higher frequency. The tubal origin of some of these tumors is suggested by a recent screening study with the use of serum CA125 assays that

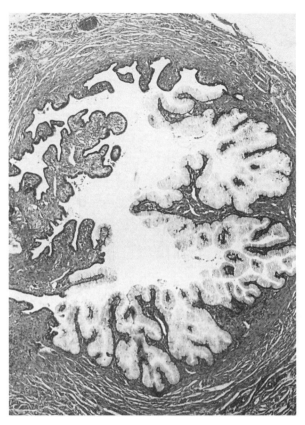

Figure 25-5
MUCINOUS METAPLASIA
Most of the tubal epithelial cells have been replaced by columnar cells filled with mucin.

detected one tubal carcinoma for every six ovarian carcinomas (69). This ratio exceeds the expected ratio of 1 to 150 based on the generally cited frequencies of the two tumors. Approximately 1500 cases of tubal carcinoma have been reported in the literature (53).

Because of its relative rarity little is known about the cause of tubal carcinoma. As in cases of ovarian carcinoma, there appears to be an abnormally high frequency of nulliparity (approximately 30 percent), but case-control studies have not been done to confirm this finding (48,54). A pathogenetic role of chronic salpingitis, particularly tuberculous salpingitis, has been suggested in the literature but appears unlikely in view of the absence of infection in most cases of carcinoma and the difference in the age incidence of patients with salpingitis and carcinoma. Also, salpingitis, including the tuberculous type, may be associated with pseudo-

carcinomatous reactive epithelial hyperplasia, sometimes resulting in a misdiagnosis of carcinoma (page 484), and the frequency of tuberculosis in patients with tubal carcinoma does not appear to exceed that in the general population (59). Nevertheless, evidence of salpingitis occasionally accompanies carcinoma, and valid cases of coexistent tubal carcinoma and salpingitis, including the tuberculous form, have been reported (27). Although fallopian tube epithelium is responsive to estrogenic stimulation there is no evidence that such stimulation increases the incidence of carcinoma, as observed in cases of endometrial carcinoma after ingestion of estrogenic hormones for treatment of the menopause (54).

An increased frequency of tubal carcinoma has been reported in patients with ovarian carcinoma, suggesting that the tubal carcinomas in such cases are independent primary tumors, reflecting a "field change" (5). This interpretation is difficult to prove because of the problem in distinguishing implants that have replaced the tubal wall from primary carcinomas; clonality studies may be helpful in making this distinction in the future. Tubal carcinoma appears to be associated with an increased frequency of endometrial and breast carcinoma (2,51).

Tubal carcinoma has been reported in women 14 to 87 years of age, with a mean of 57 years (8,48). The peak age incidence is in the early 60s, and the age-specific incidence curve is similar to those of ovarian and endometrial carcinomas. Tubal carcinoma is diagnosed preoperatively in only about 5 percent of the cases (48). The main manifestations are abnormal bleeding or discharge per vaginam, which occurs in one third to half the cases, and abdominal pain, which may be intermittent and colicky or constant and dull. Less than 10 percent of patients have a symptom complex designated "hydrops tubae profluens," which is characterized by intermittent, colicky pain relieved by the sudden discharge per vaginam of watery fluid rich in cholesterol, with relief of the pain and decrease in size of an abdominal mass (48). This rare combination of findings, however, is not specific for tubal carcinoma. Cervical-vaginal cytologic examination has been reported to be positive in as many as 60 percent of the cases (59) but the figure is 10 to 20 percent in most series (4,51,63). Occasionally, a fragment of tubal carcinoma in an endocervical or endometrial curettage specimen is the first manifestation of the disease (2,25). Elevations in the serum level of CA125 are observed commonly, and measurement of this antigen may be useful in monitoring the course of affected patients (47,48,64). Transvaginal ultrasound examination has also been effective in diagnosing tubal carcinoma (4). In one patient whose tumor secreted human chorionic gonadotropin the clinical presentation mimicked an ectopic pregnancy (2). The possibility of tubal carcinoma should be entertained in women with vaginal bleeding or discharge, or a cytologic examination positive for malignant cells that are unexplained by investigation of the lower female genital tract. Occasional patients with tubal carcinoma present with metastasis, for example, to an inguinal lymph node (25). A rare presentation is as a mass at the vaginal apex many years after a vaginal hysterectomy (20,44).

From a molecular-biologic viewpoint, tubal carcinoma has been shown to overexpress c-*erb*B-2 and p53 with frequencies similar to those encountered in cases of ovarian carcinoma (39).

Gross Findings. The tumor has been reported to be bilateral in 20 percent of the cases, but in our experience the frequency is only 3 percent (2). Right-sided and left-sided tumors are equally common when the tumor is unilateral. The ampullary portion of the tube is involved twice as frequently as the isthmic portion. Frequently, the tube is swollen, sometimes along its entire length, with closure of the fimbriated end and accumulation of watery fluid or blood in the lumen, creating an external appearance that may be indistinguishable from that of hydrosalpinx or hematosalpinx (2). For that reason, any dilated fallopian tube should be opened intraoperatively and examined carefully (4). In the presence of a large amount of fluid the consistency of the tube may be soft, but firm areas may be palpable, particularly if the wall has been invaded. Tumor may be visible on the serosal surface (fig. 25-6) or there may be obvious infiltration of adjacent viscera or the pelvic wall. Occasionally, a tubal carcinoma appears as a localized solid or partly cystic nodule involving only a portion of the tube, and rarely, as a nodular expansion of the fimbriated end. Opening the lumen of a tube involved by carcinoma usually reveals a localized or diffuse, soft, gray to pink, friable growth occupying the mucosal surface (figs. 25-7–25-9). In a few cases, multiple tumors are present; hemorrhage and yellow areas of necrosis are common.

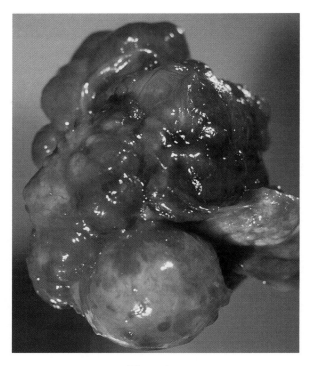

Figure 25-6
CARCINOMA
The tube is diffusely enlarged; nodular, hemorrhagic excrescences of tumor are visible on its outer surface. The ovary lies below the tube.

Usually, the tumor extends into the wall of the tube but occasionally it is loosely attached to the mucosal surface or lies free in the lumen (16).

In some cases a primary tubal carcinoma originates in the fimbriated end. Tumors of this type accounted for 8 percent of the cases in one large series (2).

Another type of carcinoma involving the tube is of uncertain origin because it is continuous with a solid ovarian mass or an ovarian cyst that communicates with the tubal lumen. The criteria for distinguishing between an ovarian and tubal origin in such cases are presented on page 471. In the occasional cases in which there is no preponderant evidence in favor of either an ovarian or tubal origin the term "tubo-ovarian carcinoma" has been suggested (25).

Microscopic Findings. Rare cases of tubal carcinoma in situ have been reported (5,26,56,59, 62), one of them after tamoxifen therapy for carcinoma of the breast (62). The diagnosis should be limited to flat or minimally papillary epithelial

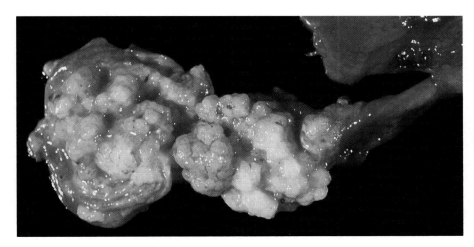

Figure 25-7
CARCINOMA
The opened tube is almost entirely filled by papillary tumor attached to its mucosa.

Figure 25-8
CARCINOMA
The lumen of the opened tube is distended by solid tumor, which was of endometrioid type.

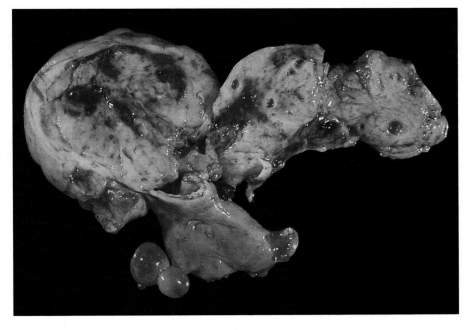

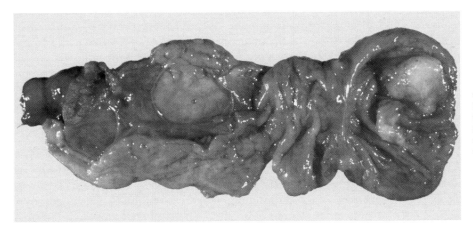

Figure 25-9
CARCINOMA
The distended, opened tube contains a solid nodule of tumor close to the obliterated fimbriated end. An uninvolved ovary is visible at the junction of the left and middle thirds of the specimen.

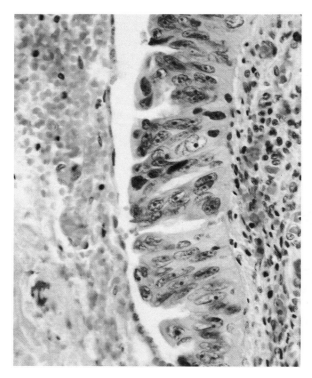

Figure 25-10
CARCINOMA IN SITU
The lesion involves the surface of a fimbria; it is covered by a hemorrhagic fibrous adhesion (left).

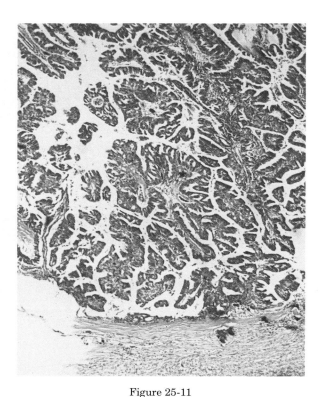

Figure 25-11
SEROUS PAPILLARY ADENOCARCINOMA
The lumen is filled with fine papillae lined by neoplastic epithelial cells. Cellular buds are visible in the lumen.

lesions that are invisible on gross examination and are characterized by replacement of tubal epithelium by obviously malignant cells (fig. 25-10) (5,49). As mentioned on page 465, lesions associated with carcinomas of similar cell type arising in other organs may be implants rather than primary tumors.

Carcinomas of all the ovarian surface epithelial cell types have been reported in the fallopian tube. The frequency of these types, however, is difficult to ascertain because in almost all large series of reported cases the tumors have been classified solely on the basis of their architecture, with designations such as papillary, adeno-, alveolar, solid, and medullary, or combinations thereof (32). Nevertheless, personal experience and analysis of microscopic descriptions and photomicrographs in the literature suggest that serous carcinoma is the most common cellular subtype. In one series of 40 cases (45), 85 percent of the tumors were serous or "poorly differentiated." In our experience over two thirds of the tumors

are serous; about 10 percent, endometrioid; 10 percent, transitional or undifferentiated; and the remainder of other epithelial cell types (2).

Tubal serous carcinomas resemble similar tumors of the ovary, and are characterized by papillarity, cellular budding, slit-like glandular spaces, and solid masses in poorly differentiated areas (figs. 25-11–25-13); psammoma bodies are occasionally seen. In our experience tubal serous carcinomas contain tumor giant cells more often than ovarian serous carcinomas (2). The tumor may extend in situ, replacing adjacent epithelium. Necrosis and vascular space invasion are common.

Over 50 endometrioid carcinomas of the fallopian tube have been documented in the literature (10,11,14,16,18,22,28,30,33,43,46,61,66,67). Approximately half of these are of an unusual type that is rare in the endometrium and is characterized in part by a resemblance to the wolffian adnexal tumor (pages 324 and 503) (16,46,61,67). Eleven of the endometrioid carcinomas contained squamous elements, which in 1 case were cytologically

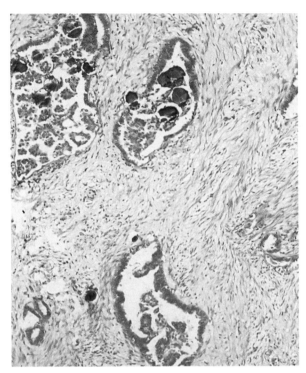

Figure 25-12
SEROUS PAPILLARY ADENOCARCINOMA
The tubal wall is infiltrated by carcinoma forming psammoma bodies and eliciting a desmoplastic stromal response.

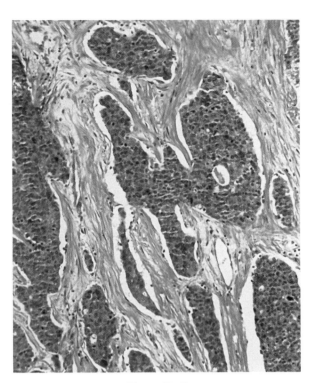

Figure 25-13
SEROUS CARCINOMA
An undifferentiated component in the tubal wall is characterized by solid islands of neoplastic epithelial cells.

malignant; 4 were associated with endometriosis, which in 2 cases lay adjacent to the tumor, suggesting an origin therein (fig. 25-14); and one tumor was oxyphilic (46). The tumors that resembled wolffian adnexal tumors formed polypoid or unattached intraluminal masses that did not infiltrate the wall of the tube except in 3 cases, in one of which the invasion was superficial (see fig. 25-8). These tumors are composed of solid masses of small, closely packed cells punctured by tubular glands that are typically small but occasionally cystic; many of the glands contain dense periodic acid–Schiff (PAS)-positive colloid-like secretion (fig. 25-15); some of the glands contain intraluminal mucin. Occasionally, the solid areas contain well differentiated spindle-shaped cells, which sometimes form focal concentric whorls (figs. 25-16–25-18). In most cases, foci of typical endometrioid carcinoma are seen as well (figs. 25-16, 25-17). Several of the tumors that were stained immunohistochemically were positive for epithelial membrane antigen, TAG72, and CA125.

One "mucinous carcinoma in situ" of the tube that was adjacent to an area of mucinous metaplasia occurred in a patient with mucinous carcinoma in situ of the cervix and mucinous carcinoma of both ovaries with peritoneal spread. Only a single case of invasive mucinous carcinoma has been reported; it was bilateral and was associated with a mucinous adenocarcinoma of the cervix (34). In one large series of tubal carcinomas, however, the mucinous type accounted for 5 percent of the cases (53).

Nine clear cell (2,28,65), 15 transitional cell (2,21,31,38), 3 squamous cell (9,12,41), 2 small cell undifferentiated (2), 1 glassy cell (29), 1 α-fetoprotein-producing hepatoid (3), and 1 lymphoepithelioma-like carcinoma (2) of the tube have been reported. Japanese investigators (64a) found that 9 of 21 tubal carcinomas (43 percent) had a predominant transitional cell pattern. Transitional cell metaplasia of the epithelium, which was detected in 3 of 10,000 specimens of fallopian tube, has been suggested as a possible source of

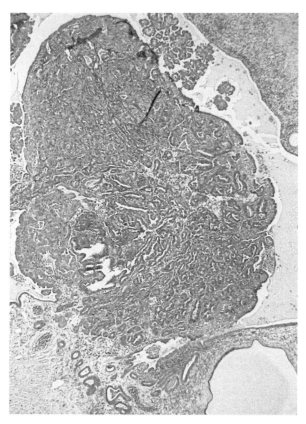

Figure 25-14
ENDOMETRIOID CARCINOMA
ARISING IN ENDOMETRIOSIS

The tumor is forming a polypoid mass protruding into the lumen. Endometriosis is seen at the base of the tumor.

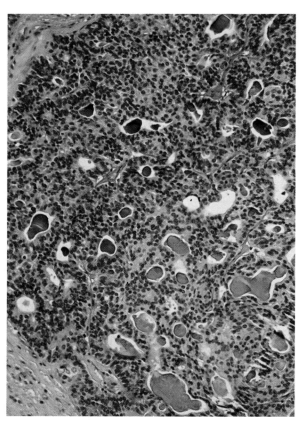

Figure 25-15
ENDOMETRIOID ADENOCARCINOMA
SIMULATING WOLFFIAN ADNEXAL TUMOR

The small glands contain densely eosinophilic hyaline material.

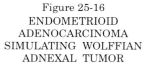
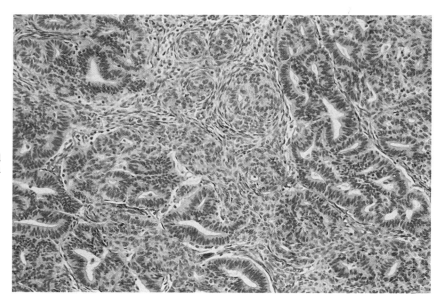

Figure 25-16
ENDOMETRIOID
ADENOCARCINOMA
SIMULATING WOLFFIAN
ADNEXAL TUMOR

The small glands are separated by spindle cells giving the tumor a biphasic appearance.

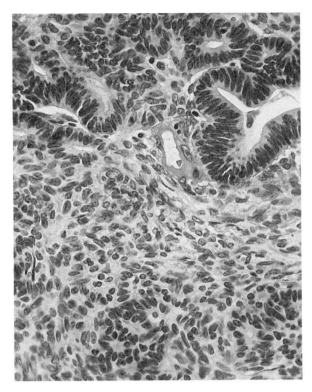

Figure 25-17
ENDOMETRIOID ADENOCARCINOMA
SIMULATING WOLFFIAN ADNEXAL TUMOR
Small glands of endometrioid type are separated by round and spindle cells suggesting biphasic differentiation.

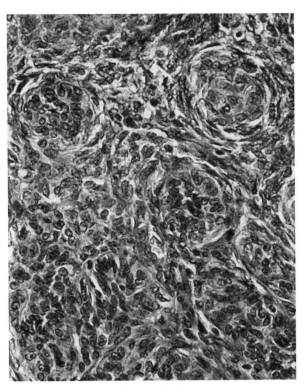

Figure 25-18
ENDOMETRIOID ADENOCARCINOMA
SIMULATING WOLFFIAN ADNEXAL TUMOR
Small, rounded whorls of neoplastic cells have arisen on a background of oval and spindle cells.

tubal carcinoma of the same cell type (19). Approximately 2 percent of tubal carcinomas are undifferentiated carcinomas of the nonsmall cell type; one of these contained giant cells that were immunoreactive for human chorionic gonadotropin (2).

In one large series of cases, 20 percent of carcinomas of all cell types were grade 1; 34 percent, grade 2; and 46 percent, grade 3 (53). In another large series, 8 percent were grade 1; 20 percent, grade 2; and 72 percent, grade 3 (2).

Spread and Metastasis. Tubal carcinoma spreads most commonly to the peritoneum, adjacent organs, and lymph nodes, mainly the para-aortic lymph nodes via the infundibulopelvic ligament, pelvic lymph nodes, and occasionally inguinal lymph nodes via the round ligament. Distant metastases are more common than in cases of ovarian carcinoma, complicating almost half the tumors that spread beyond the tube (42).

In one series of 21 cases, lymph node metastases were confined to those cases in which the tumor had extended beyond the tube and was grade 2 or 3 (37). In three large series in which FIGO staging (see Table 25-2) was performed (2,13,53), 21 to 57 percent of the tumors were stage I; 9 to 19 percent, stage II; 16 to 55 percent, stage III; and 4 to 12 percent, stage IV. In an earlier review of the literature, in which a different but comparable staging system was used, 10 of 75 grossly visible carcinomas did not invade beyond the epithelium although pathologic data were scanty in many of these cases (58). These findings indicate that tubal carcinoma in general is detected at an earlier stage than ovarian carcinoma.

Differential Diagnosis. When a carcinoma involves both the ovary and the fallopian tube, it usually predominates and is obviously primary in one or the other organ, almost always the ovary.

Occasionally, however, both organs are fused to form a solid or cystic mass with destruction of most or all landmarks. As mentioned on page 464, in such cases the tumor is almost always assumed to be a primary ovarian cancer because the latter is more frequent than tubal cancer. Microscopic examination may be helpful if the tumor is not serous or endometrioid since tubal carcinomas of clear cell or mucinous type are rare. Unfortunately, finding what appears to be in situ carcinoma adjacent to the main tumor in the tube is not a reliable criterion for a tubal origin since carcinoma that has extended into the tubal lumen from elsewhere can grow along the mucosal surface and be indistinguishable microscopically from carcinoma in situ. Cases in which a preponderance of evidence does not favor either a tubal or ovarian primary have been designated primary "tubo-ovarian carcinoma" (25). Use of this term in such cases may improve the accuracy of determining the relative frequency of tubal and ovarian carcinomas.

The most difficult problem in the microscopic differential diagnosis of tubal carcinoma involves its distinction from various forms of atypical hyperplasia, particularly those associated with chronic salpingitis. These and other rare lesions that may be confused with carcinoma are discussed on page 484.

Treatment and Prognosis. Total abdominal hysterectomy with salpingo-oophorectomy and staging similar to that performed for ovarian carcinoma is the recommended surgical approach for carcinoma of the fallopian tube. Debulking of tumor in advanced cases appears to improve the prognosis (53). Postoperative radiation therapy has been shown to be of value but the present trend is to treat patients like those with ovarian epithelial cancer, relying more on combination chemotherapy with cisplatin-containing regimens (6,8). In most cases recurrences take place within the first 2 or 3 postoperative years, but 7 to 9 year intervals have been recorded (8).

The reported 5-year survival figure for patients with stages I and II tumors is approximately 50 percent, and for stages III and IV tumors, 15 to 20 percent (8,53). In our experience (2), division of stage Ia cases into Ia-0, Ia-1, Ia-2, and I(F) (page 462) yielded important prognostic information, with increasing depth of invasion of the tubal wall associated with a decreasing length of

survival, and with a fimbrial origin associated with an outcome similar to that of stage Ic tumors. In the only other large series of cases in which depth of invasion was correlated with survival, the findings were similar to those in our series (58). The grade of the tumor has also been shown to be a prognostic indicator, but not independent of stage. Other prognostic factors are controversial or have been investigated by only one or a few authors. In our series (2) an older age (p = 0.03), a patent tubal ostium, and vascular invasion had an adverse effect on length of survival in early stage cases. Asmussen et al. (3a) also found vascular invasion to be a poor prognostic factor in stage I cases. Patients with endometrioid carcinomas resembling wolffian adnexal tumors appear to have a better prognosis than those with tubal carcinomas in general, but follow-up data are limited (16). In one such case carcinoma at the vaginal apex, assumed to be recurrent tumor, was detected 12 years after total abdominal hysterectomy with bilateral salpingo-oophorectomy and postoperative radiation therapy (61). Japanese investigators (64a) reported that carcinomas with a predominant transitional cell pattern tended to relapse later than those without such a pattern after surgical removal and postoperative chemotherapy. In one series of tubal carcinomas as a whole, the amount of residual disease after a debulking procedure was an important prognostic indicator (53).

MIXED EPITHELIAL–MESENCHYMAL TUMORS

Benign and Borderline Tumors

Adenofibromas and cystadenofibromas of the fallopian tube have been reported sporadically (71,74,75,77,80,84). These tumors resemble those encountered in the ovary. They may be intraluminal or attached to the fimbriated end or the serosal surface, and may have smooth or papillary surfaces (fig. 25-19). They range up to 3 cm in diameter; in one case the tumor was bilateral. The epithelial cell type has been serous in most of the cases (fig. 25-20) but may be endometrioid (fig. 25-21). In one nonfimbrial case the serous tumor had borderline epithelial features (74) and one fimbrial tumor of borderline endometrioid type has been described (71).

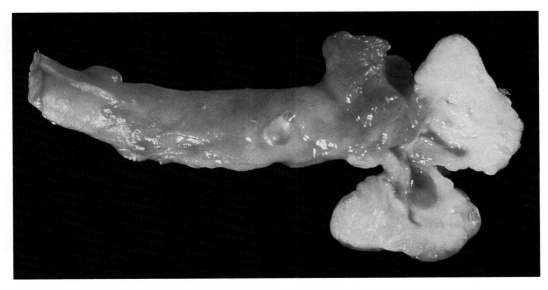

Figure 25-19
ADENOFIBROMA
The tumor is located at the fimbriated end; its sectioned surfaces are predominantly fibromatous.

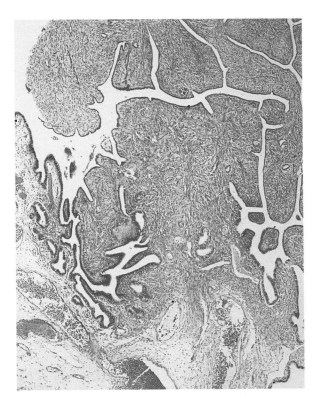

Figure 25-20
ADENOFIBROMA
The fimbriated end is focally expanded by a tumor composed largely of neoplastic stroma resembling that of an ovarian fibroma.

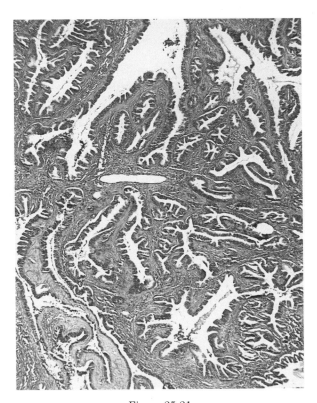

Figure 25-21
ENDOMETRIOID ADENOFIBROMA
The tumor is composed of fibromatous stroma containing numerous proliferating glands of endometrioid type.

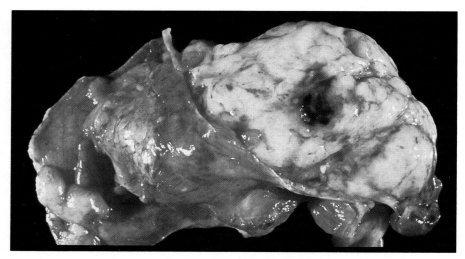

Figure 25-22
MALIGNANT MULLERIAN
MIXED TUMOR
The lumen is distended by
solid tumor tissue.

Adenosarcoma

We have seen one example of a tubal tumor of this type, which was characterized by marked adenoacanthotic atypia of its epithelial component. Another adenosarcoma that arose in the fimbriated end of the tube and recurred on the pelvic side wall has been reported (78).

Malignant Mullerian Mixed Tumor (Carcinosarcoma)

Approximately 70 cases of this tumor have been reported (72,73,79,81–83). Almost all the patients have been postmenopausal, with an average age of 60 years. They usually present with a watery or bloody vaginal discharge, abdominal pain, or both. Abdominal exploration typically reveals distension of the tube by tumor, which has spread to the pelvis, abdomen, or both in most of the cases. Opening the tube reveals neoplastic tissue that usually fills the lumen and often contains areas of hemorrhage and necrosis (fig. 25-22). The microscopic features resemble those of similar tumors that are more common elsewhere in the female genital tract (page 128). Surgical treatment is similar to that used for tubal carcinoma; postoperative chemotherapy may prolong survival. The 5-year survival rate is approximately 15 percent, and the mean length of survival is only 16 to 20 months.

This tumor is distinguished from the rare immature teratoma of the tube with use of criteria that are helpful in distinguishing those two tumors when they involve the ovary (page 130). The carcinosarcoma also must be distinguished from endometrioid carcinomas that have a prominent spindle cell epithelial component (76,85).

REFERENCES

General References

Honore LH. Pathology of the fallopian tube and broad ligament. In: Fox H, Wells M, eds. Haines and Taylor obstetrical and gynaecological pathology, 4th ed., Edinburgh: Churchill Livingstone, 1995:623–71.

Wheeler JE. Diseases of the fallopian tube. In: Kurman RJ, ed. Blaustein's pathology of the female genital tract, 4th ed. New York: Springer-Verlag, 1994:529–61.

Woodruff JD, Pauerstein CJ. The fallopian tube: structure, function, pathology, and management. Baltimore: Williams & Wilkins, 1969:237–306.

Epithelial Tumors

1. Alvarado-Cabrero I, Navani SS, Young RH, Scully RE. Tumors of the fimbriated end of the fallopian tube. A clinicopathological analysis of 20 cases, including nine carcinomas. Int J Gynecol Pathol 1997;16:189–96.
2. Alvarado-Cabrero I, Young RH, Vamvakas EC, Scully RE. Carcinoma of the fallopian tube: a clinicopatholog-ical study of 105 cases with observations on staging and prognostic factors. Gynecol Oncol 1998 (In press).
3. Aoyama T, Mizuno T, Andoh K, Takagi T, Mizuno T, Eimoto T. α-Fetoprotein-producing (hepatoid) carcinoma of the fallopian tube. Gynecol Oncol 1996;63:261–6.

3a. Asmussen M, Kaern J, Kjoerstad K, et al. Primary adenocarcinoma localized to the fallopian tubes: report on 33 cases. Gynecol Oncol 1988;30:183–6.

4. Baekelandt M, Kockx M, Wesling F, Gerris J. Primary adenocarcinoma of the fallopian tube. Review of the literature. Int J Gynecol Cancer 1993;3:65–71.

5. Bannatyne P, Russell P. Early adenocarcinoma of the fallopian tubes. A case for multifocal tumorigenesis. Diagn Gynecol Obstet 1981;3:49–60.

6. Barakat RR, Rubin SC, Saigo PE, et al. Cisplatin-based combination chemotherapy in carcinoma of the fallopian tube. Gynecol Oncol 1991;42:156–60.

7. Bartnik J, Powell WS, Moriber-Katz S, et al. Metaplastic papillary tumor of the fallopian tube. Case report, immunohistochemical features, and review of the literature. Arch Pathol Lab Med 1989;113:545–7.

8 Benedet JL, Miller DM. Tumors of fallopian tube: clinical features, staging and management. In: Coppleson M, ed. Gynecological oncology, 2nd ed., vol. 2. Edinburgh: Churchill Livingstone, 1992:853–60.

9. Block E. Squamous cell carcinoma of the fallopian tube. Acta Radiol 1947;28:49–68.

10. Case Records of the Massachusetts General Hospital (Case 53-1967). N Engl J Med 1967;277:1415–20.

11. Cheung AN, Ngan HY, Cheng D, et al. Clinicopathologic study of 16 cases of primary tubal malignancy. Int J Gynecol Cancer 1994;4:111–8.

12. Cheung AN, So KF, Ngan HY, Wong LC. Primary squamous carcinoma of the fallopian tube. Int J Gynecol Pathol 1994;13:92–5.

13. Cormio G, Maneo A, Gabriele A, Rota SM, Lissone A, Zanatta G. Primary carcinoma of the fallopian tube. A retrospective analysis of 47 patients. Ann Oncol 1996;7:271–5.

14. Czernobilsky B, Cornog JL. Squamous predominance n adenoacanthoma of adnexa: report of a patient. Obstet Gynecol 1971;37:355–9.

15. David MP, Ben-Zwi D, Langer L. Tubal intramural polyps and their relationship to infertility. Fertil Steril 1981;35:526–31.

16. Daya D, Young RH, Scully RE. Endometrioid carcinoma of the fallopian tube resembling an adnexal tumor of probable wolffian origin: a report of six cases. Int J Gynecol Pathol 1992;11:122–30.

17. Doleris A, Macrez F. Endosalpingeal papillomas. Gynecology 1988;3:289–308.

18. Eddy GL, Copeland LJ, Gershenson DM, Atkinson EN, Wharton JT, Rutledge FN. Fallopian tube carcinoma. Obstet Gynecol 1984;64:546–52.

19. Egan AJ, Russell P. Transitional (urothelial) metaplasia of the fallopian tube mucosa: morphological assessment of three cases. Int J Gynecol Pathol 1996;15:72–6.

20. Ehlen T, Randhawa G, Turko M, Clement PB. Posthysterectomy carcinoma of the fallopian tube presenting as vaginal adenocarcinoma: a case report. Gynecol Oncol 1989;33:382–5.

21. Federman Q, Toker C. Primary transitional cell tumor of the uterine adnexa. Am J Obstet Gynecol 1973;115:863–4.

22. Gaffney EF, Cornog J. Endometrioid carcinoma of the fallopian tube. Obstet Gynecol 1978;34s–6s.

23. Gatto V, Selim MA, Lankerani M. Primary carcinoma of the fallopian tube in an adolescent. J Surg Oncol 1986;33:212–4.

24. Gisser SD. Obstructing fallopian tube papilloma. Int J Gynecol Pathol 1986;5:179–82.

25. Green TH, Scully RE. Tumors of the fallopian tube. Clin Obstet Gynecol 1962;5:886–906.

26. Greene RR, Gardner GH. A preinvasive carcinoma of the uterine tube. Arch Pathol 1949;48:362–5.

27. Hameed K. Carcinoma arising in tuberculous fallopian tube. Am J Obstet Gynecol 1969;103:595–6.

28. Hellström AC, Silfverswärd C, Nilsson B, Pettersson F. Carcinoma of the fallopian tube. A clinical and histopathologic review. The Radiumhemmet series. Int J Gynecol Cancer 1994;4:395–407.

29. Herbold DR, Axelrod JH, Bobowski SJ, et al. Glassy cell carcinoma of the fallopian tube. A case report. Int J Gynecol Pathol 1988;7:384–90.

30. Hershey DW, Fennell RH, Major FJ. Primary carcinoma of the fallopian tube. Obstet Gynecol 1981;57:367–70.

31. Hovadhanakul P, Nuerenberger SP, Ritter PJ, Taylor HB, Cavanagh D. Primary transitional cell carcinoma of the fallopian tube associated with primary carcinomas of the ovary and endometrium. Gynecol Oncol 1976;4:138–43.

32. Hu CY, Taymor ML, Hertig AT. Primary carcinoma of the fallopian tube. Am J Obstet Gynecol 1950;59:58–67.

33. Imm FC. Primary adenosquamous carcinoma of the fallopian tube. South Med J 1980;73:678–80.

34. Jackson-York GL, Ramzy I. Synchronous papillary mucinous adenocarcinoma of the endocervix and fallopian tubes. Int J Gynecol Pathol 1992;11:63–7.

35. Kaspersen P, Buhl L, Moller BR. Fallopian tube papilloma in a patient with primary sterility. Acta Obstet Gynecol Scand 1988;67:93–4.

36. Keeney GL, Thrasher TV. Metaplastic papillary tumor of the fallopian tube: a case report with ultrastructure. Int J Gynecol Pathol 1988;7:86–92.

37. Klein M, Rosen A, Lahousen M, et al. Lymphogenous metastasis in the primary carcinoma of the fallopian tube. Gynecol Oncol 1994;55:336–8.

38. Koshiyama M, Konishi I, Yoshidi M, et al. Transitional cell carcinoma of the fallopian tube: a light and electron microscopic study. Int J Gynecol Pathol 1994;13:175–80.

39. Lacy MQ, Hartman LC, Keeney GL, Roche PC. C-erb-B-2 and p53 expression in fallopian tube carcinoma. Cancer 1995;75:2891–6.

40. Lisa JR, Gioia JD, Rubin IC. Observations on the interstitial portion of the fallopian tube. Surg Gynecol Obstet 1954;99:159–69.

41. Malinak LR, Miller GV, Armstrong JT. Primary squamous cell carcinoma of the fallopian tube. Am J Obstet Gynecol 1966;95:1167–8.

42. McMurray EH, Jacobs AJ, Perez CA, Camel HM, Kao MS, Godakatos A. Carcinoma of fallopian tube. Management and sites of failure. Cancer 1986;58:2070–5.

43. Moore DH, Woosley JT, Reddick RL, Walton LA, Siegal GP. Adenosquamous carcinoma of the fallopian tube. A clinicopathologic case report with verification of the diagnosis by immunohistochemical and ultrastructural studies. Am J Obstet Gynecol 1987;157:903–5.

44. Muntz HG, Goff BA, Thor AD, Tarraza HM. Post-hysterectomy carcinoma of the fallopian tube mimicking a vesicovaginal fistula. Obstet Gynecol 1992;79:853–6.

45. Muntz HG, Tarraza HM, Granai CO, Fuller AF Jr. Primary adenocarcinoma of the fallopian tube. Eur J Gynaecol Oncol 1989;10:239–49.

46. Navani SS, Alvarado-Cabrero I, Young RH, Scully RE. Endometrioid carcinoma of the fallopian tube: a clinicopathologic analysis of 26 cases. Gynecol Oncol 1996;63:371–8.

47. Niloff JM, Klug TL, Schaetzl E, Zurawski VR Jr, Knapp BC, Bast RC Jr. Elevation of serum CA125 in carcinomas of the fallopian tube, endometrium and endocervix. Am J Obstet Gynecol 1984;148:1057–8.

48. Nordin AJ. Primary carcinoma of the fallopian tube: a 20-year literature review. Obstet Gynecol Surv 1994;49:349–61.

49. Pauerstein CJ, Woodruff JD. Cellular patterns in proliferative and anaplastic disease of the fallopian tube. Am J Obstet Gynecol 1966;96:486–92.

50. Peters WA, Anderson WA, Hopkins MP. Results of chemotherapy in advanced carcinoma of the fallopian tube. Cancer 1989;63:836–8.

51. Peters WA, Andersen WA, Hopkins MP, Kumar NP, Morley GW. Prognostic features of carcinoma of the fallopian tube. Obstet Gynecol 1988;71:757–62.

52. Pettersson F. Staging rules for gestational trophoblastic tumors and fallopian tube cancer. Acta Obstet Gynecol Scand 1992;71:224–5.

53. Rosen A, Klein M, Lahousen M, Graf AH, Rainer A, Vavra N. Primary carcinoma of the fallopian tube—a retrospective analysis of 115 patients. The Austrian Cooperative Study Group for Fallopian Tube Carcinoma. Br J Cancer 1993;68:605–9.

54. Rosenblatt KA, Weiss NS, Schwartz SM. Incidence of malignant fallopian tube tumors. Gynecol Oncol 1989;35:236–9.

55. Rubin IC, Lisa JR, Trinidad S. Further observations on ectopic endometrium of the fallopian tube. Surg Gynecol Obstet 1956;103:469–74.

56. Ryan GM Jr. Carcinoma in situ of the fallopian tube. Am J Obstet Gynecol 1962;84:198.

57. Saffos RO, Rhatigan RM, Scully RE. Metaplastic papillary tumor of the fallopian tube—a distinctive lesion of pregnancy. Am J Clin Pathol 1980;74:232–6.

58. Schiller HM, Silverberg SC. Staging and prognosis in primary carcinoma of the fallopian tube. Cancer 1971;28:389–95.

59. Sedlis A. Primary carcinoma of the fallopian tube. Obstet Gynecol Surv 1961;16:209–26.

60. Seidman JD. Mucinous lesions of the fallopian tube. A report of seven cases. Am J Surg Pathol 1994;18:1205–12.

61. Seraj IM, Chase DR, King A. Endometrioid carcinoma of the oviduct. Gynecol Oncol 1991;41:152–5.

62. Sonnendecker HE, Cooper K, Kalian KN. Primary fallopian tube adenocarcinoma in situ associated with adjuvant tamoxifen therapy for breast carcinoma. Gynecol Oncol 1994;52:402–7.

63. Takashina T, Ito E, Kudo R. Cytologic diagnosis of primary tubal cancer. Acta Cytol 1985;29:367–72.

64. Tokunaga T, Miyazaki K, Matsyama S, Okamura H. Serial measurement of CA 125 in patients with primary carcinoma of the fallopian tube. Gynecol Oncol 1990;36:335–7.

64a. Uehira K, Hashimoto H, Tsuneyoshi M, Enjoji M. Transitional cell carcinoma pattern in primary carcinoma of the fallopian tube. Cancer 1993;72:2447–56.

65. Voet RL, Lifshitz S. Primary clear cell adenocarcinoma of the fallopian tube: light microscopic and ultrastructural findings. Int J Gynecol Pathol 1982;1:292–8.

66. Weiss PD, MacDougall MK, Reagan JW, Wentz WB. Primary adenosquamous carcinoma of the fallopian tube. Obstet Gynecol 1980;55:88s–9s.

67. Williamson JM, Armour A. Microcystic endometrioid carcinoma of the fallopian tube simulating an adnexal tumour of probable wolffian origin. Histopathology 1993;23:578–80.

68. Wheeler JE. Diseases of the fallopian tube. In: Kurman RJ, ed. Blaustein's pathology of the female genital tract, 4th ed. New York: Springer-Verlag, 1994:529–61.

69. Woolas R, Jacobs I, Prys Davies A, et al. What is the true incidence of primary fallopian tube carcinoma? Int J Gynecol Cancer 1994;4:384–8.

70. Zheng W, Wolf S, Kramer EE, Cox KA, Hoda SA. Borderline papillary serous tumor of the fallopian tube. Am J Surg Pathol 1996;20:30-5.

Epithelial-Mesenchymal Tumors

71. Alvarado-Cabrero I, Navani SS, Young RH, Scully RE. Tumors of the fimbriated end of the fallopian tube. A clinicopathological analysis of 20 cases, including nine carcinomas. Int J Gynecol Pathol 1997;16:189–96.

72. Benedet JL, Miller DM. Tumors of fallopian tube: clinical features, staging and management. In: Coppleson M, ed. Gynecologic oncology, 2nd ed., vol 2. Edinburgh; Churchill Livingstone, 1992:853–60.

73. Carlson JA, Ackerman BL, Wheeler JE. Malignant mixed mullerian tumor of the fallopian tube. Cancer 1993;71:187–92.

74. Casasola SV, Mindan JP. Cystadenofibroma of fallopian tube. Appl Pathol 1989;7:256–9.

75. Chen KT. Bilateral papillary adenofibroma of the fallopian tube. Am J Clin Pathol 1981;75:229–31.

76. Daya D, Young RH, Scully RE. Endometrioid carcinoma of the fallopian tube resembling an adnexal tumor of probable wolffian origin. A report of six cases. Int J Gynecol Pathol 1992;11:122–30.

77. De la Fuente AA. Benign mixed müllerian tumour-adenofibroma of the fallopian tube. Histopathology 1982;6:661–6.

78. Gollard R, Kosty M, Bordin G, Wax A, Lacey C. Two unusual presentations of mullerian adenosarcoma: case reports, literature review, and treatment considerations. Gynecol Oncol 1995;59:412–22.

79. Hellstrom AC, Auer G, Silverswärd C, Pettersson F. Malignant mixed mullerian tumor of the fallopian tube; the Radiumhemmett series 1923-1993. Int J Gynecol Oncol 1995;5(suppl):68.

80. Kanbour AI, Burgess FL, Salazar H. Intramural adenofibroma of the fallopian tube. Light and electron microscopy. Cancer 1973;31:1433–9.

81. Kinoshita M, Asano S, Yamashita M, Matsuda T. Mesodermal mixed tumor primary in the fallopian tube. Gynecol Oncol 1989;32:331–5.

82. Muntz HG, Rutgers JL, Tarraza HM, Fuller AF Jr. Carcinosarcomas and mixed mullerian tumors of the fallopian tube. Gynecol Oncol 1989;34:109–15.

83. Seraj IM, King A, Chase D. Malignant mixed mullerian tumor of the oviduct. Gynecol Oncol 1990;37:296–301.

84. Silverman AY, Artinian B, Sabin M. Serous cystadenofibroma of the fallopian tube: a case report. Am J Obstet Gynecol 1978;130:593–5.

85. Tornos C, Silva EG, McCabe KM, Ordonez NG, Gershenson DM, Scully RE. The spindle cell variant of endometrioid carcinoma. Mod Pathol 1992;5;69A.

26
OTHER TUMORS AND TUMOR-LIKE LESIONS
OF THE FALLOPIAN TUBE

TUMORS

Benign Tumors of Soft Tissue Type

Leiomyomas are the most common soft tissue tumors. Most are small; they may be mucosal, muscular, or serosal in origin (1,4,6,10), and undergo degenerative changes similar to those occurring in uterine smooth muscle tumors. Rarer benign soft tissue tumors include neurilemoma (7), angiomyolipoma (5), lipoma (2), chondroma (8a), lymphangioma (8), ganglioneuroma (11), and hemangioma (3,9). Several hemangiomas have presented with hemoperitoneum.

Malignant Tumors of Soft Tissue Type

Primary tubal sarcomas are rare, and almost all of them are leiomyosarcomas. They occur throughout adult life, with a median age incidence of 47 years (12a). The presenting symptoms are similar to those of other tubal cancers. The tumors are typically large and resemble uterine leiomyosarcomas both grossly and microscopically (fig. 26-1). Survival has been poor in the reported cases, with metastases often detected within 2 years of diagnosis (12a). One embryonal rhabdomyosarcoma was reported in a 17-year-old woman (12).

Adenomatoid Tumor

General Features. The adenomatoid tumor is the most common benign neoplasm of the fallopian tube, and is usually an incidental finding in a middle-aged or elderly woman (13–21).

Pathologic Findings. The tumors are usually 2 cm or less in diameter, circumscribed, firm, and gray, white, or yellow nodules (fig. 26-2) that replace part or all of the tube (fig. 26-3), including its fimbrial portion (15a). Rarely, they are bilateral (21).

The major microscopic patterns are, in varying proportions: irregular gland-like spaces that vary from slit-like (fig. 26-4) to moderately dilated (fig. 26-5) to cystic (fig. 26-6); oval vacuoles (fig. 26-7); small cords and clusters of cells; and

occasionally, solid areas. The neoplastic cells range from flat and endothelial-like to large with abundant eosinophilic cytoplasm (fig. 26-8). The nuclei appear bland, and mitotic figures are rare. The glandular lumens and vacuoles may contain slightly basophilic fluid, which is rich in hyaluronic acid. The stroma can be hyalinized and contain smooth muscle and lymphocytes (fig. 26-4), which may form prominent follicles. Continuity with the overlying mesothelium is occasionally seen (17), supporting an origin from this layer, which is favored by most investigators (18–20).

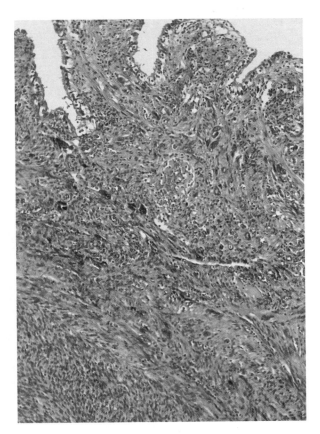

Figure 26-1
LEIOMYOSARCOMA
The inner wall is replaced by intersecting fascicles of spindle cells with marked nuclear pleomorphism.

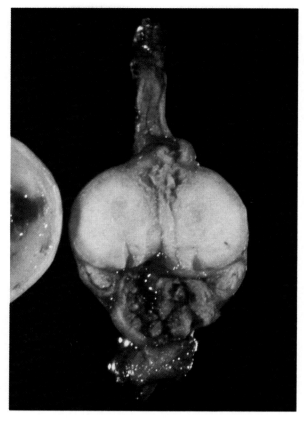

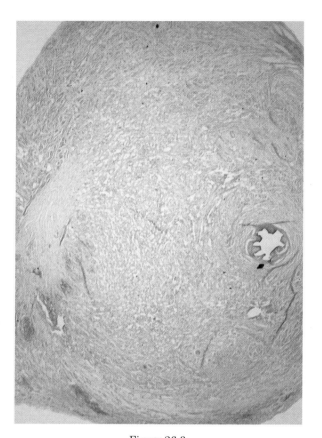

Figure 26-2
ADENOMATOID TUMOR
A well circumscribed mass occupies a segment of the tube.

Figure 26-3
ADENOMATOID TUMOR
The tubal wall is expanded by the tumor.

Figure 26-4
ADENOMATOID TUMOR
Many of the gland-like structures are slit-like. Lymphoid aggregates are evident.

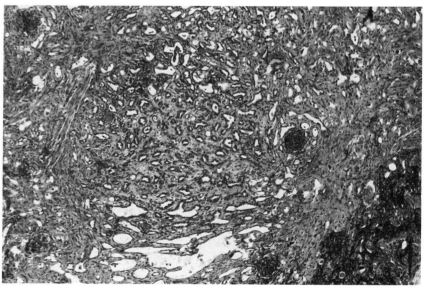

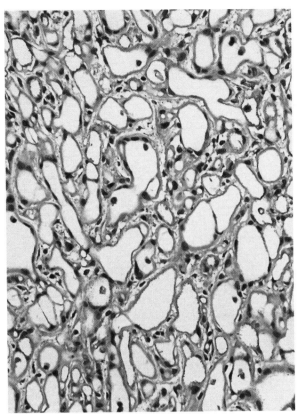

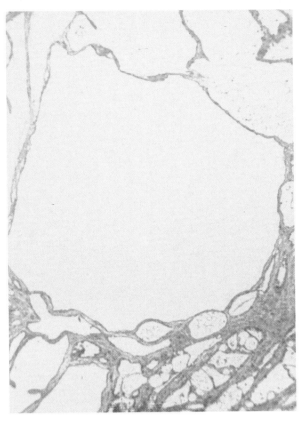

Figure 26-5
ADENOMATOID TUMOR
Vacuoles and gland-like spaces of variable shapes are separated by scanty stroma.

Figure 26-6
ADENOMATOID TUMOR
Cysts are conspicuous.

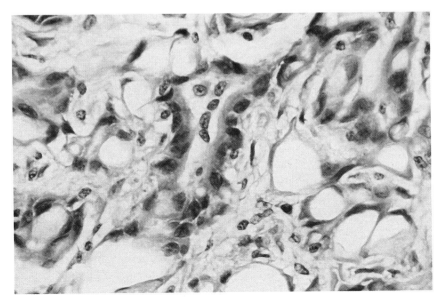

Figure 26-7
ADENOMATOID TUMOR
Characteristic vacuoles and gland-like spaces are evident.

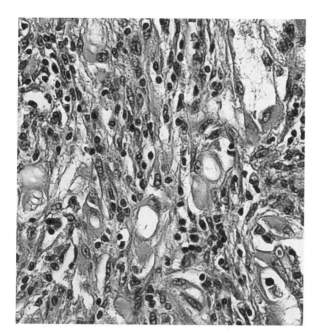

Figure 26-8
ADENOMATOID TUMOR
Some cells contain abundant eosinophilic cytoplasm; a few vacuoles are present.

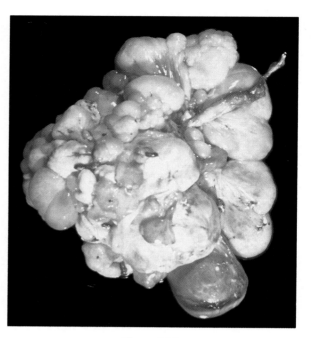

Figure 26-9
MATURE SOLID TERATOMA
A lobulated mass obscures much of the tube.

Differential Diagnosis. The adenomatoid tumor may be confused with other benign tumors, particularly lymphangiomas and leiomyomas. Careful examination of the tumor cells should permit their distinction from endothelial cells; immunoperoxidase staining for cytokeratin and *Ulex europaeus* may facilitate the diagnosis in difficult cases (19). Smooth muscle is rarely as prominent in tubal adenomatoid tumors as it is in uterine adenomatoid tumors, and the characteristic spaces of an adenomatoid tumor exclude a diagnosis of leiomyoma. Adenomatoid tumors may also be confused with malignant tumors, such as malignant mesotheliomas and adenocarcinomas, particularly those of signet-ring cell type. The circumscribed gross appearance, bland cytologic findings, and absent to low mitotic activity characteristic of adenomatoid tumors are not features of those malignant tumors.

Germ Cell Tumors

Approximately 50 teratomas of the fallopian tube have been reported (22–30). They are usually attached by a pedicle to the tubal mucosa and have ranged from 0.7 to 20 cm in diameter. Most of them have been dermoid cysts but rare examples have been solid and mature (fig. 26-9) (29) or immature (30). One solid mature teratoma had a component of insular carcinoid tumor (29). Two tumors composed entirely of thyroid tissue have been reported (24,25).

Trophoblastic Disease

Hydatidiform moles (32,36) and gestational choriocarcinomas (31,33,34,35) occur rarely in the fallopian tube and may mimic an ectopic pregnancy both clinically and on gross examination. In 1981, Ober and Maier (34) identified in the literature 22 cases reported as moles and 93 as choriocarcinomas, but accepted as valid only 4 of the moles and 58 of the choriocarcinomas. Those authors concluded that the remainder of the "moles" were ectopic pregnancies with villous hydrops. One mole was associated with an intrauterine pregnancy and complicated by pulmonary metastases, which were successfully treated with actinomycin-D (32). Differentiation of a mole from a hydropic ectopic pregnancy depends on criteria similar to those used in the uterine corpus.

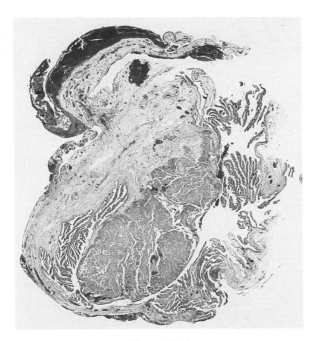

Figure 26-10
CHORIOCARCINOMA IN WALL OF
TUBE PROTRUDING INTO LUMEN
The serosa is covered by blood. (Courtesy of Dr. Robert
Maier, Augusta, GA.)

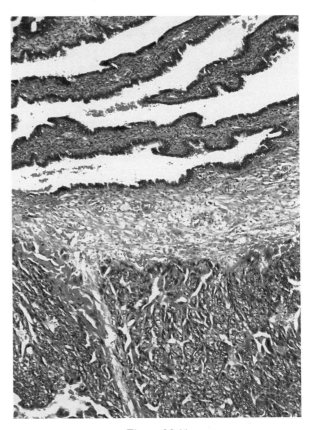

Figure 26-11
CHORIOCARCINOMA IN WALL OF TUBE
(Courtesy of Dr. Robert Maier, Augusta, GA.)

Choriocarcinomas of the fallopian tube have been reported in patients from 16 to 56 (mean, 33) years of age (34) and account for approximately 4 percent of all choriocarcinomas (35). Most of the patients have a clinical presentation similar to that of an ectopic pregnancy, but approximately 40 percent present with an enlarging adnexal mass (34). A hemorrhagic, friable mass and hemoperitoneum are usually found at laparotomy. Microscopic examination shows typical features of gestational choriocarcinoma. Although the diagnosis should be made with great caution in the presence of villi, Ober and Maier (34) concluded that villi were present in 2 of 76 (3 percent) cases. The choriocarcinoma may fill the lumen (fig. 26-10). Invasion of the muscle by trophoblast cells having the typical features of choriocarcinoma (fig. 26-11) is essential to exclude the trophoblast of an early ectopic pregnancy in which villi are not found either because they have been deported into the peritoneal cavity or are scanty and not identified microscopically. The mortality rate for patients with tubal choriocarcinoma before the advent of modern chemotherapy was close to 90 percent but in subsequently treated cases Ober and Maier reported a survival rate of 94 percent (34).

One case in which two placental site nodules were found in the tubal wall has been reported (33a).

Malignant Lymphoma and Leukemia

The fallopian tube is involved in many cases of malignant lymphoma of the female genital tract (39), including approximately one quarter of the cases in which the tumor presents as an ovarian mass (38); the tubal involvement is almost always less conspicuous on gross examination than the ovarian disease. We have seen one example of lymphoma apparently confined to the fallopian tube (fig. 26-12). The gross and microscopic features of tubal lymphoma are similar to those seen elsewhere. The tube may also be infiltrated in cases of leukemia (37).

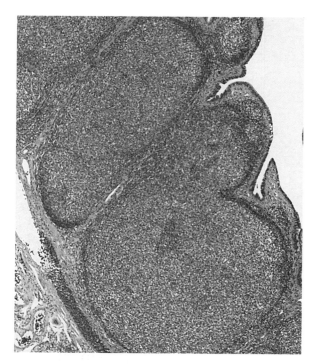

Figure 26-12
MALIGNANT LYMPHOMA, APPARENTLY PRIMARY
There is extensive involvement of the wall by follicular lymphoma.

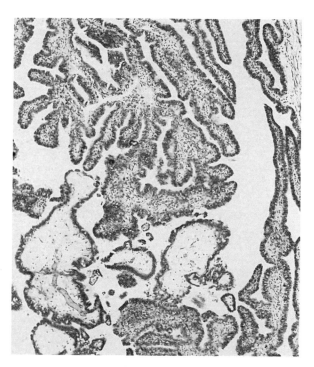

Figure 26-13
SEROUS BORDERLINE TUMOR
OF OVARY IN TUBAL LUMEN
Several fragments of serous borderline tumor with edematous stromal cores are present in the lower portion of the figure.

Secondary Tumors

Carcinoma that has spread to the fallopian tube is more common than primary tubal carcinoma, with 33 examples of the former and only 6 examples of the latter in one series (40). In another study (41), 89 percent of secondary carcinomas in the tube were of ovarian origin, and the remainder were from the endometrium. Most cases of secondary carcinoma from the ovary result from direct spread; in such cases clinical and gross pathologic findings usually aid in the pathologic interpretation. Discontinuous spread may pose a problem in determining the site of origin of the tumors, as shown in one series in which single examples of tubal spread of endometrial cancer and cervical cancer presented as possible primary tubal neoplasms (42). It is common to find implants of ovarian serous borderline tumors in the tubal lumen (fig. 26-13) or on the serosa. Both direct extension and intraluminal spread account for secondary involvement by endometrial carcinoma. Direct extension of cervical carcinoma to the tube is rare and seen usually only at autopsy

but in a small subset of cases of cervical carcinomas, some of which are in situ, spread occurs upward to the tube via the endometrium (43,43a,44). Uterine sarcomas and peritoneal mesotheliomas frequently involve the tube but are rarely the source of diagnostic difficulty.

Metastasis to the fallopian tube from sites outside the female genital tract is rare. In two combined series (40,45), only 9 of 151 metastases to the tube (6 percent) originated outside the genital tract (breast [4 cases], the gastrointestinal tract [3 cases; fig. 26-14], urinary bladder [1 case], and undetermined [1 case]). The microscopic features of secondary tubal carcinoma vary according to the morphologic features of the primary tumor and the extent and distribution of the tubal involvement. In many cases vascular invasion is observed in the plicae (fig. 26-14). In rare cases of pseudomyxoma peritonei the tubal epithelium is replaced focally by mucinous epithelium (figs. 26-15, 26-16) which characteristically is at least slightly atypical, helping to distinguish it from benign mucinous metaplasia (page 464).

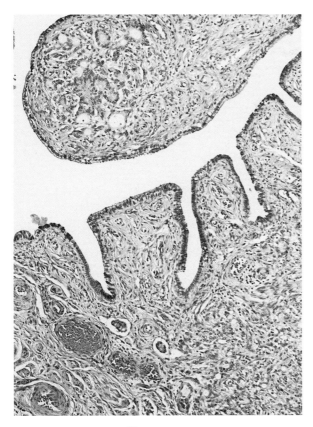

Figure 26-14
METASTATIC ADENOCARCINOMA FROM STOMACH
The lamina propria is infiltrated by glands and small solid aggregates of tumor cells. Two small vascular spaces contain tumor cells (lower center).

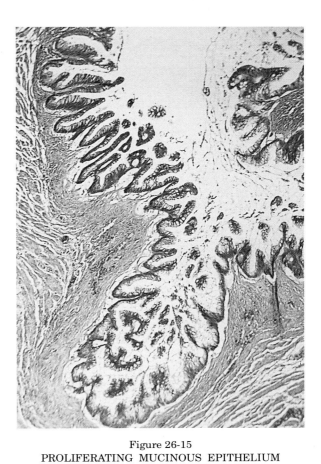

Figure 26-15
PROLIFERATING MUCINOUS EPITHELIUM LINING TUBAL LUMEN IN CASE OF PSEUDOMYXOMA PERITONEI
The proliferation resembles borderline mucinous tumors of the ovary and appendix.

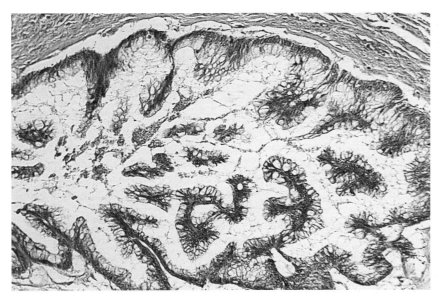

Figure 26-16
PROLIFERATING MUCINOUS EPITHELIUM LINING TUBAL LUMEN IN CASE OF PSEUDOMYXOMA PERITONEI
The epithelium resembles intestinal epithelium. (Higher power view of figure 26-15.)

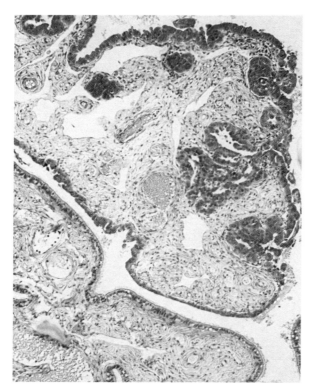

Figure 26-17
OVARIAN ADENOCARCINOMA INVOLVING TUBAL
MUCOSA AND SIMULATING CARCINOMA
IN SITU WITH MICROINVASION

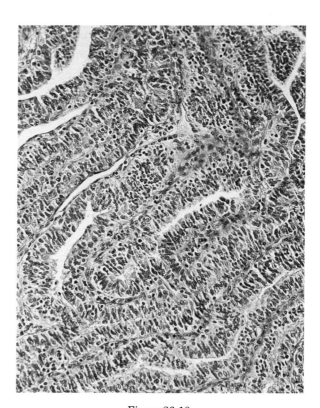

Figure 26-18
HYPERPLASIA OF TUBAL EPITHELIUM
OF UNKNOWN CAUSE
The plicae are closely packed and lined by proliferating epithelial cells with bland nuclei.

The diagnosis of a secondary tubal cancer is usually established by the clinical history, the surgical findings, or both in addition to distinctive microscopic features. It should be emphasized that epithelial involvement by secondary carcinoma may be indistinguishable microscopically from (primary) carcinoma in situ (fig. 26-17) (page 466).

TUMOR-LIKE LESIONS

Hyperplasia

Epithelial hyperplasia with stratification, a papillary or cribriform pattern, mitotic activity, or a combination of these findings may be seen in association with unopposed estrogenic stimulation (47,51) but the cellular alterations are not atypical enough to cause confusion with carcinoma in situ. Hyperplasia may occur also without any known predisposing condition (fig. 26-18): Moore and Enterline (48) reported "adenomatous hyperplasia" of the epithelium in over 18 percent of fallopian tubes

from 124 unselected hysterectomy-salpingectomy specimens. Hyperplastic changes may be associated with serous borderline tumors of the ovary (50) and tend to be more extensive than those associated with other female genital tract lesions, but are nonspecific (52).

Pseudocarcinomatous Hyperplasia

The most atypical forms of tubal hyperplasia are those associated with both tuberculous and nontuberculous salpingitis (46,49). Cases of this type have occasionally led to major diagnostic errors and unnecessary radical surgery (47). In tuberculous salpingitis (fig. 26-19) fusion of tubal plicae can result in the formation of multiple gland-like spaces (fig. 26-20), which may have a cribriform pattern (fig. 26-21) and may be lined by mildly to moderately atypical epithelium. The clues to the diagnosis of pseudocarcinomatous hyperplasia include the presence of tubercles in

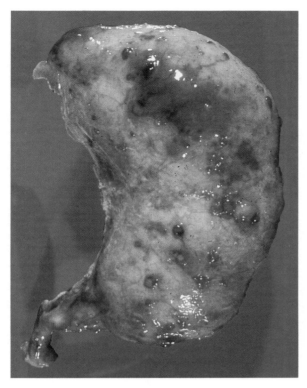

Figure 26-19
TUBERCULOUS SALPINGITIS
The tube is markedly distended. Tubercles and hemor-rhagic areas are present on the serosal surface. (Courtesy of Dr. Bradley Bigelow, New York, NY.)

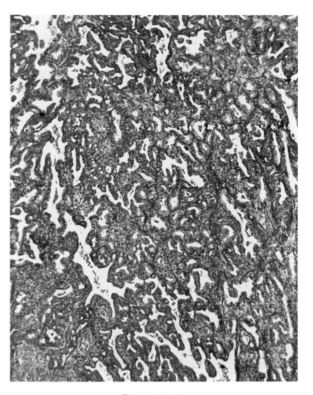

Figure 26-20
TUBERCULOUS SALPINGITIS
There is marked hyperplasia of the tubal epithelium with fusion of plicae and the formation of many crowded gland-like spaces, simulating adenocarcinoma. (Figures 26-20–26-22 are from the same patient.) (Fig. 5 from Young RH, Clement PB, Scully RE. The fallopian tube and broad ligament. In: Sternberg SS, ed. Diagnostic surgical pathology, Vol 2, 2nd ed. New York: Raven Press, 1994:2283.)

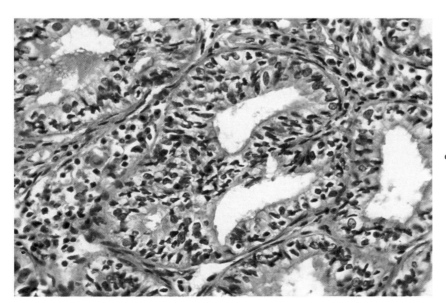

Figure 26-21
TUBERCULOUS SALPINGITIS
A cribriform pattern is present; cytologic atypia is lacking.

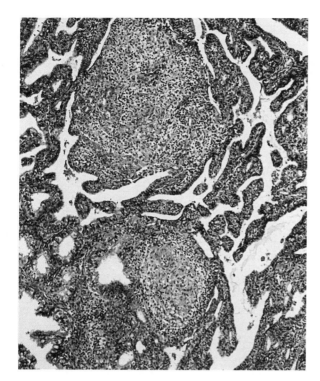

Figure 26-22
TUBERCULOUS SALPINGITIS
Two tubercles are present in the lamina propria. (Fig. 6 from Young RH, Clement PB, Scully RE. The fallopian tube and broad ligament. In: Sternberg SS, ed. Diagnostic surgical pathology, Vol 2, 2nd ed. New York: Raven Press, 1994:2283.)

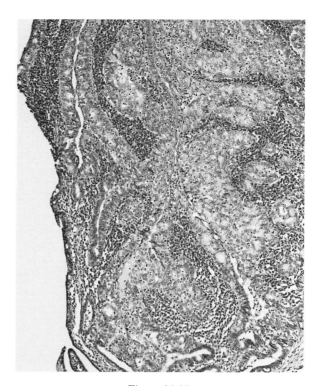

Figure 26-23
HYPERPLASIA OF TUBAL EPITHELIUM ASSOCIATED WITH NONTUBERCULOUS SALPINGITIS
Groups of closely packed gland-like structures (center) are separated by a dense inflammatory infiltrate.

the wall of the tube, particularly in its lamina propria (fig. 26-22), and a lack of cytologic malignancy of the epithelial cells. A more common problem, which has been emphasized in the literature only rarely, involves the occasional striking changes simulating those of carcinoma that may be seen in cases of chronic nontuberculous salpingitis (figs. 26-23–26-27) (46). In addition to changes of the type that can be associated with tuberculosis, there may be pseudoinvasion of the muscularis by gland-like structures (fig. 26-24); clusters of epithelial cells, which may be accompanied by psammoma bodies, within vascular spaces in the tubal wall (fig. 26-25); and a postinflammatory marked hyperplasia of overlying mesothelium that forms pseudoglandular spaces (fig. 26-27). Evidence against the diagnosis of carcinoma includes: the absence of a gross tumor; the presence of severe chronic salpingitis; a paucity of mitotic figures; a lack of severe nuclear atypia or atypical mitotic figures; and iden-

tification of the gland-like spaces in the serosa as mesothelium-lined spaces on the basis of both their architecture and their immunohistochemical staining properties (page 73). Mesothelial cell proliferation tends to be orderly, with the cells entrapped in granulation and scar tissue and arranged in interrupted parallel arrays (46). Rare tubal carcinomas, however, can be associated with marked acute or chronic salpingitis, which may cause them to be overlooked (46); the presence of epithelium that is frankly malignant cytologically is not compatible with a diagnosis of pseudocarcinoma.

Salpingitis Isthmica Nodosa

This lesion, which is of uncertain pathogenesis, is usually found in young women (mean age, 26 years), and may cause infertility or predispose to ectopic pregnancy (53–56). It typically appears as a yellow-white nodular swelling up to 2 cm in diameter (fig. 26-28) but may be grossly

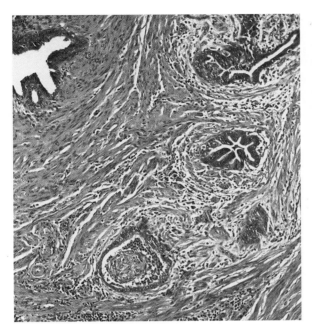

Figure 26-24
HYPERPLASIA OF TUBAL EPITHELIUM ASSOCIATED
WITH NONTUBERCULOUS SALPINGITIS
Gland-like structures are present in the muscularis,
simulating invasion. The tubal lumen is at the upper left.

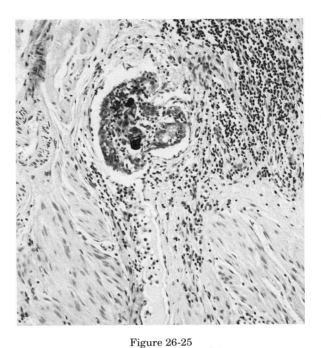

Figure 26-25
HYPERPLASIA OF TUBAL EPITHELIUM ASSOCIATED
WITH NONTUBERCULOUS SALPINGITIS
A papillary cluster of epithelial cells with psammoma bodies
lies in a vascular space.

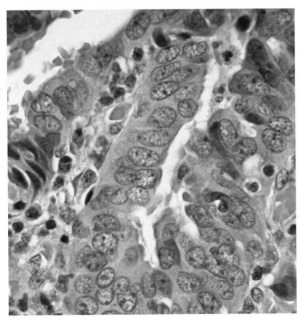

Figure 26-26
HYPERPLASIA OF TUBAL EPITHELIUM
ASSOCIATED WITH NONTUBERCULOUS SALPINGITIS
The epithelial cell nuclei are slightly atypical.

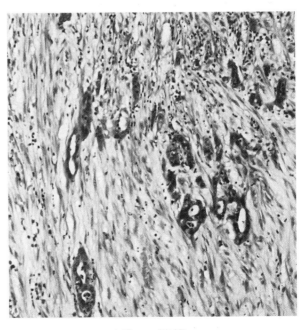

Figure 26-27
MESOTHELIAL HYPERPLASIA OVERLYING TUBE
IN CASE OF TUBAL HYPERPLASIA ASSOCIATED
WITH NONTUBERCULOUS SALPINGITIS
The gland-like structures lie in a reactive stroma, and are
oriented parallel to the mesothelial surface, which is not shown.

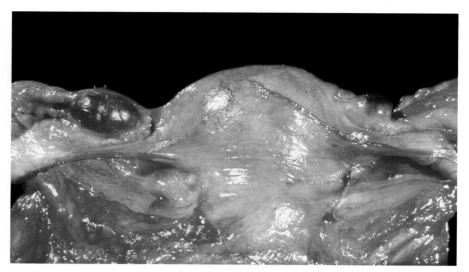

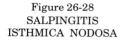

Figure 26-28
SALPINGITIS
ISTHMICA NODOSA
There are dark, nodular swellings of the isthmic portions of the tubes. The gland-like structures were distended with yellow fluid.

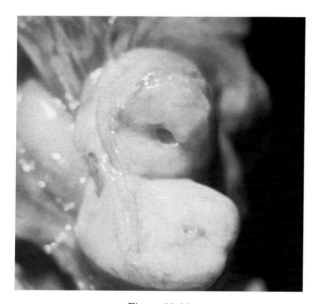

Figure 26-29
SALPINGITIS ISTHMICA NODOSA
The tube has been transected to disclose marked thickening of its wall.

inconspicuous. It usually, but not invariably, involves the isthmus, and is bilateral in approximately 85 percent of the cases (56). Sectioning shows firm, rubbery tissue (fig. 26-29). Microscopic examination reveals glands lined by tubal epithelium, usually unaccompanied by endometrial-type stroma, lying within the muscularis (fig. 26-30), which is typically thickened. In some

cases cystic dilatation of the glands is prominent. Serial sectioning has shown that the glands are diverticula that communicate with the tubal lumen. The lesion should be easily distinguished from carcinoma by the regular distribution of its widely spaced glands, the lack of significant cellular atypia, and the absence of a desmoplastic stromal response (fig. 26-31).

Heat Artifact

Operative cauterization or heating of the specimen after surgical removal may cause an appearance of cellular pseudostratification with marked elongation and dark staining of the nuclei (fig. 26-32) (57). Recognition of the distinctive appearance of this change should facilitate its differentiation from carcinoma.

Pregnancy-Related Changes

Arias-Stella Reaction. The Arias-Stella reaction has been reported as a focal finding in the fallopian tube (fig. 26-33) in 16 percent of cases of ectopic tubal pregnancy (58), and has been seen occasionally in patients with an intrauterine pregnancy (59). The concurrence with pregnancy, absence of a mass lesion, distinctive cytologic features, and lack of invasion help to differentiate this lesion from the rare clear cell carcinoma of the tube.

Clear Cell Change of Pregnancy. This change, which occurs commonly in the endometrium (60), has been described recently in a

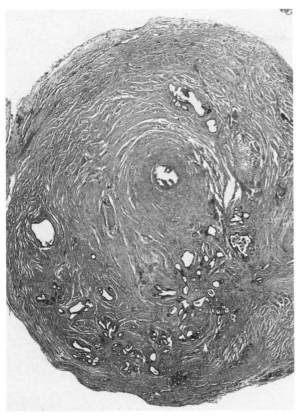

Figure 26-30
SALPINGITIS ISTHMICA NODOSA
Gland-like structures occupy much of the muscularis.

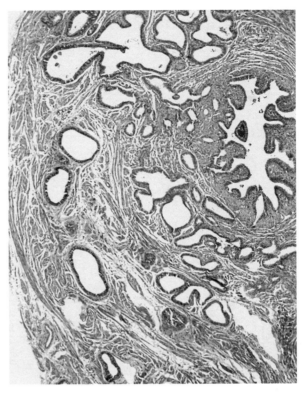

26-31
SALPINGITIS ISTHMICA NODOSA
The tubal lumen lies along the right upper margin; numerous gland-like structures unaccompanied by stroma are present in the muscularis. (Fig. 9 from Young RH, Clement PB, Scully RE. The fallopian tube and broad ligament. In: Sternberg SS, ed. Diagnostic surgical pathology, Vol 2, 2nd ed. New York: Raven Press, 1994:2285.)

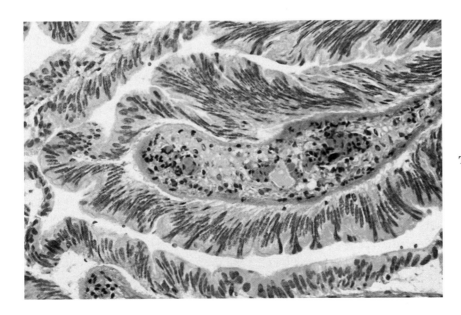

Figure 26-32
HEAT ARTIFACT
The nuclei are dark and elongated.

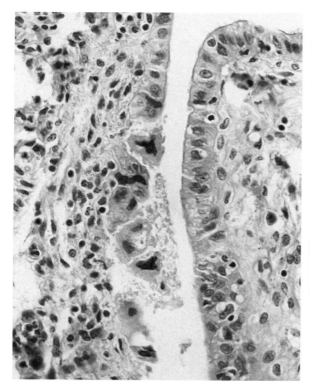

Figure 26-33
ARIAS-STELLA REACTION
Several epithelial-cell nuclei are enlarged and smudgy.

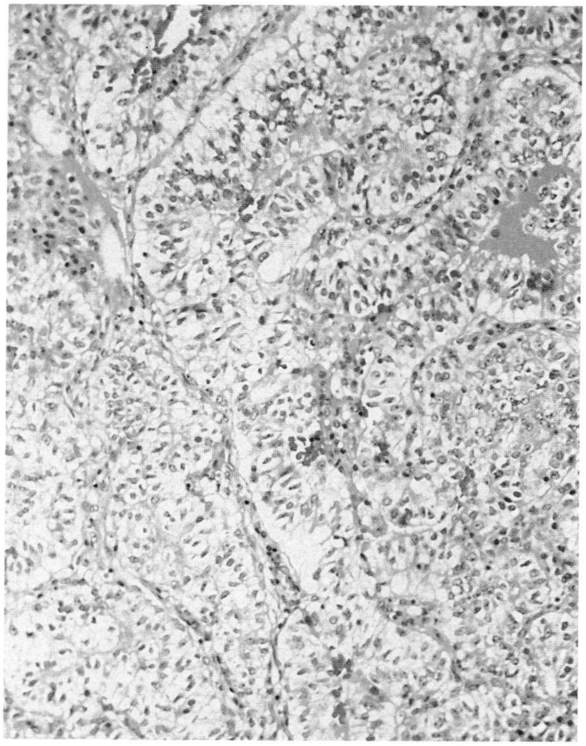

Figure 26-34
CLEAR CELL HYPERPLASIA OF PREGNANCY
The tubal epithelial cells are distended by clear cytoplasm.

fallopian tube that was the site of a tubal pregnancy (fig. 26-34) (64a). The lesion should be distinguished from clear cell carcinoma by the use of criteria similar to those applicable in the endometrium (60).

Ectopic Decidua. Decidua has been encountered in the lamina propria of the fallopian tube in 5 to 8 percent of pregnant women at term (61, 63,64), in about one third of cases of ectopic pregnancy (62a), and rarely, in women receiving progestins (62). We have seen occlusion of the lumen by decidua in one case (fig. 26-35). Decidua has also been identified in the serosal connective tissue in approximately 5 percent of a large series of tubal ligation specimens (65). These foci of decidua have always been incidental microscopic findings in the cases encountered to date. The distinctive features of decidual cells should facilitate diagnosis but potential confusion with a signet-ring cell carcinoma arises when the decidual cells contain mucin-filled in-

tracytoplasmic vacuoles (fig. 26-36). The mucin in such cells, however, is alcianophilic and unlike the mucin of most signet-ring cell carcinomas, periodic acid–Schiff (PAS) negative (60).

Endometriosis

Endometrial tissue extends directly from the uterine cornu and replaces the mucosa of the interstitial and isthmic portions of the fallopian tube in up to 25 and 10 percent of women, respectively (fig. 26-37) (72,76). This finding is considered to be a normal morphologic variation. When endometrial tissue in the interstitial and isthmic portions of the tube causes luminal occlusion (fig. 26-37), the term "endometrial colonization" has been applied (66,68,71,73) although the process may represent only an exaggeration of the normal variation described above; involvement may be bilateral. Endometrial colonization is said to account for 15 to 20 percent of cases of infertility and may be associated with tubal pregnancy. This

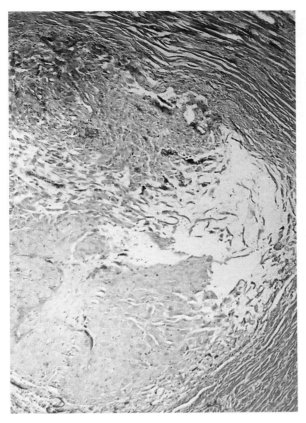

Figure 26-35
ECTOPIC DECIDUA
The tubal lumen contains a mass of decidual cells and a pool of mucin. (Mucicarmine stain)

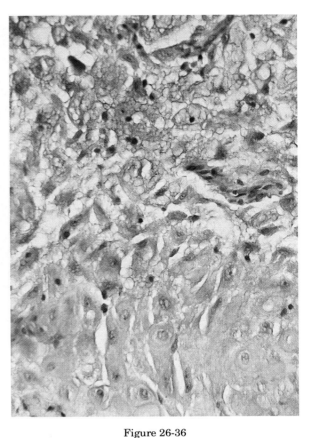

Figure 26-36
ECTOPIC DECIDUA
A high-power view of figure 26-35 shows cytoplasmic mucin in many decidual cells. (Mucicarmine stain)

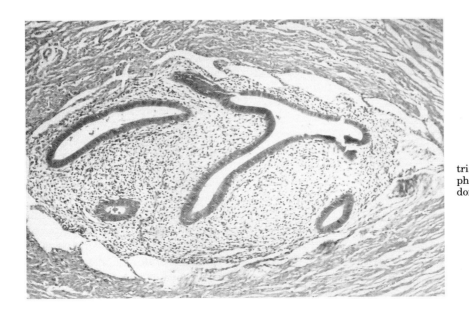

Figure 26-37
ENDOMETRIOSIS
(COLONIZATION) OF
THE FALLOPIAN TUBE
The lumen is occluded by endometrial glands and stroma. Dilated lymphatics lie at the junction of the endometrial tissue and muscle layer.

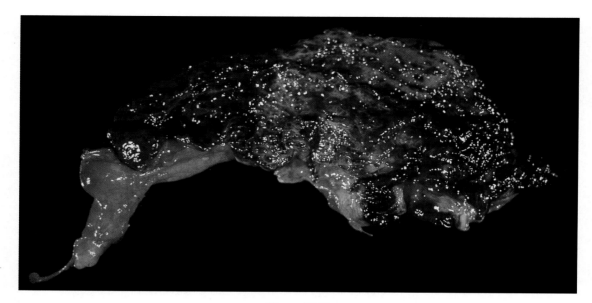

Figure 26-38
PSEUDOXANTHOMATOUS SALPINGITIS
There is brown discoloration of the mucosa.

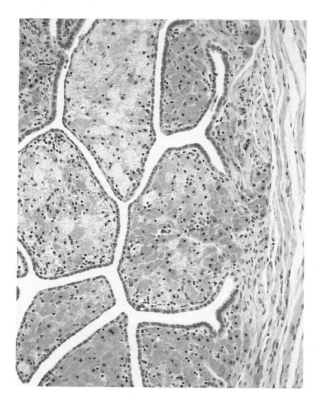

Figure 26-39
PSEUDOXANTHOMATOUS SALPINGITIS

Pseudoxanthoma cells with brown lipofuscin pigment expand the tubal plicae.

ectopic endometrial tissue may be the site of origin of some tubal polyps (page 462) (67,70,74).

True tubal endometriosis is most commonly serosal and associated with endometriosis elsewhere in the pelvis; the myosalpinx is not involved in most of the cases (79); rarely, prominent mucosal involvement is seen. In some cases of pelvic endometriosis the mucosal surface appears brown because of an accumulation of old blood pigment in pseudoxanthoma cells in the lamina propria (figs. 26-38, 26-39).

Another type of endometriosis of the fallopian tube is postsalpingectomy endometriosis (69,77, 78,80), which has been found in 20 to 50 percent of tubes examined after ligation. The frequency of this complication is increased if electrocautery was used, if the proximal stumps are short, and if the postligation interval is long. The lesion occurs at the tip of the proximal tubal stump, typically 1 to 4 years after the ligation. It may be associated with salpingitis isthmica nodosa. The lesion is histologically similar to uterine adenomyosis, consisting of endometrial glands and stroma that have extended from the endosalpinx into the muscularis, and often to the serosal surface. Hysterosalpingography or India ink injection of the specimen may show tuboperitoneal fistulas (75) in which postligation ectopic pregnancies may occur.

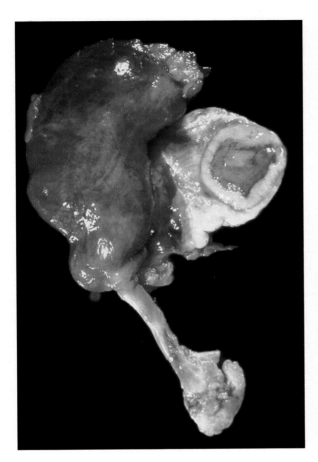

Figure 26-40
ECTOPIC PREGNANCY
The ampullary portion of the tube is markedly distended by blood. A corpus luteum of pregnancy is present in the adjacent ovary.

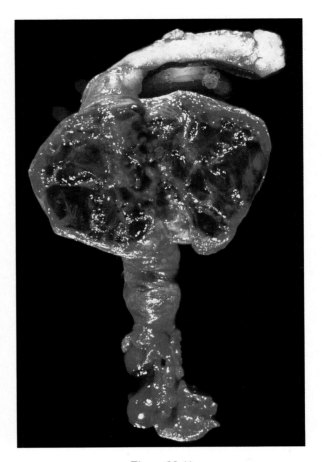

Figure 26-41
ECTOPIC PREGNANCY
A portion of tubal lumen is distended with blood.

Ectopic Pregnancy

In approximately half the cases of tubal pregnancy there is a sausage-shaped distension of the ampullary portion of the tube (83,84), which typically has a thinned wall and a dusky red serosal surface (figs. 26-40, 26-41); the tube may be ruptured. Less commonly, the isthmic portion is involved, and least often, the interstitial portion or fimbriated end. Microscopic examination may reveal fetal parts, villi, which are frequently degenerated, and trophoblast in varying combinations, as well as blood clot, which accounts for the marked luminal distension (81). There may be evidence of an underlying disorder that predisposes to ectopic pregnancy, such as chronic salpingitis, salpingitis isthmica nodosa, endometriosis, or a small tumor.

In chronic ectopic pregnancy a densely adherent, palpable mass may form (82a). Although the hemorrhagic mass resulting from the ectopic pregnancy is usually limited to the fallopian tube and adjacent tissue, in rare chronic cases it dissects into the broad ligament and may even extend to the contralateral adnexa (82).

Rarely, a clinically unsuspected remnant of an involuted ectopic pregnancy, either a placental site nodule (page 481) or hyalinized remains of chorionic villi, is encountered on microscopic examination of a fallopian tube (83a).

Torsion

Tubal torsion (fig. 26-42) usually accompanies torsion of the adjacent ovary (page 441) but occasionally, only the tube is involved (86). On gross

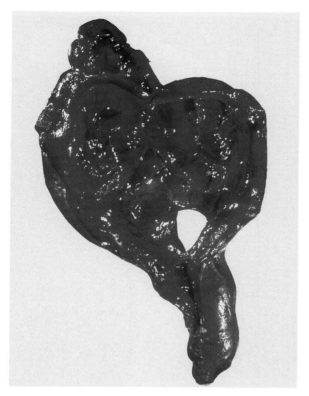

Figure 26-42
HEMORRHAGIC INFARCTION OF
TUBE DUE TO TORSION

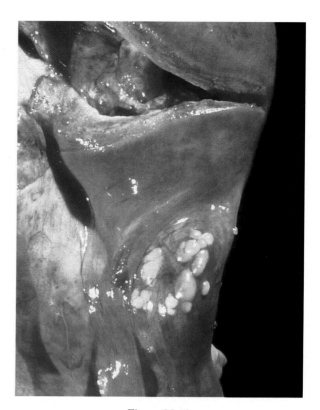

Figure 26-43
WALTHARD NESTS
Several small yellow nodules are clustered on the serosa of the isthmic portion of the tube.

inspection the tube is swollen and typically dusky red-blue (fig. 26-42). Rarely, there is synchronous or metachronous involvement of the contralateral tube (85,87).

Prolapse

In approximately 80 percent of the reported cases, prolapse of the fallopian tube occurs after a hysterectomy performed by the vaginal approach (88–91). On clinical examination a lesion simulating granulation tissue is visible at the vaginal apex. Microscopic examination of a biopsy specimen may result in an erroneous diagnosis of papillary adenocarcinoma (see page 466) unless the "papillae" are recognized as tubal plicae lined by bland tubal epithelium.

Walthard Nests

These nests of transitional epithelium are common on the serosal surfaces of the fallopian

tubes, mesosalpinx, and mesovarium (92,93). They are often visible grossly as one or more white to yellow cysts or nodules a few millimeters in diameter (fig. 26-43), and are occasionally mistaken for granulomas or tumor implants. Microscopic examination reveals well-circumscribed, small cysts (fig. 26-44) or solid nests (fig. 26-45), or less often, surface plaques that focally replace the normal mesothelium. The solid nests are composed of cytologically benign, mitotically inactive, transitional-type cells (fig. 26-45); their nuclei contain fine chromatin and one or two small nucleoli, and are often grooved. Sometimes the cells have a squamous appearance, but keratinization is absent. The cysts are lined by transitional cells, which may be flattened; inspissated eosinophilic secretion is typically and mucin occasionally present within the lumens. The bland cytologic features of this lesion should facilitate its distinction from implants of carcinoma.

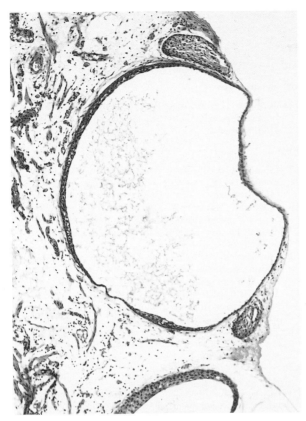

Figure 26-44
WALTHARD NESTS
Two nests are cystic.

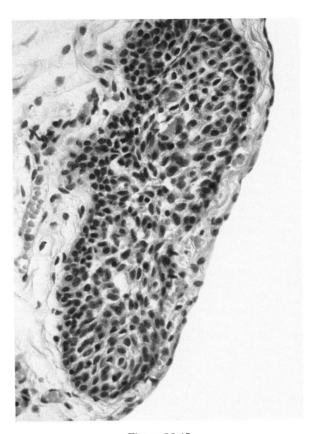

Figure 26-45
WALTHARD NEST
An aggregate of bland-appearing transitional cells is present in the tubal serosa.

Ectopic Tissue in Fallopian Tube

Ectopic tissue includes nests of hilus cells in the fallopian tube and paratubal tissue (94,95,97). In a thorough examination of over 2,000 tubes or segments thereof, Honore and O'Hara (94) found hilus cells in 0.5 percent of the cases. The cells were found only in the endosalpinx and paratubal connective tissue, most commonly in the fimbriae. A single case of ectopic pancreas in the fallopian tube has been reported (96).

REFERENCE

Benign Tumors of Soft Tissue Type

1. Crissman JD, Handwerker D. Leiomyoma of the uterine tube: report of a case [Letter]. Am J Obstet Gynecol 1976;126:1046.
2. Dede JA, Janovski NA. Lipoma of the uterine tube—a gynecologic rarity. Obstet Gynecol 1963;22:461–7.
3. Ebrahimi T, Okagaki T. Hemangioma of the fallopian tube. Am J Obstet Gynecol 1973;115:864–5.
4. Honore LH. Parauterine leiomyomas in women: a clinicopathologic study of 22 cases. Eur J Obstet Gynec Reprod Biol 1981;11:273–9.
5. Katz DA, Thom D, Bogard P, Dermer MS. Angiomyolipoma of the fallopian tube. Am J Obstet Gynecol 1984;148:341–3.
6. Moore OA, Waxman M, Udoffia C. Leiomyoma of the fallopian tube: a cause of tubal pregnancy. Am J Obstet Gynecol 1979;134:101–2.
7. Okagaki T, Richart RM. Neurilemoma of the fallopian tube. Am J Obstet Gynecol 1970;106:929.
8. Sanes S, Warner R. Primary lymphangioma of the fallopian tube. Am J Obstet Gynecol 1939;37:316–21.

8a. Spanta R, Lawrence WD. Soft tissue chondroma of the fallopian tube. Differential diagnosis and histogenetic considerations. Path Res Pract 1995;190:174–6.

9. Talerman A. Haemangioma of the fallopian tube. J Obstet Gynaec Brit Cmwlth 1969;76:559–60.

10. Talerman A. Leiomyoma of the fallopian tube. Int J Gynaecol Obstet 1974;12:145–7.

11. Weber DL, Fazzini E. Ganglioneuroma of the fallopian tube. A hitherto unreported finding. Acta Neuropathol (Berl) 1970;16:173–5.

Malignant Tumors of Soft Tissue Type

12. Buchwalter CL, Jenison EL, Fromm M, Mehta VT, Hart WR. Case report. Pure embryonal rhabdomyosarcoma of the fallopian tube. Gynecol Oncol 1997;67:95–101.

12a. Jacoby AF, Fuller AF Jr, Thor AD, Muntz HG. Primary leiomyosarcoma of the fallopian tube. Gynecol Oncol 1993;51:404–7.

Adenomatoid Tumor

13. Bolton RN, Hunter WC. Adenomatoid tumors of the uterus and adnexa. Report of eleven cases. Am J Obstet Gynecol 1958;76:647–52.

14. Evans N. Mesotheliomas of the uterine and tubal serosa and the tunica vaginalis testis. Am J Pathol 1943;19:461–71.

15. Golden A, Ash JE. Adenomatoid tumors of the genital tract. Am J Pathol 1945;21:63–73.

15a. Honore LH, O'Hara KE. Adenomatoid tumor of the fimbrial endosalpinx: report of two cases with discussion of histogenesis. Eur J Obs Gyn Reprod Biol 1979; 9:335–9.

16. Jackson JR. The histogenesis of the "adenomatoid" tumor of the genital tract. Cancer 1958;11:337–50.

17. Pauerstein CJ, Woodruff JD, Quinton SW. Developmental patterns in "adenomatoid lesions" of the fallopian tube. Am J Obstet Gynecol 1968;100:1000–7.

18. Salazar H, Kanbour A, Burgess F. Ultrastructure and observations on the histogenesis of mesotheliomas "adenomatoid tumors" of the female genital tract. Cancer 1972;29:141–52.

19. Stephenson TJ, Mills PM. Adenomatoid tumors: an immunohistochemical and ultrastructural appraisal of their histogenesis. J Pathol 1986;148:327–35.

20. Taxy JB, Battifora H, Oyasu R. Adenomatoid tumors: a light microscopic, histochemical, and ultrastructural study. Cancer 1974;34:306–16.

21. Youngs LA, Taylor HB. Adenomatoid tumors of the uterus and fallopian tube. Am J Clin Pathol 1967;48:537–45.

Germ Cell Tumors

22. Aaron JB. Dermoid cyst in the uterine tube: a case report with a review of the literature. Am J Obstet Gynecol 1941;42:1080–6.

23. Grimes HG, Kornmesser JG. Benign cystic teratoma of the oviduct: report of a case and review of the literature. Obstet Gynecol 1960;16:85–8.

24. Henricksen E. Struma salpingi. Report of a case. Obstet Gynecol 1955;5:833–5.

25. Hoda SA, Huvos AG. Struma salpingis associated with struma ovarii. Am J Surg Pathol 1993;17:1187–9.

26. Horn T, Jao W, Keh PC. Benign cystic teratoma of the fallopian tube [Letter]. Arch Pathol Lab Med 1983;107:48.

27. Kutteh WH, Albert T. Mature cystic teratoma of the fallopian tube associated with an ectopic pregnancy. Obstet Gynecol 1991;78:984–6.

28. Mazzarella P, Okagaki T, Richart RM. Teratoma of the uterine tube. A case report and review of the literature. Obstet Gynecol 1972;39:381–8.

29. Scully RE. Germ cell tumors of the ovary and fallopian tube. In: Meigs JV, Strugis SH, eds. Progress in gynecology, vol 4. New York: Grune & Stratton, 1963:335–47.

30. Sweet RL, Selinger HE, McKay DG. Malignant teratoma of the uterine tube. Obstet Gynecol 1975;45:553–6.

Trophoblastic Disease

31. Dekel A, van Iddekinge B, Isaacson C, Dicker D, Feldberg D, Goldman J. Primary choriocarcinoma of the fallopian tube. Report of a case with survival and postoperative delivery. Review of the literature. Obstet Gynec Surv 1986;41:142–8.

32. Govender NS, Goldstein DP. Metastatic tubal mole and coexisting intrauterine pregnancy. Obstet Gynecol 1977;49:67s–9s.

33. Muto MG, Lage JM, Berkowitz RS, Goldstein DP, Bernstein MR. Gestational trophoblastic disease of the fallopian tube. J Reprod Med 1991;36:57–60.

33a. Nayar R, Snell J, Silverberg SG, Lage JM. Placental site nodule occurring in a fallopian tube. Hum Pathol 1996;27:1243–5.

34. Ober WB, Maier RC. Gestational choriocarcinoma of the fallopian tube. Diagn Gynecol Obstet 1982;3:213–31.

35. Park WW, Lees JC. Choriocarcinoma, a general review with review of 516 cases. Arch Pathol 1950;49:205–41.

36. Westerhout FC Jr. Ruptured tubal hydatidiform mole. Report of a case. Obstet Gynecol 1964;23:138–9.

Malignant Lymphoma and Leukemia

37. Cecalupo AJ, Frankel LS, Sullivan MP. Pelvic and ovarian extramedullary leukemic relapse in young girls: a report of four cases and review of the literature. Cancer 1982;50:587–93.

38. Osborne BM, Robboy SJ. Lymphomas or leukemia presenting as ovarian tumors. An analysis of 42 cases. Cancer 1983;52:1933–43.

39. Rosenberg SA, Diamond HD, Jaslowitz B, Craver LF. Lymphosarcoma—a review of 1269 cases. Medicine 1961;40:31–84.

Secondary Tumors of the Fallopian Tube

40. Finn WF, Javert CT. Primary and metastatic cancer of the fallopian tube. Cancer 1949;2:803–14.
41. Holland WM. Primary carcinoma of the fallopian tubes. Surg Gynecol Obstet 1930;51:683–91.
42. Mazur MT, Hsueh S, Gersell DJ. Metastases to the female genital tract. Analysis of 325 cases. Cancer 1984;53:1978–84.
43. Motoyama T, Watanabe H. Squamous cell carcinoma of the cervix with extensive superficial spreading to almost whole genital tract and associated with endometrial stromal sarcoma. Acta Pathol Jpn 1988;38:1445–52.
43a. Pins MR, Young RH, Crum CP, Leach IH, Scully RE. Cervical squamous cell carcinoma in situ with intraepithelial extension to the upper genital tract and invasion of tubes and ovaries: report of a case with human papilloma virus analysis. Int J Gynecol Pathol 1997;16:272–8.
44. Punnonen R, Gronroos M, Vaajalahti P. Squamous cell carcinoma in situ from the uterine cervix to the distal end of the fallopian tube. Acta Obstet Gynecol Scand 1979;58:101–4.
45. Woodruff JD, Julian CG. Multiple malignancy in the upper genital canal. Am J Obstet Gynecol 1969;103:810–22.

Hyperplasia including Pseudocarcinomatous Hyperplasia

46. Cheung AN, Young RH, Scully RE. Pseudocarcinomatous hyperplasia of the fallopian tube associated with salpingitis. A report of 14 cases. Am J Surg Pathol 1994;8:1125–30.
47. Dougherty CM, Cotten NM. Proliferative epithelial lesions of the uterine tube. I. Adenomatous hyperplasia. Obstet Gynecol 1964;24:849–54.
48. Moore SW, Enterline HT. Significance of proliferative epithelial lesions of the uterine tube. Obstet Gynecol 1975;45:385–90.
49. Pauerstein CJ, Woodruff JD. Cellular patterns in proliferative and anaplastic disease of the fallopian tube. Am J Obstet Gynecol 1966;96:486–92.
50. Robey SS, Silva EG. Epithelial hyperplasia of the fallopian tube. Its association with serous borderline tumors of the ovary. Int J Gynecol Pathol 1989;8:214–20.
51. Stern J, Buscema J, Parmley T, Woodruff JD, Rosenshein NB. Atypical epithelial proliferations in the fallopian tube. Am J Obstet Gynecol 1981;140:309–12.
52. Yanai-Inbar I, Siriaunkgul S, Silverberg SG. Mucosal epithelial proliferation of the fallopian tube: a particular association with ovarian serous tumor of low malignant potential? Int J Gynecol Pathol 1995;14:107–13.

Salpingitis Isthmica Nodosa

53. Benjamin CL, Beaver DC. Pathogenesis of salpingitis isthmica nodosa. Am J Clin Pathol 1951;21:212–22.
54. Majmudar B, Henderson PH III, Sample E. Salpingitis isthmica nodosa: a high-risk factor for tubal pregnancy. Obstet Gynecol 1983;62:73–8.
55. Schenken JR, Burns EL. A study and classification of nodular lesions of the fallopian tubes. "Salpingitis isthmica nodosa." Am J Obstet Gynecol 1943;45:624–36.
56. Wrork OH, Broders AC. Adenomyosis of the fallopian tubes. Am J Obstet Gynecol 1942;44:412–32.

Heat Artifact

57. Cornog JL, Currie JL, Rubin A. Heat artifact simulating adenocarcinoma of fallopian tube. JAMA 1970;214:1118–9.

Arias-Stella Reaction

58. Birch HW, Collins CG. Atypical changes of genital epithelium associated with ectopic pregnancy. Am J Obstet Gynecol 1961;81:1198–208.
59. Milchgrub S, Sandstad J. Arias-Stella reaction in fallopian tube epithelium. A light and electron microscopic study with a review of the literature. Am J Clin Pathol 1991;95:892–5.

Ectopic Decidua and Clear Cell Change of Pregnancy

60. Clement PB, Young RH, Scully RE. Nontrophoblastic pathology of the female genital tract and peritoneum associated with pregnancy. Semin Diagn Pathol 1989;6:372–406.
61. Hellman LM. The morphology of the human fallopian tube in the early puerperium. Am J Obstet Gynecol 1949;57:154–65.
62. Mills SE, Fechner RE. Stromal and epithelial changes in the fallopian tube following hormonal therapy. Hum Pathol 1983;11:583–5.
62a. Pauerstein CJ, Croxatto HB, Eddy CA, Ramzy I, Walters MD. Anatomy and pathology of tubal pregnancy. Obstet Gynecol 1986;67:301–8.
63. Rewell RE. Extra-uterine decidua. J Pathol 1972;105:219–22.
64. Tilden IL, Winstedt R. Decidual reactions in fallopian tubes. Histologic study of tubal segments from 144 postpartum sterilizations. Am J Pathol 1943;19:1043–51.
64a. Tziortziotis DV, Bouros AC, Ziogas VS, Young RH. Clear cell hyperplasia of the fallopian tube epithelium associated with ectopic pregnancy. Report of a case. Int J Gynecol Pathol 1997;16:79–80.
65. Zaytsev P, Taxy JB. Pregnancy-associated ectopic decidua. Am J Surg Pathol 1987;11:526–30.

Endometriosis

66. Cioltei A, Tasca L, Titiriga L, Maakaron G, Calciu V. Nodular salpingitis and tubal endometriosis. I. Comparative clinical study. Acta Eur Fertil 1979;10:135–41.

67. David MP, Ben-Zwi D, Langer L. Tubal intramural polyps and their relationship to infertility. Fertil Steril 1981;35:526–31.

68. De Brux J. The contribution of pathological anatomy to the diagnosis and prognosis of different forms of tubal sterility. Acta Eur Fertil 1975;6:185–95.

69. Donnez J, Casanas-Roux F, Ferin J, Thomas K. Tubal polyps, epithelial inclusions, and endometriosis after tubal sterilization. Fertil Steril 1984;41:564–8.

70. Fernstrom I, Lagerlof B. Polyps in the intramural part of the fallopian tubes. A radiographic and clinical study. Br J Obstet Gynaecol 1964;71:681–91.

71. Fortier KJ, Haney AF. The pathologic spectrum of uterotubal junction obstruction. Obstet Gynecol 1985;65:93–8.

72. Lisa JR, Gioia JD, Rubin IC. Observations on the interstitial portion of the fallopian tube. Surg Gynecol Obstet 1954;99:159–69.

73. Madelenat P, De Brux J, Palmer R. L'etiologie des obstructions tubaires proximales et son role dan le pronostic des implantations. Gynecologie 1977;28:47–53.

74. McLaughlin DS. Successful pregnancy outcome following removal of bilateral cornual polyps by microsurgical linear salpingostomy with the aid of the CO2 laser. Fertil Steril 1984;42:939–41.

75. Rock JA, Parmley TH, King TM, Laufe LE, Su BC. Endometriosis and the development of tuboperitoneal fistulas after tubal ligation. Fertil Steril 1981;35:16–20.

76. Rubin IC, Lisa JR, Trinidad S. Further observations on ectopic endometrium of the fallopian tube. Surg Gynecol Obstet 1956;103:469–74.

77. Sampson JA. Postsalpingectomy endometriosis (endosalpingiosis). Am J Obstet Gynecol 1930;20:443–80.

78. Sampson JA. Pathogenesis of postsalpingectomy endometriosis in laparotomy scars. Am J Obstet Gynecol 1945;50:597–620.

79. Sheldon RS, Wilson RB, Dockerty MB. Serosal endometriosis of fallopian tubes. Am J Obstet Gynecol 1967;99:882–4.

80. Stock RJ. Postsalpingectomy endometriosis: a reassessment. Obstet Gynecol 1982;60:560–70.

Ectopic Pregnancy

81. Budowick M, Johnson TR, Genadry R, Parmley TH, Woodruff JD. The histopathology of the developing tubal ectopic pregnancy. Fertil Steril 1980;34:169–71.

82. Case records of the Massachusetts General Hospital (case 11-1976). N Engl J Med 1976;294:600–5.

82a. Cole T, Corlett RC. Chronic ectopic pregnancy. Obstet Gynecol 1982;59:63–8.

83. Fox H, Buckley CH, Randall S. Ectopic pregnancy. In: Fox H, ed. Haines and Taylor obstetrical and gynecological pathology, 3rd ed, Vol 2. Churchill Livingstone: New York, 1987.

83a. Jacques SM, Qureshi F, Ramirez NC, Lawrence WD. Retained trophoblastic tissue in fallopian tubes: a consequence of unsuspected ectopic pregnancies. Int J Gynecol Pathol 1997;16:219–24.

84. Pauerstein CJ, Croxatto HB, Eddy CA, Ramzy I, Walters MD. Anatomy and pathology of tubal pregnancy. Obstet Gynecol 1986;67:301–8.

Torsion

85. Dunnihoo DR, Wolff J. Bilateral torsion of the adnexa: a case report and a review of the world literature. Obstet Gynecol 1984;64:55–9.

86. Filtenborg TA, Hertz JB. Torsion of the fallopian tube. Eur J Obstet Gyn Reprod Biol 1981;12:177–81.

87. Lewis AC. Bilateral torsion of fallopian tubes. A case report. J Obstet Gynaecol Brit Cmwlth 1971;78:93–4.

Prolapse

88. Ellsworth HS, Harris JW, McQuarrie HG, Stone RA, Anderson AE. Prolapse of the fallopian tube following vaginal hysterectomy. JAMA 1973;224:891–2.

89. Sapan IP, Solberg NS. Prolapse of the uterine tube after abdominal hysterectomy. Obstet Gynecol 1973;42:26–32.

90. Silverberg SG, Frable WJ. Prolapse of fallopian tube into vaginal vault after hysterectomy. Histopathology, cytopathology, and differential diagnosis. Arch Pathol 1974;97:100–3.

91. Wheelock JB, Schneider V, Goplerud DR. Prolapsed fallopian tube masquerading as adenocarcinoma of the vagina in a postmenopausal woman. Gynecol Oncol 1985;21:369–75.

Walthard Nests

92. Teoh TB. The structure and development of Walthard nests. J Pathol Bacteriol 1953;66:433–9.

93. Bransilver BR, Ferenczy A, Richart RM. Brenner tumors and Walthard cell nests. Arch Pathol 1974;98:76–86.

Ectopic Tissue in Fallopian Tube

94. Honore LH, O'Hara KE. Ovarian hilus cell heterotopia. Obstet Gynecol 1979;53:461–4.

95. Lewis JD. Hilus-cell hyperplasia of ovaries and tubes. Report of a case. Obstet Gynecol 1964;24:728–31.

96. Mason TE, Quagliarello JR. Ectopic pancreas in the fallopian tube. Report of a first case. Obstet Gynecol 1976;48:70s–5s.

97. Palomaki JF, Blair OM. Hilus cell rest of the fallopian tube. A case report. Obstet Gynecol 1971;37:60–2.

27
TUMORS OF THE BROAD LIGAMENT
AND OTHER UTERINE LIGAMENTS

The broad ligament, which includes the mesosalpinx and mesovarium, contains a variety of structures and tissues from which neoplasms and tumor-like lesions can arise, including normal embryonic remnants, embryonic remnants created by minor disorders of development, and nonspecific tissues such as blood vessels, lymphatic vessels, connective tissue, and nerves. Normal embryonic remnants comprise those of the mesonephric duct and tubules (fig. 27-1). Remnants associated with minor disorders of embryonic development include pedunculated and sessile structures that are usually of mullerian duct origin, such as hydatids of Morgagni (figs. 27-2, 27-3) and accessory fallopian tubes (fig. 27-4). Adrenocortical rests have been identified in 23 percent of carefully sectioned broad ligaments (fig. 27-1) (5), and collections of hilus cells are occasionally encountered.

Accessory ovarian tissue (page 3) may account for the origin of some of the unusual tumors of ovarian type seen at this site. Finally, a tumor arising in the ovarian hilus or outer wall of the uterus or fallopian tube may extend into the broad ligament and even lose its connection with its parent organ, presenting as a tumor of the broad ligament. The World Health Organization (WHO) classification of tumors of the broad ligament is presented in Table 27-1.

In a retrospective review of adnexal tumors spanning a recent decade, tumors of the broad ligament were one fifth to one sixth as common as ovarian tumors (6). The frequency of borderline or invasive epithelial tumors among the broad ligament tumors, however, was only 2 percent in contrast to a 25 percent frequency among the ovarian tumors. Seventy-eight percent of the broad ligament tumors occurred in

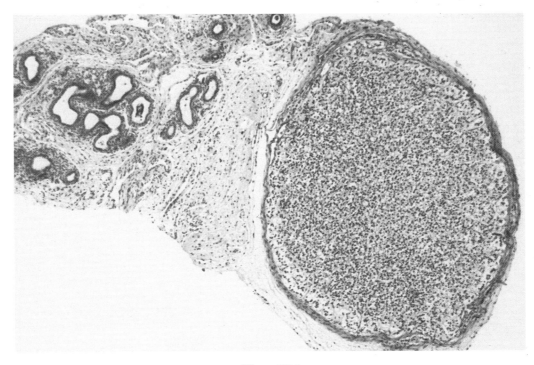

Figure 27-1
MESONEPHRIC (WOLFFIAN) REMNANTS (LEFT) AND ADRENAL CORTICAL REST (RIGHT)

Figure 27-2
HYDATID OF MORGAGNI
The tiny hydatid is pedunculated from the fimbriated end of the right fallopian tube. The left ovary contains a serous cystadenoma.

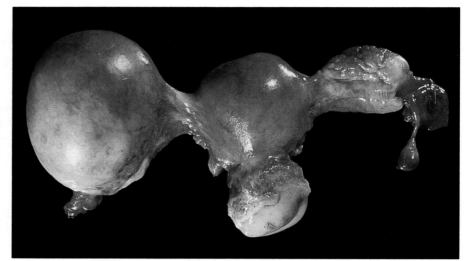

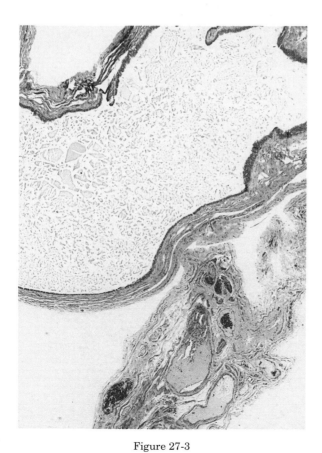

Figure 27-3
HYDATID OF MORGAGNI
The pedunculated cyst is lined by thick and thin epithelium (of mullerian type).

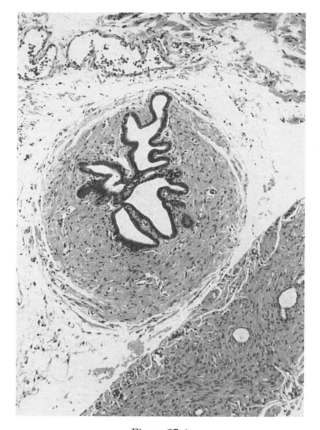

Figure 27-4
ACCESSORY FALLOPIAN TUBE
The irregular lumen is surrounded by a thick layer of smooth muscle.

Table 27-1

WORLD HEALTH ORGANIZATION CLASSIFICATION OF TUMORS OF THE BROAD LIGAMENT AND OTHER UTERINE LIGAMENTS

EPITHELIAL TUMORS
  Mullerian
    Serous tumors
      Cystadenoma
      Cystic tumor of borderline malignancy
      Carcinoma
    Endometrioid tumors
    Clear cell carcinoma
    Mucinous carcinoma
    Brenner tumor and transitional cell carcinoma
  Wolffian and probable wolffian tumors
    Papillary cystadenoma*
    Adnexal tumor of probable wolffian origin
  Ependymoma
MIXED EPITHELIAL-MESENCHYMAL TUMORS
  Adenomyoma
  Adenosarcoma
  Others
SOFT TISSUE TUMORS
  Benign
    Leiomyoma
    Others
  Malignant
    Leiomyosarcoma
    Others
MISCELLANEOUS TUMORS
  Germ cell tumors
  Granulosa cell tumor
  Thecoma
  Fibroma
  Steroid cell tumor
  Adenomatoid tumor
  Pheochromocytoma
  Others
SECONDARY TUMORS
  Carcinoma
  Lymphoma and leukemia
  Others
TUMOR-LIKE LESIONS
  Cysts
    Mullerian
    Wolffian
    Mesothelial
  Endometriosis
  Adrenal cortical rest hyperplasia (Nelson's syndrome)
  Infectious masses
  Fibroxanthoma (inflammatory pseudotumor)
  Malakoplakia
  Foreign body granulomas
  Nodular fasciitis
  Others

*This tumor may be associated with von Hippel-Lindau disease.

patients between the ages of 20 and 50 years, 10 percent in older women, and 12 percent during the second decade. The tumors ranged from 3 to 40 cm in greatest diameter, with 72 percent of them, 5 to 12 cm; 16 percent of the tumors were bilateral. The clinical manifestations of tumors of the broad ligament are similar to those of ovarian tumors. Like the latter, they can be identified on ultrasound examination. Other ligamentous sites of neoplasia are the round ligament and the uterosacral ligament, which contain considerable smooth muscle. Tumors of the round ligament may present intra-abdominally, in the inguinal canal, or in the labium, where the ligament inserts.

EPITHELIAL TUMORS

Epithelial tumors of mullerian type are the most common of the epithelial neoplasms of the broad ligament, where tumors of almost every mullerian cell type have been encountered at least once. The second most frequently reported category of epithelial tumors at this site comprise those that are probably or definitely derived from wolffian remnants.

Epithelial Tumors of Mullerian Type

Although only a few cases have been reported in detail (21,22), in one large series of neoplasms of the broad ligament the serous cystadenoma was by far the most common type of mullerian tumor (17a). The authors distinguished serous cystadenomas from non-neoplastic cysts of serous type by the presence in the former of a thick wall composed of cellular stroma resembling ovarian stroma and the absence of folds or plicae. Approximately 35 cases of serous cystic tumor of borderline malignancy of the broad ligament have been reported in women 19 to 67 years of age (average, 33 years). All the tumors were unilateral and confined to the broad ligament (7,8). One serous borderline tumor that contained mucinous cells and may have been of mixed epithelial type (30), and one mucinous borderline tumor of intestinal type (23) have also been reported. One cystadenofibroma, best interpreted as endometrioid, was reported in a patient with von Hippel-Lindau disease (33a) (see below). Five benign Brenner tumors of the broad ligament have been described (20,28);

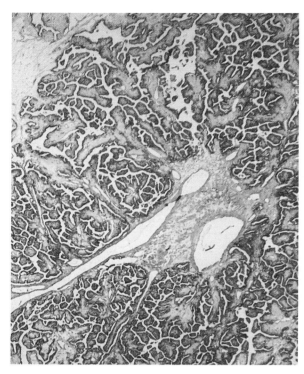

Figure 27-5
PAPILLARY CYSTADENOMA ASSOCIATED
WITH VON HIPPEL-LINDAU DISEASE
The intricate papillary proliferation simulates that of a
serous papillary tumor.

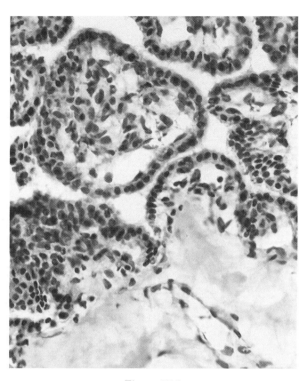

Figure 27-6
PAPILLARY CYSTADENOMA ASSOCIATED
WITH VON HIPPEL-LINDAU DISEASE
The papillae are lined by a mostly single layer of bland
cuboidal epithelial cells.

these tumors were found in women 30 to 64 years of age and ranged from 0.8 to 16 cm in greatest diameter. One of the Brenner tumors was associated with a mucinous cystadenoma and another with a serous cystadenoma (28).

Fourteen cases of carcinoma of mullerian type have been reported. The patients ranged from 23 to 75 years of age (9). Four tumors were endometrioid carcinomas, four were clear cell carcinomas, three were serous carcinomas (7,31), one a probable mucinous carcinoma, one a transitional cell carcinoma (33), and one a probable transitional cell carcinoma (26). In two of the four cases of endometrioid carcinoma and one of the four cases of clear cell carcinoma endometriosis was also present, suggesting the possibility of an origin of the tumor therein. All the carcinomas were unilateral. Because of a limited period of follow-up in many of the cases, the prognosis associated with these tumors is uncertain, but several of them had spread beyond the broad ligament. Therapy similar to that used for ovarian carcinomas of similar cell types is indicated.

Epithelial Tumors of Definite or Probable Wolffian Origin

Four cases of papillary cystadenoma of mesonephric origin in the broad ligament have been reported in patients with von Hippel-Lindau disease (an autosomal dominant disorder characterized by a variety of lesions, including hemangioblastomas of the retina and central nervous system, hepatic and renal adenomas, renal cell carcinoma, paragangliomas, cysts of the pancreas and kidney, papillary cystadenomas of the epididymis in the male, and a number of rarer cysts, tumors, and congenital abnormalities) (16–18,25). The tumors were bilateral in two cases, and in one of these cases was the first recognized manifestation of the disease (25). The tumors were cystic and ranged up to 3 cm in diameter. Microscopic examination revealed the presence

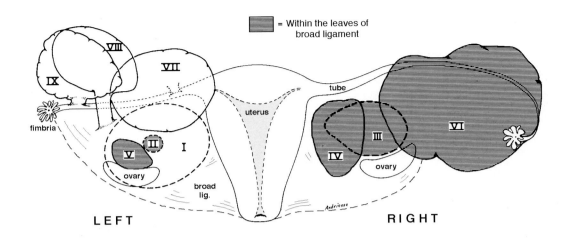

Figure 27-7
DIAGRAM SHOWING LOCATIONS OF NINE EXTRAOVARIAN
ADNEXAL TUMORS OF PROBABLE WOLFFIAN ORIGIN
The shapes and relative sizes of the tumors are shown. (Fig. 1 from Kariminejad MH, Scully RE. Female adnexal tumor of probable Wolffian origin. A distinctive pathologic entity. Cancer 1973;31:671–7.)

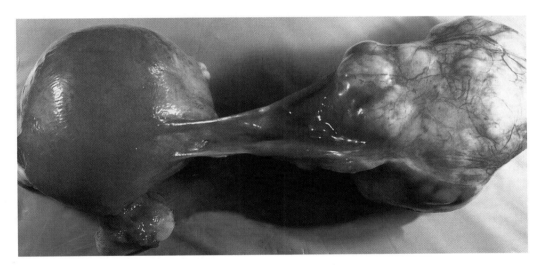

Figure 27-8
BROAD LIGAMENT TUMOR OF PROBABLE WOLFFIAN ORIGIN
The tumor lies within the broad ligament and has a lobulated, smooth external surface. (Fig. 2 from Kariminejad MH, Scully RE. Female adnexal tumor of probable Wolffian origin. A distinctive pathologic entity. Cancer 1973;31:671–7.)

of complex papillae lined by cuboidal, nonciliated cells with bland nuclei (figs. 27-5, 27-6).

A more common tumor of the broad ligament, for which there is very strong evidence of a wolffian origin, is the female adnexal tumor of probable wolffian origin; approximately 40 cases have been reported (12,24). Similar tumors occur in the ovary (page 324) and the retroperitoneum

(11,13). The patients ranged in age from 15 to 81 years. All the tumors were unilateral, with diameters of 0.5 to 18 cm, and were situated mainly within the leaves of the broad ligament or pedunculated from it or from the serosa of the fallopian tube (figs. 27-7, 27-8). The sectioned surfaces (fig. 27-9) were entirely or predominantly solid, often containing small cysts. The solid tissue varied from

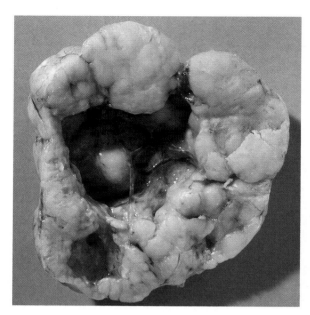

Figure 27-9
SECTIONED SURFACE OF BROAD LIGAMENT
TUMOR OF PROBABLE WOLFFIAN ORIGIN
The tissue is mostly solid and lobulated but contains a few cysts. (Fig. 3 from Kariminejad MH, Scully RE. Female adnexal tumor of probable Wolffian origin. A distinctive pathologic entity. Cancer 1973;31:671–7.)

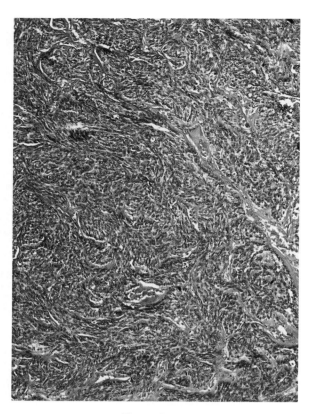

Figure 27-10
BROAD LIGAMENT TUMOR
OF PROBABLE WOLFFIAN ORIGIN
The tumor has a solid architecture.

grayish white to tan or yellow, and was typically firm or rubbery; hemorrhage and necrosis were present only occasionally. The microscopic features of the tumor are described on page 325 (figs. 27-10–27-12).

The wolffian origin of these tumors is supported by their relatively common occurrence in the broad ligament, where wolffian remnants are located; their lack of a close resemblance to tumors of known mullerian type on light microscopic examination; and their ultrastructural and immunohistochemical features, which also differ from those of mullerian neoplasms. Electron microscopic examination of several tumors has revealed an absence or paucity of cilia, Golgi apparatus, secretory granules, and glycogen, and the presence of a thick peritubular basal lamina (11,14). Immunohistochemical staining has been negative for epithelial membrane antigen (EMA), TAG72, and carcinoembryonic antigen (CEA) in contrast to typically opposite findings in tumors of mullerian type (29,32).

Four of the broad ligament tumors of probable wolffian origin have had a malignant behavior,

with either evidence of spread to the peritoneum at the time of diagnosis or recurrence 6 or more years after removal of the primary tumor (12). Many of the patients whose tumors have not been clinically malignant had short follow-up periods. Although some of the clinically malignant tumors contained pleomorphic nuclei and numerous mitotic figures, others had a bland appearance, indicating the necessity for long-term follow-up in all the cases regardless of the microscopic features of the tumor.

Ependymoma

Three ependymomas of the broad ligament and one of the uterosacral ligament have been reported in patients 13, 45, 47, and 48 years of age, respectively (10,15,19). They varied from 1 cm in diameter to a large mass filling the pelvis and extending to the umbilicus. The microscopic

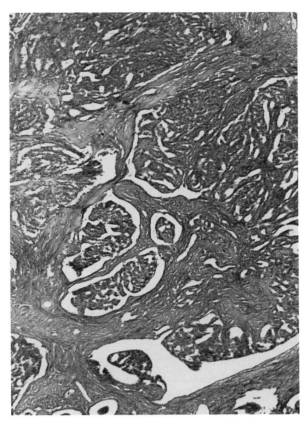

Figure 27-11
BROAD LIGAMENT TUMOR OF PROBABLE
WOLFFIAN ORIGIN
The tumor has a papillary adenomatous architecture.

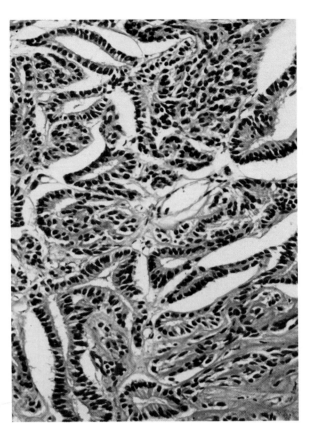

Figure 27-12
BROAD LIGAMENT TUMOR OF PROBABLE
WOLFFIAN ORIGIN
The tumor is characterized by hollow empty tubules.

features were similar to those of ependymomas of the central nervous system. In one case the presence of cysts containing papillae with psammoma body formation simulated closely the appearance of serous papillary carcinoma; the tumor was distinguished from the latter only by finding the characteristic perivascular rosettes of the ependymoma and staining for glial fibrillary acidic protein, which was observed in all the reported cases. One tumor contained an island of cartilage, but its presence did not establish the diagnosis of teratoma since cartilage has been described in ependymomas of the central nervous system. In two patients the tumor had spread beyond the broad ligament or uterosacral ligament at the time of operation; a third patient had two retroperitoneal recurrences of tumor over a period of 24 years. Except for that case the duration of follow-up has been relatively short.

MIXED EPITHELIAL–MESENCHYMAL TUMORS

The adenomyoma, which is composed of endometrial-type glands (with or without endometrioid stroma) and proliferating smooth muscle, is the most common mixed epithelial-mesenchymal tumor of the broad ligament, round ligament, and uterosacral ligament (fig. 27-13). It is difficult to determine the frequency of these tumors because the terms "adenomyoma" and "endometriosis" have often been used interchangeably in these areas. One high-grade mullerian adenosarcoma reported to have arisen in the round ligament was fatal within a year after its discovery (40).

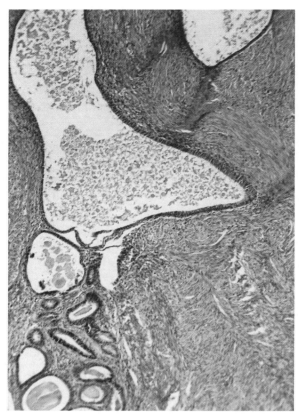

Figure 27-13
ADENOMYOMA OF ROUND LIGAMENT
Endometrioid glands with scanty adjacent stroma are separated by smooth muscle.

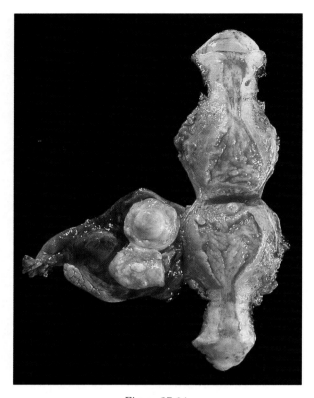

Figure 27-14
LEIOMYOMA OF BROAD LIGAMENT
The small tumor, which has been bisected, is clearly separate from the ovary and the uterus.

SOFT TISSUE TUMORS

Benign Tumors

Leiomyomas and lipomas are the most common benign mesenchymal tumors of the broad and round ligaments (34,36a,38a). Because of their proximity to the fallopian tube and uterus it is often difficult to determine the site of origin of leiomyomas, causing Gardner et al. (36b) to designate them as ligamentous tumors only when they were small and clearly separated from the myometrium (fig. 27-14). Lipomas are usually small and lie below the tube or in its serosa along the distal portion of the ampulla; rarely, they are large and cause symptoms (38a). Occasional cases of many other varieties of soft tissue tumor of the broad and round ligaments have been reported (34,39), including a fibroma with heterotopic bone formation (46) and two benign mesenchymomas composed of adipocytes, smooth muscle cells, and thin-walled blood vessels (42).

Malignant Tumors

The most common sarcoma of the broad ligament is the leiomyosarcoma, of which only 10 reported cases are acceptable if strict diagnostic criteria are used (35,38). Like their uterine counterparts these tumors are associated with a poor prognosis. At least two embryonal rhabdomyosarcomas of the broad ligament have been reported in children 3 and 6 years of age, both of which were fatal (37). One endometrioid stromal sarcoma arising in endometriosis in the broad ligament has been described (43). Other reported broad ligament sarcomas have included a malignant fibrous histiocytoma (36), a mixed mesenchymal sarcoma (45), a myxoid liposarcoma (44), and a Ewing's sarcoma (41).

MISCELLANEOUS AND SECONDARY TUMORS

A variety of miscellaneous tumors, many of them of ovarian type, have been reported in the literature. Others are undoubtedly hidden or are inadequately documented within series of tumors of the pelvis or series of specific neoplasms in which a broad ligament location is not included in the title of the paper.

The occurrence of ovarian-type tumors in the broad ligament always raises the question of an origin in an accessory ovary, but in almost all the reported cases the tumor was large enough to replace the accessory ovarian tissue if it had been present originally. Dermoid cysts (49) and a yolk sac tumor (52) have been reported in the broad ligament; the dermoid cysts arose bilaterally in accessory ovaries. A dermoid cyst containing pituitary tissue was found in the uterosacral ligament (50). A choriocarcinoma presented as a mass in the mesosalpinx of a 45-year-old woman, and tumor was also found within vessels in the wall of the adjacent fallopian tube; the origin of the tumor was in doubt (53).

At least four tumors that were designated "granulosa cell tumor" originated in the broad ligament (49a,56,57), but some of those in the older literature may have been female adnexal tumors of probable wolffian origin misinterpreted as granulosa cell tumors. The literature contains at least three broad ligament tumors in the thecoma-fibroma category (54,55); in one 70-year-old woman (54) the tumor was associated with an elevated estradiol level and cystic hyperplasia of the endometrium. At least three steroid cell tumors have arisen in the broad ligament (58–60). In two cases (58,60) the tumor was virilizing, and in one of them was demonstrated to have arisen in an accessory ovary (58); that tumor was clinically malignant. The common adrenal-cortical rests of the broad ligament are another possible source of tumors of this type.

An adenomatoid tumor has been reported in the broad ligament (61). Two pheochromocytomas of the broad ligament have been described (47,48); in one case, in a 51-year-old woman, the tumor was only 3 cm in diameter and was associated with hypertension and an elevated vanillylmandelic acid level; both manifestations reverted to normal postoperatively (48).

Any type of malignant tumor arising in the uterus, fallopian tube, elsewhere in the pelvis or abdomen, or outside the abdomen may spread by direct extension, lymphatic vessels, or blood vessels to the broad ligament. Intravenous leiomyomatosis and endometrial stromal sarcoma of the uterus may present at operation as a mass within the broad ligament.

TUMOR-LIKE LESIONS

Among the most common tumor-like lesions are cysts of mullerian, mesonephric, and mesothelial origin (62a–64,66). These cysts vary in size from barely recognizable grossly to relatively rare examples 20 cm or more in diameter (figs. 27-15, 27-16). Pedunculated cysts (hydatids of Morgagni), which are very common, are situated close to the fimbriated end of the fallopian tube (see fig. 27-2). They are lined most often by fallopian tube–type epithelium and may contain branching folds within their lumens, resembling the plicae of the fallopian tube and suggesting an origin in an accessory tube (see fig. 27-3). Cysts with a similar lining are less often sessile within the leaves of the broad ligament (fig. 27-17). Occasional cysts are lined by cuboidal cells of mesothelial type or by cuboidal epithelium resembling that of mesonephric remnants of the broad ligament; the latter cysts may have a prominent basement membrane like the remnants from which they arise. It may not be possible in every case to determine the subtype of a broad ligament cyst, especially when it is large; in some cases it may be difficult to distinguish a cyst of mullerian origin from a cystadenoma, although the latter typically has a prominent stromal component resembling the stroma of an ovarian cystadenoma. Mesothelial cysts are typically lined by flattened cells and may be unilocular or multilocular (fig. 27-18). Sizable broad ligament cysts are subject to the same complications as ovarian cysts, including torsion, infarction, and rarely, infection. Endometriosis often involves the broad ligament, typically in association with involvement of other pelvic organs and tissues. In one case (61a) a uterus-like cystic mass lined by endometrioid tissue surrounded by smooth muscle was connected to the broad ligament (see page 421). The adrenal cortical rest hyperplasia that has been

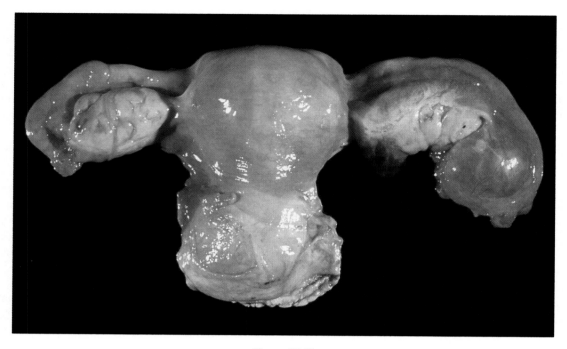

Figure 27-15
BROAD LIGAMENT CYST
The cyst is between the ovary and fallopian tube.

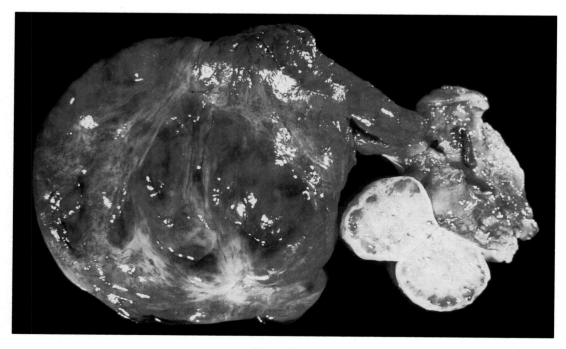

Figure 27-16
BROAD LIGAMENT CYST
The cyst and tube are twisted, with a hemorrhagic surface.

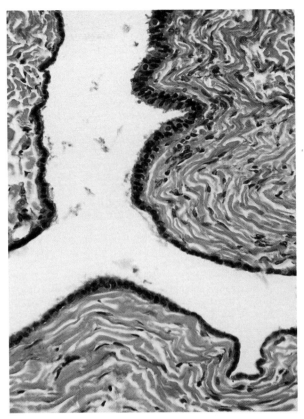

Figure 27-17
MULLERIAN CYST OF BROAD LIGAMENT
The cyst is lined by a thin, focally ciliated epithelium with underlying nonspecific collagenous tissue.

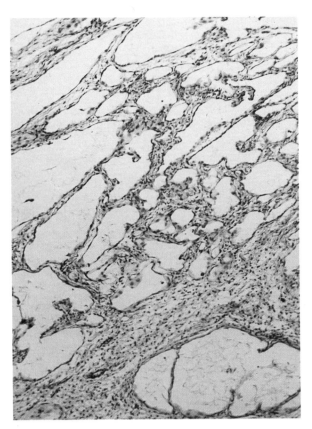

Figure 27-18
MULTILOCULAR PERITONEAL INCLUSION CYST
(BENIGN CYSTIC MESOTHELIOMA)
OF BROAD LIGAMENT

reported in cases of Nelson's syndrome has been discussed on page 453. A wide variety of inflammatory lesions caused by specific organisms or due to foreign bodies can involve the broad ligament, usually having spread from an adjacent pelvic organ. We have seen one example of an inflammatory pseudotumor confined to the broad ligament. One case of malakoplakia involved the broad ligament and inguinal canal (65) and there was one report of nodular fasciitis of the round ligament presenting as a small nodule in a labium (62).

REFERENCES

General References

1. Gardner GH, Greene RR, Peckham BM. Normal and cystic structures of the broad ligament. Am J Obstet Gynecol 1948;55:917–39.
2. Gardner GH, Greene RR, Peckham BM. Tumors of the broad ligament. Am J Obstet Gynecol 1957;73:536–55.
3. Janovski NA, Paramanandhan TL. Ovarian tumors. Tumors and tumor-like conditions of the ovaries, fallopian tubes and ligaments of the uterus. Major problems in obstetrics and gynecology, Vol 4, Philadelphia: WB Saunders, 1973:182–203.
4. Samaha M, Woodruff JD. Paratubal cysts: frequency, histogenesis and associated clinical features. Obstet Gynecol 1985;65:691–4.

5. Falls JL. Accessory adrenal cortex in the broad ligament. Incidence and functional significance. Cancer 1955;8:143–50.

6. Stein AL, Koonings PP, Schlaerth JB, Grimes DA, dAblaing G III. Relative frequency of malignant parovarian tumors: should parovarian tumors be aspirated? Obstet Gynecol 1990;75:1029–31.

Epithelial Tumors

7. Altaras MM, Jaffe R, Corduba M, Holtzinger M, Bahary C. Primary paraovarian cystadenocarcinoma: clinical and management aspects and literature review. Gynecol Oncol 1990;38:268–72.

8. Aslani M, Ahn GH, Scully RE. Serous papillary cystadenoma of broad ligament: a report of 25 cases. Int J Gynecol Pathol 1988;7:131–8.

9. Aslani M, Scully RE. Primary carcinoma of the broad ligament. Report of four cases and review of the literature. Cancer 1989;64:1640–5.

10. Bell DA, Woodruff JM, Scully RE. Ependymoma of the broad ligament. A report of two cases. Am J Surg Pathol 1984;8:203–9.

11. Brescia RJ, Cardoso de Almeida PC, Fuller AF, Dickersin GR, Robboy SJ. Female adnexal tumor of probable wolffian origin with multiple recurrences over 16 years. Cancer 1985;56:1456–61.

12. Daya D. Malignant female adnexal tumor of probable wolffian origin with review of the literature. Arch Pathol Lab Med 1994;118:310–2.

13. Daya D, Murphy J, Simon G. Paravaginal female adnexal tumor of probable wolffian origin. Am J Clin Pathol 1994;101:275–8.

14. Demopoulos RI, Sitelman A, Flotte T, Bigelow B. Ultrastructural study of a female adnexal tumor of probable wolffian origin. Cancer 1980;46:2273–80.

15. Duggan MA, Hugh J, Nation JG, Robertson DJ, Stuart GC. Ependymoma of uterosacral ligament. Cancer 1989;64:2565–71.

16. Funk KC, Heiken JP. Papillary cystadenoma of the broad ligament in a patient with von Hippel-Lindau disease. AJR Am J Roentgenol 1989;153:527–8.

17. Gaffey MJ, Mills SE, Boyd JC. Aggressive papillary tumor of middle ear/temporal bone and adnexal papillary cystadenoma. Manifestations of von Hippel-Lindau disease. Am J Surg Pathol 1994;18:1254–60.

17a. Gardner GH, Greene RR, Peckham BM. Normal and cystic structures of the broad ligament. Am J Obstet Gynecol 1948;55:917–39.

18. Gersell DJ, King TC. Papillary cystadenoma of the mesosalpinx in von Hippel-Lindau disease. Am J Surg Pathol 1988;12:145–9.

19. Grody WW, Nieberg RK, Bhuta S. Ependymoma-like tumor of the mesovarium. Arch Pathol Lab Med 1985;109:291–3.

20. Hampton HL, Huffman HT, Meeks GR. Extraovarian Brenner tumor. Obstet Gynecol 1992;79:844–6.

21. Honore LH, Nickerson KG. Papillary serous cystadenoma arising in a paramesonephric cyst of the parovarium. Am J Obstet Gynecol 1976;125:870–1.

22. Janovski N, Bozzetti LP. Serous papillary cystadenoma arising in paramesonephric rest of the mesosalpinx. Obstet Gynecol 1963;22:684–7.

23. Jensen ML, Nielsen MN. Broad ligament mucinous cystadenoma of borderline malignancy. Histopathology 1990;16:89–103.

24. Kariminejad MH, Scully RE. Female adnexal tumor of probable wolffian origin. A distinctive pathologic entity. Cancer 1973;31:671–7.

25. Korn WT, Schatzki SC, Disciullo AJ, Scully RE. Papillary cystadenoma of the broad ligament in von Hippel-Lindau disease. Am J Obstet Gynecol 1990;163:596–8.

26. Merrill JA. Carcinoma of the broad ligament. Obstet Gynecol 1959;13:472–6.

27. Prasad CJ, Ray JA, Kessler S. Female adnexal tumor of wolffian origin. Arch Pathol Lab Med 1992;116:189–91.

28. Pschera H, Wikstrom B. Extraovarian Brenner tumor coexisting with serous cystadenoma. Case report. Gynecol Obstet Invest 1991;31:185–7.

29. Rahilly MA, Williams AR, Krausz T, Al-Nafussi AL. Female adnexal tumour of probable wolffian origin: a clinicopathological and immunohistochemical study of three cases. Histopathology 1995;26:69–74.

30. Seltzer VL, Molho L, Fougner A, et al. Parovarian cystadenocarcinoma of low-malignant potential. Gynecol Oncol 1988;30:216–21.

31. Stapleton JJ, Holser MH, Linder LE. Paramesonephric papillary serous cystadenocarcinoma. A case report with scanning electron microscopy. Acta Cytol 1981; 25:310–6.

32. Tavassoli FA, Andrade R, Merino M. Retiform wolffian adenoma. In: Fenoglio-Preiser CM, Wolffe M, Rilke F, eds. Progress in surgical pathology. New York: Field & Wood Medical Publishers, 1990;11:121–36.

33. Thomason RN, Rush W, Dave H. Transitional cell carcinoma arising within a paratubal cyst: report of a case. Int J Gynecol Pathol 1995;14:270–3.

33a. Werness BA, Guccion JG. Tumor of the broad ligament in von Hippel-Lindau disease of probable mullerian origin. Int J Gynecol Oncol 1997;16:282–5.

Mesenchymal and Mixed Epithelial-Mesenchymal Tumors

34. Breen JL, Neubecker RD. Tumors of the round ligament. A review of the literature and a report of 25 cases. Obstet Gynecol 1962;19:771–80.

35. Cheng WF, Lin HH, Chen CK, Chang DY, Huang SC. Leiomyosarcoma of the broad ligament: a case report and literature review. Gynecol Oncol 1995;56:85–9.

36. Dieste MC, Lynch GR, Gordon A, Estrada R, Lane M. Malignant fibrous histiocytoma of the broad ligament:

a case report and literature review. Gynecol Oncol 1987;28:225–9.

36a. Gardner GH, Greene RR, Peckham BM. Normal and cystic structures of the broad ligament. Am J Obstet Gynecol 1948;55:917–39.

36b. Gardner GH, Greene RR, Peckham BM. Tumors of the broad ligament. Am J Obstet Gynecol 1957;73:536–55.

37. Ghazali S. Embryonic rhabdomyosarcoma of the urogenital tract. Brit J Surg 1973;60:124–8.

38. Herbold DR, Fu YS, Silbert SW. Leiomyosarcoma of the broad ligament. A case report and literature review with follow-up. Am J Surg Pathol 1983;7:285–92.

38a.Honoré LH. Pathology of the fallopian tube and broad ligament. In: Fox H, Wells M, eds. Haines and Taylor obstetrical and gynaecological pathology, 4th ed. Edinburgh: Churchill Livingstone, 1995:623–71.

39. Janovski NA, Paramanandhan TL. Ovarian tumors. Tumors and tumor-like conditions of the ovaries, fallopian tubes and ligaments of the uterus. Major problems in obstetrics and gynecology, vol 4, Philadelphia: WB Saunders, 1973:182–203.

40. Kao GF, Norris HS. Benign and low grade variants of mixed mesodermal tumors (adenosarcoma) of the ovary and adnexal region. Cancer 1978;42:1314–24.

41. Longway SR, Lind HM, Haghighi P. Extraskeletal Ewing's sarcoma arising in the broad ligament. Arch Pathol Lab Med 1986;110:1058–61.

42. Nuovo MA, Nuovo GJ, Smith D, Lewis SH. Benign mesenchymoma of the round ligament. A report of two cases with immunohistochemistry. Am J Clin Pathol 1990;93:421–4.

43. Persad V, Anderson MF. Endometrial stromal sarcoma of the broad ligament arising in the area of endometriosis in a paramesonephric cyst. Case report. Br J Obstet Gynaecol 1977;84:149–52.

44. Singh TT, Hopkins MP, Price J, Schuen R. Myxoid liposarcoma of the broad ligament. Int J Gynecol Cancer 1992;2:220–3.

45. Sworn MJ, Hammond GT, Buchanan R. Mixed mesenchymal sarcoma of the broad ligament. Brit J Obstet Gynaecol 1979;86:403–6.

46. Terada S, Suzuki N, Uchide K, Shozu M, Akasofu K. Parovarian fibroma with heterotopic bone formation of probable wolffian origin. Gynecol Oncol 1993;50:115–8.

Miscellaneous Tumors

47. Al-Jafari MS, Panton HM, Gradwell E. Phaeochromocytoma of the broad ligament. Case report. Brit J Obstet Gynaecol 1985;92:649–51.

48. Aron DC, Marks WM, Alper PR, Karam JH. Phaeochromocytoma of the broad ligament. Localization by computerized tomography and ultrasonography. Arch Int Med 1980;140:550–2.

49. Gabbay-Mor M, Ovadia Y, Neri A. Accessory ovaries with bilateral dermoid cysts. Eur J Obstet Gynecol Reprod Biol 1982;14:171–3.

49a.Gardner GH, Greene RR, Peckham BM. Normal and cystic structures of the broad ligament. Am J Obstet Gynecol 1948;55:917–39.

50. Heller DS, Keohane M, Bessim S, Jagirdar J, Deligdisch L. Pituitary-containing benign cystic teratoma arising from the uterosacral ligament. Arch Pathol Lab Med 1989;113:802–4.

51. Honoré LH. Pathology of the fallopian tube and broad ligament. In: Fox H, Wells M, eds. Haines and Taylor obstetrical and gynaecological pathology, 4th ed. Edinburgh: Churchill Livingstone, 1995:623–71.

52. Huntington RW, Bullock WK. Yolk sac tumors of extragonadal origin. Cancer 1970;25:1368–76.

53. Kay S, Schneider V, Litt J. Choriocarcinoma of the mesosalpinx masquerading as congestive heart failure:

ultrastructural observations of the tumor. Int J Gynecol Pathol 1983;2:72–87.

54. Lin HH, Chen YP, Lee TY. A hormone-producing thecoma of broad ligament. Acta Obstet Gynecol Scand 1987;66:725–7.

55. Merino MJ, LiVolsi VA, Trepeta RW. Fibrothecoma of the broad ligament. Diagn Gynecol Obstet 1980;2:51–4.

56. Morris JM, Scully RE. Granulosa-theca cell tumors. In: Endocrine pathology of the ovary. St. Louis: CV Mosby, 1958:65–81.

57. Reddy DB, Rao DB, Sarojini JS. Extra-ovarian granulosa cell tumour. J Indian Med Ass 1963;41:254–7.

58. Roth LM, Davis MM, Sutton GP. Steroid cell tumor of the broad ligament arising in an accessory ovary. Arch Pathol Lab Med. 1996;120:405–9.

59. Sasano H, Sato S, Yajima A, Akama J, Nagura H. Adrenal rest tumor of the broad ligament: case report with immunohistochemical study of steroidogenic enzymes. Pathol Int 1997;47:493–6.

60. Van Ingen G, Schoemaker J, Baak JA. A testosterone-producing tumour in the mesovarium. Path Res Pract 1991;187:362–70.

61. Williamson HO, Moore MP. Ovarian and paraovarian adenomatoid tumors: case reports. Am J Obstet Gynecol 1964;90:388–94.

Tumor-Like Lesions

61a.Ahmed AA, Swan RW, Owen A, Kraus FT, Patrick F. Uterus-like mass arising in the broad ligament: a metaplasia or mullerian duct anomaly? Int J Gynecol Pathol 1997;16:279–81.

62. Breen JL, Lukeman JM, Neubecker RD. Nodular fasciitis of the round ligament. Report of a case. Gynecol Oncol 1962;19:397–400.

62a.Gardner GH, Greene RR, Peckham BM. Tumors of the broad ligament. Am J Obstet Gynecol 1957;73:536–55.

63. Genadry R, Parmley T, Woodruff JD. The origin and clinical behavior of the parovarian tumor. Am J Obstet Gynecol 1977;129:873–80.

64. MacDonald CJ, Pratt JH. Twisted parovarian cysts. Obstet Gynecol 1967;29:113–7.

65. Rao NR. Malacoplakia of broad ligament, inguinal region, and endometrium. Arch Pathol 1969;88:85–8.

66. Samaha M, Woodruff JD. Paratubal cysts: frequency, histogenesis and associated clinical features. Obstet Gynecol 1985;65:691–4.

Index*

---

*Numbers in boldface indicate table and figure pages.